WinkingSkull.com

A study aid for must-know anatomy

Register for WinkingSkull.com PLUS!

Your study aid for must-know anatomy

Gain a solid foundation in human anatomy with WinkingSkull.com, a study aid that is ideal for supplementing course study and for exam preparation. This user-friendly website features more than 200 stunning images derived from *Atlas of Anatomy*.

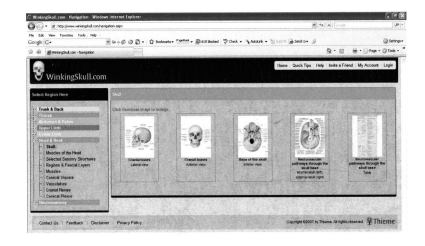

FEATURES

- Must-know concepts for the study of anatomy
- An intuitive design that simplifies navigation
- Stunning, full-color illustrations—art of the 21st century!
- Timed tests to assess comprehension
- Test scores that are instantly available for viewing

Buyers of *Atlas of Anatomy* gain exclusive access to additional clinical content that builds on the highly practical scope of the book to prepare students for the clinical setting. This exclusive material includes:

- MRIs
- CT scans
- Sectional anatomy with explanatory schematics

Scratch the panel below to reveal the unique access code that will enable you to register for WinkingSkull.com PLUS. Log on to www.WinkingSkull.com to get started.

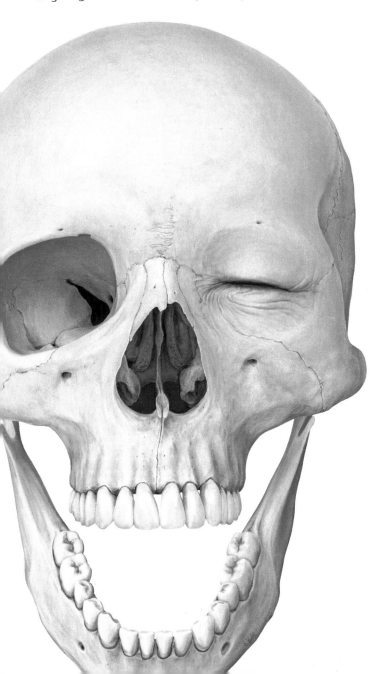

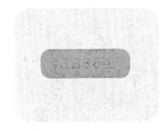

Atlas of Anatomy

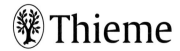

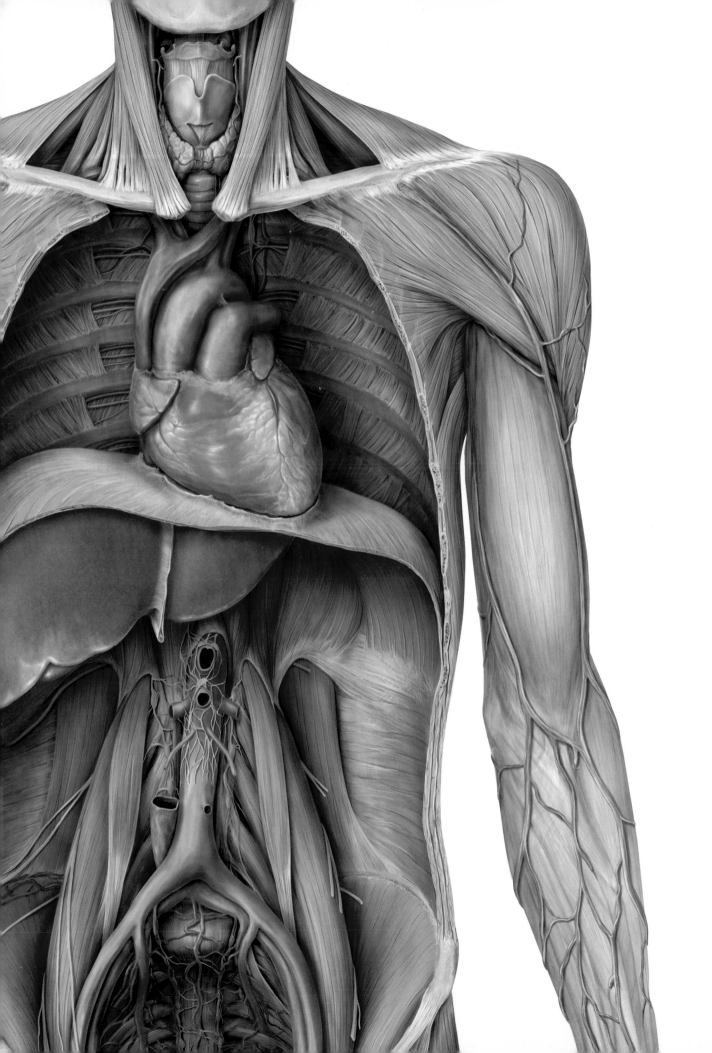

Atlas of Anatomy

Anne M. Gilroy

University of Massachusetts, Worcester, MA

Brian R. MacPherson

University of Kentucky Medical School, Lexington, KY

Lawrence M. Ross

University of Texas Medical School at Houston

Contributing Authors

Michael Schuenke

Erik Schulte

Udo Schumacher

Illustrations by

Markus Voll

Karl Wesker

Thieme

Stuttgart · New York

Thieme Medical Publishers, Inc.
333 Seventh Avenue
New York, New York 10001

Developmental Editor: Bridget N. Queenan
Editorial Director, Educational Products: Cathrin E. Schulz, M.D.
Senior Production Editor: Adelaide Elsie Starbecker
Director of Sales: Ross Lumpkin
National Sales Manager: James Nunn
Vice President, Production and Electronic Publishing: Anne T. Vinnicombe
Vice President, International Marketing and Sales: Cornelia Schulze
Chief Financial Officer: Peter van Woerden
President: Brian D. Scanlan

Illustrators
Markus Voll
Karl Wesker

Compositor: Compset, Beverly, MA
Printer: Appl, Wemding, Germany

Library of Congress Cataloging-in-Publication Data is available
from the publisher.

References: Detailed references are available from the publisher
upon request.

Important note: Medical knowledge is ever-changing. As new research and clinical experience broaden our knowledge, changes in treatment and drug therapy may be required. The authors and editors of the material herein have consulted sources believed to be reliable in their efforts to provide information that is complete and in accord with the standards accepted at the time of publication. However, in view of the possibility of human error by the authors, editors, or publisher of the work herein or changes in medical knowledge, neither the authors, editors, nor publisher, nor any other party who has been involved in the preparation of this work, warrants that the information contained herein is in every respect accurate or complete, and they are not responsible for any errors or omissions or for the results obtained from use of such information. Readers are encouraged to confirm the information contained herein with other sources. For example, readers are advised to check the product information sheet included in the package of each drug they plan to administer to be certain that the information contained in this publication is accurate and that changes have not been made in the recommended dose or in the contraindications for administration. This recommendation is of particular importance in connection with new or infrequently used drugs.

Some of the product names, patents, and registered designs referred to in this book are in fact registered trademarks or proprietary names even though specific reference to this fact is not always made in the text. Therefore, the appearance of a name without designation as proprietary is not to be construed as a representation by the publisher that it is in the public domain.

Softcover: ISBN 978-1-60406-062-1
Hardcover: ISBN 978-1-60406-151-2

Dedication

To my father, Francis Gilroy, whose dedication to medicine has been a greater inspiration to me than he has ever realized; to my students who lovingly tolerate, and sometimes share, my passion for human anatomy; and most of all to my sons, Colin & Bryan, whose love and support I treasure beyond all else.

To my friend and mentor, Dr. Ken McFadden of the Division of Anatomy at the University of Alberta, who ensured I received the training in gross anatomy instruction required to be successful, and to the thousands of professional students who I have taught over the past 30 years honing these skills. However, none of the success I've enjoyed during my time in academia would have been possible without the constant support, participation and encouragement of my wife, Cynthia Long.

To my wife, Irene; to the children, Chip, Jennifer, Jocelyn & Barry, Tricia, Scott, Katie & Snapper, and Trey; and to my students who have taught me so well.

Acknowledgments

We cordially thank the members of the Advisory Board
for their contributions.

- Bruce M. Carlson, MD, PhD
  University of Michigan
  Ann Arbor, Michigan

- Derek Bryant (Class of 2011)
  University of Toronto Medical School
  Burlington, Ontario

- Peter Cole, MD
  Glamorum Healing Centre
  Orangeville, Ontario

- Michael Droller, MD
  The Mount Sinai Medical Center
  New York, New York

- Anthony Firth, PhD
  Imperial College London
  London

- Mark H. Hankin, PhD
  University of Toledo, College of Medicine
  Toledo, Ohio

- Katharine Hudson (Class of 2010)
  McGill Medical School
  Montreal, Quebec

- Christopher Lee (Class of 2010)
  Harvard Medical School
  Cambridge, Massachusetts

- Francis Liuzzi, PhD
  Lake Erie College of Osteopathic Medicine
  Bradenton, Florida

- Graham Louw, PhD
  University of Cape Town Medical School
  University of Cape Town

- Estomih Mtui, MD
  Weill Cornell Medical College
  New York, New York

- Srinivas Murthy, MD
  Harvard Medical School
  Boston, Massachusetts

- Jeff Rihn, MD
  The Rothman Institute
  Philadelphia, Pennsylvania

- Lawrence Rizzolo, PhD
  Yale University
  New Haven, Connecticut

- Mikel Snow, PhD
  University of Southern California
  Los Angeles, California

- Kelly Wright (Class of 2010)
  Wayne State University School of Medicine
  Detroit, Michigan

Foreword

This Atlas of Anatomy is, in my opinion, the finest single volume atlas of human anatomy that has ever been created. Two factors make it so: the images and the way they have been organized.

The artists, Markus Voll and Karl Wesker, have created a new standard of excellence in anatomical art. Their graceful use of transparency and their sensitive representation of light and shadow give the reader an accurate three-dimensional understanding of every structure.

The authors have organized the images so that they give just the flow of information a student needs to build up a clear mental image of the human body. Each two-page spread is a self-contained lesson that un-obtrusively shows the hand of an experienced and thoughtful teacher. I wish I could have held this book in my hands when I was a student; I envy any student who does so now.

Robert B. Acland
Louisville, KY   March 2008

Preface

Each of the authors was amazed and impressed with the extraordinary detail, accuracy, and beauty of the illustrations that were created for the Thieme Atlas of Anatomy. We felt these images were one of the most significant additions to anatomical education in the past 50 years. It was our intent to use these exceptional illustrations as the cornerstone of our effort to create a concise single volume Atlas of Anatomy for the curious and eager health science student.

Our challenge was first to select from this extensive collection those images that are most instructive and illustrative of current dissection approaches. Along the way, however, we realized that creating a single volume atlas was much more than choosing images: each image had to convey a significant amount of detail while the appeal and labeling needed to be clean and soothing to the eye. Therefore, hundreds of illustrations were drawn new or modified to fit the approach of this new atlas. In addition, key schematic diagrams and simplified summary-form tables were added wherever needed. Dozens of applicable radiographic images and important clinical correlates have been added where appropriate. Additionally, surface anatomy illustrations are accompanied by questions designed to direct the student's attention to anatomic detail that is most relevant in conducting the physical exam. Elements from each of these features are arranged in a regional format to facilitate common dissection approaches. Within each region the various components are examined systemically, followed by topographical images to tie the systems within the region together. In all of this, a clinical perspective on the anatomical structures is taken. The unique two facing pages "spread" format focuses the user to the area/topic being explored.

We hope these efforts, the results of close to 100 combined years of experience teaching the discipline of anatomy to bright, enthusiastic students, has resulted in a comprehensive, easy-to-use resource and reference.

We would like to thank our colleagues at Thieme Publishers who so professionally facilitated this effort. We cannot thank enough, Cathrin E. Schulz, M.D., Editorial Director Educational Products, who so graciously reminded us of deadlines, while always being available to troubleshoot problems. More importantly, she encouraged, helped, and complimented our efforts.

We also wish to extend very special thanks and appreciation to Bridget Queenan, Developmental Editor, who edited and developed the manuscript with an outstanding talent for visualization and intuitive flow of information. We are very grateful to her for catching many details along the way while always patiently responding to requests for artwork and labeling changes.

Cordial thanks to Elsie Starbecker, Senior Production Editor, who with great care and speed produced this atlas with its over 2,200 illustrations. Finally thanks to Rebecca McTavish, Developmental Editor, for joining the team in the correction phase. Their hard work has made the Atlas of Anatomy a reality.

Anne M. Gilroy
Brian R. MacPherson
Lawrence M. Ross

March 2008,
Worcester, MA, Lexington, KY, and Houston, TX

Table of Contents

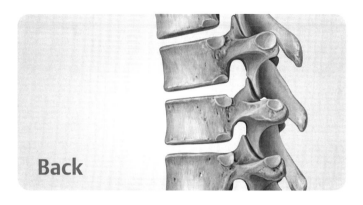

Back

Thorax

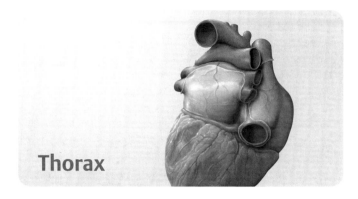

Abdomen & Pelvis

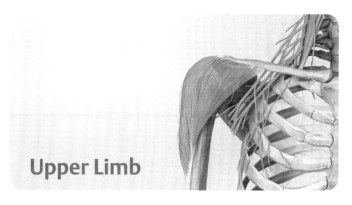

Upper Limb

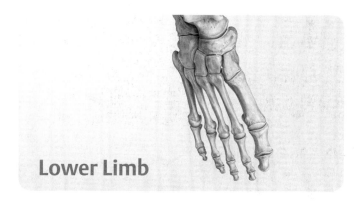

Lower Limb

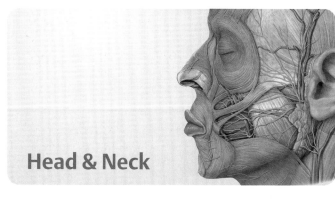

Head & Neck

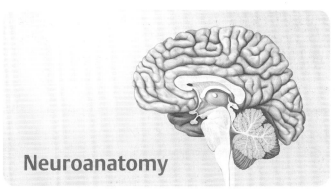

Neuroanatomy

Appendix

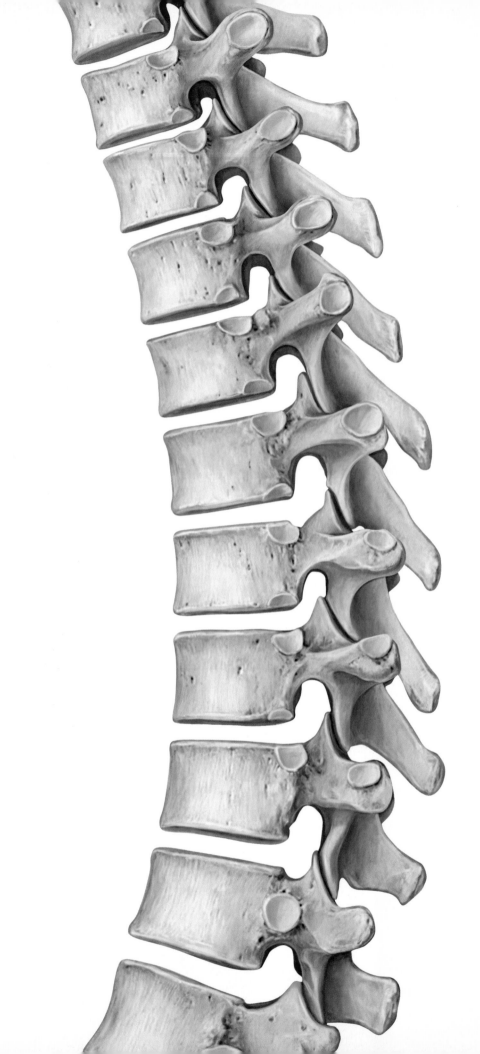

Back

Vertebral Column: Overview

 The vertebral column (spine) is divided into four regions: the cervical, thoracic, lumbar, and sacral spines. Both the cervical and lumbar spines demonstrate lordosis (inward curvature); the thoracic and sacral spines demonstrate kyphosis (outward curvature).

Fig. 1.1 Vertebral column
Left lateral view.

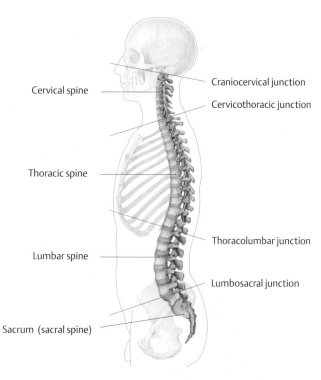

Cervical spine

Craniocervical junction

Cervicothoracic junction

Thoracic spine

Thoracolumbar junction

Lumbar spine

Lumbosacral junction

Sacrum (sacral spine)

A Regions of the spine.

🩺 *Clinical*

Spinal development

The characteristic curvatures of the adult spine appear over the course of postnatal development, being only partially present in a newborn. The newborn has a "kyphotic" spinal curvature (**A**); lumbar lordosis develops later and becomes stable at puberty (**C**).

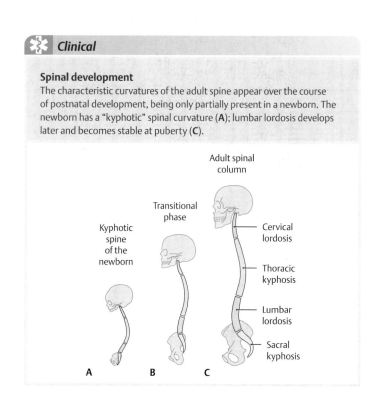

Adult spinal column

Transitional phase

Kyphotic spine of the newborn

Cervical lordosis

Thoracic kyphosis

Lumbar lordosis

Sacral kyphosis

A   B   C

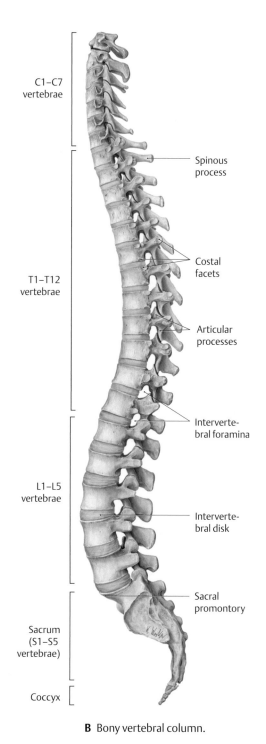

C1–C7 vertebrae

Spinous process

Costal facets

T1–T12 vertebrae

Articular processes

Intervertebral foramina

L1–L5 vertebrae

Intervertebral disk

Sacrum (S1–S5 vertebrae)

Sacral promontory

Coccyx

B Bony vertebral column.

Fig. 1.2 **Normal anatomical position of the spine**

Left lateral view.

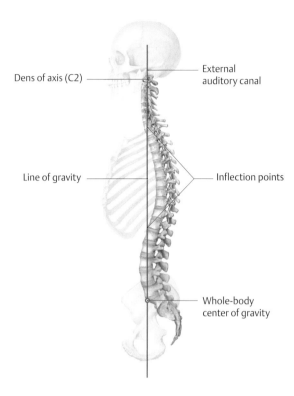

A Line of gravity. The line of gravity passes through certain anatomical landmarks, including the inflection points at the cervicothoracic and thoracolumbar junctions. It continues through the center of gravity (anterior to the sacral promontory) before passing through the hip joint, knee, and ankle.

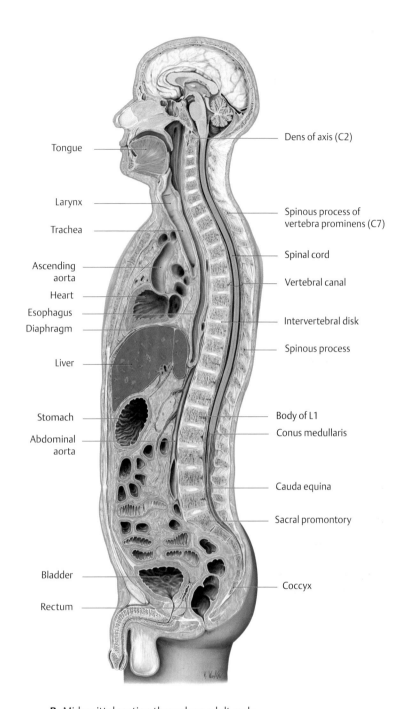

B Midsagittal section through an adult male.

Vertebral Column: Elements

***Fig. 1.3* Bones of the vertebral column**

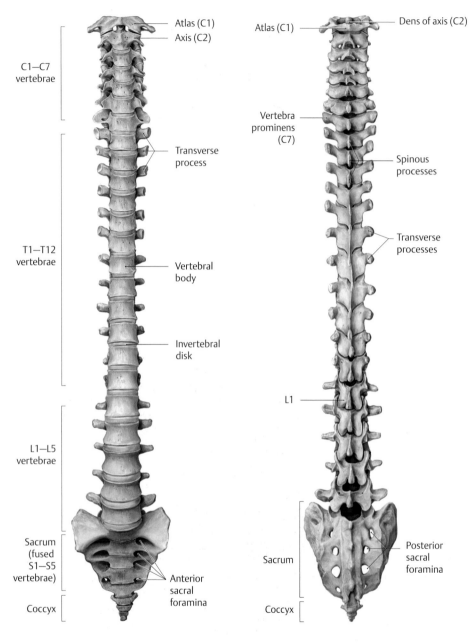

A Anterior view. **B** Posterior view.

***Fig. 1.4* Palpable spinous processes as landmarks**

Posterior view. The easily palpated spinous processes provide important landmarks during physical examination.

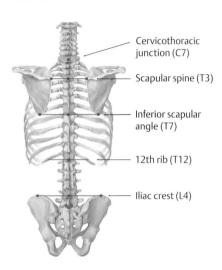

Fig. 1.5 Structural elements of a vertebra

Left posterosuperior view. With the exception of the atlas (C1) and axis (C2), all vertebrae consist of the same structural elements.

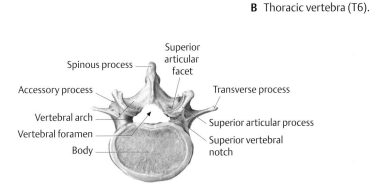

Fig. 1.6 Typical vertebrae

Superior view.

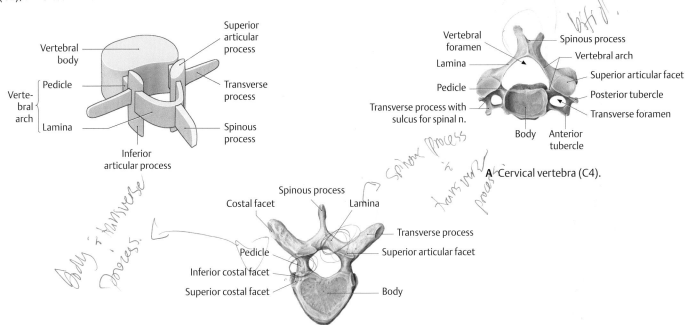

A Cervical vertebra (C4).

B Thoracic vertebra (T6).

C Lumbar vertebra (L4).

D Sacrum.

Table 1.1	Structural elements of vertebrae				
Vertebrae	Body	Vertebral foramen	Transverse processes	Articular processes	Spinous process
Cervical vertebrae C3*–C7	Small (kidney-shaped)	Large (triangular)	Small (may be absent in C7); anterior and posterior tubercles enclose transverse foramen	Superoposteriorly and inferoanteriorly; oblique facets: most nearly horizontal	Short (C3–C5); bifid (C3–C6); long (C7)
Thoracic vertebrae T1–T12	Medium (heart-shaped); includes costal facets	Small (circular)	Large and strong; length decreases T1–T12; costal facets (T1–T10)	Posteriorly (slightly laterally) and anteriorly (slightly medially); facets in coronal plane	Long, sloping postero-inferiorly; tip extends to level of vertebral body below
Lumbar vertebrae L1–L5	Large (kidney-shaped)	Medium (triangular)	Long and slender; accessory process on posterior surface	Posteromedially (or medially) and anterolaterally (or laterally); facets nearly in sagittal plane; mammillary process on posterior surface of each superior articular process	Short and broad
Sacral vertebrae (sacrum) S1–S5 (fused)	Decreases from base to apex	Sacral canal	Fused to rudimentary rib (ribs, see pp. 44–47)	Superoposteriorly (SI) superior surface of lateral sacrum-auricular surface	Median sacral crest

*C1 (atlas) and C2 (axis) are considered atypical (see pp. 6–7).

Cervical Vertebrae

 The seven vertebrae of the cervical spine differ most conspicuously from the common vertebral morphology. They are specialized to bear the weight of the head and allow the neck to move in all directions. C1 and C2 are known as the atlas and axis, respectively. C7 is called the vertebra prominens for its long, palpable spinous process.

Fig. 1.7 Cervical spine
Left lateral view.

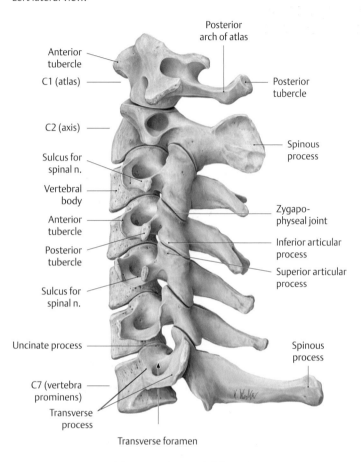

A Bones of the cervical spine, left lateral view.

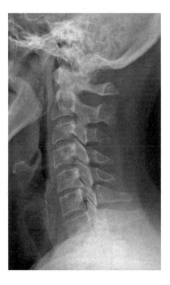

B Radiograph of the cervical spine, left lateral view.

Fig. 1.8 Atlas (C1)

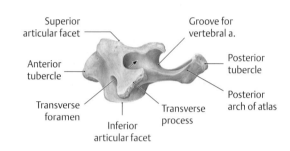

A Left lateral view.

Fig. 1.9 Axis (C2)

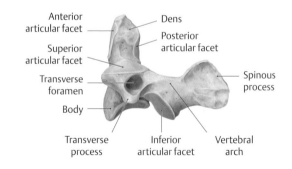

A Left lateral view.

Fig. 1.10 Typical cervical vertebra (C4)

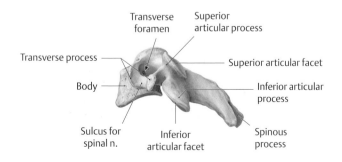

A Left lateral view.

Injuries in the cervical spine
The cervical spine is prone to hyperextension injuries, such as "whiplash," which can occur when the head extends back much farther than it normally would. The most common injuries of the cervical spine are fractures of the dens of the axis, traumatic spondylolisthesis (ventral slippage of a vertebral body), and atlas fractures. Patient prognosis is largely dependent on the spinal level of the injuries (see p. 600).

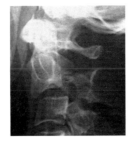

This patient hit the dashboard of his car while not wearing a seat belt. The resulting hyperextension caused the traumatic spondylolisthesis of C2 (axis) with fracture of the vertebral arch of C2, as well as tearing of the ligaments between C2 and C3. This injury is often referred to as "hangman's fracture."

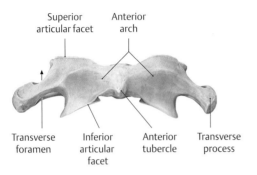

B Anterior view.

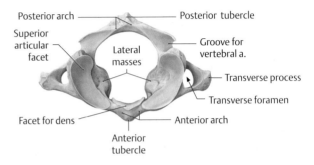

C Superior view.

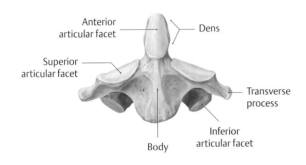

B Anterior view.

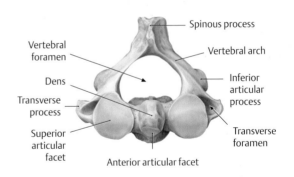

C Superior view.

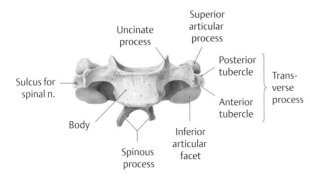

B Anterior view.

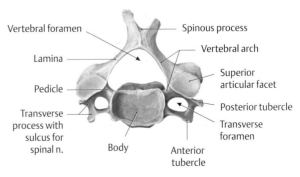

C Superior view.

Thoracic & Lumbar Vertebrae

Fig. 1.11 Thoracic spine
Left lateral view.

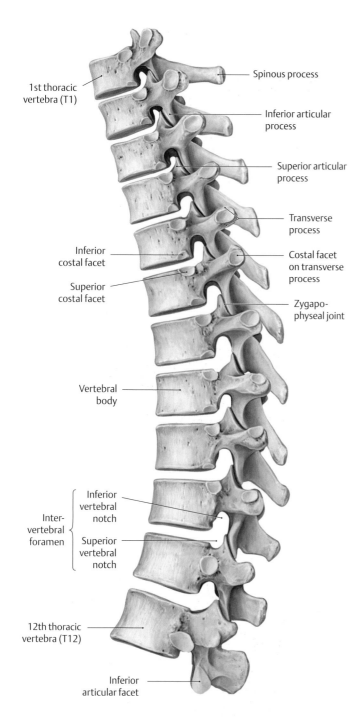

1st thoracic vertebra (T1)

Spinous process

Inferior articular process

Superior articular process

Transverse process

Inferior costal facet

Costal facet on transverse process

Superior costal facet

Zygapo- physeal joint

Vertebral body

Inter- vertebral foramen

Inferior vertebral notch

Superior vertebral notch

12th thoracic vertebra (T12)

Inferior articular facet

Fig. 1.12 Typical thoracic vertebra (T6)

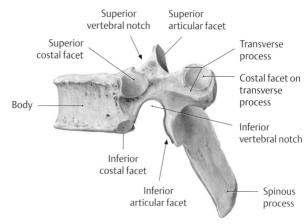

Superior vertebral notch

Superior articular facet

Superior costal facet

Transverse process

Body

Costal facet on transverse process

Inferior vertebral notch

Inferior costal facet

Inferior articular facet

Spinous process

A Left lateral view.

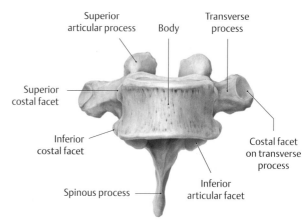

Superior articular process

Body

Transverse process

Superior costal facet

Inferior costal facet

Costal facet on transverse process

Spinous process

Inferior articular facet

B Anterior view.

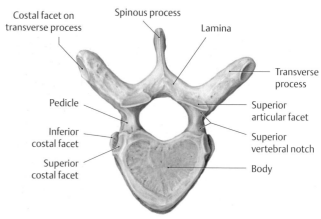

Costal facet on transverse process

Spinous process

Lamina

Transverse process

Pedicle

Superior articular facet

Inferior costal facet

Superior vertebral notch

Superior costal facet

Body

C Superior view.

Fig. 1.13 Lumbar spine

Left lateral view.

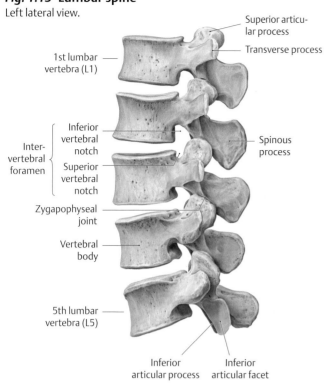

- 1st lumbar vertebra (L1)
- Superior articular process
- Transverse process
- Inferior vertebral notch
- Intervertebral foramen
- Superior vertebral notch
- Spinous process
- Zygapophyseal joint
- Vertebral body
- 5th lumbar vertebra (L5)
- Inferior articular process
- Inferior articular facet

 Clinical

Osteoporosis

The spine is the structure most affected by degenerative diseases of the skeleton, such as arthrosis and osteoporosis. In osteoporosis, more bone material gets reabsorbed than built up, resulting in a loss of bone mass. Symptoms include compression fractures and resulting back pain.

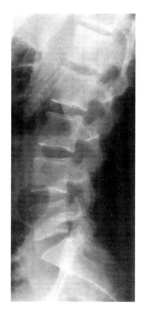

A Radiograph of a normal lumbar spine, left lateral view.

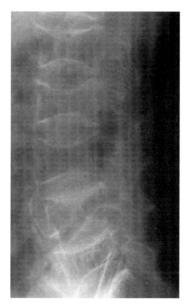

B Radiograph of an osteoporotic spine. The vertebral bodies are decreased in density, and the internal trabecular structure is coarse. Lower and upper end plates are fractured.

Fig. 1.14 Typical lumbar vertebra (L4)

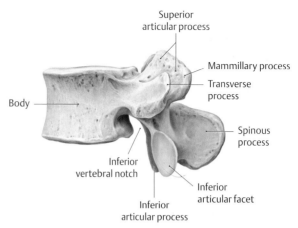

- Superior articular process
- Mammillary process
- Transverse process
- Body
- Spinous process
- Inferior vertebral notch
- Inferior articular process
- Inferior articular facet

A Left lateral view.

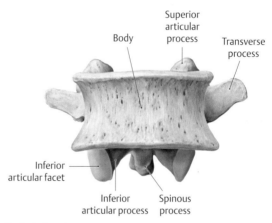

- Superior articular process
- Body
- Transverse process
- Inferior articular facet
- Inferior articular process
- Spinous process

B Anterior view.

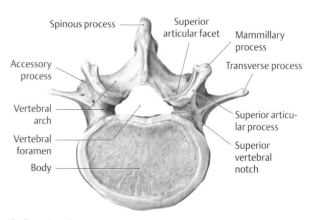

- Spinous process
- Superior articular facet
- Mammillary process
- Accessory process
- Transverse process
- Vertebral arch
- Superior articular process
- Vertebral foramen
- Superior vertebral notch
- Body

C Superior view.

Sacrum & Coccyx

 The sacrum is formed from five postnatally fused sacral vertebrae. The base of the sacrum articulates with the fifth lumbar vertebra, and the apex articulates with the coccyx, a series of three or four rudimentary vertebrae.

Fig. 1.15 **Sacrum and coccyx**

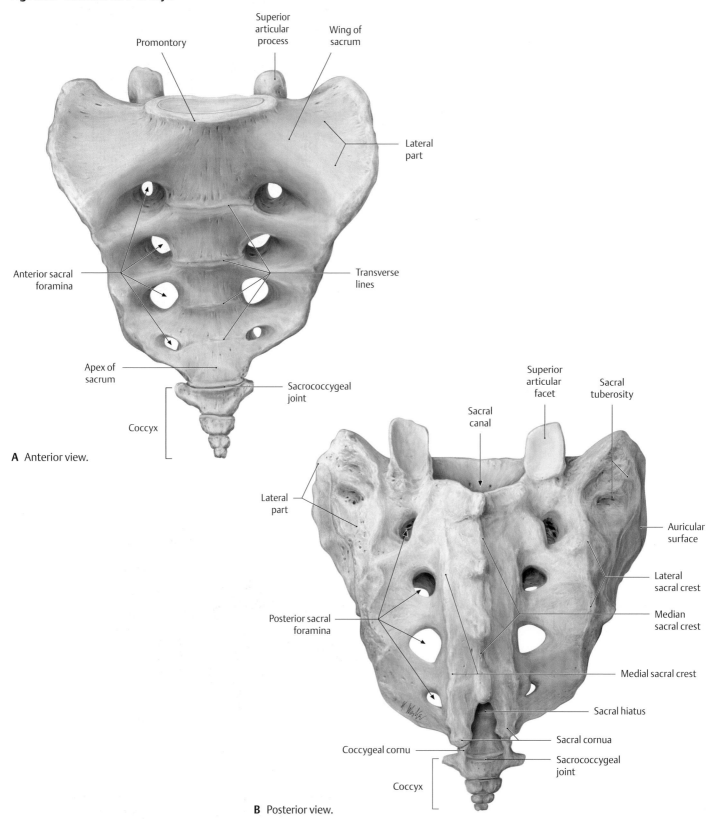

A Anterior view.

B Posterior view.

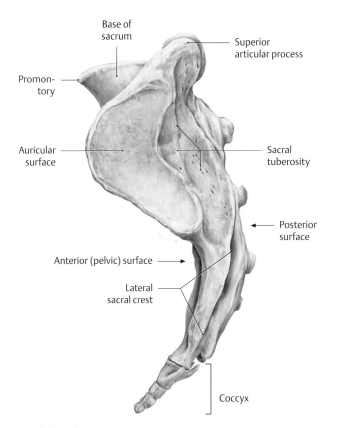

C Left lateral view.

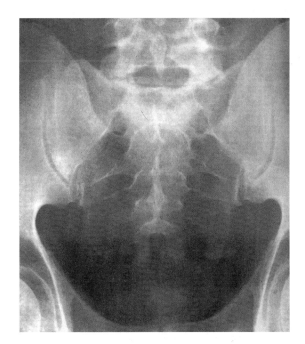

D Radiograph of sacrum, anteroposterior view.

Fig. 1.16 **Sacrum**
Superior view.

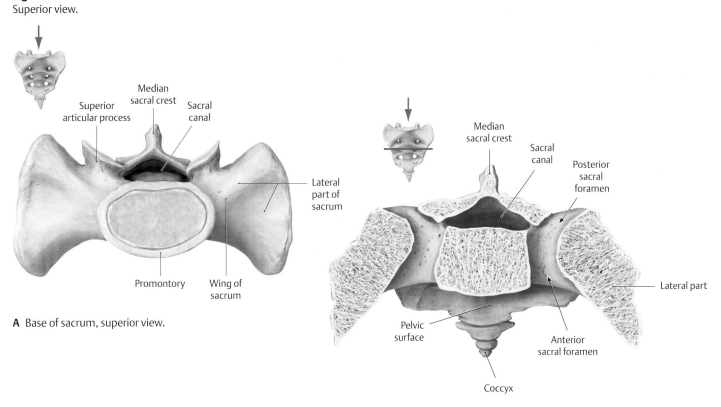

A Base of sacrum, superior view.

B Transverse section through second sacral vertebra demonstrating anterior and posterior sacral foramina, superior view.

Intervertebral Disks

Fig. 1.17 Intervertebral disk in the vertebral column

Sagittal section of T11–T12, left lateral view. The intervertebral disks occupy the spaces between vertebrae (intervertebral joints, see p. 14).

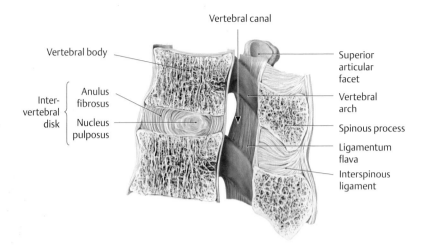

Vertebral canal

Vertebral body

Inter-vertebral disk — Anulus fibrosus
Nucleus pulposus

Superior articular facet

Vertebral arch

Spinous process

Ligamentum flava

Interspinous ligament

Fig. 1.18 Structure of intervertebral disk

Anterosuperior view with the anterior half of the disk and the right half of the end plate removed. The intervertebral disk consists of an external fibrous ring (anulus fibrosus) and a gelatinous core (nucleus pulposus).

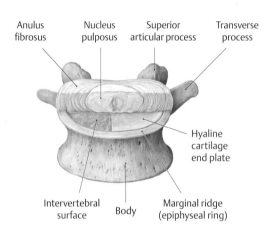

Anulus fibrosus

Nucleus pulposus

Superior articular process

Transverse process

Hyaline cartilage end plate

Intervertebral surface

Body

Marginal ridge (epiphyseal ring)

Fig. 1.19 Relation of intervertebral disk to vertebral canal

Fourth lumbar vertebra, superior view.

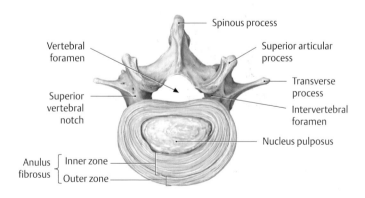

Spinous process

Vertebral foramen

Superior articular process

Transverse process

Intervertebral foramen

Superior vertebral notch

Nucleus pulposus

Anulus fibrosus — Inner zone
Outer zone

Fig. 1.20 Outer zone of the anulus fibrosus

Anterior view of L3–L4 with intervertebral disk.

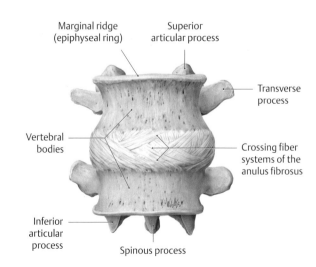

Marginal ridge (epiphyseal ring)

Superior articular process

Transverse process

Vertebral bodies

Crossing fiber systems of the anulus fibrosus

Inferior articular process

Spinous process

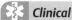
Disk herniation in the lumbar spine

As the stress resistance of the anulus fibrosus declines with age, the tissue of the nucleus pulposus may protrude through weak spots under loading. If the fibrous ring of the anulus ruptures completely, the herniated material may compress the contents of the intervertebral foramen (nerve roots and blood vessels). These patients often suffer from severe local back pain. Pain is also felt in the associated dermatome (see p. 600). When the motor part of

the spinal nerve is affected, the muscles served by that spinal nerve will show weakening. It is an important diagnostic step to test the muscles innervated by a nerve from a certain spinal segment, as well as the sensitivity in the specific dermatome. Example: The first sacral nerve root innervates the gastrocnemius and soleus muscles; thus, standing or walking on toes can be affected (see p. 398).

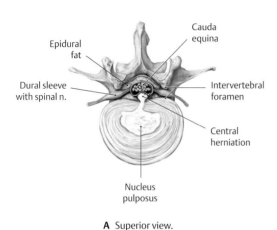

A Superior view.

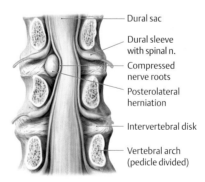

B Midsagittal T2-weighted MRI (magnetic resonance image).

Posterior herniation (A, B) In the MRI, a conspicuously herniated disk at the level of L3–L4 protrudes posteriorly (transligamentous herniation). The dural sac is deeply indented at that level. *CSF (cerebrospinal fluid).

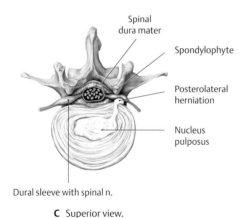

C Superior view.

D Posterior view, vertebral arches removed.

Posterolateral herniation (C, D) A posterolateral herniation may compress the spinal nerve as it passes through the intervertebral foramen. If more medially positioned, the herniation may spare the nerve at that level, but impact nerves at inferior levels.

Joints of the Vertebral Column: Overview

Table 1.2   **Joints of the vertebral column**

Craniovertebral joints		
①	Atlanto-occipital joints	Occiput–C1
②	Atlantoaxial joints	C1–C2
Joints of the vertebral bodies		
③	Uncovertebral joints	C3–C7
④	Intervertebral joints	C1–S1
Joints of the vertebral arch		
⑤	Zygapophyseal joints	C1–S1

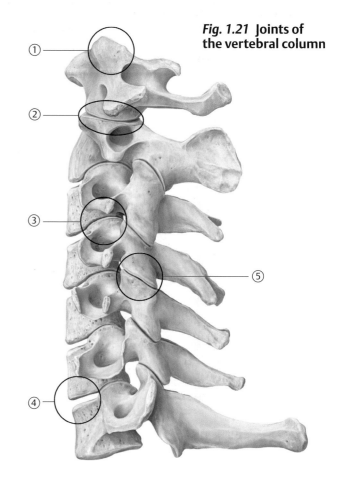

Fig. 1.21 **Joints of the vertebral column**

Fig. 1.22 Zygapophyseal (intervertebral facet) joints

The orientation of the zygapophyseal joints differs between the spinal regions, influencing the degree and direction of movement.

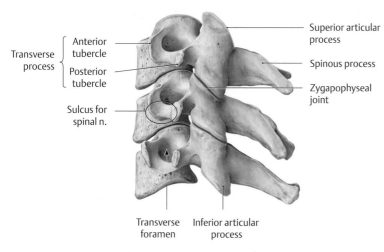

A Cervical region, left lateral view. The zygapophyseal joints lie 45 degrees from the horizontal.

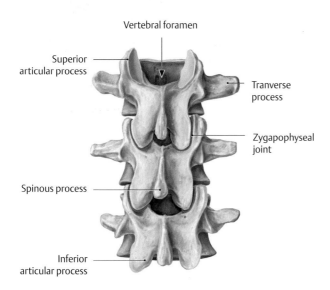

C Lumbar region, posterior view. The joints lie in the sagittal plane.

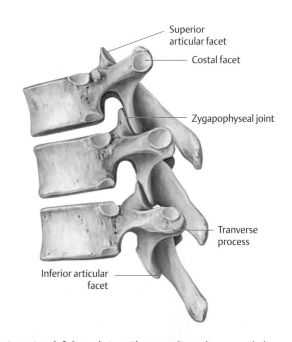

B Thoracic region, left lateral view. The joints lie in the coronal plane.

Fig. 1.23 Uncovertebral joints

Anterior view. Uncovertebral joints form during childhood between the uncinate processes of C3–C6 and the vertebral bodies immediately superior. The joints may result from fissures in the cartilage of the disks that assume an articular character. If the fissures become complete tears, the risk of pulposus herniation is increased (see p. 13).

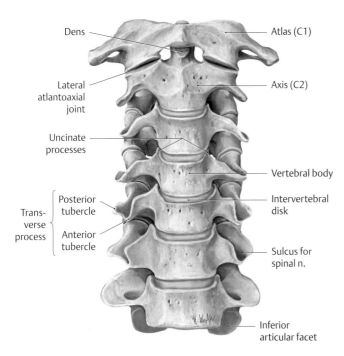

A Uncovertebral joints in the cervical spine of an 18-year-old man, anterior view.

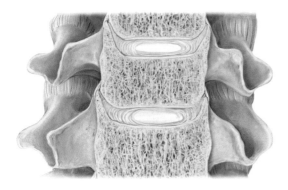

B Uncovertebral joint (enlarged), anterior view of coronal section.

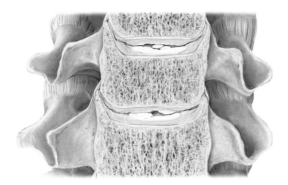

C Split intervertebral disk, anterior view of coronal section.

✚ Clinical

Proximity of spinal nerve and vertebral artery to the uncinate process

The spinal nerve and vertebral artery pass through the intervertebral and transverse foramina, respectively. Bony outgrowths (osteophytes) resulting from uncovertebral arthrosis may compress both the nerve and the artery and can lead to chronic pain in the neck.

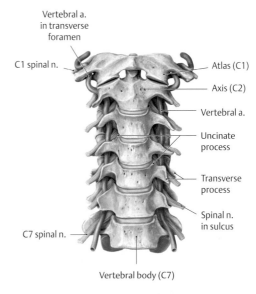

A Cervical spine, anterior view.

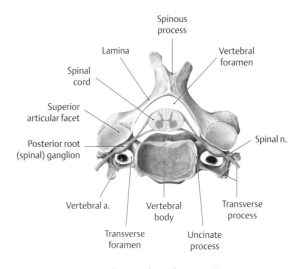

B Fourth cervical vertebra, superior view.

Joints of the Vertebral Column: Craniovertebral Region

Fig. 1.24 **Craniovertebral joints**

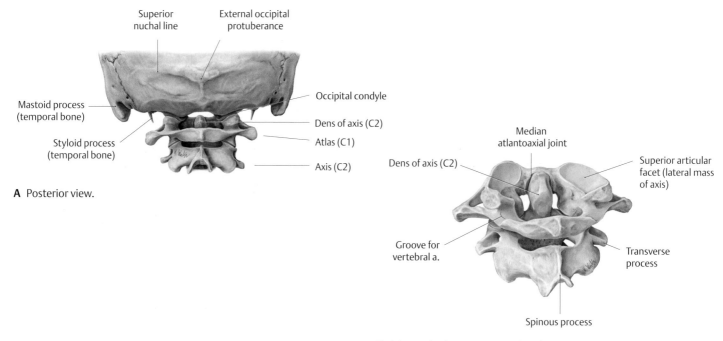

A Posterior view.

B Atlas and axis, posterosuperior view.

Fig. 1.25 **Dissection of the craniovertebral joint ligaments**
Posterior view.

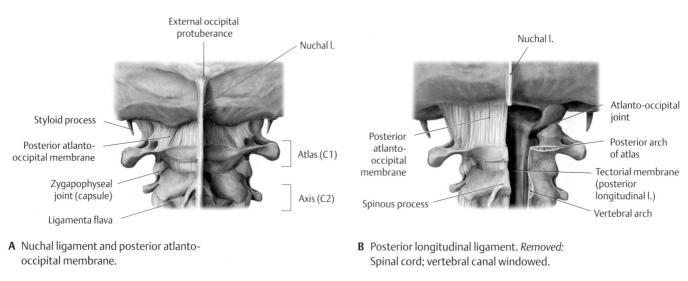

A Nuchal ligament and posterior atlanto-occipital membrane.

B Posterior longitudinal ligament. *Removed:* Spinal cord; vertebral canal windowed.

The atlanto-occipital joints are the two articulations between the convex occipital condyles of the occipital bone and the slightly concave superior articular facets of the atlas (C1). The atlanto-axial joints are the two lateral and one medial articulations between the atlas (C1) and axis (C2).

Fig. 1.26 Ligaments of the craniovertebral joints

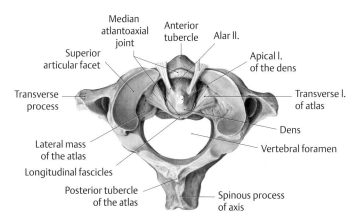

A Ligaments of the median atlantoaxial joint, superior view. The fovea of the atlas is hidden by the joint capsule.

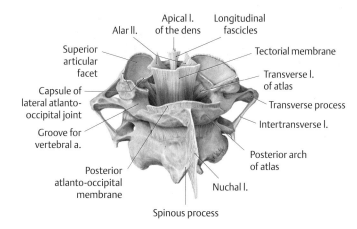

B Ligaments of the craniovertebral joints, posterosuperior view. The dens of the axis is hidden by the tectorial membrane.

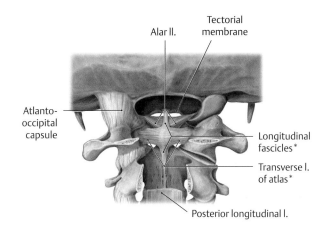

C Cruciform ligament of atlas (*). *Removed:* Tectorial membrane.

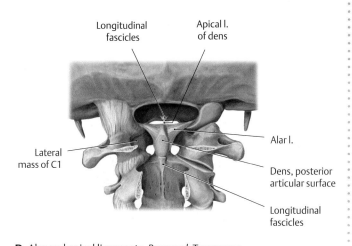

D Alar and apical ligaments. *Removed:* Transverse ligament of atlas, longitudinal fascicles.

Vertebral Ligaments: Overview & Cervical Spine

The ligaments of the spinal column bind the vertebrae and enable the spine to withstand high mechanical loads and shearing stresses and limit the range of motion. The ligaments are subdivided into vertebral body ligaments and vertebral arch ligaments.

Fig. 1.27 Vertebral ligaments
Viewed obliquely from the left posterior view.

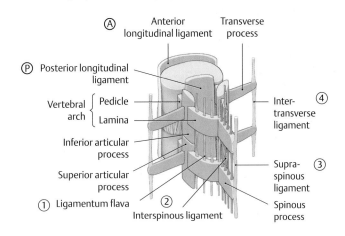

Table 1.3		Vertebral ligaments	
Ligament			**Location**
Vertebral body ligaments			
Ⓐ	Anterior longitudinal ligament		Along anterior surface of vertebral body
Ⓟ	Posterior longitudinal ligament		Along posterior surface of vertebral body
Vertebral arch ligaments			
①	Ligamenta flava		Between laminae
②	Interspinous ligaments		Between spinous process
③	Supraspinous ligaments		Along posterior ridge of spinous processes
④	Intertransverse ligaments		Between transverse processes
	Nuchal ligament*		Between external occipital protuberance and spinous process of C7

*Corresponds to a supraspinous ligament that is broadened superiorly.

Fig. 1.28 Anterior longitudinal ligament
Anterior longitudinal ligament. Anterior view with base of skull removed.

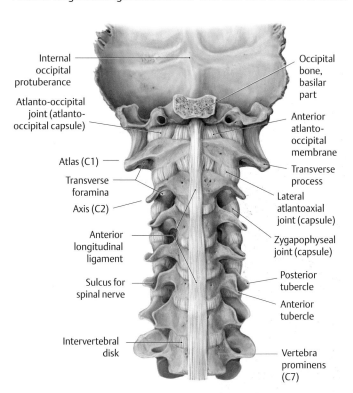

Fig. 1.29 Posterior longitudinal ligament
Posterior view with vertebral canal windowed and spinal cord removed. The tectorial membrane is a broadened expansion of the posterior longitudinal ligament.

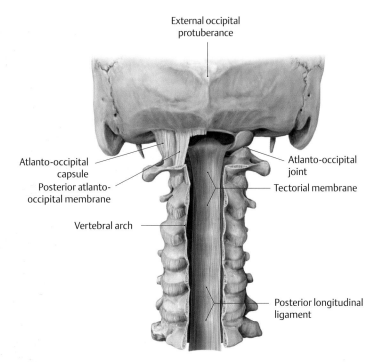

Fig. 1.30 Ligaments of the cervical spine

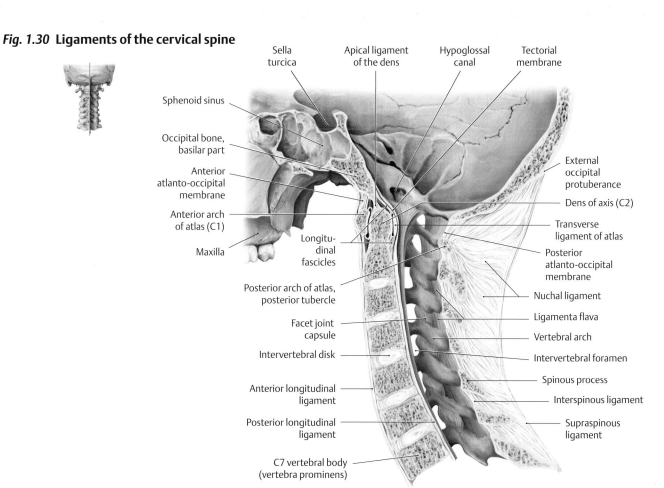

A Midsagittal section, left lateral view. The nuchal ligament is the broadened, sagittally oriented part of the supraspinous ligament that extends from the vertebra prominens (C7) to the external occipital protuberance.

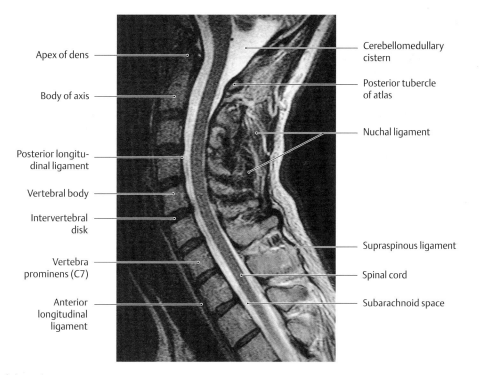

B Midsagittal T2-weighted MRI, left lateral view.

Vertebral Ligaments: Thoracolumbar Spine

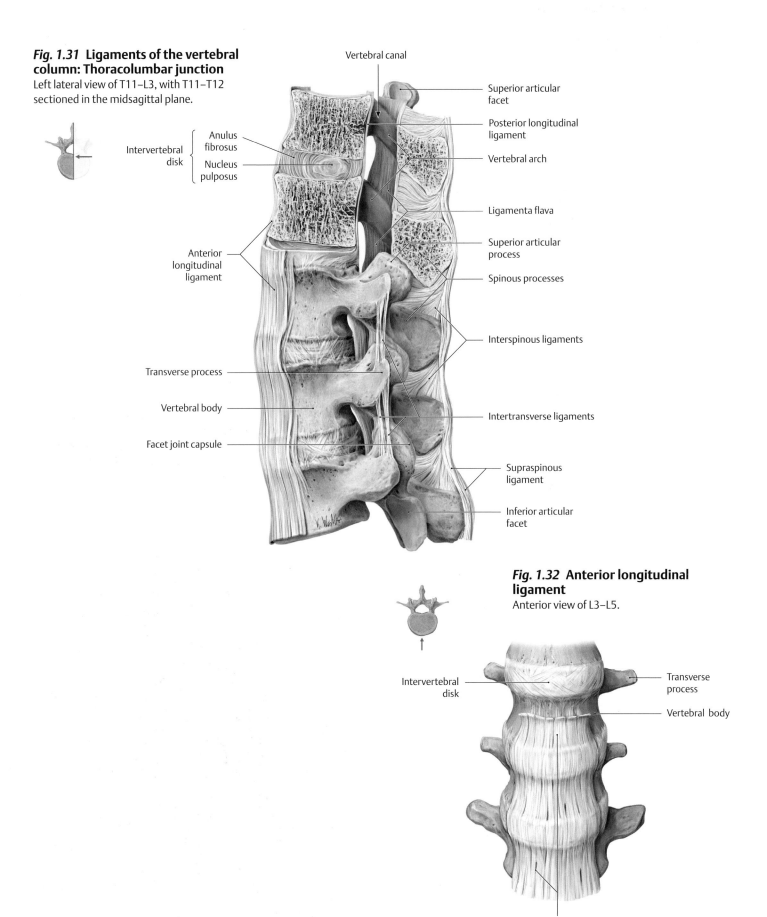

Fig. 1.31 Ligaments of the vertebral column: Thoracolumbar junction
Left lateral view of T11–L3, with T11–T12 sectioned in the midsagittal plane.

Intervertebral disk
Anulus fibrosus
Nucleus pulposus

Anterior longitudinal ligament

Transverse process

Vertebral body

Facet joint capsule

Vertebral canal

Superior articular facet

Posterior longitudinal ligament

Vertebral arch

Ligamenta flava

Superior articular process

Spinous processes

Interspinous ligaments

Intertransverse ligaments

Supraspinous ligament

Inferior articular facet

Fig. 1.32 Anterior longitudinal ligament
Anterior view of L3–L5.

Intervertebral disk

Transverse process

Vertebral body

Anterior longitudinal ligament

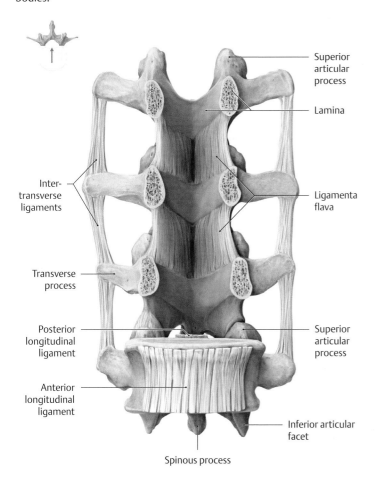

Fig. 1.33 Ligamentum flavum and intertransverse ligament

Anterior view of opened vertebral canal at level of L2–L5. *Removed:* L2–L4 vertebral bodies.

Superior articular process

Lamina

Inter-transverse ligaments

Ligamenta flava

Transverse process

Posterior longitudinal ligament

Superior articular process

Anterior longitudinal ligament

Inferior articular facet

Spinous process

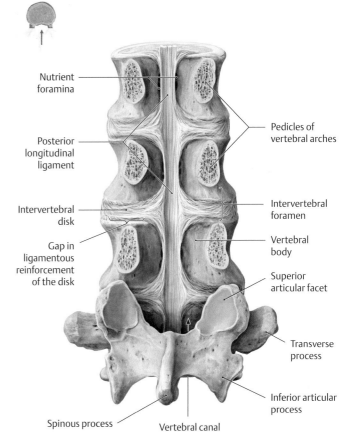

Fig. 1.34 Posterior longitudinal ligament

Posterior view of opened vertebral canal at level of L2–L5. *Removed:* L2–L4 vertebral arches at pedicular level.

Nutrient foramina

Pedicles of vertebral arches

Posterior longitudinal ligament

Intervertebral disk

Intervertebral foramen

Gap in ligamentous reinforcement of the disk

Vertebral body

Superior articular facet

Transverse process

Inferior articular process

Spinous process

Vertebral canal

Muscles of the Back: Overview

 The muscles of the back are divided into two groups, the extrinsic and the intrinsic muscles, which are separated by the superficial layer of the thoracolumbar fascia. The superficial extrinsic muscles are considered muscles of the upper limb that have migrated to the back; these muscles are discussed in Unit 4.

Fig. 2.1 **Superficial (extrinsic) muscles of the back**

Posterior view. *Removed:* Trapezius and latissimus dorsi (right). *Revealed:* Thoracolumbar fascia. *Note:* The superficial layer of the thoracolumbar fascia is reinforced by the aponeurotic origin of the latissimus dorsi.

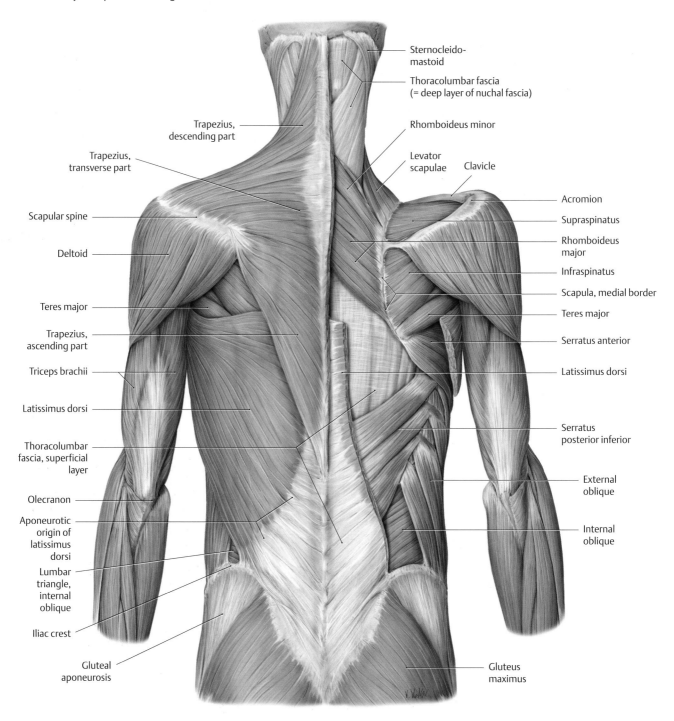

Fig. 2.2 Thoracolumbar fascia

Transverse section, superior view. The intrinsic back muscles are seques-
tered in an osseofibrous canal, formed by the thoracolumbar fascia, the
vertebral arches, and the spinous and transverse processes of associated
vertebrae. The thoracolumbar fascia consists of a superficial and a deep
layer that unite at the lateral margin of the intrinsic back muscles. In the
neck, the superficial layer blends with the nuchal fascia (deep layer),
becoming continuous with the cervical fascia (prevertebral layer).

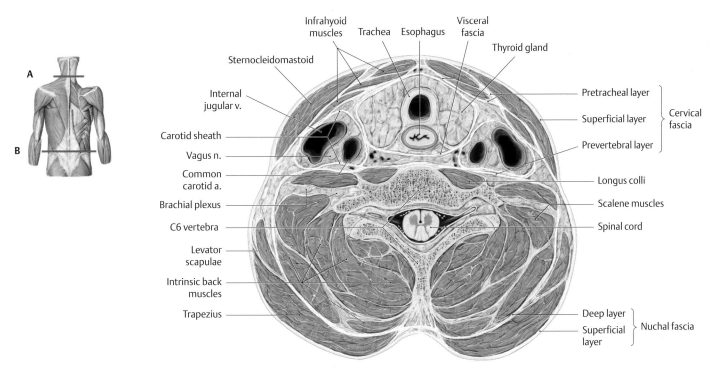

A Transverse section at level of C6 vertebra, superior view.

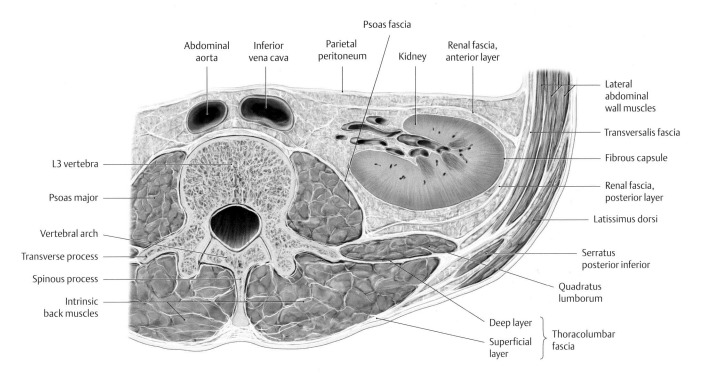

B Transverse section at level of L3, superior view.
Removed: Cauda equina and anterior trunk wall.

Intrinsic Muscles of the Cervical Spine

***Fig. 2.3* Muscles in the nuchal region**
Posterior view. *Removed:* Trapezius, sternocleidomastoid, splenius, and semispinalis muscles (right). *Revealed:* Nuchal muscles (right).

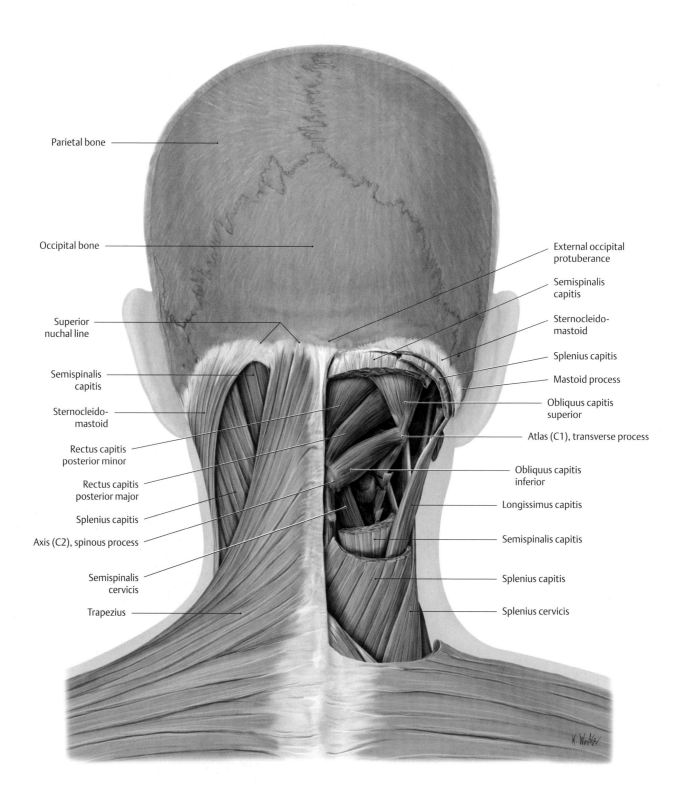

Parietal bone

Occipital bone

External occipital protuberance

Semispinalis capitis

Sternocleidomastoid

Superior nuchal line

Splenius capitis

Semispinalis capitis

Mastoid process

Sternocleidomastoid

Obliquus capitis superior

Rectus capitis posterior minor

Atlas (C1), transverse process

Rectus capitis posterior major

Obliquus capitis inferior

Splenius capitis

Longissimus capitis

Axis (C2), spinous process

Semispinalis capitis

Semispinalis cervicis

Splenius capitis

Trapezius

Splenius cervicis

Fig. 2.4 Short nuchal muscles
Posterior view. See Fig. 2.6.

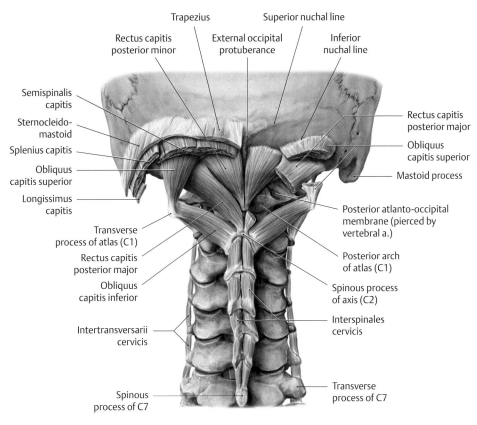

A Course of the short nuchal muscles.

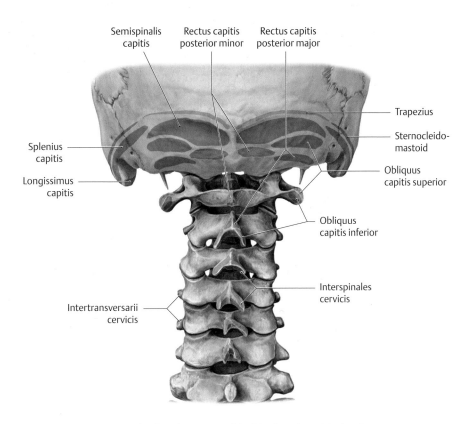

B Origins (red) and insertions (blue) in the suboccipital region.

Intrinsic Muscles of the Back

 The extrinsic muscles of the back (trapezius, latissimus dorsi, levator scapulae, and rhomboids) are discussed in Unit 4. The serratus posterior, considered an intermediate extrinsic back muscle, has been included with the superficial intrinsic muscles in this unit.

Fig. 2.5 **Intrinsic muscles of the back**

Posterior view. Sequential dissection of the thoracolumbar fascia, superficial intrinsic muscles, intermediate intrinsic muscles, and deep intrinsic muscles of the back.

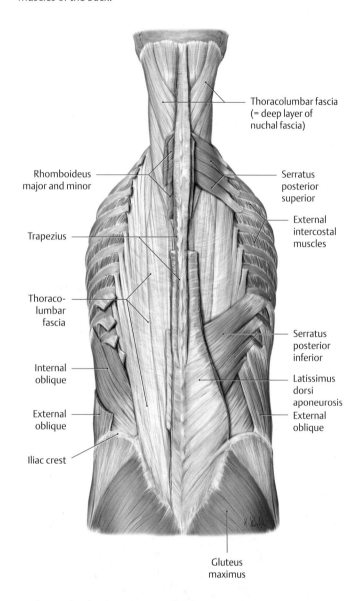

A Thoracolumbar fascia. *Removed:* Shoulder girdles and extrinsic back muscles (except serratus posterior and aponeurotic origin of latissimus dorsi). *Revealed:* Superficial layer of thoracolumbar fascia.

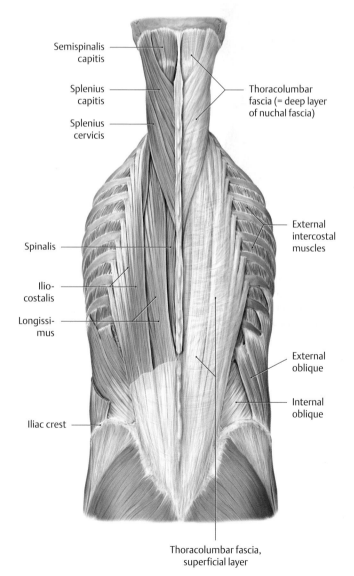

B Superficial and intermediate intrinsic back muscles. *Removed:* Thoracolumbar fascia (left). *Revealed:* Erector spinae and splenius muscles.

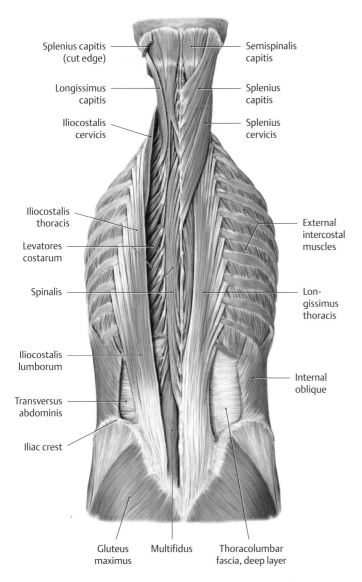

Splenius capitis (cut edge)
Semispinalis capitis
Longissimus capitis
Splenius capitis
Iliocostalis cervicis
Splenius cervicis
Iliocostalis thoracis
External intercostal muscles
Levatores costarum
Spinalis
Longissimus thoracis
Iliocostalis lumborum
Internal oblique
Transversus abdominis
Iliac crest
Gluteus maximus
Multifidus
Thoracolumbar fascia, deep layer

C Intermediate and deep intrinsic back muscles. *Removed:* Longissimus thoracis and cervicis, splenius muscles (left); iliocostalis (right). *Note:* The deep layer of the thoracolumbar fascia gives origin to the internal oblique and transversus abdominus. *Revealed:* Deep muscles of the back.

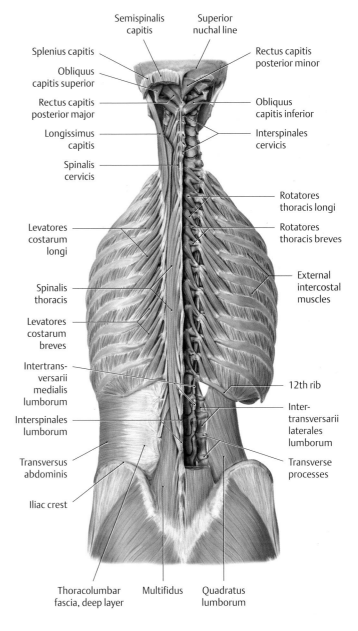

Semispinalis capitis
Superior nuchal line
Splenius capitis
Obliquus capitis superior
Rectus capitis posterior minor
Rectus capitis posterior major
Obliquus capitis inferior
Longissimus capitis
Interspinales cervicis
Spinalis cervicis
Rotatores thoracis longi
Rotatores thoracis breves
Levatores costarum longi
External intercostal muscles
Spinalis thoracis
Levatores costarum breves
Intertransversarii medialis lumborum
12th rib
Interspinales lumborum
Intertransversarii laterales lumborum
Transversus abdominis
Transverse processes
Iliac crest
Thoracolumbar fascia, deep layer
Multifidus
Quadratus lumborum

D Deep intrinsic back muscles. *Removed:* Superficial and intermediate intrinsic back muscles (all); deep fascial layer and multifidus (right). *Revealed:* Intertransversarii and quadratus lumborum (right).

27

Muscle Facts (I)

Fig. 2.6 **Short nuchal and craniovertebral joint muscles**

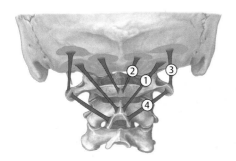

A Posterior view.

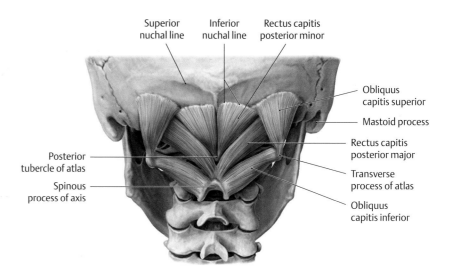

B Suboccipital muscles, posterior view.

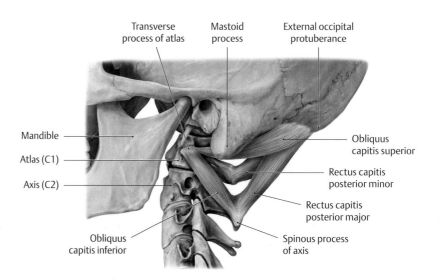

C Suboccipital muscles, left lateral view.

Table 2.1		Short nuchal and craniovertebral joint muscles			
Muscle		**Origin**	**Insertion**	**Innervation**	**Action**
Rectus capitis posterior	① Rectus capitis posterior major	C2 (spinous process)	Occipital bone (inferior nuchal line, middle third)	C1 (posterior ramus = suboccipital n.)	*Bilateral:* Extends head *Unilateral:* Rotates head to same side
	② Rectus capitis posterior minor	C1 (posterior tubercle)	Occipital bone (inferior nuchal line, inner third)		
Obliquus capitis	③ Obliquus capitis superior	C1 (transverse process)	Occipital bone (inferior nuchal line, middle third; above rectus capitis posterior major)		*Bilateral:* Extends head *Unilateral:* Tilts head to same side; rotates to opposite side
	④ Obliquus capitis inferior	C2 (spinous process)	C1 (transverse process)		*Bilateral:* Extends head *Unilateral:* Rotates head to same side

Fig. 2.7 **Prevertebral muscles**

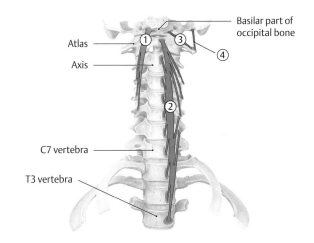

A Anterior view.

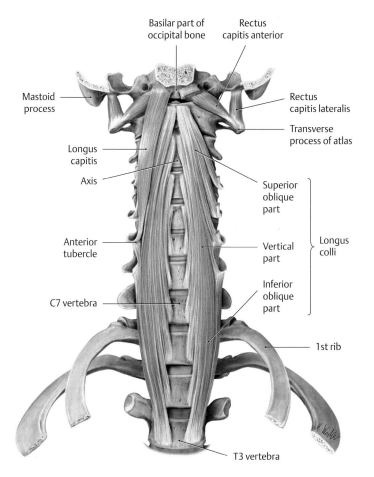

B Prevertebral muscles, anterior view.
Removed: Longus capitis (left); cervical viscera.

Table 2.2		Prevertebral muscles			
Muscle		**Origin**	**Insertion**	**Innervation**	**Action**
① Longus capitis		C3–C6 (transverse processes, anterior tubercles)	Occipital bone (basilar part)	Direct branches from cervical plexus (C1–C3)	*Bilateral:* Flexes head *Unilateral:* Tilts and slightly rotates head to same side
② Longus colli (cervicis)	Vertical (medial) part	C5–T3 (anterior sides of vertebral bodies)	C2–C4 (anterior sides of vertebral bodies)	Direct branches from cervical plexus (C2–C6)	*Bilateral:* Flexes cervical spine *Unilateral:* Tilts and rotates cervical spine to same side
	Superior oblique part	C3–C5 (transverse processes, anterior tubercles)	C1 (transverse process, anterior tubercle)		
	Inferior oblique part	T1–T3 (anterior sides of vertebral bodies)	C5–C6 (transverse processes, anterior tubercles)		
Rectus capitis	③ Rectus capitis anterior	C1 (lateral mass)	Occipital bone (basilar part)	C1 (anterior ramus)	*Bilateral:* Flexion at atlanto-occipital joint *Unilateral:* Lateral flexion at atlanto-occipital joint
	④ Rectus capitis lateralis	C1 (transverse process)	Occipital bone (basilar part, lateral to occipital condyles)		

Muscle Facts (II)

 The intrinsic back muscles are divided into superficial, intermediate, and deep layers. The posterior serratus muscles are extrinsic back muscles, innervated by the ventral rami of intercostal nerves, not the dorsal rami, which innervate the intrinsic back muscles. They are included here as they are encountered in dissection of the back musculature.

Table 2.3		Superficial intrinsic back muscles			
Muscle		**Origin**	**Insertion**	**Innervation**	**Action**
Posterior serratus	① Posterior serratus superior	Ligamentum nuchae; C7–T3 (spinous processes)	2nd–4th ribs (superior borders)	2nd–5th intercostal nn.	Elevates ribs
	② Posterior serratus inferior	T11–L2 (spinous processes)	8th–12th ribs (inferior borders, near angles)	Spinal nn. T9–T12 (anterior rami)	Depresses ribs
Splenius	③ Splenius capitis	Ligamentum nuchae; C7–T3 (spinous processes)	Occipital bone (lateral superior nuchal line; mastoid process)	Spinal nn. C1–C6 (posterior rami, lateral branches)	*Bilateral:* Extends cervical spine and head *Unilateral:* Flexes and rotates head to the same side
	④ Splenius cervicis	T3–T6 (spinous processes)	C1–C2 (transverse processes)		

Fig. 2.8 Superficial intrinsic back muscles (schematic)
Right side, posterior view.

Fig. 2.9 Intermediate intrinsic back muscles (schematic)
Right side, posterior view. These muscles are collectively known as the erector spinae.

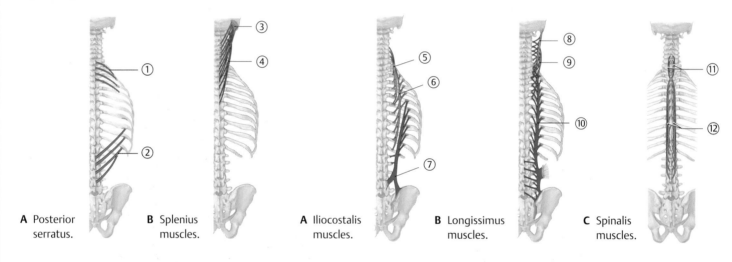

A Posterior serratus. **B** Splenius muscles. **A** Iliocostalis muscles. **B** Longissimus muscles. **C** Spinalis muscles.

Table 2.4		Intermediate intrinsic back muscles			
Muscle		**Origin**	**Insertion**	**Innervation**	**Action**
Iliocostalis	⑤ Iliocostalis cervicis	3rd–7th ribs	C4–C6 (transverse processes)	Spinal nn. C8–L1 (posterior rami, lateral branches)	*Bilateral:* Extends spine *Unilateral:* Bends spine laterally to same side
	⑥ Iliocostalis thoracis	7th–12th ribs	1st–6th ribs		
	⑦ Iliocostalis lumborum	Sacrum; iliac crest; thoracolumbar fascia	6th–12th ribs; thoracolumbar fascia (deep layer); upper lumbar vertebrae (transverse processes)		
Longissimus	⑧ Longissimus capitis	T1–T3 (transverse processes); C4–C7 (transverse and articular processes)	Temporal bone (mastoid process)	Spinal nn. C1–L5 (posterior rami, lateral branches)	*Bilateral:* Extends head *Unilateral:* Flexes and rotates head to same side
	⑨ Longissimus cervicis	T1–T6 (transverse processes)	C2–C5 (transverse processes)		*Bilateral:* Extends spine *Unilateral:* Bends spine laterally to same side
	⑩ Longissimus thoracis	Sacrum; iliac crest; lumbar vertebrae (spinous processes); lower thoracic vertebrae (transverse processes)	2nd–12th ribs; lumbar vertebrae (costal processes); thoracic vertebrae (transverse processes)		
Spinalis	⑪ Spinalis cervicis	C5–T2 (spinous processes)	C2–C5 (spinous processes)	Spinal nn. (posterior rami)	*Bilateral:* Extends cervical and thoracic spine *Unilateral:* Bends cervical and thoracic spine to same side
	⑫ Spinalis thoracis	T10–L3 (spinous processes, lateral surfaces)	T2–T8 (spinous processes, lateral surfaces)		

Fig. 2.10 Superficial and intermediate intrinsic back muscles
Posterior view.

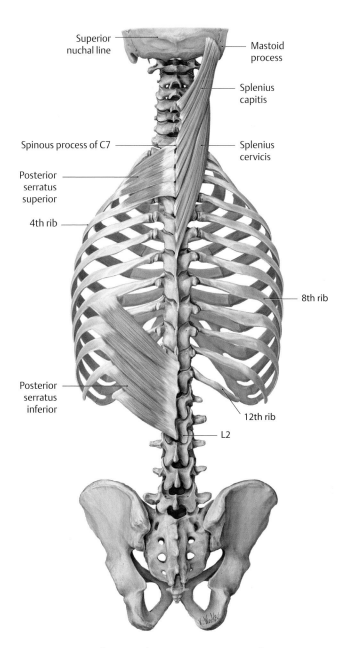

Superior nuchal line

Mastoid process

Splenius capitis

Spinous process of C7

Splenius cervicis

Posterior serratus superior

4th rib

8th rib

Posterior serratus inferior

12th rib

L2

A Splenius and posterior serratus muscles.

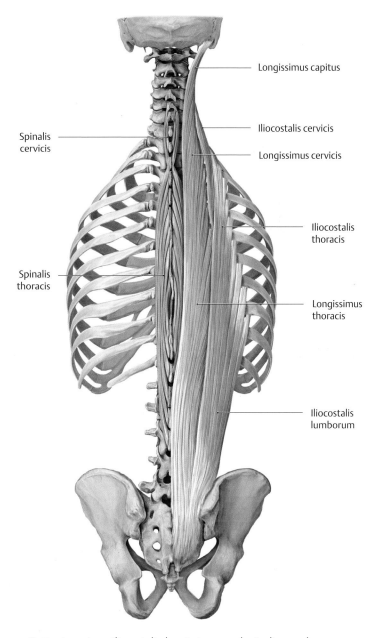

Longissimus capitus

Iliocostalis cervicis

Spinalis cervicis

Longissimus cervicis

Iliocostalis thoracis

Spinalis thoracis

Longissimus thoracis

Iliocostalis lumborum

B Erector spinae: Iliocostalis, longissimus, and spinalis muscles.

Muscle Facts (III)

 The deep intrinsic back muscles are divided into two groups: transversospinal and deep segmental muscles. The transverso-spinalis muscles pass between the transverse and spinous processes of the vertebrae.

Table 2.5		Transversospinalis muscles			
Muscle		**Origin**	**Insertion**	**Innervation**	**Action**
Rotatores	① Rotatores brevis	T1–T12 (between transverse and spinous processes of adjacent vertebrae)		Spinal nn. (posterior rami)	*Bilateral:* Extends throacic spine *Unilateral:* Rotates spine to opposite side
	② Rotatores longi	T1–T12 (between transverse and spinous processes, skipping one vertebra)			
Multifidus ③		C2–sacrum (between transverse and spinous processes, skipping two to four vertebrae)			*Bilateral:* Extends spine *Unilateral:* Flexes spine to same side, rotates to opposite side
Semispinalis	④ Semispinalis capitis	C4–T7 (transverse and articular processes)	Occipital bone (between superior and inferior nuchal lines)		*Bilateral:* Extends thoracic and cervical spines and head (stabilizes craniovertebral joints) *Unilateral:* Bends head, cervical and thoracic spines to same side, rotates to opposite side
	⑤ Semispinalis cervicis	T1–T6 (transverse processes)	C2–C5 (spinous processes)		
	⑥ Semispinalis thoracis	T6–T12 (transverse processes)	C6–T4 (spinous processes)		

Fig. 2.11 Transversospinalis muscles (schematic)
Posterior view.

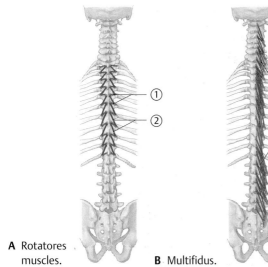

A Rotatores muscles. **B** Multifidus. **C** Semispinalis.

Fig. 2.12 Deep segmental muscles (schematic)
Posterior view.

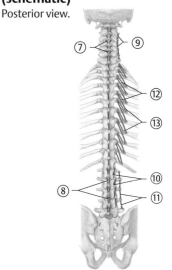

Table 2.6		Deep segmental back muscles			
Muscle		**Origin**	**Insertion**	**Innervation**	**Action**
Interspinales*	⑦ Interspinales cervicis	C1–C7 (between spinous processes of adjacent vertebrae)		Spinal nn. (posterior rami)	Extends cervical and lumbar spines
	⑧ Interspinales lumborum	L1–L5 (between spinous processes of adjacent vertebrae)			
Inter-transversarii*	Intertransversarii anteriores cervicis	C2–C7 (between anterior tubercles of adjacent vertebrae)		Spinal nn. (anterior rami)	*Bilateral:* Stabilizes and extends the cervical and lumbar spines *Unilateral:* Bends the cervical and lumbar spines laterally to same side
	⑨ Intertransversarii posteriores cervicis	C2–C7 (between posterior tubercles of adjacent vertebrae)			
	⑩ Intertransversarii mediales lumborum	L1–L5 (between mammillary processes of adjacent vertebrae)		Spinal nn. (posterior rami)	
	⑪ Intertransversarii laterales lumborum	L1–L5 (between transverse processes of adjacent vertebrae)			
Levatores costarum	⑫ Levatores costarum breves	C7–T11 (transverse processes)	Costal angle of next lower rib		*Bilateral:* Extends thoracic spine *Unilateral:* Bends thoracic spine to same side, rotates to opposite side
	⑬ Levatores costarum longi		Costal angle of rib two vertebrae below		

*Both the interspinales and intertransversarii muscles traverse the entire spine; only their clinically relevant components have been included.

Fig. 2.13 Deep intrinsic back muscles
Posterior view.

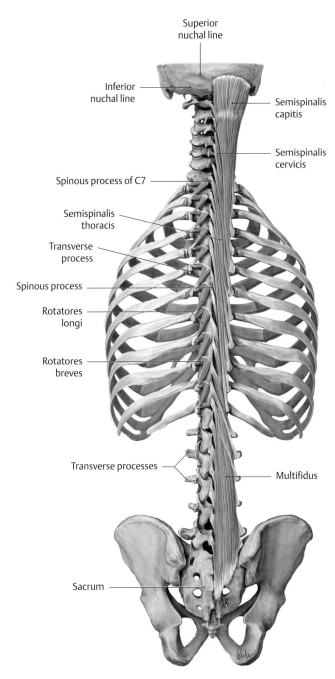

Superior
nuchal line

Inferior
nuchal line

Semispinalis
capitis

Semispinalis
cervicis

Spinous process of C7

Semispinalis
thoracis

Transverse
process

Spinous process

Rotatores
longi

Rotatores
breves

Transverse processes

Multifidus

Sacrum

A Transversospinalis muscles: Rotatores,
multifidus, and semispinalis.

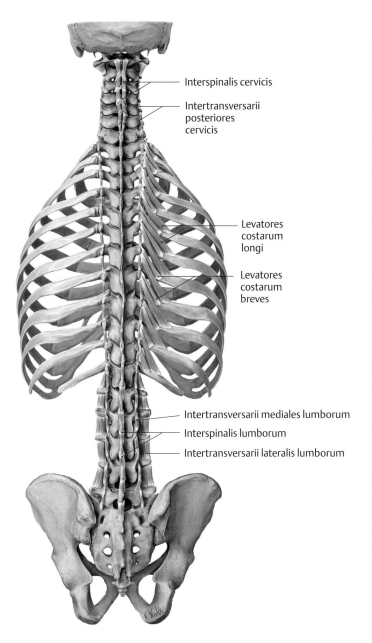

Interspinalis cervicis

Intertransversarii
posteriores
cervicis

Levatores
costarum
longi

Levatores
costarum
breves

Intertransversarii mediales lumborum

Interspinalis lumborum

Intertransversarii lateralis lumborum

B Deep segmental muscles: Interspinales,
intertransversarii, and levatores costarum.

Arteries & Veins of the Back

Fig. 3.1 Arteries of the back

The structures of the back are supplied by branches of the posterior intercostal arteries, which arise from the thoracic aorta or directly from the subclavian artery.

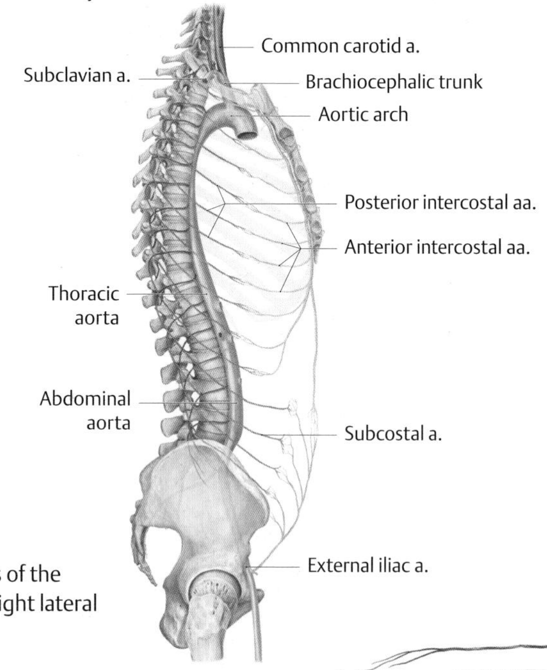

Common carotid a.

Subclavian a.

Brachiocephalic trunk

Aortic arch

Posterior intercostal aa.

Anterior intercostal aa.

Thoracic aorta

Abdominal aorta

Subcostal a.

External iliac a.

A Arteries of the trunk, right lateral view.

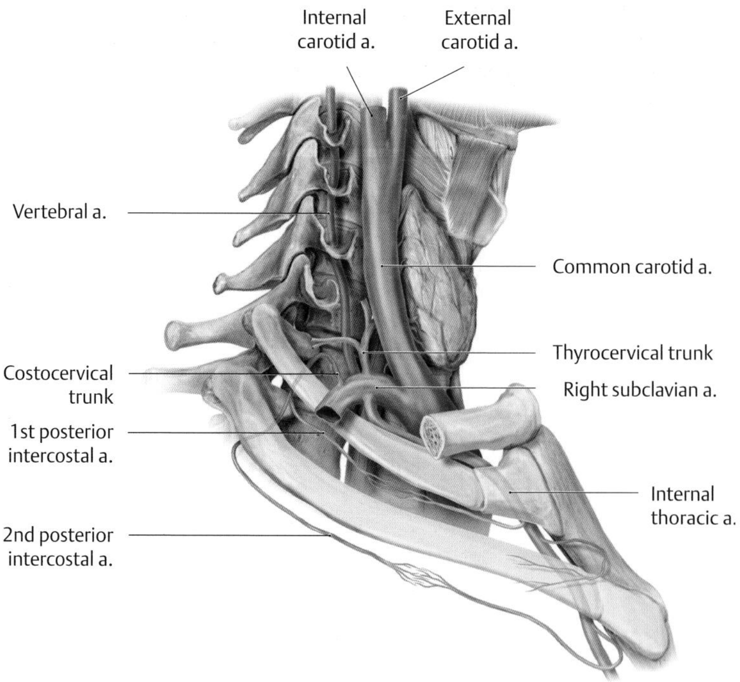

Internal carotid a.

External carotid a.

Vertebral a.

Common carotid a.

Costocervical trunk

Thyrocervical trunk

Right subclavian a.

1st posterior intercostal a.

2nd posterior intercostal a.

Internal thoracic a.

B Vascular supply to the nuchal region, posterolateral view. *Note:* The first and second posterior intercostal arteries arise from the costo-cervical trunk, a branch of the subclavian artery.

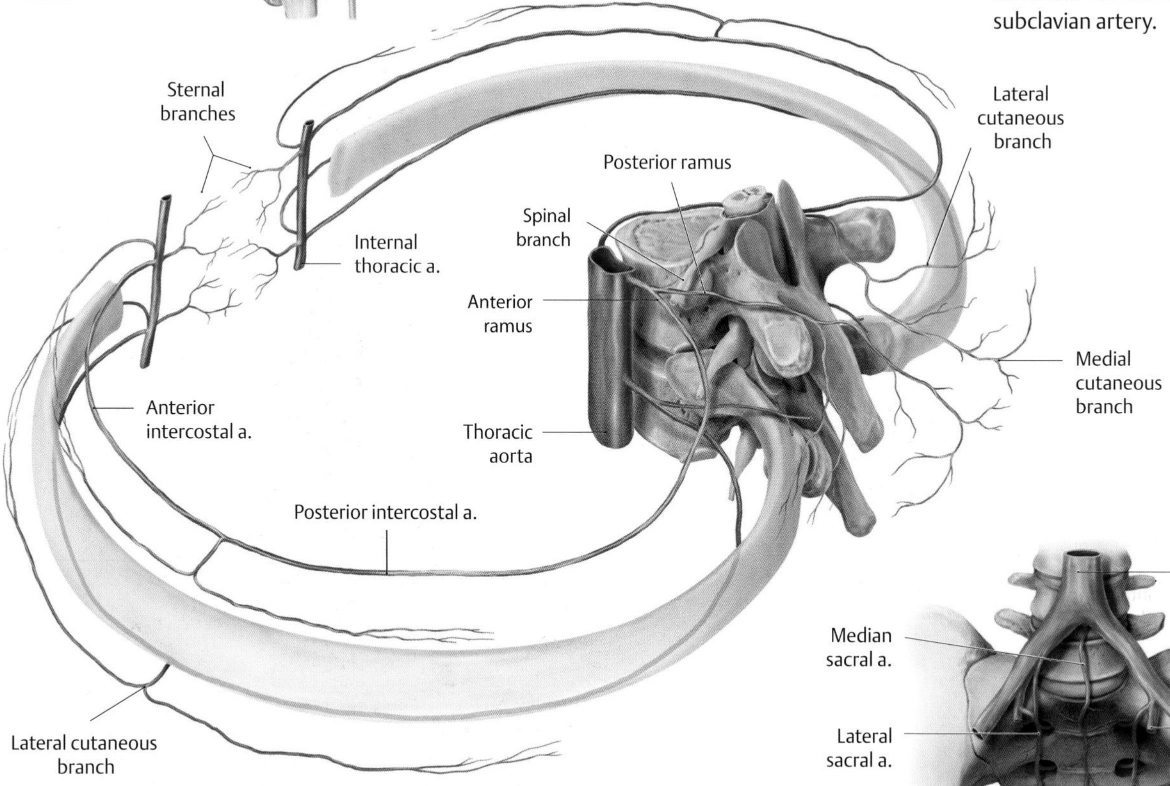

Sternal branches

Lateral cutaneous branch

Posterior ramus

Spinal branch

Internal thoracic a.

Anterior ramus

Medial cutaneous branch

Anterior intercostal a.

Thoracic aorta

Posterior intercostal a.

Lateral cutaneous branch

C Posterior intercostal arteries, oblique posterosuperior view. The posterior intercostal arteries give rise to cutaneous and muscular branches, as well as spinal branches that supply the spinal cord.

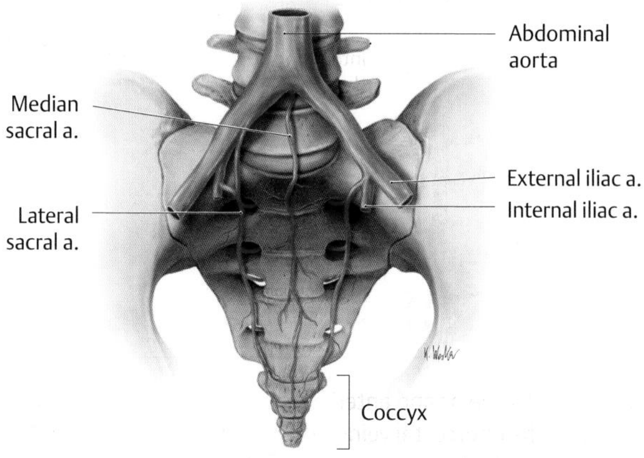

Abdominal aorta

Median sacral a.

External iliac a.

Internal iliac a.

Lateral sacral a.

Coccyx

D Vascular supply to the sacrum, anterior view.

Fig. 3.2 Veins of the back

The veins of the back drain into the azygos vein via the superior intercostal veins, hemiazygos veins, and ascending lumbar veins. The interior of the spinal column is drained by the vertebral venous plexus that runs the length of the spine.

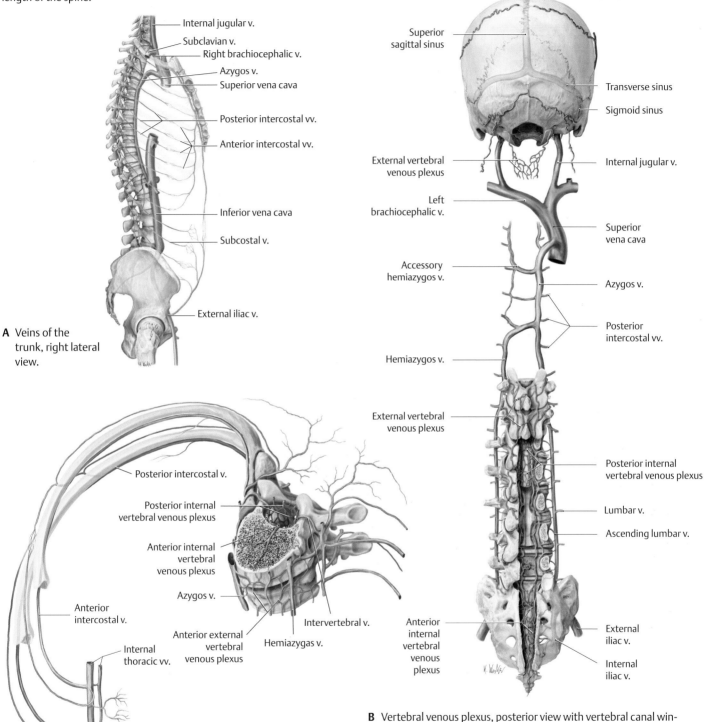

A Veins of the trunk, right lateral view.

Labels in A:
- Internal jugular v.
- Subclavian v.
- Right brachiocephalic v.
- Azygos v.
- Superior vena cava
- Posterior intercostal vv.
- Anterior intercostal vv.
- Inferior vena cava
- Subcostal v.
- External iliac v.

Labels in B:
- Superior sagittal sinus
- Transverse sinus
- Sigmoid sinus
- External vertebral venous plexus
- Internal jugular v.
- Left brachiocephalic v.
- Superior vena cava
- Accessory hemiazygos v.
- Azygos v.
- Posterior intercostal vv.
- Hemiazygos v.
- External vertebral venous plexus
- Posterior internal vertebral venous plexus
- Lumbar v.
- Ascending lumbar v.
- Anterior internal vertebral venous plexus
- External iliac v.
- Internal iliac v.

Labels in C:
- Posterior intercostal v.
- Posterior internal vertebral venous plexus
- Anterior internal vertebral venous plexus
- Azygos v.
- Anterior intercostal v.
- Anterior external vertebral venous plexus
- Hemiazygas v.
- Intervertebral v.
- Internal thoracic vv.

B Vertebral venous plexus, posterior view with vertebral canal windowed in the lumbar and sacral spine. The external vertebral venous plexus communicates with the sigmoid sinus through emissary veins in the skull. The *external* vertebral venous plexus is divided into an anterior and a posterior portion that run along the exterior of the spinal column. The anterior and posterior *internal* vertebral venous plexus run in the vertebral foramen and drain the spinal cord.

C Intercostal veins and anterior vertebral venous plexus, anterosuperior view. The intercostal veins follow a similar course as the intercostal nerves and arteries (see pp. 34, 36). *Note:* The anterior external vertebral venous plexus can be seen communicating with the azygos vein.

Nerves of the Back

 The back receives its innervation from branches of the spinal nerves. The *posterior* rami of the spinal nerves supply most of the intrinsic muscles of the back. The extrinsic muscles of the back are supplied by the *anterior* rami of the spinal nerves.

Fig. 3.3 Nerves of the back

The anterior rami of spinal nerves T1–T11 form the intercostal nerves, which course along the ribs and give rise to lateral and anterior cutaneous branches.

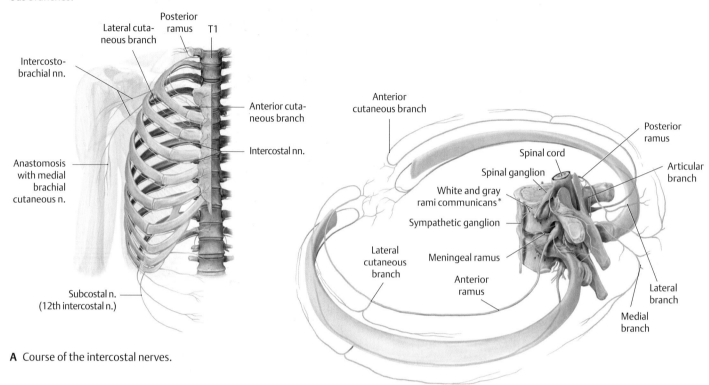

A Course of the intercostal nerves.

B Spinal nerve branches, superior view. The *posterior* rami of the spinal nerves give rise to muscular and cutaneous branches, as well as articular branches to the zygapophyseal joints. The *anterior* rami of spinal nerves T1–T11 produce the intercostal nerves (T12 produces the subcostal nerve).

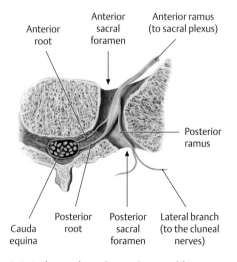

C Spinal nerve branches in the sacral foramina. Superior view of transverse section through right half of sacrum.

Table 3.1	Branches of a spinal nerve		
Branches			**Territory**
Meningeal ramus			Spinal meninges; ligaments of spinal column
Posterior ramus	Medial branches	Articular branch	Zygapophyseal joints
		Muscular branch	Intrinsic back muscles
		Cutaneous branch	Skin of posterior head, neck, back, and buttocks
	Lateral branches	Cutaneous branch	
		Muscular branch	Intrinsic back muscles
Anterior ramus	Lateral cutaneous branches		Skin of lateral chest wall
	Anterior cutaneous branches		Skin of anterior chest wall
*The white and gray rami communicans carry pre- and postganglionic fibers between the sympathetic trunk and spinal nerve. They are shown on p. 622.			

Fig. 3.4 Nerves of the nuchal region

Right side, posterior view. Like the back, the nuchal region receives most of its motor and sensory innervation from the *posterior* rami of the spinal nerves. The posterior rami of C1–C3 have specific names: suboccipital nerve (C1), greater occipital nerve (C2), and third occipital nerve (C3). The lesser occipital and great auricular nerves arise from the *anterior* rami of the C1–C4 spinal nerves and innervate the skin of the anterolateral head and neck. The anterior rami of C1–C4 also give rise to the *ansa cervicalis,* which innervates the infrahyoid muscles (see p. 562).

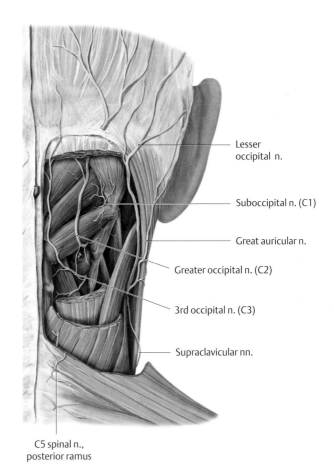

Lesser occipital n.

Suboccipital n. (C1)

Great auricular n.

Greater occipital n. (C2)

3rd occipital n. (C3)

Supraclavicular nn.

C5 spinal n., posterior ramus

Fig. 3.5 Cutaneous innervation of the back

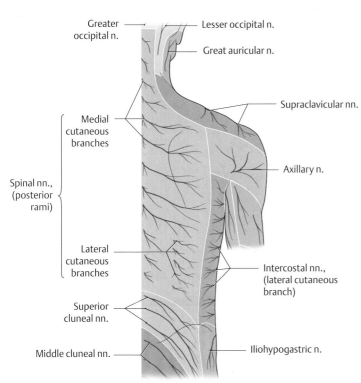

Greater occipital n.

Lesser occipital n.

Great auricular n.

Supraclavicular nn.

Medial cutaneous branches

Axillary n.

Spinal nn., (posterior rami)

Lateral cutaneous branches

Intercostal nn., (lateral cutaneous branch)

Superior cluneal nn.

Middle cluneal nn.

Iliohypogastric n.

A Peripheral sensory cutaneous innervation of the back.

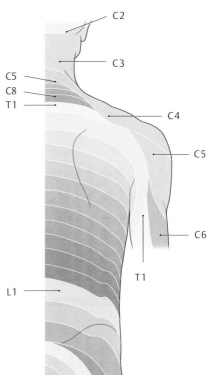

C2

C3

C5

C8

T1

C4

C5

C6

T1

L1

B Dermatomes: Segmental (radicular) cutaneous innervation of the back. *Note*: The posterior ramus of C1 is purely motor; there is consequently no C1 dermatome.

Neurovascular Topography of the Back

Fig. 3.6 Neurovasculature of the nuchal region

Posterior view. *Removed:* Trapezius, sternocleidomastoid, splenius capitis, and semispinalis capitis. *Revealed:* Suboccipital region. See p. 60 for the course of the intercostal vessels.

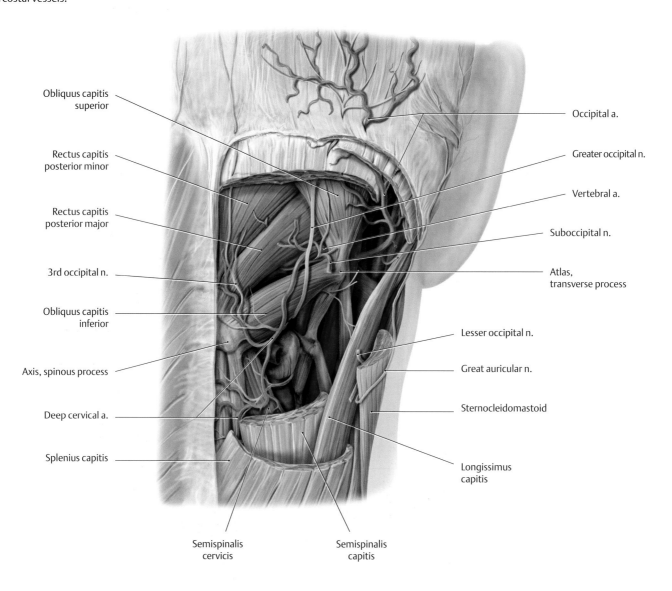

Obliquus capitis superior

Rectus capitis posterior minor

Rectus capitis posterior major

3rd occipital n.

Obliquus capitis inferior

Axis, spinous process

Deep cervical a.

Splenius capitis

Occipital a.

Greater occipital n.

Vertebral a.

Suboccipital n.

Atlas, transverse process

Lesser occipital n.

Great auricular n.

Sternocleidomastoid

Longissimus capitis

Semispinalis cervicis

Semispinalis capitis

Fig. 3.7 **Neurovasculature of the back**

Posterior view. *Removed:* Muscle fascia (except superficial layer of thoracolumbar fascia); latissimus dorsi (right). *Reflected:* Trapezius (right). *Revealed:* Transverse cervical artery in the deep scapular region.

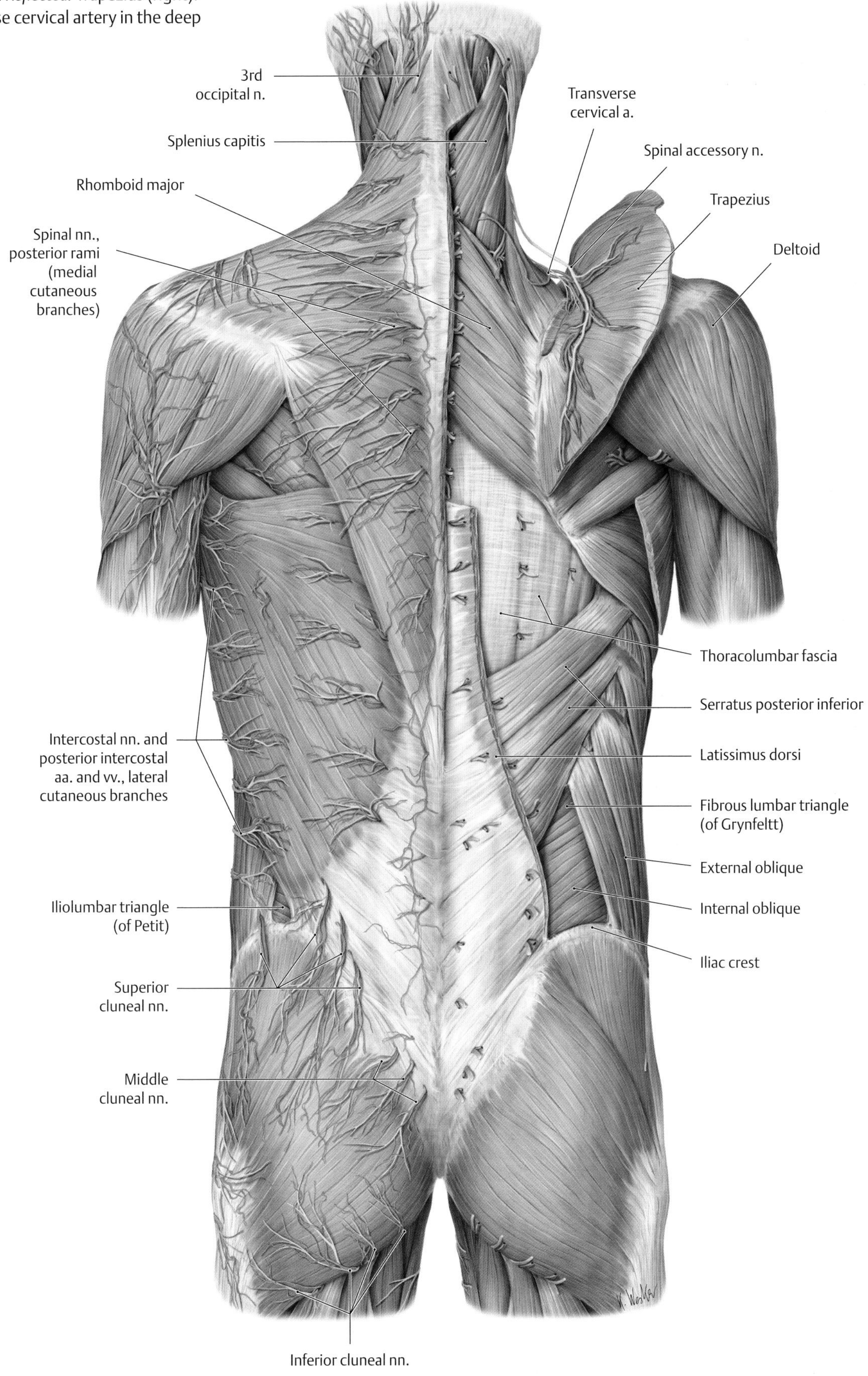

3rd occipital n.

Splenius capitis

Rhomboid major

Spinal nn., posterior rami (medial cutaneous branches)

Transverse cervical a.

Spinal accessory n.

Trapezius

Deltoid

Thoracolumbar fascia

Serratus posterior inferior

Latissimus dorsi

Fibrous lumbar triangle (of Grynfeltt)

External oblique

Internal oblique

Iliac crest

Intercostal nn. and posterior intercostal aa. and vv., lateral cutaneous branches

Iliolumbar triangle (of Petit)

Superior cluneal nn.

Middle cluneal nn.

Inferior cluneal nn.

Surface Anatomy

Fig. 4.1 **Palpable structures in the back**
Posterior view.

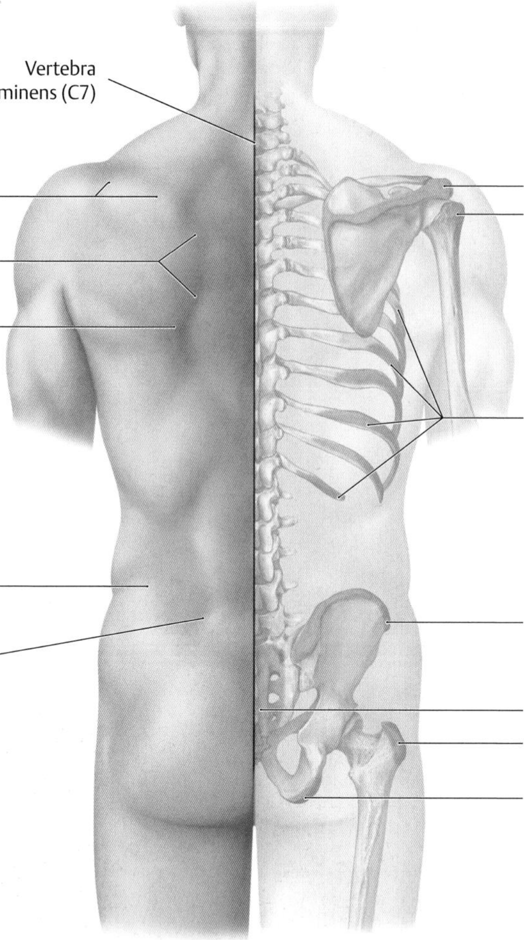

Vertebra prominens (C7)

Scapular spine

Medial border

Inferior angle

Iliac crest

Posterior superior iliac spine

Acromion

Greater tuberosity

6th through 12th ribs

Anterior superior iliac spine

Sacrum

Greater trochanter

Ischial tuberosity

A Bony prominences.

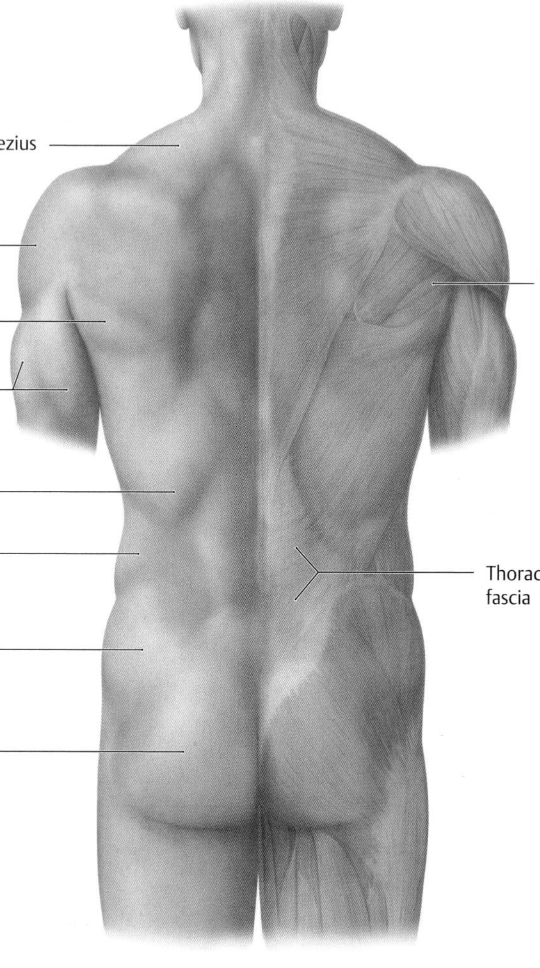

Trapezius

Deltoid

Teres major

Triceps brachii

Latissimus dorsi

External oblique

Gluteus medius

Gluteus maximus

Teres minor

Thoracolumbar fascia

B Musculature.

Fig. 4.2 **Surface anatomy of the back**
Posterior view.

Q1: Michaelis' rhomboid can be used as an indicator of the width of the female pelvis. What are its boundaries?

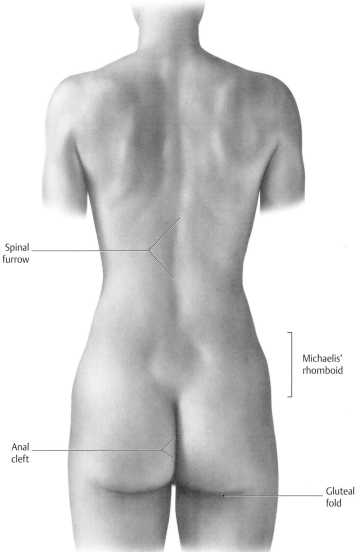

Spinal furrow

Michaelis' rhomboid

Anal cleft

Gluteal fold

A Female back.

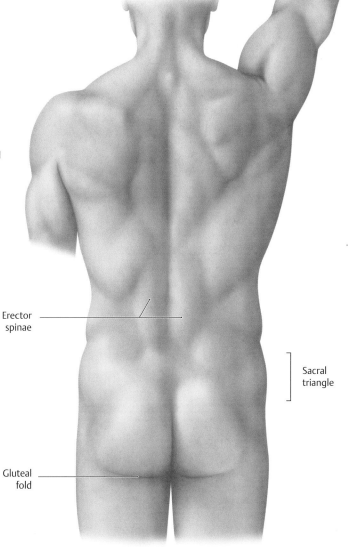

Erector spinae

Sacral triangle

Gluteal fold

Q2: The limb girdles are reliable indicators of specific vertebral levels. What level corresponds to the inferior angle of the scapula? What level corresponds to the iliac crest?

See answers beginning on p. 626.

B Male back.

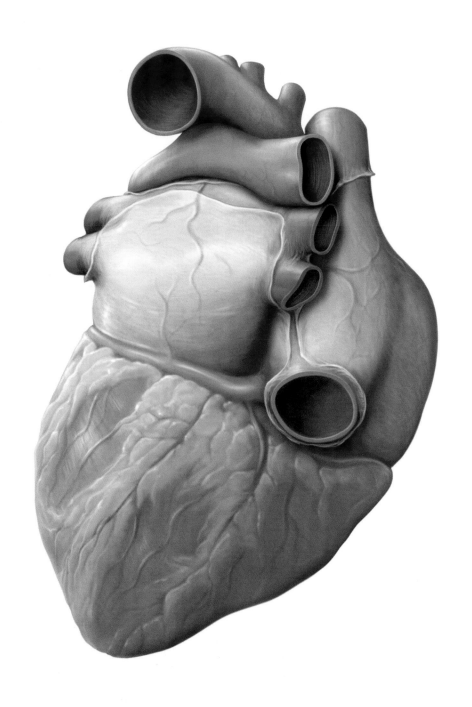

Thorax

Thoracic Skeleton

 The thoracic skeleton consists of 12 thoracic vertebrae (p. 8), 12 pairs of ribs with costal cartilages, and the sternum. In addition to participating in respiratory movements, it provides a measure of protection to vital organs. The female thorax is generally narrower and shorter than the male equivalent.

Fig. 5.1 **Thoracic skeleton**

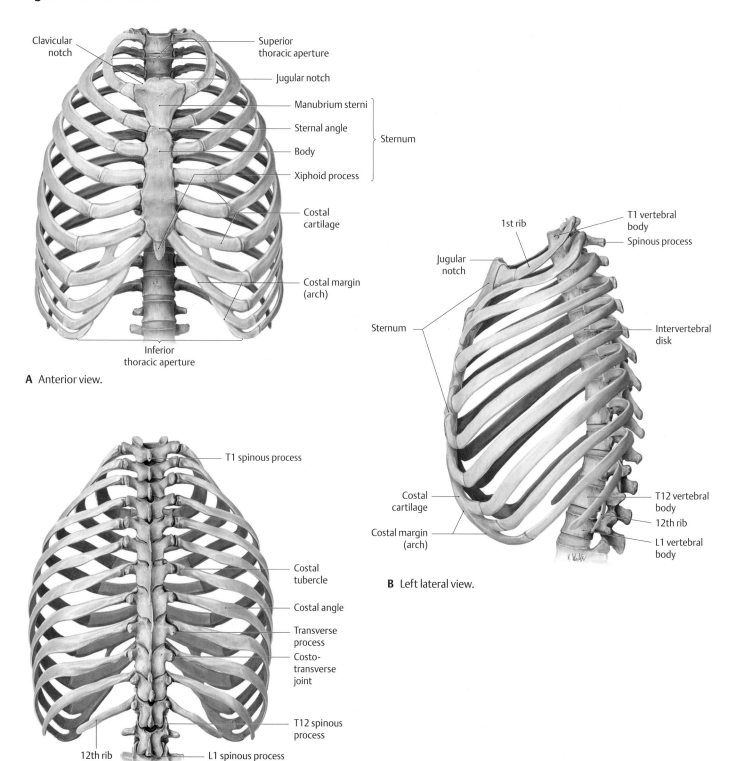

A Anterior view.

B Left lateral view.

C Posterior view.

Fig. 5.2 **Structure of a thoracic segment**
Superior view of 6th rib pair.

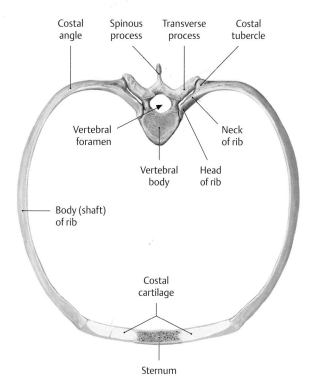

| Costal angle | Spinous process | Transverse process | Costal tubercle |

Vertebral foramen

Neck of rib

Vertebral body

Head of rib

Body (shaft) of rib

Costal cartilage

Sternum

Table 5.1	**Elements of a thoracic segment**		
Vertebra			
Rib	Bony part (costal bone)	Head	
		Neck	
		Costal tubercle	
		Body (including costal angle)	
	Costal part (costal cartilage)		
Sternum (articulates with costal cartilage of true ribs only; see Fig. 5.3)			

Fig. 5.3 **Types of ribs**
Left lateral view.

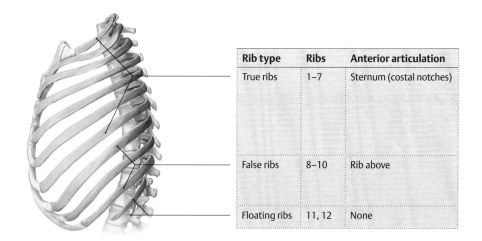

Rib type	Ribs	Anterior articulation
True ribs	1–7	Sternum (costal notches)
False ribs	8–10	Rib above
Floating ribs	11, 12	None

Sternum & Ribs

Fig. 5.4 **Sternum**

The sternum is a bladelike bone consisting of the manubrium, body, and xiphoid process. The junction of the manubrium and body (the sternal angle) is typically elevated and marks the articulation of the second rib. The sternal angle is an important landmark for internal structures.

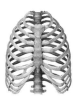

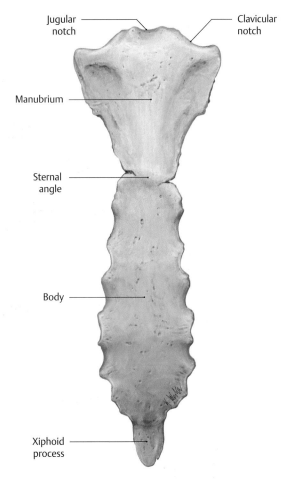

Jugular notch

Clavicular notch

Manubrium

Sternal angle

Body

Xiphoid process

A Anterior view.

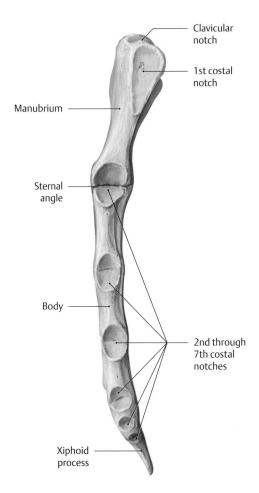

Clavicular notch

1st costal notch

Manubrium

Sternal angle

Body

2nd through 7th costal notches

Xiphoid process

B Left lateral view. The costal notches are sites of articulation with the costal cartilage of the true ribs (see Fig. 5.3).

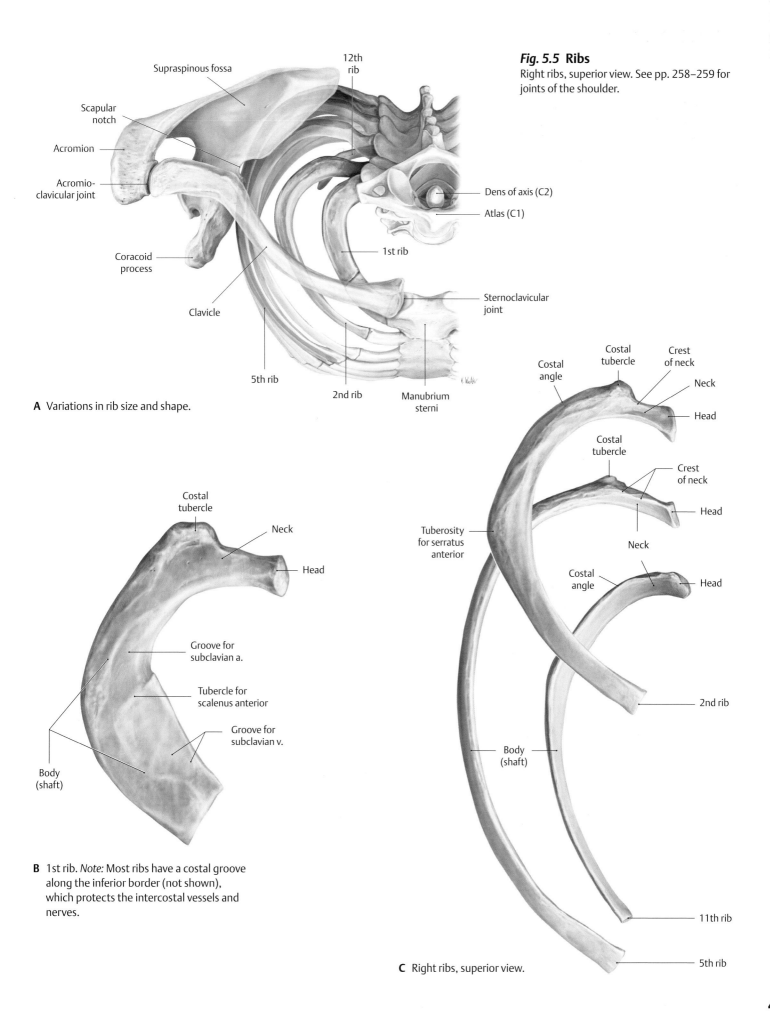

***Fig. 5.5* Ribs**
Right ribs, superior view. See pp. 258–259 for joints of the shoulder.

Supraspinous fossa

Scapular notch

Acromion

Acromio-clavicular joint

Coracoid process

Clavicle

12th rib

Dens of axis (C2)

Atlas (C1)

1st rib

Sternoclavicular joint

5th rib

2nd rib

Manubrium sterni

A Variations in rib size and shape.

Costal tubercle

Neck

Head

Groove for subclavian a.

Tubercle for scalenus anterior

Groove for subclavian v.

Body (shaft)

B 1st rib. *Note:* Most ribs have a costal groove along the inferior border (not shown), which protects the intercostal vessels and nerves.

Costal angle

Costal tubercle

Crest of neck

Neck

Head

Costal tubercle

Crest of neck

Head

Tuberosity for serratus anterior

Neck

Costal angle

Head

Body (shaft)

2nd rib

11th rib

5th rib

C Right ribs, superior view.

47

Joints of the Thoracic Cage

 The diaphragm is the chief muscle for quiet respiration (see p. 52). The muscles of the thoracic wall (see p. 50) contribute to deep (forced) inspiration.

Fig. 5.6 Rib cage movement

Full inspiration (red); full expiration (blue). In deep inspiration, there is an increase in transverse and sagittal thoracic diameters, as well as the infrasternal angle. The descent of the diaphragm further increases the volume of the thoracic cavity.

Inspiration

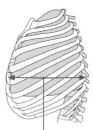

Infrasternal angle

Transverse thoracic diameter

Sagittal thoracic diameter

Expiration

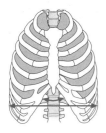

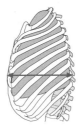

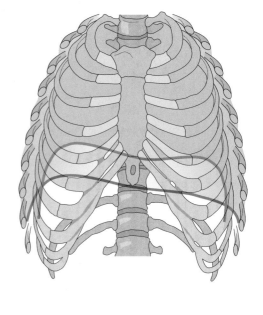

A Anterior view.

B Left lateral view.

C Position of diaphragm during respiration.

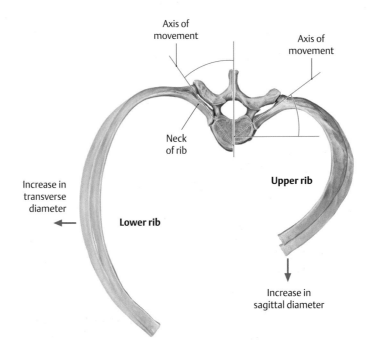

Axis of movement

Axis of movement

Neck of rib

Upper rib

Increase in transverse diameter

Lower rib

Increase in sagittal diameter

D Axes of rib movement, superior view.

Fig. 5.7 **Sternocostal joints**

Anterior view with right half of sternum sectioned frontally. True joints are generally found only at ribs 2 to 5; ribs 1, 6, and 7 attach to the sternum by synchondroses.

Fig. 5.8 **Costovertebral joints**

Two synovial joints make up the costovertebral articulation of each rib. The costal tubercle of each rib articulates with the costal facet of its accompanying vertebra (**A**). The head of most ribs articulates with the vertebra of its own number and the vertebra immediately superior. Ribs 1, 11, and 12 typically articulate only with their own vertebrae.

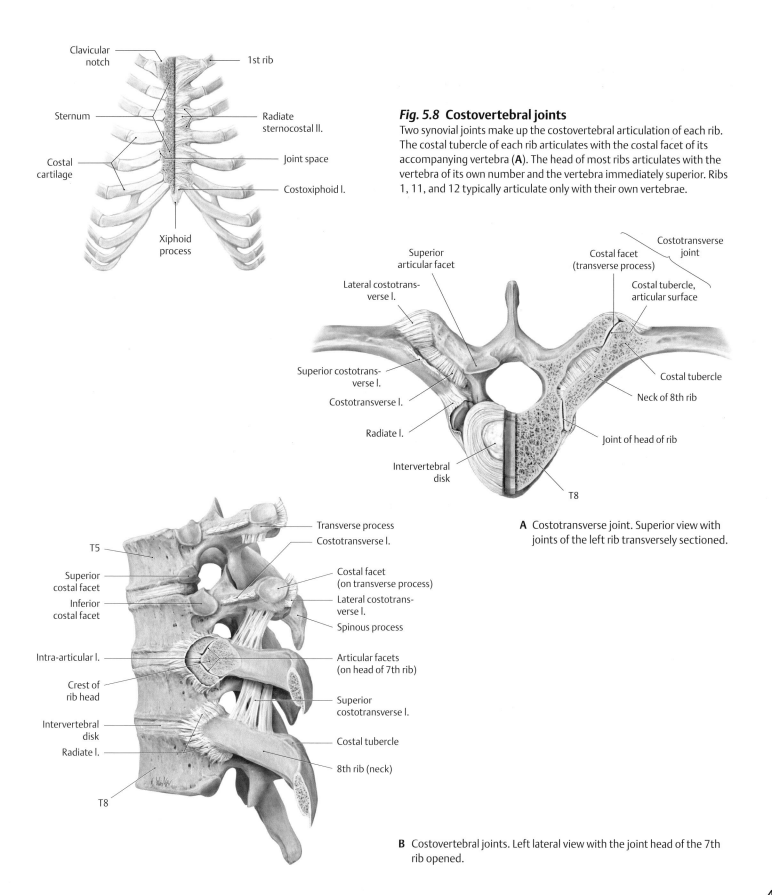

A Costotransverse joint. Superior view with joints of the left rib transversely sectioned.

B Costovertebral joints. Left lateral view with the joint head of the 7th rib opened.

Thoracic Wall Muscle Facts

 The muscles of the thoracic wall are primarily responsible for chest respiration, although other muscles aid in *deep* inspiration: the pectoralis major and serratus anterior are discussed with the shoulder (see pp. 264–267), and the serratus posterior is discussed with the back (see p. 30).

Fig. 5.9 **Muscles of the thoracic wall**

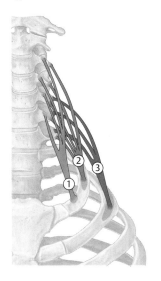

A Scalene muscles, anterior view.

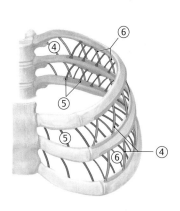

B Intercostal muscles, anterior view.

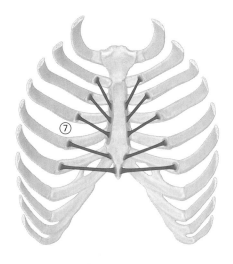

C Transversus thoracis, posterior view.

Table 5.2		Muscles of the thoracic wall			
Muscle		**Origin**	**Insertion**	**Innervation**	**Action**
Scalene	① Anterior scalene	C3–C6 (transverse processes, anterior tubercles)	1st rib (scalene tubercle)	Direct branches from cervical and brachial plexus (C3–C6)	*With ribs mobile*: Raises upper ribs (inspiration) *With ribs fixed*: Bends cervical spine to same side (unilateral); flexes neck (bilateral)
	② Middle scalene	C4–C6 (transverse processes, posterior tubercles)	1st rib (posterior to groove for subclavian a.)		
	③ Posterior scalene		2nd rib (outer surface)		
Intercostal	④ External intercostal	Lower margin of rib to upper margin of next lower rib (courses obliquely forward and downward from costal tubercle to chondro-osseous junction)		1st to 11th intercostal nn.	Raises ribs (inspiration); supports intercostal spaces; stabilizes chest wall
	⑤ Internal intercostal ⑥ Innermost intercostal	Lower margin of rib to lower margin of next lower rib (courses obliquely forward and upward from costal angle to sternum)			Lowers ribs (expiration); supports intercostal spaces, stabilizes chest wall
Subcostal		Lower margin of lower ribs to inner surface of ribs two to three ribs below		Variable lower intercostal nn.	Raises ribs (inspiration)
⑦ Transversus thoracis		Sternum and xiphoid process (inner surface)	2nd to 6th ribs (costal cartilage, inner surface)	2nd to 7th intercostal nn.	Weakly lowers ribs (expiration)

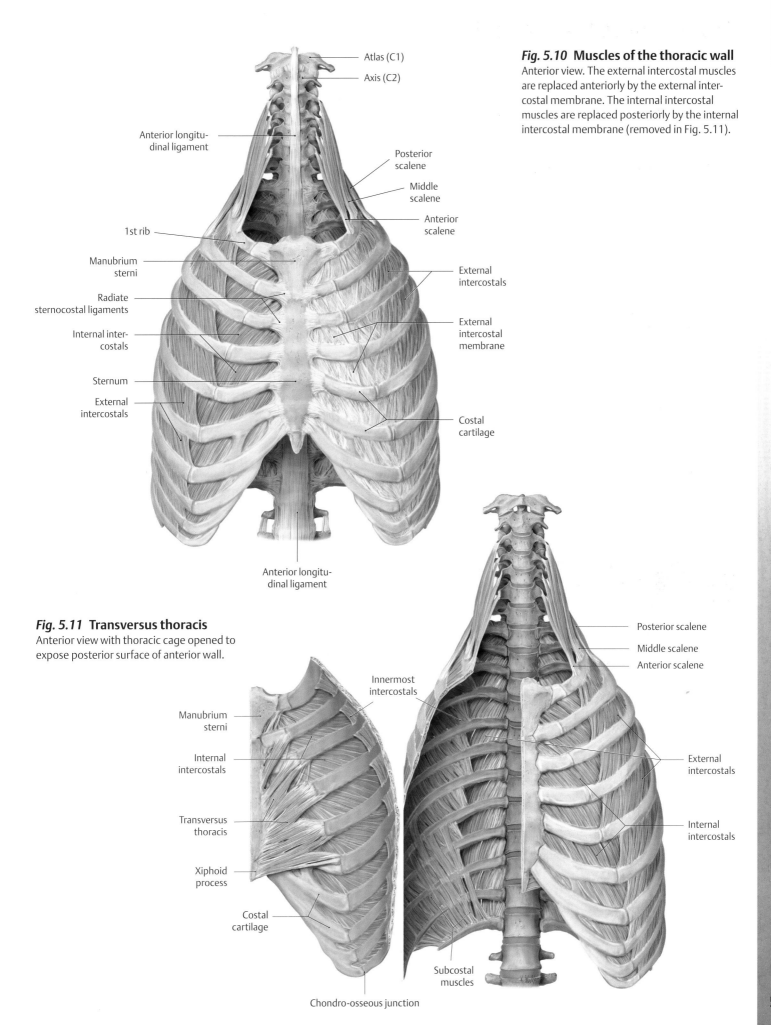

Atlas (C1)

Axis (C2)

Anterior longitu-
dinal ligament

Posterior
scalene

Middle
scalene

Anterior
scalene

1st rib

Manubrium
sterni

Radiate
sternocostal ligaments

Internal inter-
costals

Sternum

External
intercostals

External
intercostals

External
intercostal
membrane

Costal
cartilage

Anterior longitu-
dinal ligament

Fig. 5.10 Muscles of the thoracic wall
Anterior view. The external intercostal muscles
are replaced anteriorly by the external intercostal membrane. The internal intercostal
muscles are replaced posteriorly by the internal
intercostal membrane (removed in Fig. 5.11).

Fig. 5.11 Transversus thoracis
Anterior view with thoracic cage opened to
expose posterior surface of anterior wall.

Manubrium
sterni

Internal
intercostals

Transversus
thoracis

Xiphoid
process

Costal
cartilage

Innermost
intercostals

Posterior scalene

Middle scalene

Anterior scalene

External
intercostals

Internal
intercostals

Subcostal
muscles

Chondro-osseous junction

Diaphragm

Fig. 5.12 Diaphragm

The diaphragm, which separates the thorax from the abdomen, has two asymmetric domes and three apertures (for the aorta, vena cava, and esophagus; see Fig. 5.13B).

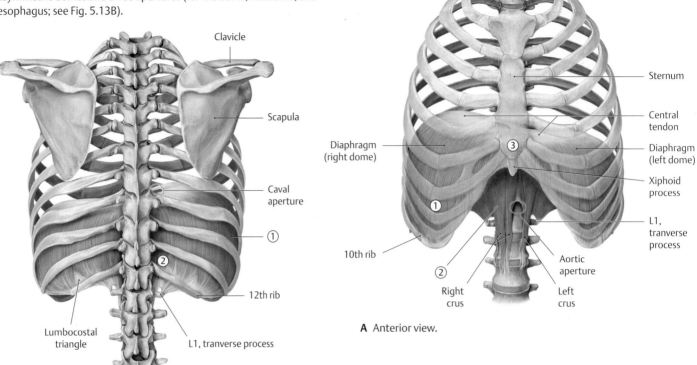

B Posterior view.

A Anterior view.

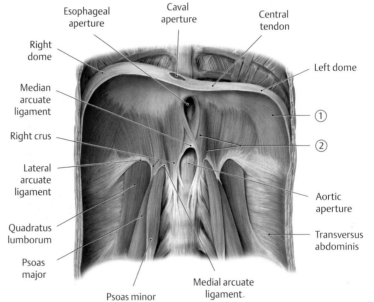

C Coronal section with diaphragm in intermediate position.

Table 5.3		Diaphragm			
Muscle		**Origin**	**Insertion**	**Innervation**	**Action**
Diaphragm	① Costal part	7th to 12th ribs (inner surface; lower margin of costal arch)	Central tendon	Phrenic n. (C3–C5, cervical plexus)	Principal muscle of respiration (diaphragmatic and thoracic breathing); aids in compressing abdominal viscera (abdominal press)
	② Lumbar part	Medial part: L1–L3 vertebral bodies, intervertebral disks, and anterior longitudinal ligament as right and left crura			
		Lateral parts: lateral and medial arcuate ligaments			
	③ Sternal part	Xiphoid process (posterior surface)			

Fig. 5.13 **Diaphragm in situ**

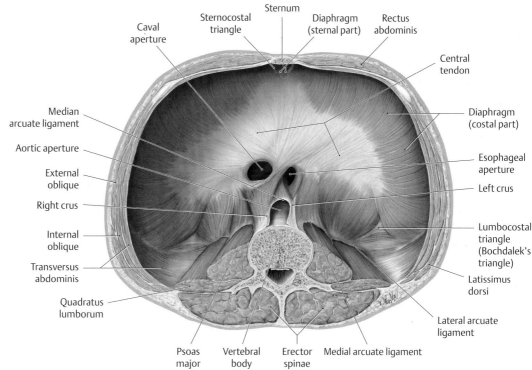

Sternum
Diaphragm (sternal part)
Central tendon
Caval aperture
Diaphragm (costal part)
Intercostal muscles
Esophageal aperture
Aortic aperture
T8
Rib
Endothoracic fascia
Intrinsic back muscles

A Superior view.

Caval aperture
Sternocostal triangle
Sternum
Diaphragm (sternal part)
Rectus abdominis
Central tendon
Median arcuate ligament
Diaphragm (costal part)
Aortic aperture
Esophageal aperture
External oblique
Left crus
Right crus
Lumbocostal triangle (Bochdalek's triangle)
Internal oblique
Latissimus dorsi
Transversus abdominis
Lateral arcuate ligament
Quadratus lumborum
Psoas major
Vertebral body
Erector spinae
Medial arcuate ligament

B Inferior view.

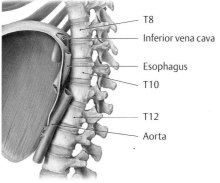

T8
Inferior vena cava
Esophagus
T10
T12
Aorta

C Diaphragmatic apertures, left lateral view.

Neurovasculature of the Diaphragm

***Fig. 5.14* Neurovasculature of the diaphragm**
Anterior view of opened thoracic cage.

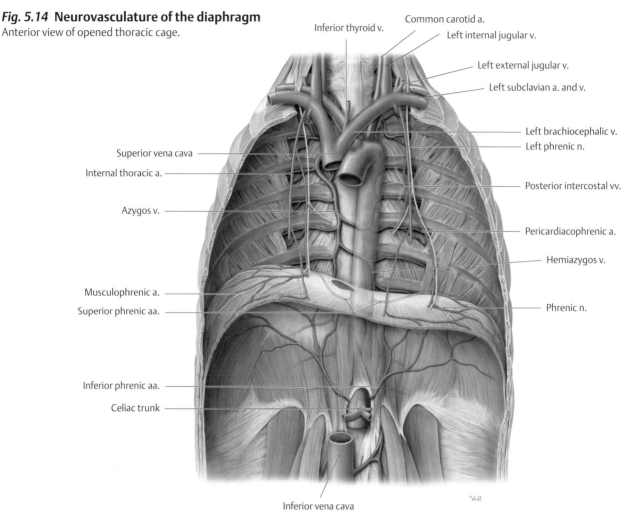

Inferior thyroid v.

Common carotid a.

Left internal jugular v.

Left external jugular v.

Left subclavian a. and v.

Left brachiocephalic v.

Left phrenic n.

Superior vena cava

Internal thoracic a.

Posterior intercostal vv.

Azygos v.

Pericardiacophrenic a.

Hemiazygos v.

Musculophrenic a.

Superior phrenic aa.

Phrenic n.

Inferior phrenic aa.

Celiac trunk

Inferior vena cava

***Fig. 5.15* Innervation of the diaphragm**
Anterior view. The phrenic nerve lies on the lateral surface of the fibrous pericardium together with the pericardiacophrenic arteries and veins. *Note*: The phrenic nerve also innervates the pericardium.

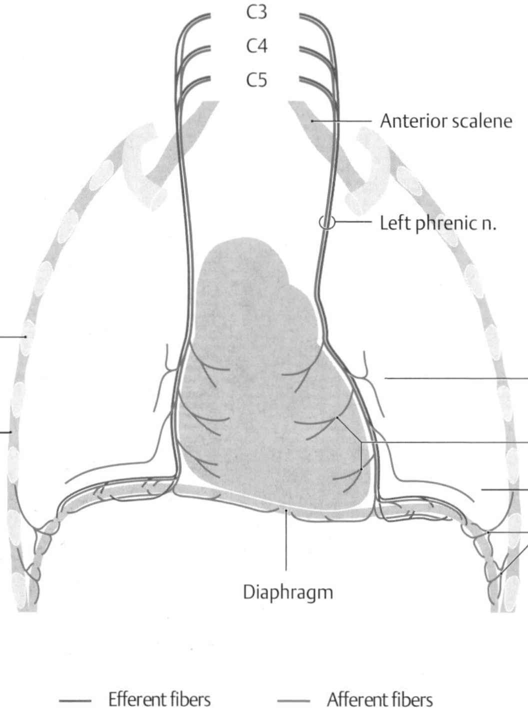

C3
C4
C5

Anterior scalene

Left phrenic n.

Rib

Intercostal muscles

To parietal pleura, mediastinal part

Pericardial branches

To parietal pleura, diaphragmatic part

Intercostal nn.

Diaphragm

— Efferent fibers   — Afferent fibers

Table 5.4	Blood vessels of the diaphragm		
Artery	**Origin**	**Vein**	**Drainage**
Inferior phrenic aa. (chief blood supply)	Abdominal aorta; occasionally from celiac trunk	Posterior intercostal vv.	
Superior phrenic aa.	Thoracic aorta	Superior phrenic vv.	Right side: Azygos v.; Left side: Hemiazygos v.
Pericardiacophrenic aa.	Internal thoracic a.	Right superior intercostal v.	
Musculophrenic aa.			

Fig. 5.16 **Arteries and nerves of the diaphragm**

Note: The margins of the diaphragm receive sensory innervation from the lowest intercostal nerves.

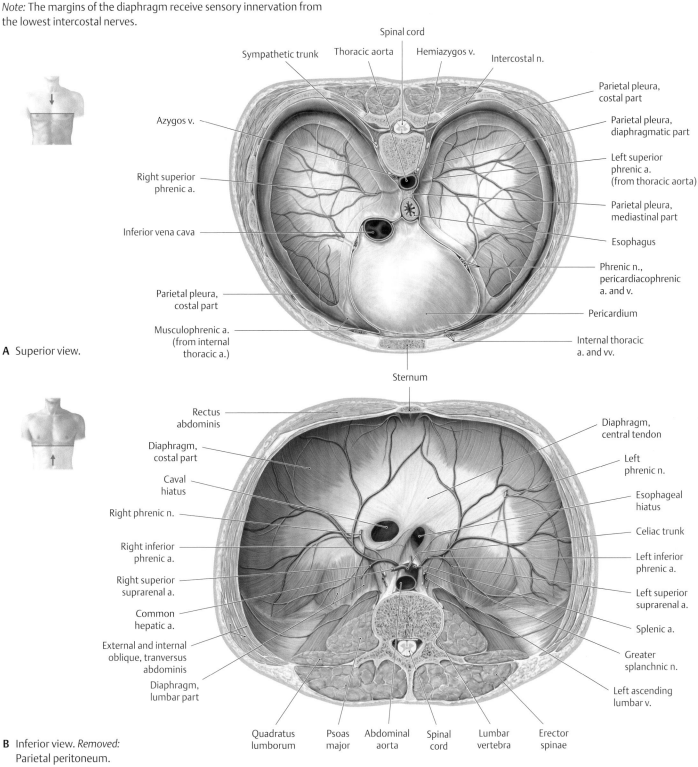

A Superior view.

B Inferior view. *Removed:* Parietal peritoneum.

Arteries & Veins of the Thoracic Wall

 The posterior intercostal arteries anostomose with the anterior intercostal arteries to supply the structures of the thoracic wall. The posterior intercostal arteries branch from the thoracic aorta, with the exception of the 1st and 2nd, which arise from the superior intercostal artery (a branch of the costocervical trunk).

Fig. 5.17 Arteries of the thoracic wall
Anterior view.

Table 5.5	Arteries of the thoracic wall
Origin	**Branch**
Subclavian a.	Superior thoracic a.
	Lateral thoracic a.
	Thoracoacromial a.
	Posterior intercostal aa. (1st and 2nd; see p. 34)
Thoracic aorta	Posterior intercostal aa. (3rd through 12th)
Internal thoracic a.	Anterior intercostal aa.
	Musculophrenic a.
	Superior epigastric a.

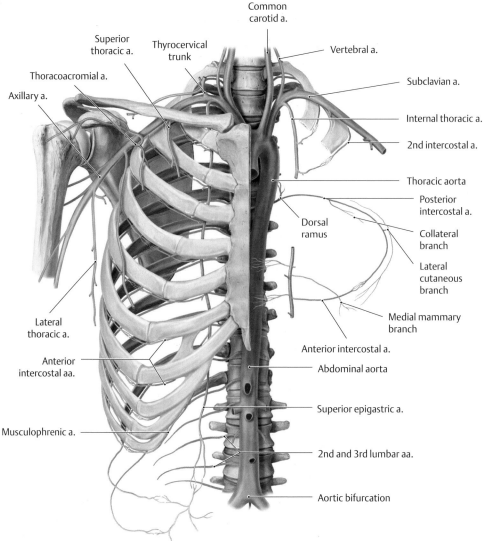

Fig. 5.18 Branches of the posterior intercostal arteries
Superior view.

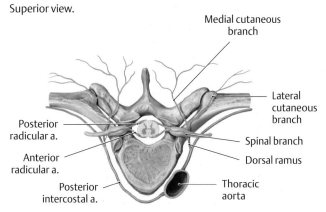

Table 5.6	Branches of the intercostal arteries		
Artery	**Branches**		**Supplies**
Posterior intercostal aa.	Dorsal branch	Spinal branch	Spinal cord
		Medial cutaneous branch	Posterior thoracic wall
		Lateral cutaneous branch	
	Collateral branch		Lateral thoracic wall
Anterior intercostal aa.	Lateral cutaneous branch*		Anterior thoracic wall

*The lateral mammary branch from the lateral cutaneous branch supplies the breast along with the medial mammary branch from the internal thoracic artery.

The intercostal veins drain primarily into the azygos system, but also into the internal thoracic vein. This blood ultimately returns to the heart via the superior vena cava. The intercostal veins follow a similar course to their arterial counterparts. However, the veins of the vertebral column form an external vertebral venous plexus that traverses the entire length of the spine (see p. 35).

Fig. 5.19 Veins of the thoracic wall
Anterior view.

A Anterior view with rib cage opened.

B Vertebral venous plexus.

Fig. 5.20 Superficial veins
Anterior view. The thoracoepigastric veins are a potential superficial collateral venous drainage route in the event of superior or inferior vena cava obstruction.

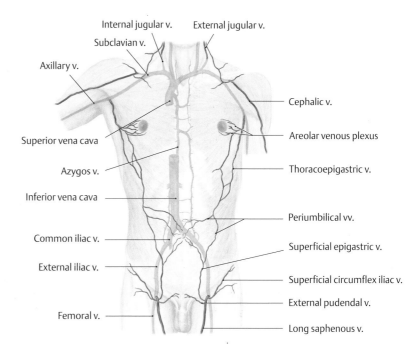

Nerves of the Thoracic Wall

***Fig. 5.21* Intercostal nerves**

Anterior view. The 1st rib has been removed to reveal the 1st and 2nd intercostal nerves.

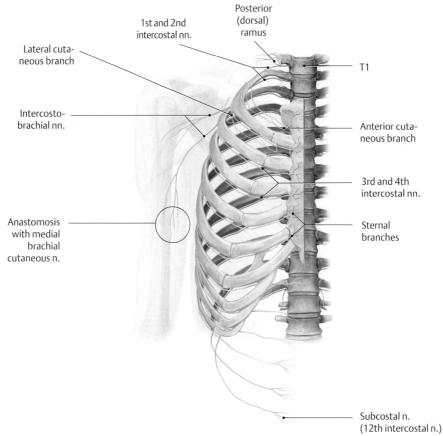

***Fig. 5.22* Thoracic wall: Peripheral sensory cutaneous innervation**

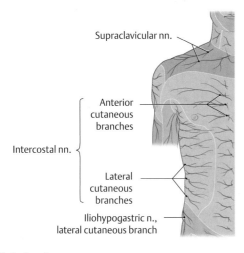

A Anterior view.

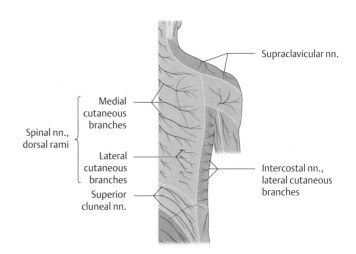

B Posterior view.

Fig. 5.23 Spinal nerve branches

Superior view. Formed by the union of the posterior (sensory) and anterior (motor) roots, the at-most 1 cm-long spinal nerve courses through the intervertebral foramen and exits the vertebral canal. Its posterior ramus innervates the skin and intrinsic muscles of the back; its anterior ramus forms the intercostal nerves. See p. 36 for more details.

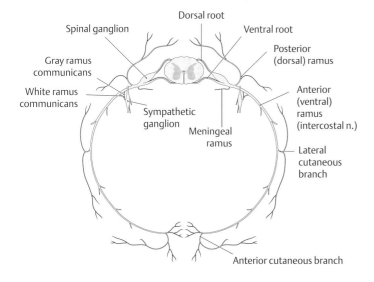

Fig. 5.24 Course of the intercostal nerves

Coronal section, anterior view.

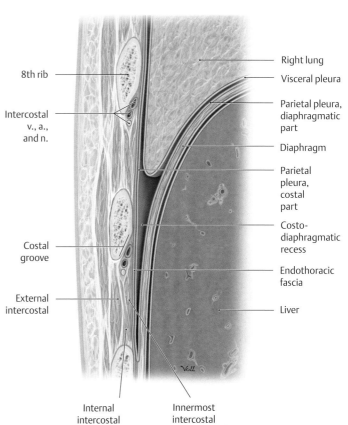

Fig. 5.25 Thoracic wall: Dermatomes

Landmarks: T4 generally includes the nipple; T6 innervates the skin over the xiphoid.

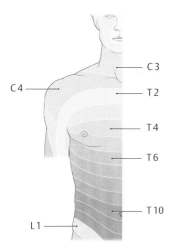

A Anterior view.

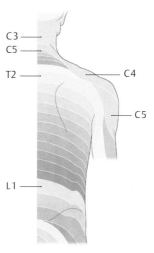

B Posterior view.

Neurovascular Topography of the Thoracic Wall

Fig. 5.26 Anterior structures
Anterior view (see pp. 34–39 for neurovasculature of the back).

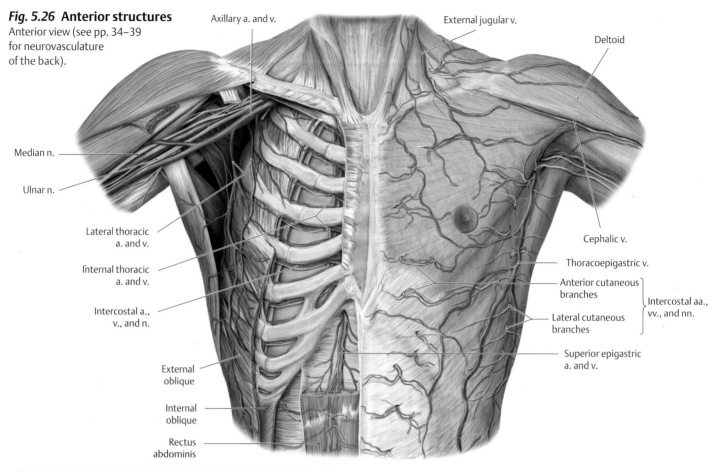

Axillary a. and v.

External jugular v.

Deltoid

Median n.

Ulnar n.

Lateral thoracic a. and v.

Internal thoracic a. and v.

Intercostal a., v., and n.

External oblique

Internal oblique

Rectus abdominis

Cephalic v.

Thoracoepigastric v.

Anterior cutaneous branches

Lateral cutaneous branches

Intercostal aa., vv., and nn.

Superior epigastric a. and v.

✚ Clinical

Insertion of a chest tube

Abnormal fluid collection in the pleural space (e.g., pleural effusion due to bronchial carcinoma) may necessitate the insertion of a chest tube. Generally, the optimal puncture site in a sitting patient is at the level of the 7th or 8th intercostal space on the posterior axillary line. The drain should always be introduced at the upper margin of a rib to avoid injuring the intercostal vein, artery, and nerve. See p. 113 for details on collapsed lungs.

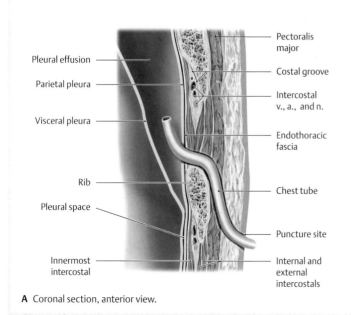

Pleural effusion

Parietal pleura

Visceral pleura

Rib

Pleural space

Innermost intercostal

Pectoralis major

Costal groove

Intercostal v., a., and n.

Endothoracic fascia

Chest tube

Puncture site

Internal and external intercostals

A Coronal section, anterior view.

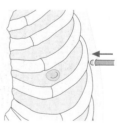

B Drainage tube is inserted perpendicular to chest wall.

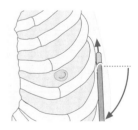

C At ribs, the tube is angled and advanced parallel to the chest wall in the subcutaneous plane.

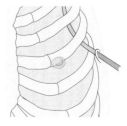

D At the superior margin of the rib, the tube is passed through the intercostal muscles and advanced into the pleural cavity.

Fig. 5.27 Intercostal structures in cross section

Transverse section, anterosuperior view.

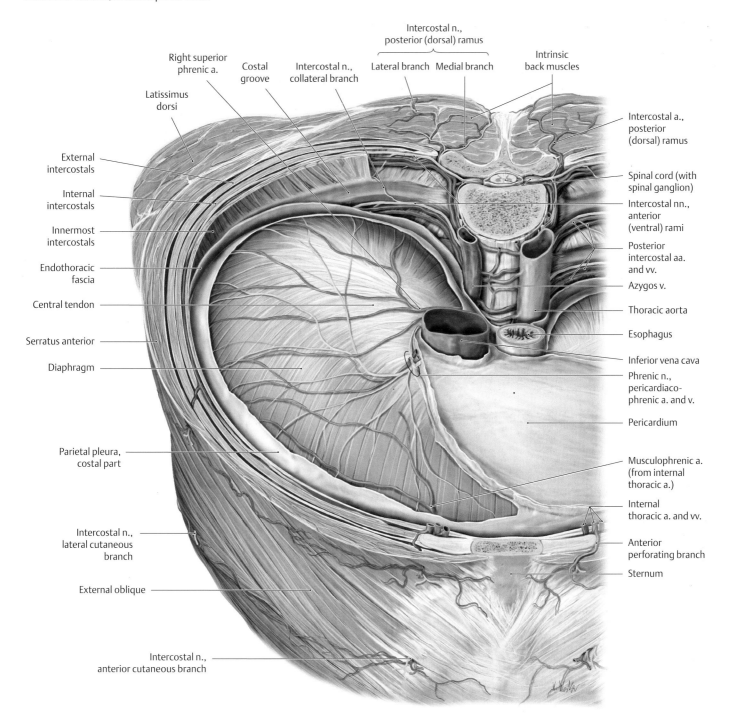

Right superior phrenic a.

Latissimus dorsi

External intercostals

Internal intercostals

Innermost intercostals

Endothoracic fascia

Central tendon

Serratus anterior

Diaphragm

Parietal pleura, costal part

Intercostal n., lateral cutaneous branch

External oblique

Intercostal n., anterior cutaneous branch

Costal groove

Intercostal n., collateral branch

Intercostal n., posterior (dorsal) ramus

Lateral branch Medial branch

Intrinsic back muscles

Intercostal a., posterior (dorsal) ramus

Spinal cord (with spinal ganglion)

Intercostal nn., anterior (ventral) rami

Posterior intercostal aa. and vv.

Azygos v.

Thoracic aorta

Esophagus

Inferior vena cava

Phrenic n., pericardiaco-phrenic a. and v.

Pericardium

Musculophrenic a. (from internal thoracic a.)

Internal thoracic a. and vv.

Anterior perforating branch

Sternum

Female Breast

 The female breast, a modified sweat gland in the subcutaneous tissue layer, consists of glandular tissue, fibrous stroma, and fat. The breast extends from the 2nd to the 6th rib and is loosely attached to the pectoral, axillary, and superficial abdominal fascia by connective tissue. The breast is additionally supported by suspensory ligaments. An extension of the breast tissue into the axilla, the axillary tail, is often present.

Fig. 5.28 Female breast
Right breast, anterior view.

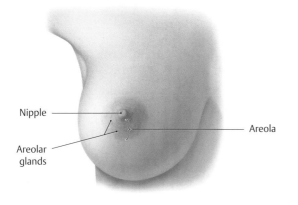

Nipple

Areolar glands

Areola

Fig. 5.29 Mammary ridges
Rudimentary mammary glands form in both sexes along the mammary ridges. Occasionally, these may persist in humans to form accessory nipples (*polythelia*), although only the thoracic pair normally remains.

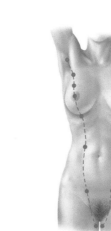

Fig. 5.30 Blood supply to the breast

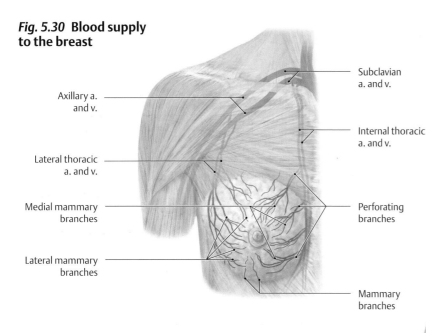

Axillary a. and v.

Lateral thoracic a. and v.

Medial mammary branches

Lateral mammary branches

Subclavian a. and v.

Internal thoracic a. and v.

Perforating branches

Mammary branches

Fig. 5.31 Sensory innervation of the breast

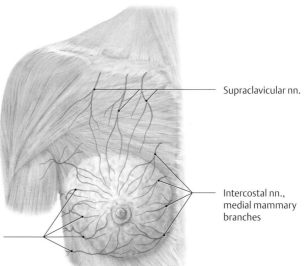

Supraclavicular nn.

Intercostal nn., medial mammary branches

Intercostal nn., lateral mammary branches

The glandular tissue is composed of 10 to 20 individual lobes, each with its own lactiferous duct. The gland ducts open on the elevated nipple at the center of the pigmented areola. Just proximal to the duct opening is a dilated portion called the lactiferous sinus. Areolar elevations are the openings of the areolar glands (sebaceous). The glands and lactiferous ducts are surrounded by firm, fibrofatty tissue with a rich blood supply.

Fig. 5.32 Structures of the breast

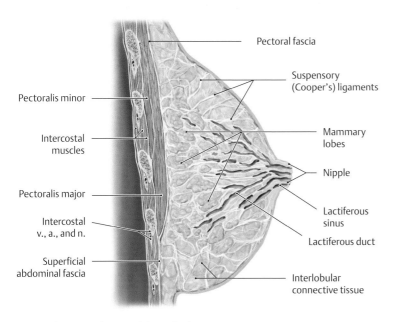

A Sagittal section along midclavicular line.

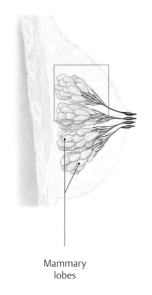

B Duct system and portions of a lobe, sagittal section. In the nonlactating breast (shown here), the lobules contain clusters of rudimentary acini.

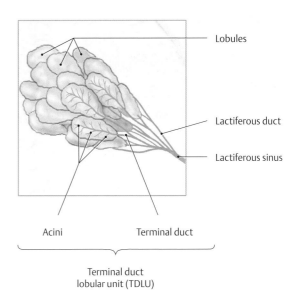

C Terminal duct lobular unit (TDLU). The clustered acini composing the lobule empty into a terminal ductule; these structures are collectively known as the TDLU.

Lymphatics of the Female Breast

 The lymphatic vessels of the breast (not shown) are divided into three systems: superficial, subcutaneous, and deep. These drain primarily into the axillary lymph nodes, which are classified based on their relationship to the pectoralis minor (Table 5.7). The medial portion of the breast is drained by the parasternal lymph nodes, which are associated with the internal thoracic vessels.

Fig. 5.33 **Axillary lymph nodes**

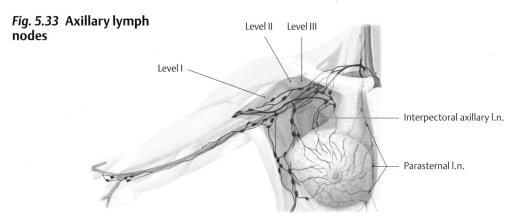

Level I

Level II   Level III

Interpectoral axillary l.n.

Parasternal l.n.

A Lymphatic drainage of the breast.

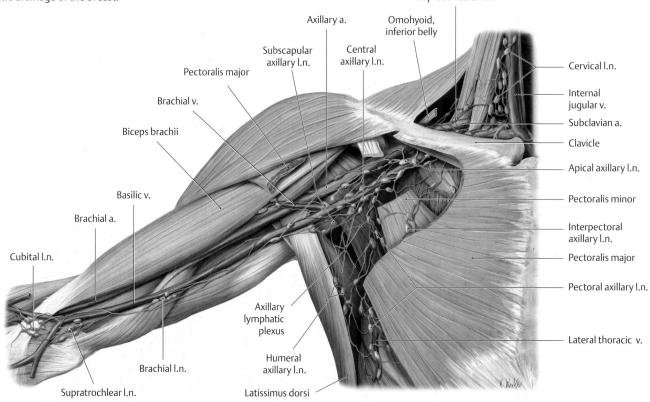

Supraclavicular l.n.

Axillary a.

Subscapular axillary l.n.

Central axillary l.n.

Omohyoid, inferior belly

Pectoralis major

Cervical l.n.

Brachial v.

Internal jugular v.

Biceps brachii

Subclavian a.

Clavicle

Basilic v.

Apical axillary l.n.

Brachial a.

Pectoralis minor

Cubital l.n.

Interpectoral axillary l.n.

Pectoralis major

Pectoral axillary l.n.

Axillary lymphatic plexus

Lateral thoracic v.

Humeral axillary l.n.

Brachial l.n.

Supratrochlear l.n.

Latissimus dorsi

B Anterior view.

Table 5.7	Levels of axillary lymph nodes	
Level	**Position**	**Lymph nodes (l.n.)**
I	Lower axillary group	Lateral to pectoralis minor	Pectoral axillary l.n.
			Subscapular axillary l.n.
			Humeral axillary l.n.
			Central l.n.
II	Middle axillary group	Along pectoralis minor	Interpectoral axillary l.n.
III	Upper infraclavicular group	Medial to pectoralis minor	Apical axillary l.n.

Breast cancer

Stem cells in the intralobular connective tissue give rise to tremendous cell growth, necessary for duct system proliferation and acini differentiation. This makes the terminal duct lobular unit (TDLU) the most common site of origin of malignant breast tumors.

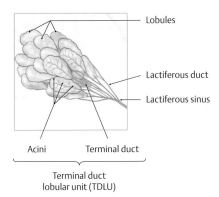

Lobules

Lactiferous duct

Lactiferous sinus

Acini   Terminal duct

Terminal duct lobular unit (TDLU)

A Terminal duct lobular unit.

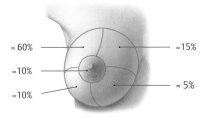

≈ 60%   ≈ 15%

≈ 10%

≈ 10%   ≈ 5%

B Origin of malignant tumors by quadrant.

Tumors originating in the breast spread via the lymphatic vessels. The deep system of lymphatic drainage (level III) is of particular importance, although the parasternal lymph nodes provide a route by which tumor cells may spread across the midline. The survival rate in breast cancer correlates most strongly with the number of lymph nodes involved at the axillary nodal level. Metastatic involvement is gauged through scintigraphic mapping with radiolabeled colloids (technetium [Tc] 99m sulfur microcolloid). The downstream sentinel node is the first to receive lymphatic drainage from the tumor and is therefore the first to be visualized with radiolabeling. Once identified, it can then be removed (via *sentinel lymphadenectomy*) and histologically examined for tumor cells. This method is 98% accurate in predicting the level of axillary nodal involvement.

Metastatic involvement	5-year survival rate
Level I	65%
Level II	31%
Level III	~0%

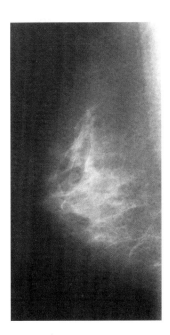

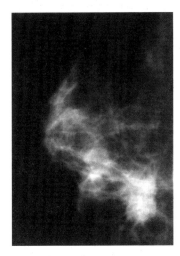

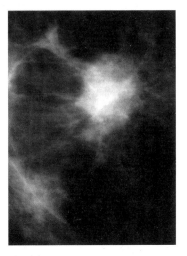

C Normal mammogram.

D Mammogram of invasive ductal carcinoma. The large lesion has changed the architecture of the neighboring breast tissue.

Divisions of the Thoracic Cavity

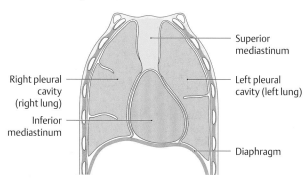

The thoracic cavity is divided into three large spaces: the mediastinum (p. 76) and the two pleural cavities (p. 102).

Fig. 6.1 **Thoracic cavity**
Coronal section, anterior view.

Superior
mediastinum

Right pleural
cavity
(right lung)

Left pleural
cavity (left lung)

Inferior
mediastinum

Diaphragm

A Divisions of the thoracic cavity.

Table 6.1	Major structures of the thoracic cavity		
Mediastinum	Superior mediastinum		Thymus, great vessels, trachea, esophagus, and thoracic duct
	Inferior mediastinum	Anterior	Thymus
		Middle	Heart, pericardium, and roots of great vessels
		Posterior	Thoracic aorta, thoracic duct, esophagus, and azygos venous system
Pleural cavities	Right pleural cavity		Right lung
	Left pleural cavity		Left lung

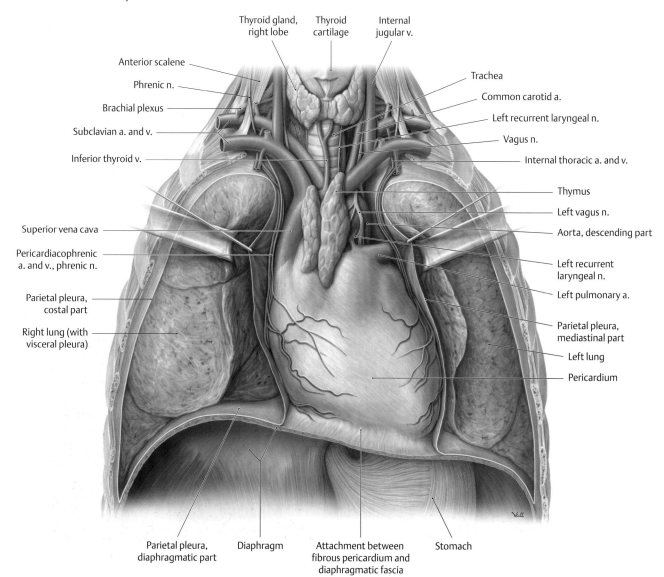

Thyroid gland, right lobe — Thyroid cartilage — Internal jugular v.

Anterior scalene — Trachea

Phrenic n. — Common carotid a.

Brachial plexus — Left recurrent laryngeal n.

Subclavian a. and v. — Vagus n.

Inferior thyroid v. — Internal thoracic a. and v.

Thymus

Superior vena cava — Left vagus n.

Aorta, descending part

Pericardiacophrenic a. and v., phrenic n. — Left recurrent laryngeal n.

Left pulmonary a.

Parietal pleura, costal part — Parietal pleura, mediastinal part

Right lung (with visceral pleura) — Left lung

Pericardium

Parietal pleura, diaphragmatic part — Diaphragm — Attachment between fibrous pericardium and diaphragmatic fascia — Stomach

B Opened thoracic cavity. *Removed:* Thoracic wall; connective tissue of anterior mediastinum.

Fig. 6.2 Divisions of the mediastinum

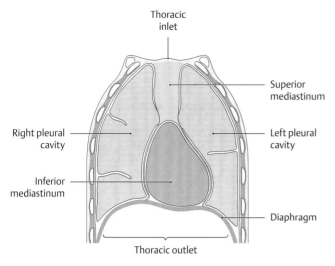

A Anterior view (coronal section).

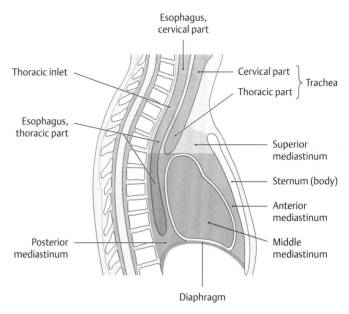

B Lateral view (midsagittal section).

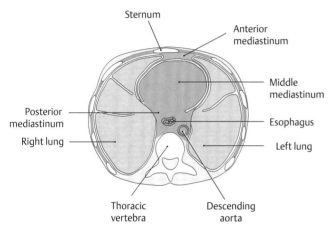

C Inferior view (transverse section).

Fig. 6.3 Transverse sections of the thorax

Computed tomography (CT) scan of thorax, inferior view.

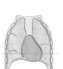

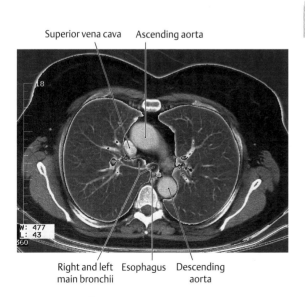

A Superior mediastinum.

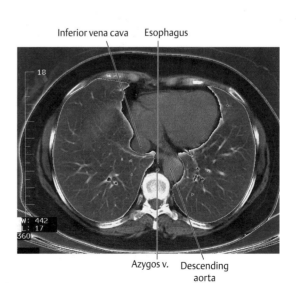

B Inferior mediastinum.

Arteries of the Thoracic Cavity

 The arch of the aorta has three major branches: the brachioce-phalic trunk, left common carotid artery, and left subclavian artery. After the aortic arch, the aorta begins its descent, becoming the thoracic aorta at the level of the sternal angle and the abdominal aorta once it passes through the aortic hiatus in the diaphragm.

Fig. 6.4 Thoracic aorta

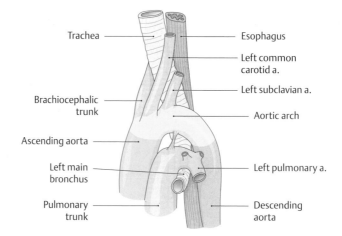

A Parts of the aorta, left lateral view. *Note:* The aortic arch begins and ends at the level of the sternal angle (see p. 46).

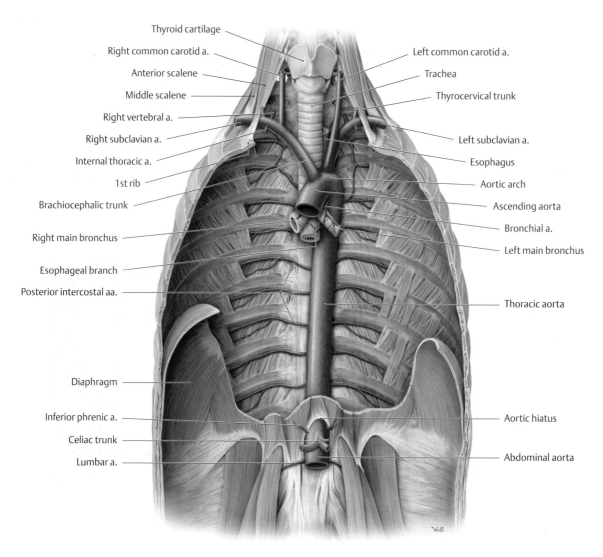

B Thoracic aorta in situ, anterior view. *Removed:* Heart, lungs, portions of diaphragm.

Table 6.2	Branches of the thoracic aorta			

The thoracic organs are supplied by direct branches from the thoracic aorta, as well as indirect branches from the subclavian arteries.

Branches				Region supplied
Brachiocephalic trunk	Right subclavian a.			See left subclavian a.
	Right common carotid a.			Head and neck
Left common carotid a.				
Left subclavian a.	Vertebral a.			
	Internal thoracic a.	Anterior intercostal aa.		Anterior chest wall
		Thymic branches		Thymus
		Mediastinal branches		Posterior mediastinum
		Pericardiacophrenic a.		Pericardium, diaphragm
	Thyrocervical trunk	Inferior thyroid a.		Esophagus, trachea, thyroid gland
	Costocervical trunk	Superior intercostal a.		Chest wall
Descending thoracic aorta	Visceral branches			Heart, pericardium, bronchi, trachea, esophagus
	Parietal branches	Posterior intercostal aa.		Posterior chest wall
		Superior phrenic aa.		Diaphragm

Clinical

Aortic dissection

A tear in the inner wall (intima) of the aorta allows blood to separate the layers of the aortic wall, creating a "false lumen" and potentially resulting in life-threatening aortic rupture. Symptoms are dyspnea (shortness of blood) and sudden onset of excruciating pain. Acute aortic dissections occur most often in the ascending aorta and generally require surgery. More distal aortic dissections may be treated conservatively, provided there are no complications (e.g., obstruction of blood supply to the organs, in which case a stent may be inserted to restore perfusion). Aortic dissections occurring at the base of a coronary artery may cause myocardial infarction.

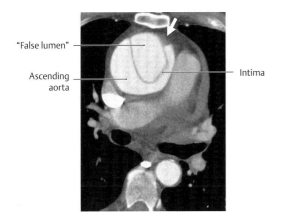

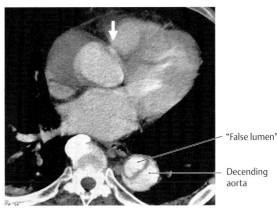

A Aortic dissection. Parts of the intima are still attached to the connective tissue in the wall of the aorta (*arrow*).

B The flow in the coronary arteries is intact (*arrow*).

Veins of the Thoracic Cavity

The superior vena cava is formed by the union of the two brachio-cephalic veins at the level of the T2–T3 junction. It receives blood drained by the azygos system (the inferior vena cava has no tributaries in the thorax).

Fig. 6.5 Superior vena cava and azygos system

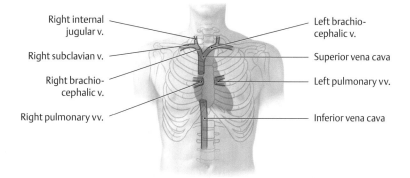

Right internal jugular v.
Right subclavian v.
Right brachio-cephalic v.
Right pulmonary vv.

Left brachio-cephalic v.
Superior vena cava
Left pulmonary vv.
Inferior vena cava

A Projection of venae cavae onto chest, anterior view.

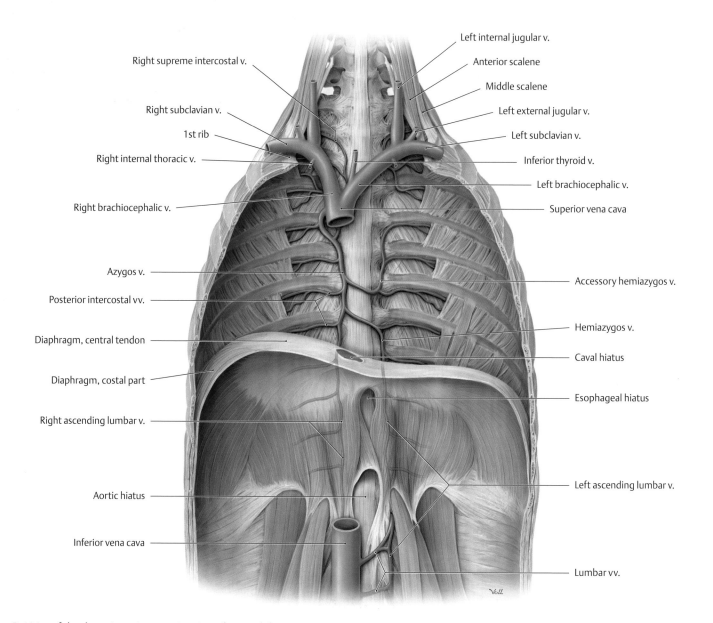

Right supreme intercostal v.
Right subclavian v.
1st rib
Right internal thoracic v.
Right brachiocephalic v.
Azygos v.
Posterior intercostal vv.
Diaphragm, central tendon
Diaphragm, costal part
Right ascending lumbar v.
Aortic hiatus
Inferior vena cava

Left internal jugular v.
Anterior scalene
Middle scalene
Left external jugular v.
Left subclavian v.
Inferior thyroid v.
Left brachiocephalic v.
Superior vena cava
Accessory hemiazygos v.
Hemiazygos v.
Caval hiatus
Esophageal hiatus
Left ascending lumbar v.
Lumbar vv.

B Veins of the thoracic cavity, anterior view of opened thorax.

Table 6.3	Thoracic tributaries of the superior vena cava			
Major vein	**Tributaries**			**Region drained**
Brachiocephalic vv.	Inferior thyroid v.			Esophagus, trachea, thyroid gland
	Internal jugular vv.			Head, neck, upper limb
	External jugular vv.			
	Subclavian vv.			
	Supreme intercostal vv.			
	Pericardial vv.			
	Left superior intercostal v.			
Azygos system (left side: accessory hemiazygos v.; right side: azygos v.)	Visceral branches			Trachea, bronchi, esophagus
	Parietal branches	Posterior intercostal vv.		Inner chest wall and diaphragm
		Superior phrenic vv.		
		Right superior intercostal v.		
Internal thoracic v.	Thymic vv.			Thymus
	Mediastinal tributaries			Posterior mediastinum
	Anterior intercostal vv.			Anterior chest wall
	Pericardiacophrenic v.			Pericardium
	Musculophrenic v.			Diaphragm

Note: Structures of the superior mediastinum may also drain directly to the brachiocephalic veins via the tracheal, esophageal, and mediastinal veins.

Fig. 6.6 Azygos system
Anterior view.

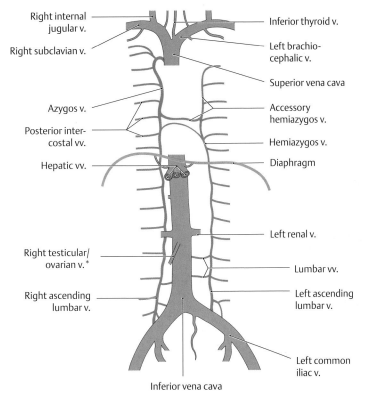

*The left testicular/ovarian vein arises from the left renal vein.

Lymphatics of the Thoracic Cavity

 The body's chief lymph vessel is the thoracic duct. Beginning in the abdomen at the level of L1 as the *cisterna chyli*, the thoracic duct empties into the junction of the left internal jugular and subclavian veins. The right lymphatic duct drains to the right junction of the internal jugular and subclavian veins.

***Fig. 6.7* Lymphatic trunks in the thorax**
Anterior view of opened thorax.

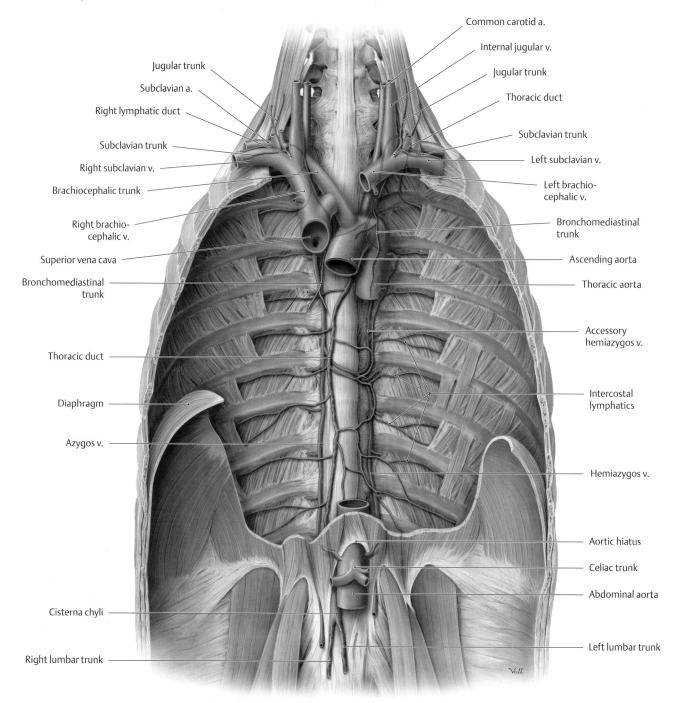

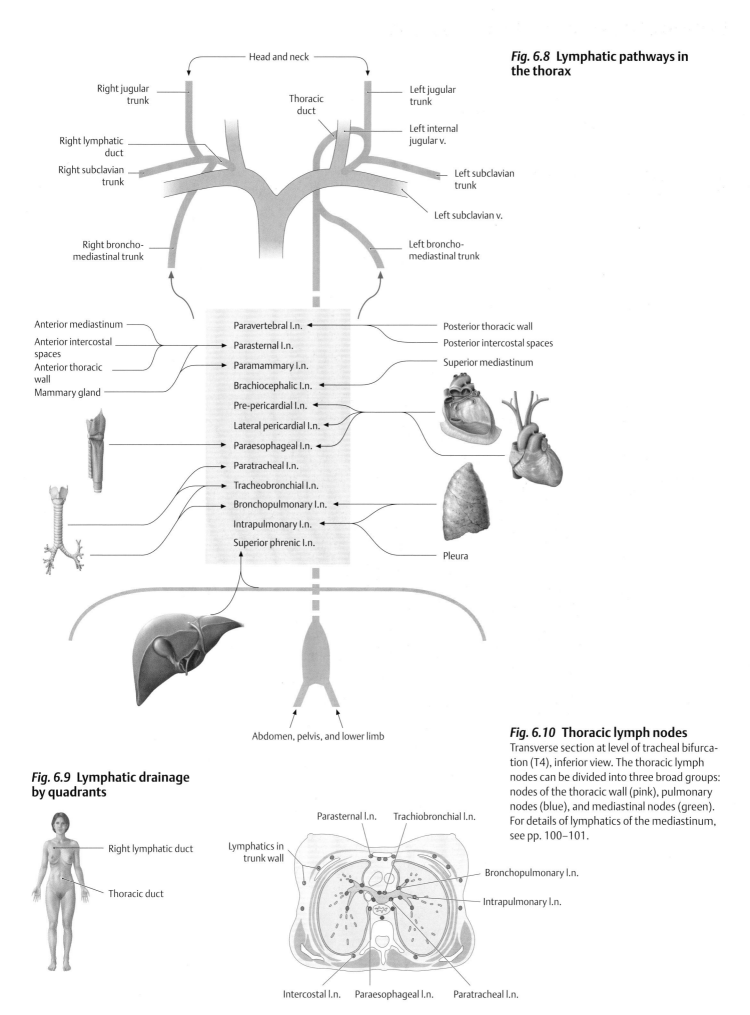

Fig. 6.8 Lymphatic pathways in the thorax

Head and neck

Right jugular trunk

Thoracic duct

Left jugular trunk

Left internal jugular v.

Right lymphatic duct

Right subclavian trunk

Left subclavian trunk

Left subclavian v.

Right broncho-mediastinal trunk

Left broncho-mediastinal trunk

Anterior mediastinum

Anterior intercostal spaces

Anterior thoracic wall

Mammary gland

Paravertebral l.n.

Parasternal l.n.

Paramammary l.n.

Brachiocephalic l.n.

Pre-pericardial l.n.

Lateral pericardial l.n.

Paraesophageal l.n.

Paratracheal l.n.

Tracheobronchial l.n.

Bronchopulmonary l.n.

Intrapulmonary l.n.

Superior phrenic l.n.

Posterior thoracic wall

Posterior intercostal spaces

Superior mediastinum

Pleura

Abdomen, pelvis, and lower limb

Fig. 6.9 Lymphatic drainage by quadrants

Right lymphatic duct

Thoracic duct

Fig. 6.10 Thoracic lymph nodes

Transverse section at level of tracheal bifurcation (T4), inferior view. The thoracic lymph nodes can be divided into three broad groups: nodes of the thoracic wall (pink), pulmonary nodes (blue), and mediastinal nodes (green). For details of lymphatics of the mediastinum, see pp. 100–101.

Parasternal l.n.

Trachiobronchial l.n.

Lymphatics in trunk wall

Bronchopulmonary l.n.

Intrapulmonary l.n.

Intercostal l.n.

Paraesophageal l.n.

Paratracheal l.n.

Nerves of the Thoracic Cavity

 Thoracic innervation is mostly autonomic, arising from the paravertebral sympathetic trunks and parasympathetic vagus nerves. There are two exceptions: the phrenic nerves innervate the pericardium and diaphragm (p. 54), and the intercostal nerves innervate the thoracic wall (p. 58).

Fig. 6.11 **Nerves in the thorax**
Anterior view of opened thorax.

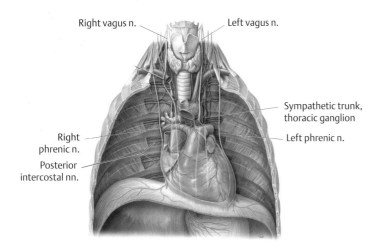

Right vagus n.

Left vagus n.

Sympathetic trunk, thoracic ganglion

Right phrenic n.

Left phrenic n.

Posterior intercostal nn.

A Thoracic innervation.

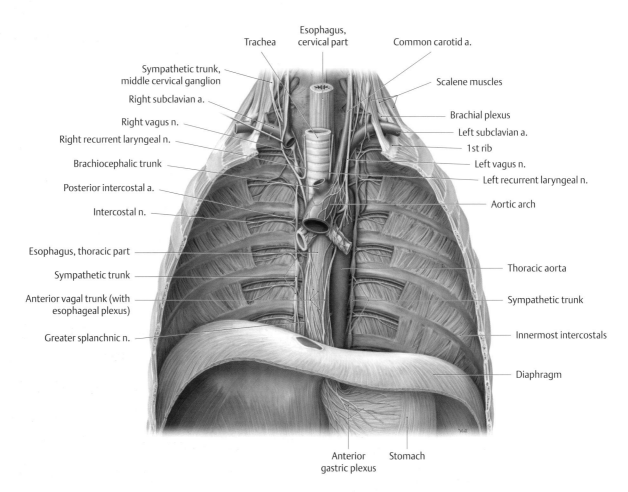

Trachea

Esophagus, cervical part

Common carotid a.

Sympathetic trunk, middle cervical ganglion

Scalene muscles

Right subclavian a.

Brachial plexus

Right vagus n.

Left subclavian a.

Right recurrent laryngeal n.

1st rib

Brachiocephalic trunk

Left vagus n.

Posterior intercostal a.

Left recurrent laryngeal n.

Intercostal n.

Aortic arch

Esophagus, thoracic part

Thoracic aorta

Sympathetic trunk

Anterior vagal trunk (with esophageal plexus)

Sympathetic trunk

Greater splanchnic n.

Innermost intercostals

Diaphragm

Anterior gastric plexus

Stomach

B Nerves of the thorax in situ. *Note:* The recurrent laryngeal nerves have been slightly anteriorly retracted; normally, they occupy the groove between the trachea and the esophagus, making them vulnerable during thyroid gland surgery.

The autonomic nervous system innervates smooth muscle, cardiac muscle, and glands. It is subdivided into the sympathetic (red) and parasympathetic (blue) nervous systems, which together regulates blood flow, secretions, and organ function.

Fig. 6.12 Sympathetic and parasympathetic nervous systems in the thorax

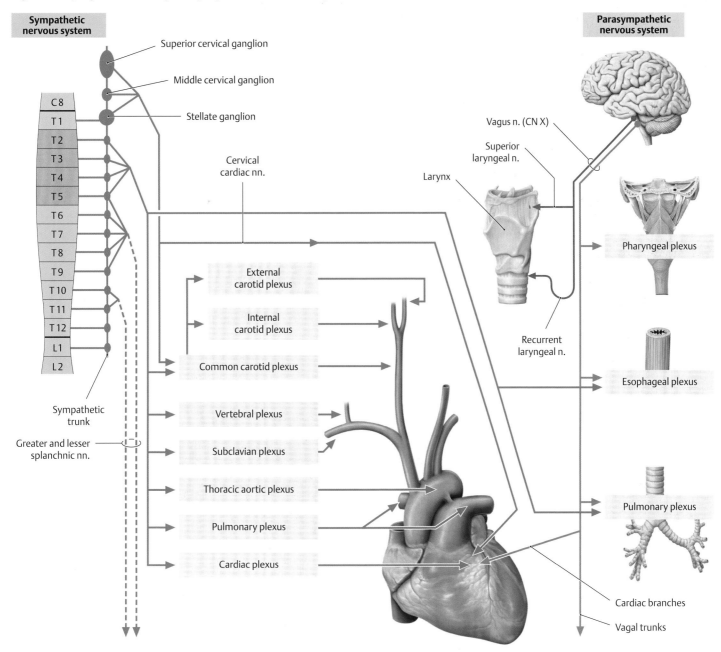

Table 6.4	Peripheral sympathetic nervous system		
Origin of presynaptic fibers *	**Ganglion cells**	**Course of postsynaptic fibers**	**Target**
Spinal cord	Sympathetic trunk	Follow intercostal nn.	Blood vessels and glands in chest wall
		Accompany intrathoracic aa.	Visceral targets
		Gather in greater and lesser splanchnic nn.	Abdomen

*The axons of presynaptic neurons exit the spinal cord via the anterior roots and synapse with *post*synaptic neurons in the sympathetic ganglia.

Table 6.5	Peripheral parasympathetic nervous system		
Origin of presynaptic fibers	**Course of presynaptic motor axons** *		**Target**
Brainstem	Vagus n. (CN X)	Cardiac branches	Cardiac plexus
		Esophageal branches	Esophageal plexus
		Tracheal branches	Trachea
		Bronchial branches	Pulmonary plexus (bronchi, pulmonary vessels)

*The ganglion cells of the parasympathetic nervous system are scattered in microscopic groups in their target organs. The vagus nerve thus carries the *pre*synaptic motor axons to these targets.
CN = cranial nerve.

Mediastinum: Overview

 The mediastinum is the space in the thorax between the pleural sacs of the lungs. It is divided into two parts: superior and inferior.

The inferior mediastinum is further divided into anterior, middle, and posterior portions.

Fig. 7.1 Divisions of the mediastinum

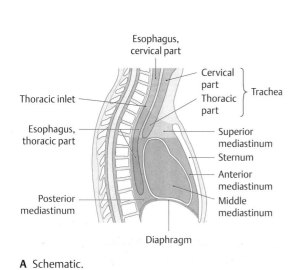

A Schematic.

Table 7.1	Contents of the mediastinum			
	Superior mediastinum	**Inferior mediastinum**		
		Anterior	*Middle*	*Posterior*
Organs	• Thymus • Trachea • Esophagus • Thoracic duct	• Thymus (in children, see Fig. 7.5)	• Heart • Pericardium	• Esophagus
Arteries	• Aortic arch • Brachiocephalic trunk • Left common carotid a. • Left subclavian a.	• Smaller vessels	• Ascending aorta • Pulmonary trunk and branches • Pericardiacophrenic aa. and vv.	• Thoracic aorta and branches • Thoracic duct
Veins and lymph vessels	• Superior vena cava • Brachiocephalic vv. • Thoracic duct	• Smaller vessels, lymphatics, and lymph nodes	• Superior vena cava • Azygos v. • Pulmonary vv. • Pericardiacophrenic aa. and vv.	• Azygos v. • Hemiazygos v. • Thoracic duct
Nerves	• Vagus nn. • Left recurrent laryngeal n. • Cardiac nn. • Phrenic nn.	• None	• Phrenic nn.	• Vagus nn.

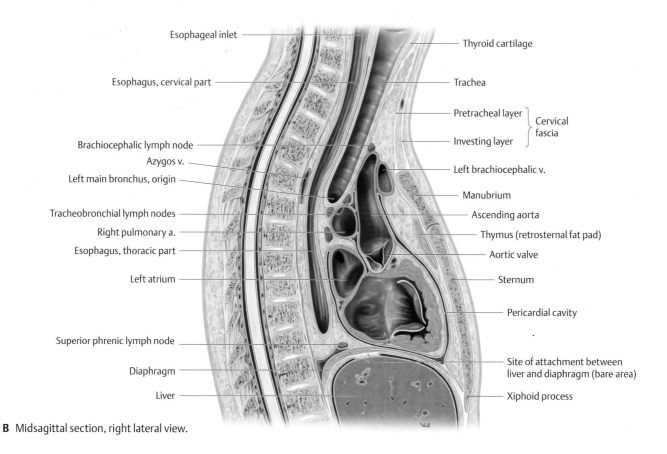

B Midsagittal section, right lateral view.

Fig. 7.2 Contents of the mediastinum

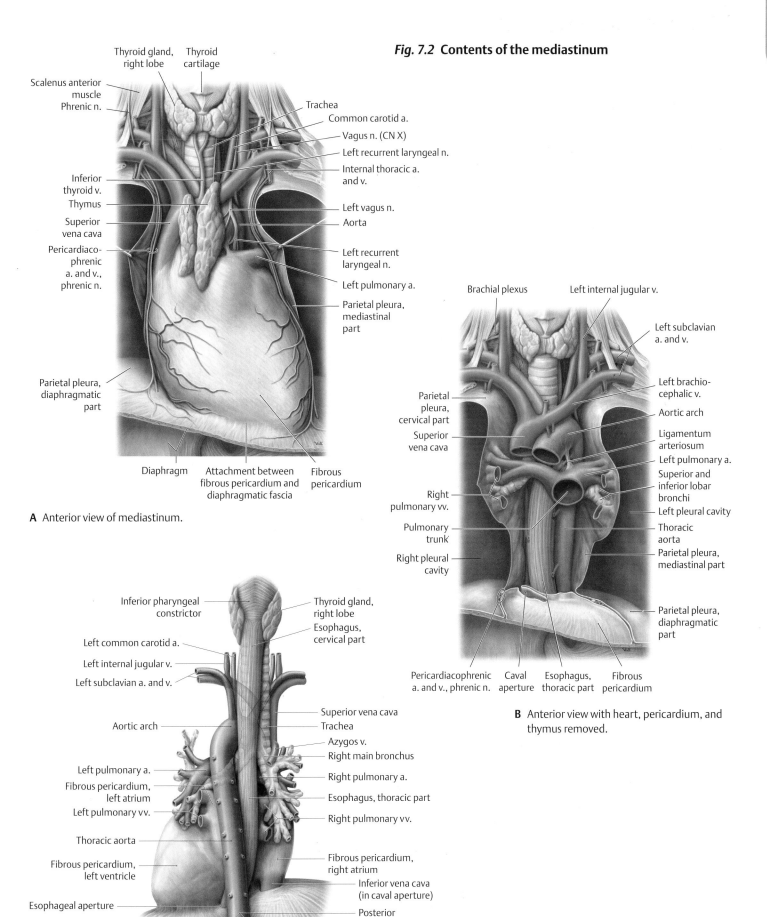

A Anterior view of mediastinum.

Thyroid gland, right lobe
Thyroid cartilage
Scalenus anterior muscle
Phrenic n.
Trachea
Common carotid a.
Vagus n. (CN X)
Left recurrent laryngeal n.
Internal thoracic a. and v.
Inferior thyroid v.
Thymus
Left vagus n.
Superior vena cava
Aorta
Pericardiaco-phrenic a. and v., phrenic n.
Left recurrent laryngeal n.
Left pulmonary a.
Parietal pleura, mediastinal part
Parietal pleura, diaphragmatic part
Diaphragm
Attachment between fibrous pericardium and diaphragmatic fascia
Fibrous pericardium

B Anterior view with heart, pericardium, and thymus removed.

Brachial plexus
Left internal jugular v.
Left subclavian a. and v.
Parietal pleura, cervical part
Left brachio-cephalic v.
Aortic arch
Superior vena cava
Ligamentum arteriosum
Left pulmonary a.
Right pulmonary vv.
Superior and inferior lobar bronchi
Left pleural cavity
Thoracic aorta
Pulmonary trunk
Right pleural cavity
Parietal pleura, mediastinal part
Parietal pleura, diaphragmatic part
Pericardiacophrenic a. and v., phrenic n.
Caval aperture
Esophagus, thoracic part
Fibrous pericardium

C Posterior view.

Inferior pharyngeal constrictor
Thyroid gland, right lobe
Esophagus, cervical part
Left common carotid a.
Left internal jugular v.
Left subclavian a. and v.
Superior vena cava
Trachea
Aortic arch
Azygos v.
Right main bronchus
Left pulmonary a.
Right pulmonary a.
Fibrous pericardium, left atrium
Esophagus, thoracic part
Left pulmonary vv.
Right pulmonary vv.
Thoracic aorta
Fibrous pericardium, left ventricle
Fibrous pericardium, right atrium
Inferior vena cava (in caval aperture)
Esophageal aperture
Posterior intercostal aa.
Diaphragm

Mediastinum: Structures

Fig. 7.3 **Mediastinum**

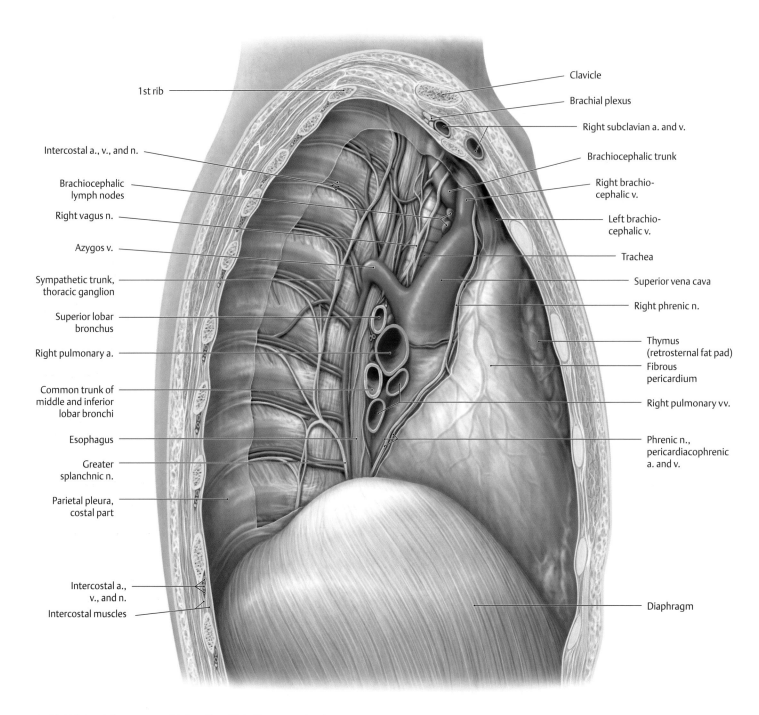

1st rib

Intercostal a., v., and n.

Brachiocephalic
lymph nodes

Right vagus n.

Azygos v.

Sympathetic trunk,
thoracic ganglion

Superior lobar
bronchus

Right pulmonary a.

Common trunk of
middle and inferior
lobar bronchi

Esophagus

Greater
splanchnic n.

Parietal pleura,
costal part

Intercostal a.,
v., and n.

Intercostal muscles

Clavicle

Brachial plexus

Right subclavian a. and v.

Brachiocephalic trunk

Right brachio-
cephalic v.

Left brachio-
cephalic v.

Trachea

Superior vena cava

Right phrenic n.

Thymus
(retrosternal fat pad)

Fibrous
pericardium

Right pulmonary vv.

Phrenic n.,
pericardiacophrenic
a. and v.

Diaphragm

A Right lateral view, parasagittal section. Note the many structures
passing between the superior and inferior (middle and posterior)
mediastinum.

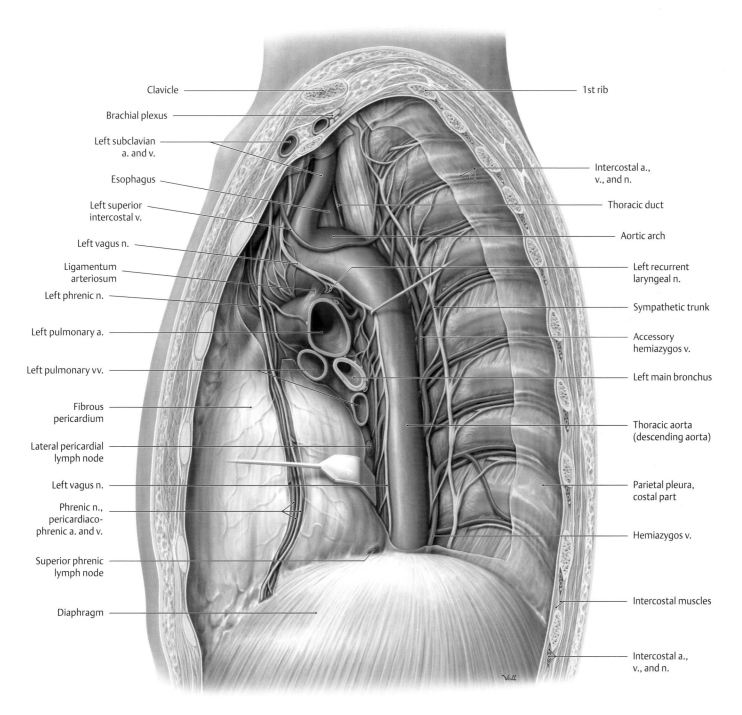

Clavicle

Brachial plexus

Left subclavian a. and v.

Esophagus

Left superior intercostal v.

Left vagus n.

Ligamentum arteriosum

Left phrenic n.

Left pulmonary a.

Left pulmonary vv.

Fibrous pericardium

Lateral pericardial lymph node

Left vagus n.

Phrenic n., pericardiaco-phrenic a. and v.

Superior phrenic lymph node

Diaphragm

1st rib

Intercostal a., v., and n.

Thoracic duct

Aortic arch

Left recurrent laryngeal n.

Sympathetic trunk

Accessory hemiazygos v.

Left main bronchus

Thoracic aorta (descending aorta)

Parietal pleura, costal part

Hemiazygos v.

Intercostal muscles

Intercostal a., v., and n.

B Left lateral view, parasagittal section. *Removed:* Left lung and parietal pleura. *Revealed:* Posterior mediastinal structures.

Thymus & Pericardium

Fig. 7.4 **Thymus and pericardium in situ**

Anterior view of coronal section. The thymus lies in the superior mediastinum.

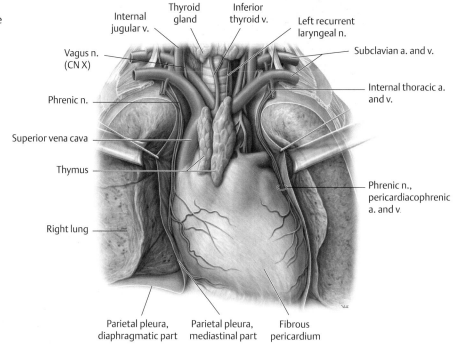

Internal jugular v.
Thyroid gland
Inferior thyroid v.
Left recurrent laryngeal n.
Vagus n. (CN X)
Subclavian a. and v.
Phrenic n.
Internal thoracic a. and v.
Superior vena cava
Thymus
Phrenic n., pericardiacophrenic a. and v.
Right lung
Parietal pleura, diaphragmatic part
Parietal pleura, mediastinal part
Fibrous pericardium

Fig. 7.5 **Thymus**

Anterior view of opened thorax of a 2-year-old child. The thymus is well developed at this age, extending inferiorly into the anterior mediastinum (compare with Fig. 7.4). The thymus grows throughout childhood; at puberty, high levels of circulating sex hormones cause the thymus to atrophy.

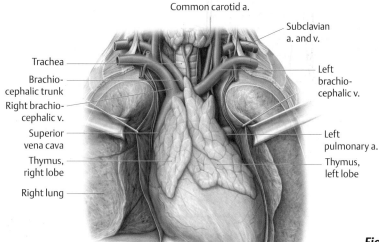

Common carotid a.
Subclavian a. and v.
Trachea
Brachio-cephalic trunk
Right brachio-cephalic v.
Left brachio-cephalic v.
Superior vena cava
Left pulmonary a.
Thymus, right lobe
Thymus, left lobe
Right lung

Fig. 7.6 **Pericardium**

Anterior view of opened thorax with flaps of fibrous pericardium reflected.

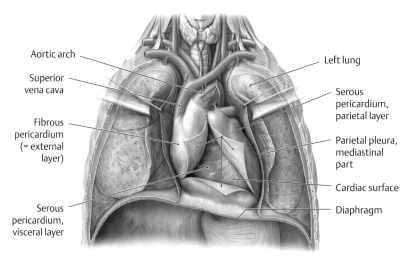

Aortic arch
Left lung
Superior vena cava
Serous pericardium, parietal layer
Fibrous pericardium (= external layer)
Parietal pleura, mediastinal part
Cardiac surface
Serous pericardium, visceral layer
Diaphragm

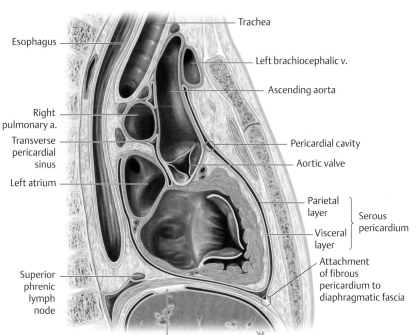

A Sagittal section through the mediastinum. Note the continuity of the parietal serous and visceral serous pericardia.

Fig. 7.7 Serous pericardial reflections

Anterior view. The parietal and visceral serous pericardium are continuous with one another around the great vessels of the heart. The passage between the arterial- and venous-associated reflections is the transverse pericardial sinus (see **B**).

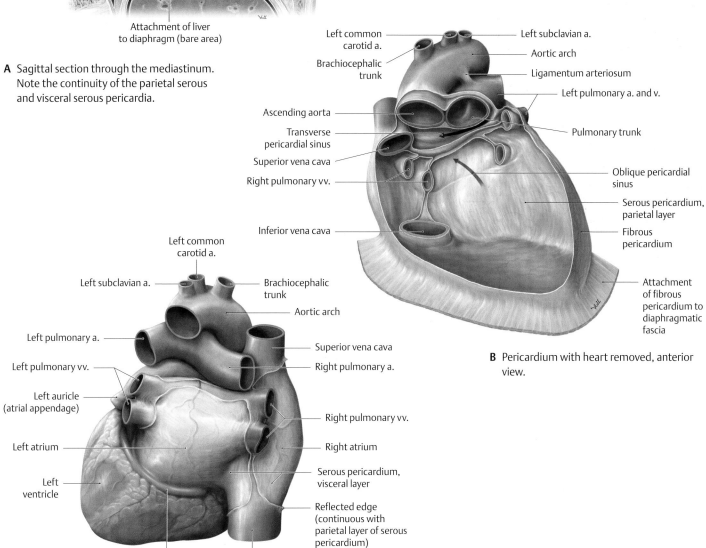

B Pericardium with heart removed, anterior view.

C Heart removed from fibrous pericardium, posterior view. Note the reflection of the visceral layer of serous pericardium (cut edges).

Heart in Situ

 The heart is located posterior to the sternum in the middle portion of the inferior mediastinum. The heart projects into the left side of the thoracic cavity.

Fig. 7.8 Topographical relations of the heart

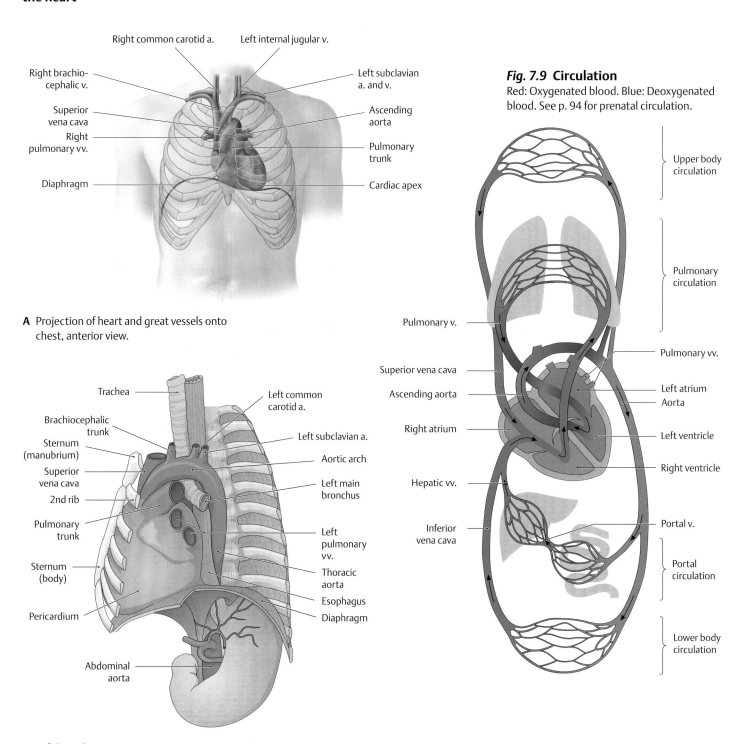

Right common carotid a.

Left internal jugular v.

Right brachio-cephalic v.

Left subclavian a. and v.

Superior vena cava

Ascending aorta

Right pulmonary vv.

Pulmonary trunk

Diaphragm

Cardiac apex

A Projection of heart and great vessels onto chest, anterior view.

Trachea

Left common carotid a.

Brachiocephalic trunk

Left subclavian a.

Sternum (manubrium)

Aortic arch

Superior vena cava

Left main bronchus

2nd rib

Pulmonary trunk

Left pulmonary vv.

Sternum (body)

Thoracic aorta

Esophagus

Pericardium

Diaphragm

Abdominal aorta

B Left lateral view.

Fig. 7.9 Circulation

Red: Oxygenated blood. Blue: Deoxygenated blood. See p. 94 for prenatal circulation.

Pulmonary v.

Upper body circulation

Pulmonary circulation

Pulmonary vv.

Superior vena cava

Left atrium

Ascending aorta

Aorta

Right atrium

Left ventricle

Hepatic vv.

Right ventricle

Inferior vena cava

Portal v.

Portal circulation

Lower body circulation

***Fig. 7.10* Heart in situ**
Anterior view.

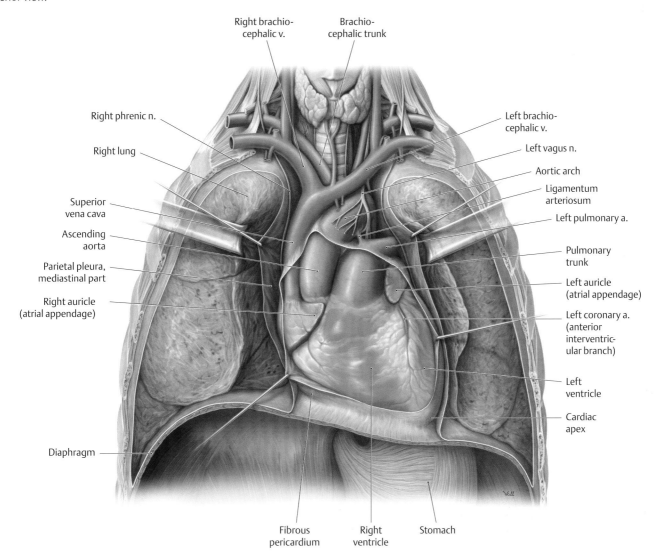

Right brachio-cephalic v.

Brachio-cephalic trunk

Right phrenic n.

Right lung

Superior vena cava

Ascending aorta

Parietal pleura, mediastinal part

Right auricle (atrial appendage)

Diaphragm

Left brachio-cephalic v.

Left vagus n.

Aortic arch

Ligamentum arteriosum

Left pulmonary a.

Pulmonary trunk

Left auricle (atrial appendage)

Left coronary a. (anterior interventric-ular branch)

Left ventricle

Cardiac apex

Fibrous pericardium

Right ventricle

Stomach

Heart: Surfaces & Chambers

 Note the reflection of visceral serous pericardium to become parietal serous pericardium.

Fig. 7.11 **Surfaces of the heart**
The heart has three surfaces: anterior (sternocostal), posterior (base), and inferior (diaphragmatic).

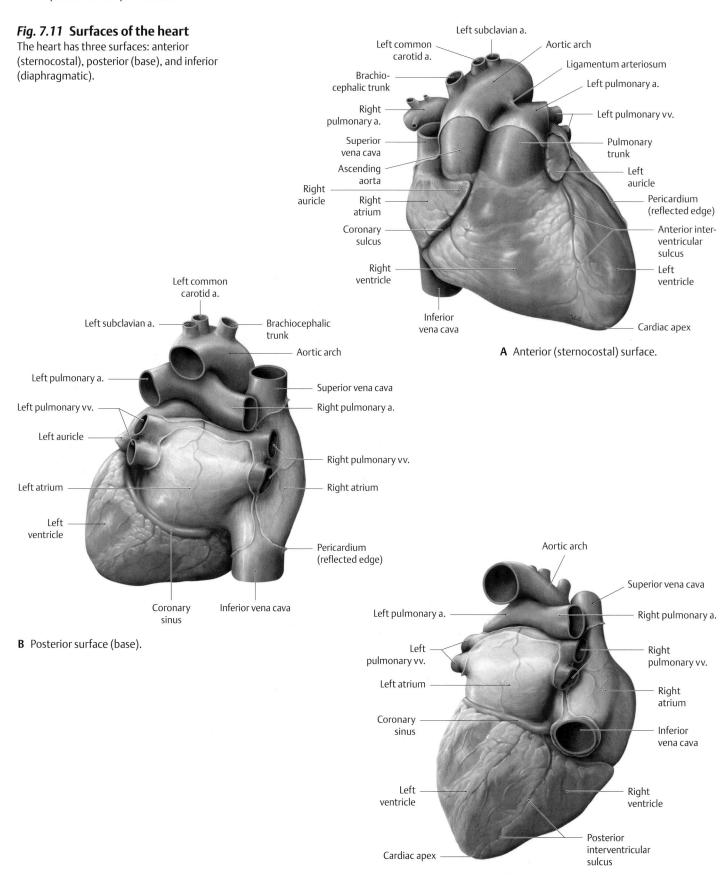

A Anterior (sternocostal) surface.

B Posterior surface (base).

C Inferior (diaphragmatic) surface.

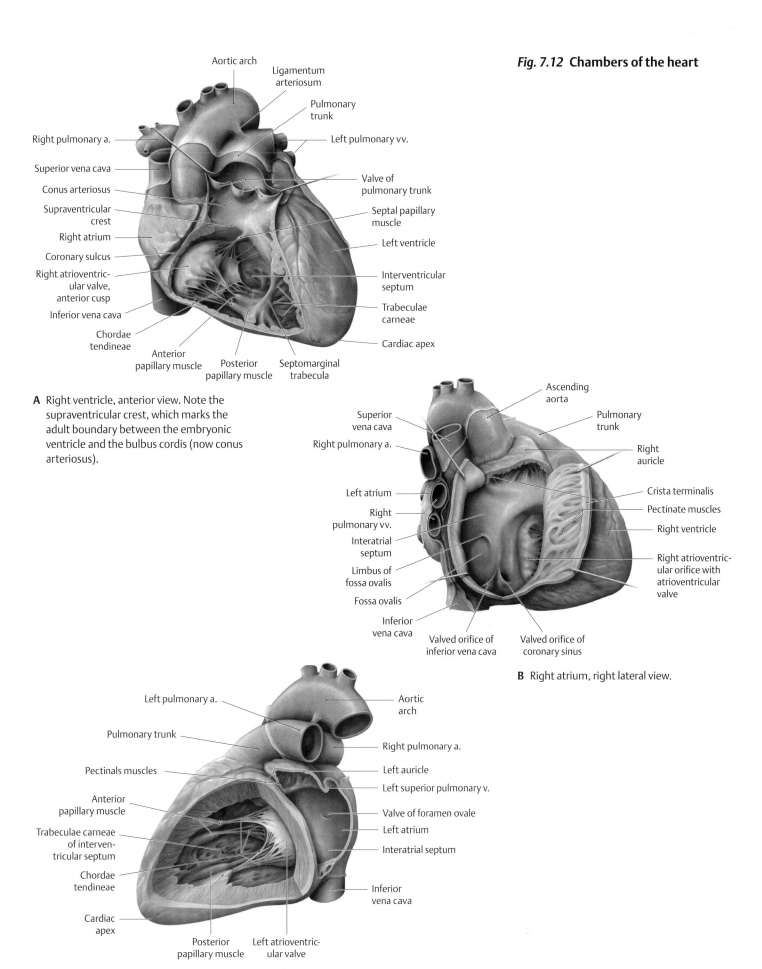

Fig. 7.12 Chambers of the heart

Aortic arch

Ligamentum arteriosum

Pulmonary trunk

Right pulmonary a.

Left pulmonary vv.

Superior vena cava

Valve of pulmonary trunk

Conus arteriosus

Supraventricular crest

Septal papillary muscle

Right atrium

Left ventricle

Coronary sulcus

Right atrioventricular valve, anterior cusp

Interventricular septum

Inferior vena cava

Trabeculae carneae

Chordae tendineae

Cardiac apex

Anterior papillary muscle

Posterior papillary muscle

Septomarginal trabecula

A Right ventricle, anterior view. Note the supraventricular crest, which marks the adult boundary between the embryonic ventricle and the bulbus cordis (now conus arteriosus).

Ascending aorta

Superior vena cava

Pulmonary trunk

Right pulmonary a.

Right auricle

Left atrium

Crista terminalis

Right pulmonary vv.

Pectinate muscles

Interatrial septum

Right ventricle

Limbus of fossa ovalis

Right atrioventricular orifice with atrioventricular valve

Fossa ovalis

Inferior vena cava

Valved orifice of inferior vena cava

Valved orifice of coronary sinus

B Right atrium, right lateral view.

Left pulmonary a.

Aortic arch

Pulmonary trunk

Right pulmonary a.

Pectinals muscles

Left auricle

Anterior papillary muscle

Left superior pulmonary v.

Trabeculae carneae of interventricular septum

Valve of foramen ovale

Left atrium

Chordae tendineae

Interatrial septum

Cardiac apex

Inferior vena cava

Posterior papillary muscle

Left atrioventricular valve

C Left atrium and ventricle, left lateral view. Note the irregular trabeculae carneae characteristic of the ventricular wall.

Heart: Valves

The cardiac valves are divided into two groups: semilunar and atrioventricular. The two semilunar valves (aortic and pulmonary) located at the base of the two great arteries of the heart regulate passage of blood from the ventricles to the aorta and pulmonary trunk. The two atrioventricular valves (left and right) lie at the interface between the atria and ventricles.

Fig. 7.13 Cardiac valves
Plane of cardiac valves, superior view. *Removed:* Atria and great arteries.

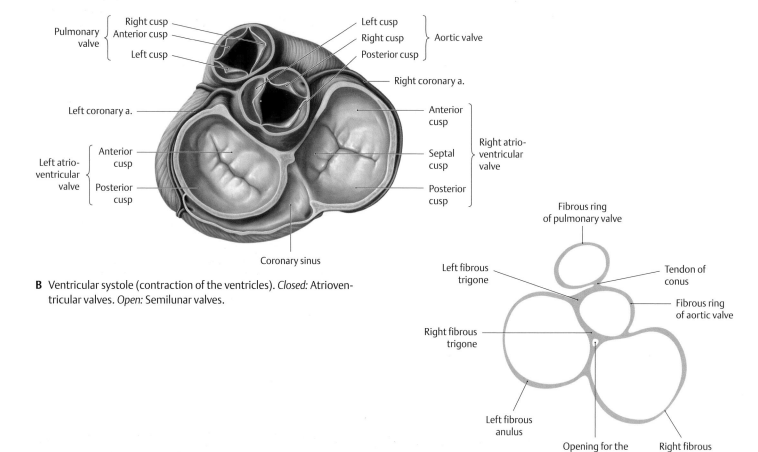

A Ventricular diastole (relaxation of the ventricles). *Closed:* Semilunar valves. *Open:* Atrioventricular valves.

B Ventricular systole (contraction of the ventricles). *Closed:* Atrioventricular valves. *Open:* Semilunar valves.

C Cardiac skeleton. The cardiac skeleton is formed by dense fibrous connective tissue. The fibrous anuli (rings) and intervening trigones separate the atria from the ventricles. This provides mechanical stability, electrical insulation (see p. 90 for cardiac conduction system), and an attachment point for the cardiac muscles and valve cusps.

Fig. 7.14 Semilunar valves

Valves have been longitudinally sectioned and opened.

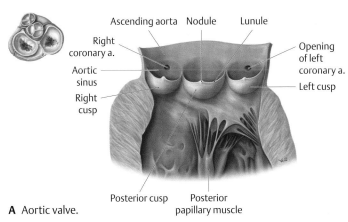

A Aortic valve.

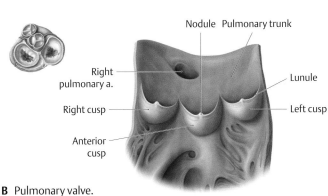

B Pulmonary valve.

Fig. 7.15 Atrioventricular valves

Anterior view during ventricular systole.

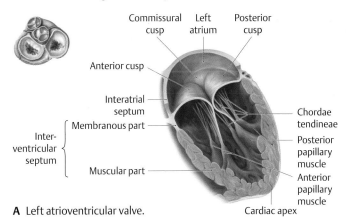

A Left atrioventricular valve.

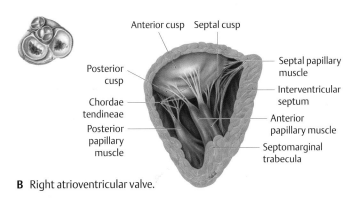

B Right atrioventricular valve.

✱ Clinical

Auscultation of the cardiac valves

Heart sounds, produced by closure of the semilunar and atrioventricular valves, are carried by the blood flowing through the valve. The resulting sounds are therefore best heard "downstream," at defined auscultation sites (dark circles). Valvular heart disease causes turbulent blood flow through the valve; this produces a murmur that may be detected in the colored regions.

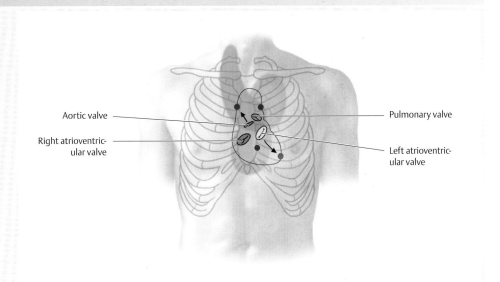

Table 7.2	Position and auscultation sites of cardiac valves	
Valve	**Anatomical projection**	**Auscultation site**
Aortic valve	Left sternal border (at level of 3rd rib)	Right 2nd intercostal space (at sternal margin)
Pulmonary valve	Left sternal border (at level of 3rd costal cartilage)	Left 2nd intercostal space (at sternal margin)
Left atrioventricular valve	Left 4th/5th costal cartilage	Left 5th intercostal space (at midclavicular line) or cardiac apex
Right atrioventricular valve	Sternum (at level of 3rd costal cartilage)	Left 5th intercostal space (at sternal margin)

Arteries & Veins of the Heart

Fig. 7.16 Coronary arteries and cardiac veins

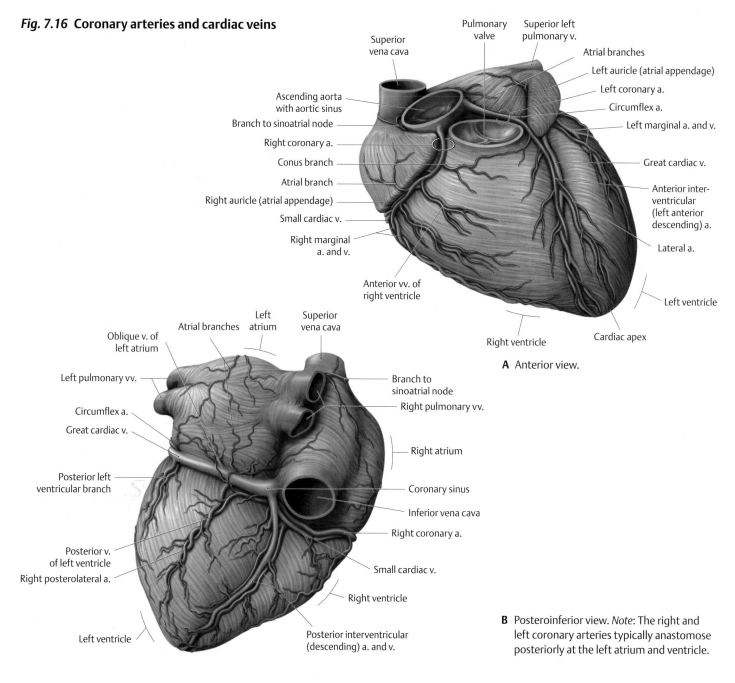

A Anterior view.

B Posteroinferior view. *Note:* The right and left coronary arteries typically anastomose posteriorly at the left atrium and ventricle.

Table 7.3	Branches of the coronary arteries
Left coronary artery	**Right coronary artery**
Circumflex a. • Atrial branch • Left marginal a. • Posterior left ventricular a.	Branch to SA node
	Conus branch
	Atrial branch
	Right marginal a.
Anterior interventricular a. (left anterior descending a.) • Conus branch • Lateral branch • Interventricular septal branches	Posterior interventricular (descending) a. • Interventricular septal branches
	Branch to AV node
	Right posterolateral a.
AV = atrioventricular; SA = sinoatrial.	

Table 7.4	Divisions of the cardiac veins	
Vein	**Tributaries**	**Drainage**
Anterior cardiac vv. (not shown)		Right atrium
Great cardiac v.	Anterior interventricular v.	Coronary sinus
	Left marginal v.	
	Oblique v. of left atrium	
Left posterior ventricular v.		
Posterior interventricular v. (middle cardiac v.)		
Small cardiac v.	Anterior vv. of right ventricle	
	Right marginal v.	

Fig. 7.17 Distribution of the coronary arteries

Anterior and posterior views of the heart, with superior views of transverse sections through the ventricles. The distribution of the coronary arteries differs from person to person. Right coronery artery and branches (green); left coronary artery and branches (red).

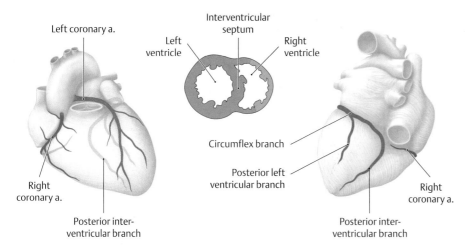

A Left coronary dominance (~15%).

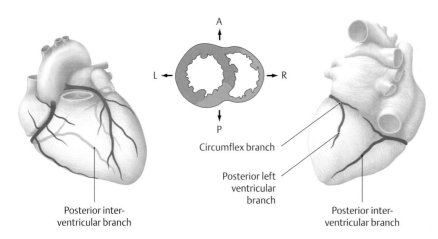

B Balanced distribution (~70%).

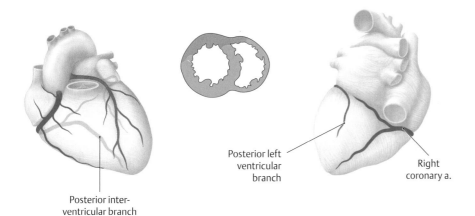

C Right coronary dominance (~15%).

Disturbed coronary blood flow

Although the coronary arteries are connected by structural anastomoses, they are end arteries from a functional standpoint. The most frequent cause of deficient blood flow is *atherosclerosis*, a narrowing of the coronary lumen due to plaque-like deposits on the vessel wall. When the decrease in luminal size (stenosis) reaches a critical point, coronary blood flow is restricted, causing chest pain (*angina pectoris*). Initially, this pain is induced by physical effort, but eventually it persists at rest, often radiating to characteristic sites (e.g., left arm, left side of head and neck). A myocardial infarction occurs when deficient blood supply causes myocardial tissue to die (necrosis). The location and extent of the infarction depends on the stenosed vessel (see **A–E**, after Heinecker).

A Supra-apical anterior infarction.

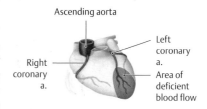

B Apical anterior infarction.

C Anterior lateral infarction.

D Posterior lateral infarction.

E Posterior infarction.

Conduction & Innervation of the Heart

Contraction of cardiac muscle is modulated by the cardiac conduction system. This system of specialized myocardial cells generates and conducts excitatory impulses in the heart. The conduction system contains two nodes, both located in the atria: the sinoatrial (SA) node, known as the pacemaker, and the atrioventricular (AV) node.

Fig. 7.18 Cardiac conduction system

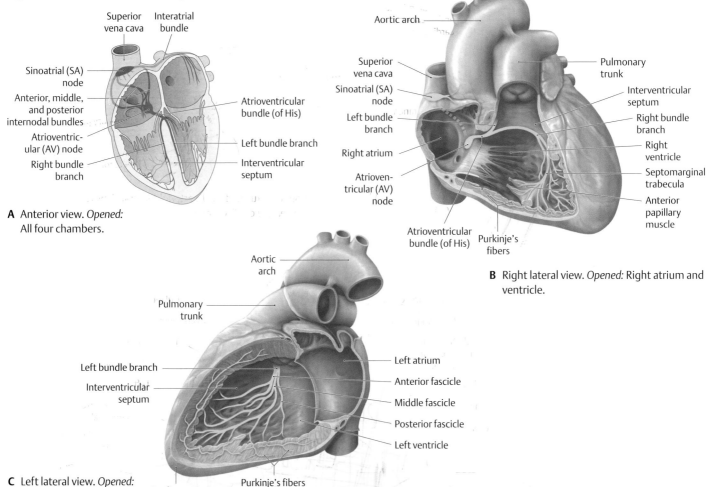

A Anterior view. *Opened:* All four chambers.

B Right lateral view. *Opened:* Right atrium and ventricle.

C Left lateral view. *Opened:* Left atrium and ventricle.

⚕ Clinical

Electrocardiogram (ECG)

The cardiac impulse (a physical dipole) travels across the heart and may be detected with electrodes. The use of three electrodes that separately record electrical activity of the heart along three axes or vectors (Einthoven limb leads) generates an electrocardiogram (ECG). The ECG graphs the cardiac cycle ("heartbeat"), reducing it to a series of waves, segments, and intervals. These ECG components can be used to determine whether cardiac impulses are normal or abnormal (e.g., myocardial infarction, chamber enlargement). *Note:* Although only three leads are required, a standard ECG examination includes at least two others (Goldberger, Wilson leads).

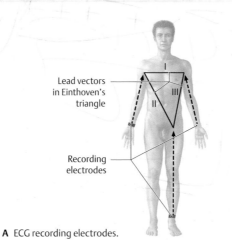

A ECG recording electrodes.

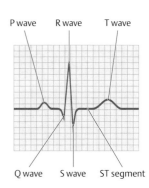

B ECG.

Sympathetic innervation: Presynaptic neurons from T1 to T6 spinal cord segments send fibers to synapse on postsynaptic neurons in the cervical and upper thoracic sympathetic ganglia. The three cervical cardiac nerves and thoracic cardiac branches contribute to the cardiac plexus. Parasympathetic innervation: Presynaptic neurons and fibers reach the heart via cardiac branches, some of which also arise in the cervical region. They synapse on postsynaptic neurons near the SA node and along the coronary arteries.

Fig. 7.19 Autonomic innervation of the heart

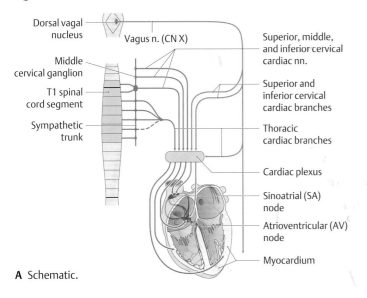

A Schematic.

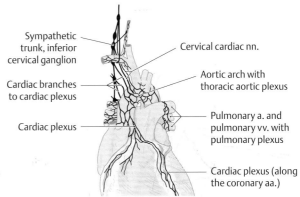

B Autonomic plexuses of the heart, right lateral view. Note the continuity between the cardiac, aortic, and pulmonary plexuses.

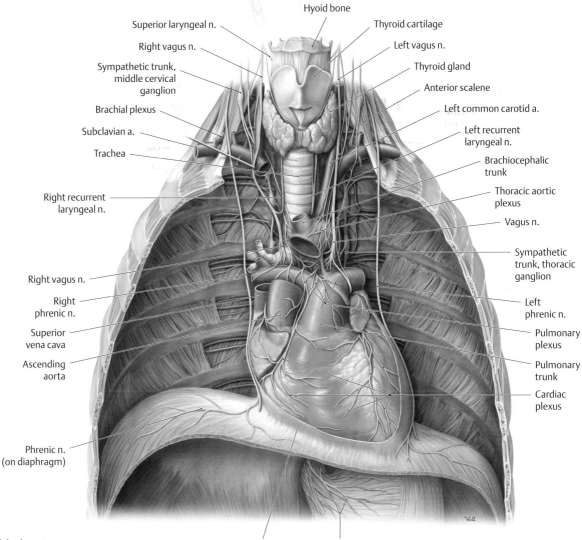

C Autonomic nerves of the heart. Anterior view of opened thorax.

Heart: Radiology

Table 7.5	Borders of the heart
Border	**Defining structures**
Right cardiac border	Right atrium
	Superior vena cava
Apex	Left ventricle
Left cardiac border	Aortic arch ("aortic knob")
	Pulmonary trunk
	Left atrium
	Left ventricle
Inferior cardiac border	Left ventricle
	Right ventricle

Fig. 7.20 Cardiac borders and configurations

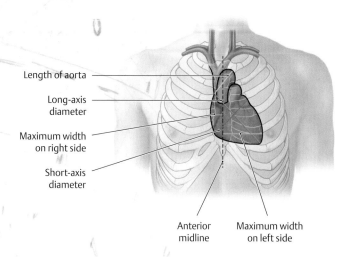

Length of aorta
Long-axis diameter
Maximum width on right side
Short-axis diameter
Anterior midline
Maximum width on left side

Fig. 7.21 Radiographic appearance of the heart

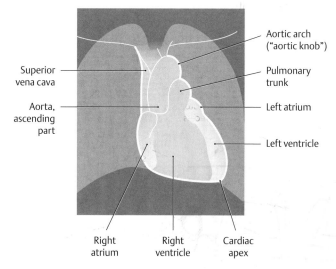

Aortic arch ("aortic knob")
Superior vena cava
Pulmonary trunk
Aorta, ascending part
Left atrium
Left ventricle
Right atrium
Right ventricle
Cardiac apex

A Anterior view.

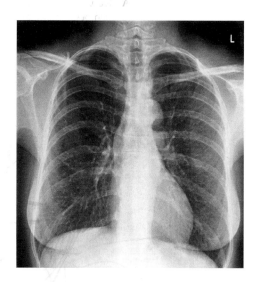

B Anteroposterior chest radiograph.

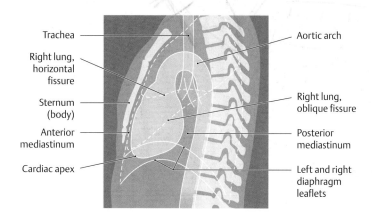

Trachea
Aortic arch
Right lung, horizontal fissure
Sternum (body)
Right lung, oblique fissure
Anterior mediastinum
Posterior mediastinum
Cardiac apex
Left and right diaphragm leaflets

C Lateral view. *Visible:* Diaphragm leaflets and lungs. The aortic arch forms a sling over the left main bronchus. Note the narrowness of the anterior mediastinum relative to the posterior mediastinum.

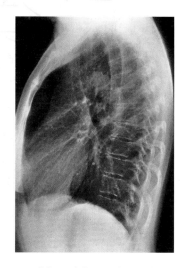

D Left lateral chest radiograph.

Fig. 7.22 **Heart in transverse section**

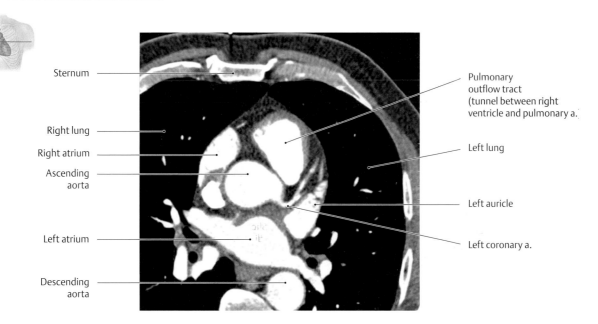

Sternum

Right lung

Right atrium

Ascending aorta

Left atrium

Descending aorta

Pulmonary outflow tract (tunnel between right ventricle and pulmonary a.)

Left lung

Left auricle

Left coronary a.

A Heart in normal chest magnetic resonance imaging (MRI). The cardiac chambers are clearly displayed owing to the high signal intensity, and the lungs are not visualized.

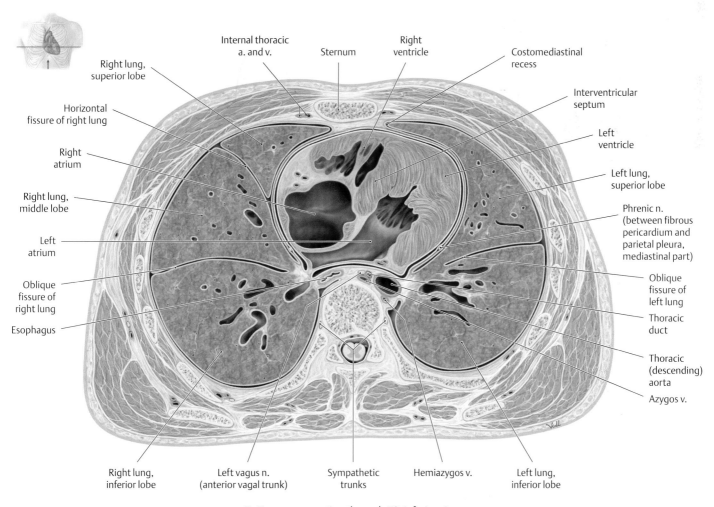

Right lung, superior lobe

Horizontal fissure of right lung

Right atrium

Right lung, middle lobe

Left atrium

Oblique fissure of right lung

Esophagus

Internal thoracic a. and v.

Sternum

Right ventricle

Costomediastinal recess

Interventricular septum

Left ventricle

Left lung, superior lobe

Phrenic n. (between fibrous pericardium and parietal pleura, mediastinal part)

Oblique fissure of left lung

Thoracic duct

Thoracic (descending) aorta

Azygos v.

Right lung, inferior lobe

Left vagus n. (anterior vagal trunk)

Sympathetic trunks

Hemiazygos v.

Left lung, inferior lobe

B Transverse section through T8, inferior view.

Pre- & Postnatal Circulation

***Fig. 7.23* Prenatal circulation**
After Fritsch and Kühnel.

① Oxygenated and nutrient-rich fetal blood from the placenta passes to the fetus via the umbilical *vein*.

② Approximately half of this blood bypasses the liver (via the ductus venosus) and enters the inferior vena cava. The remainder enters the portal vein to supply the liver with nutrients and oxygen.

③ Blood entering the right atrium from the inferior vena cava bypasses the right ventricle (as the lungs are not yet functioning) to enter the left atrium via the foramen ovale, a right-to-left shunt.

④ Blood from the superior vena cava enters the right atrium, passes to the right ventricle, and moves into the pulmonary trunk. Most of this blood enters the aorta via the ductus arteriosus, a right-to-left shunt.

⑤ The partially oxygenated blood in the aorta returns to the placenta via the paired umbilical arteries that arise from the internal iliac arteries.

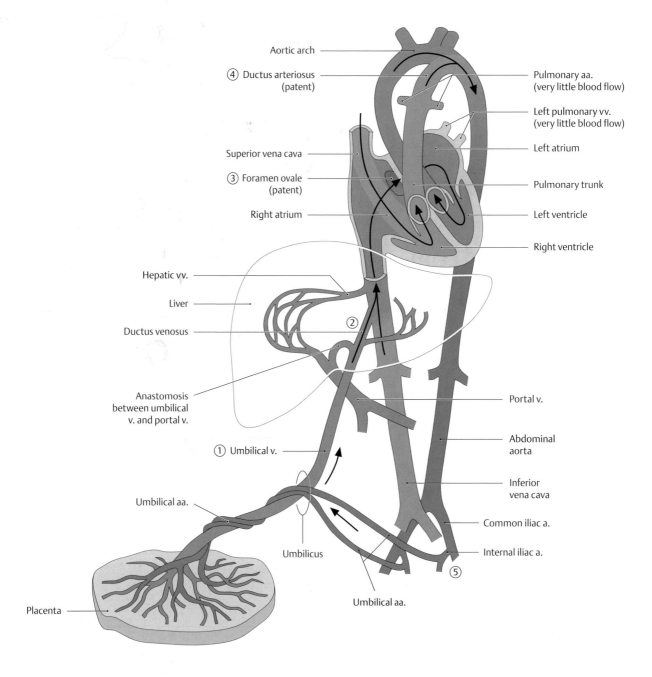

Aortic arch
④ Ductus arteriosus (patent)
Pulmonary aa. (very little blood flow)
Left pulmonary vv. (very little blood flow)
Superior vena cava
Left atrium
③ Foramen ovale (patent)
Pulmonary trunk
Right atrium
Left ventricle
Right ventricle
Hepatic vv.
Liver
Ductus venosus
②
Anastomosis between umbilical v. and portal v.
Portal v.
① Umbilical v.
Abdominal aorta
Umbilical aa.
Inferior vena cava
Common iliac a.
Umbilicus
Internal iliac a.
⑤
Umbilical aa.
Placenta

① As pulmonary respiration begins at birth, pulmonary blood pressure falls, causing blood from the right pulmonary trunk to enter the pulmonary veins.

② The foramen ovale and ductus arteriosus close, eliminating the fetal right-to-left shunts. The pulmonary and systemic circulations in the heart are now separate.

③ As the infant is separated from the placenta, the umbilical arteries occlude (except for the proximal portions), along with the umbilical vein and ductus venosus.

④ Blood to be metabolized now passes through the liver.

Fig. 7.24 **Postnatal circulation**
After Fritsch and Kühnel.

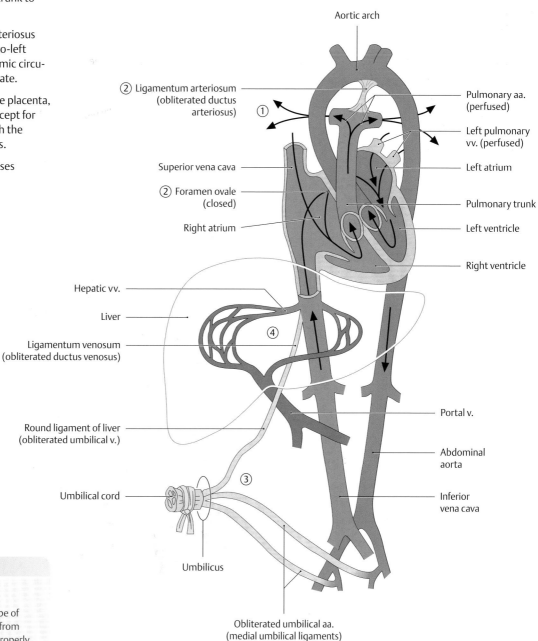

Aortic arch

② Ligamentum arteriosum (obliterated ductus arteriosus)

①

Pulmonary aa. (perfused)

Left pulmonary vv. (perfused)

Superior vena cava

② Foramen ovale (closed)

Right atrium

Left atrium

Pulmonary trunk

Left ventricle

Right ventricle

Hepatic vv.

Liver

Ligamentum venosum (obliterated ductus venosus)

④

Round ligament of liver (obliterated umbilical v.)

Portal v.

Abdominal aorta

Umbilical cord

③

Inferior vena cava

Umbilicus

Obliterated umbilical aa. (medial umbilical ligaments)

 Clinical

Septal defects
Septal defects, the most common type of congenital heart defect, allow blood from the left chambers of the heart to improperly pass into the right chambers during systole. Ventrical septal defect (VSD, shown below) is the most common form. Patent foramen ovale, the most prevalent form of *atrial* septal defect (ASD), results from improper closure of the fetal shunt.

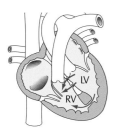

Table 7.6	**Derivatives of fetal circulatory structures**
Fetal structure	**Adult remnant**
Ductus arteriosus	Ligamentum arteriosum
Foramen ovale	Fossa ovalis
Ductus venosus	Ligamentum venosum
Umbilical v.	Round ligament of the liver (ligamentum teres)
Umbilical a.	Medial umbilical ligament

Esophagus

 The esophagus is divided into three parts: cervical (C6–T1), thoracic (T1 to the esophageal hiatus of the diaphragm), and abdominal (the diaphragm to the cardiac orifice of the stomach).

It descends slightly to the right of the thoracic aorta and pierces the diaphragm slightly to the left, just below the xiphoid process of the sternum.

Fig. 7.25 Esophagus: Location and constrictions

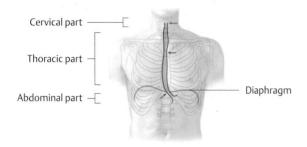

A Projection of esophagus onto chest wall. Esophageal constrictions are indicated with arrows.

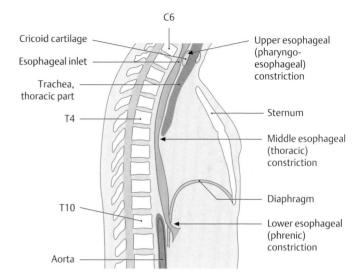

B Esophageal constrictions, right lateral view.

Fig. 7.26 Esophagus in situ
Anterior view.

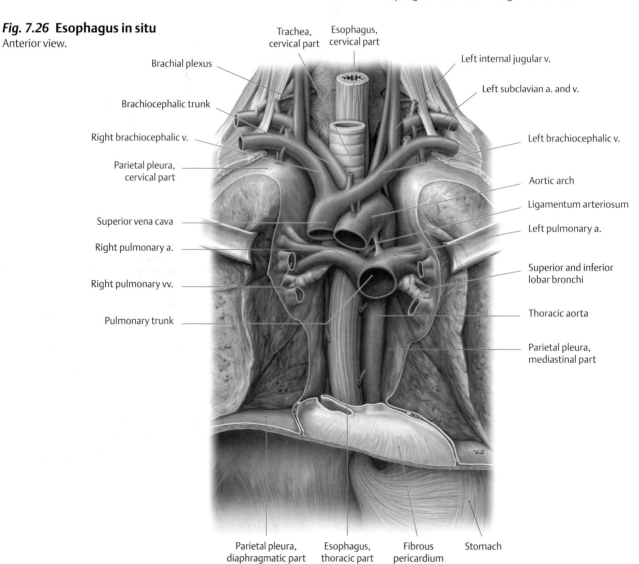

Fig. 7.27 Structure of the esophagus

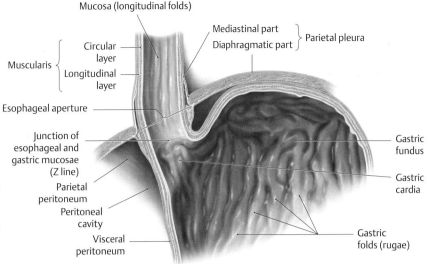

B Esophagogastric junction, anterior view. A true sphincter is not identifiable at this junction; instead, the diaphragmatic muscle of the esophageal aperture functions as a sphincter. It is often referred to as the "Z line" because of its zigzag form.

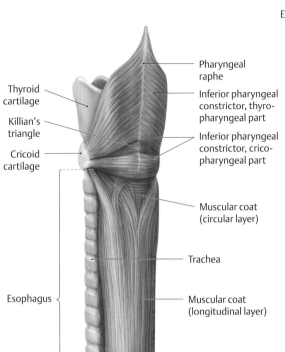

A Esophageal wall, oblique left posterior view. Pharynx (p. 552); trachea (p. 110).

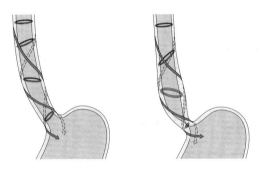

C Functional architecture of esophageal muscle.

✦ Clinical

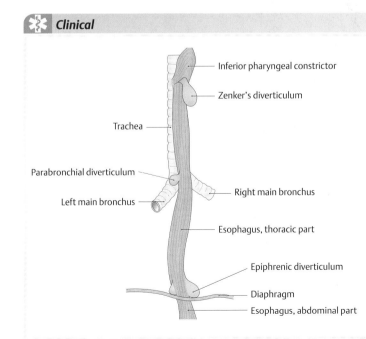

Esophageal diverticula

Diverticula (abnormal outpouchings or sacs) generally develop at weak spots in the esophageal wall. There are three main types of esophageal diverticula:

- Hypopharyngeal (pharyngo-esophageal) diverticula: Outpouchings occurring at the junction of the pharynx and the esophagus. These include Zenker's diverticula (70% of cases).

- "True" traction diverticula: Protrusion of all wall layers, not typically occurring at characteristic weak spots. However, they generally result from an inflammatory process (e.g., lymphangitis) and are thus common at sites where the esophagus closely approaches the bronchi and bronchial lymph nodes (thoracic or parabronchial diverticula).

- "False" pulsion diverticula: Herniations of the mucosa and submucosa through weak spots in the muscular coat due to a rise in esophageal pressure (e.g., during normal swallowing). These include parahiatal and epiphrenic diverticula occurring above the esophageal aperture of the diaphragm (10% of cases).

Neurovasculature of the Esophagus

 Sympathetic innervation: Presynaptic fibers arise from the T2–T6 spinal cord segments. Postsynaptic fibers arise from the sympathetic chain to join the esophageal plexus. Parasympathetic innervation: Presynaptic fibers arise from the dorsal vagal nucleus and travel in the vagus nerves to form the extensive esophageal plexus. *Note:* The postsynaptic neurons are in the wall of the esophagus. Fibers to the cervical portion of the esophagus travel in the recurrent laryngeal nerves.

Fig. 7.28 Autonomic innervation of the esophagus

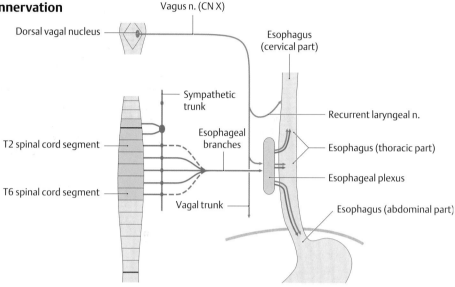

Fig. 7.29 Esophageal plexus

The left and right vagus nerves initially descend on the left and right sides of the esophagus. As they begin to contribute to the esophageal plexus, they shift to anterior and posterior positions, respectively. As the vagus nerves continue into the abdomen, they are named the anterior and posterior vagal trunks.

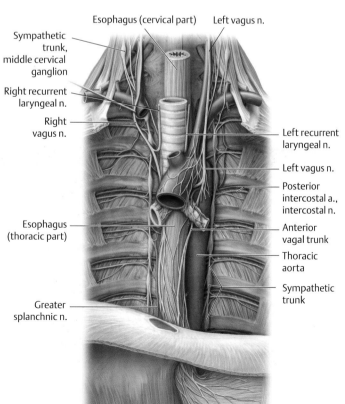

A Esophageal plexus in situ. Anterior view.

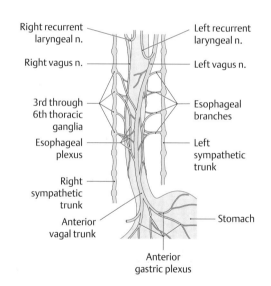

B Anterior view. Note the postsynaptic sympathetic contribution to the esophageal plexus.

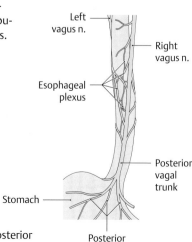

C Posterior view.

Fig. 7.30 Esophageal arteries
Anterior view.

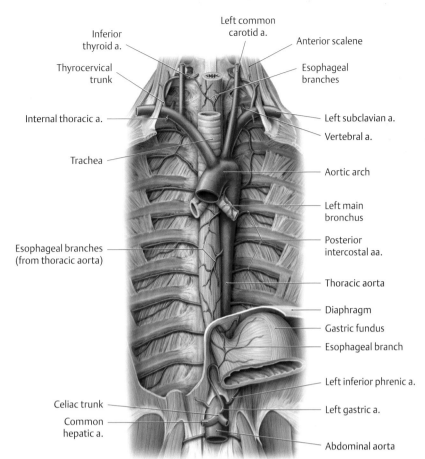

Fig. 7.31 Esophageal veins
Anterior view.

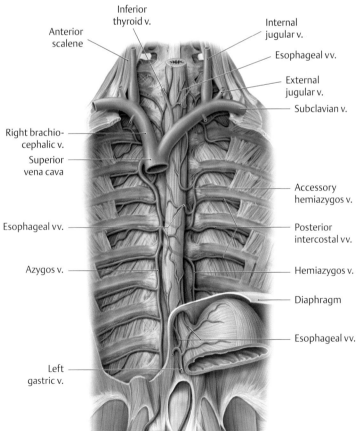

Table 7.7	Blood vessels of the esophagus	
Part	**Origin of esophageal arteries**	**Drainage of esophageal veins**
Cervical	Inferior thyroid a.	Inferior thyroid v.
	Rarely direct branches from thyrocervical trunk or common carotid a.	Left brachiocephalic v.
Thoracic	Aorta (four or five esophageal aa.)	Upper left: Accessory hemiazygos v. or left brachiocephalic v.
		Lower left: Hemiazygos v.
		Right side: Azygos v.
Abdominal	Left gastric a.	Left gastric v.

Lymphatics of the Mediastinum

 The superior phrenic lymph nodes drain lymph from the diaphragm, pericardium, lower esophagus, lung, and liver into the bronchomediastinal trunk. The inferior phrenic lymph nodes, found in the abdomen, collect lymph from the diaphragm and lower lobes of the lung and convey it to the lumbar trunk. *Note:* The pericardium may also drain superiorly to the brachiocephalic lymph nodes.

***Fig. 7.32* Lymph nodes of the mediastinum and thoracic cavity**
Left anterior oblique view.

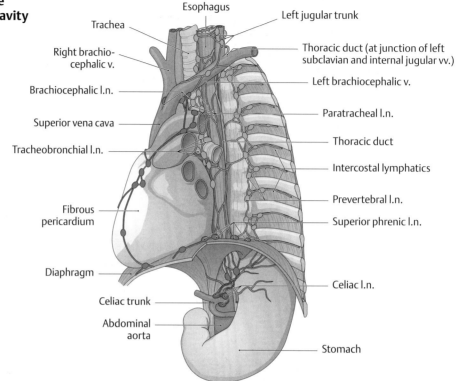

***Fig. 7.33* Lymphatic drainage of the heart**
A unique "crossed" drainage pattern exists in the heart: lymph from the left atrium and ventricle drains to the right venous junction, whereas lymph from the right atrium and ventricle drains to the left venous junction.

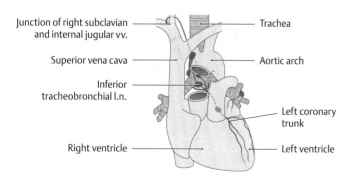

A Lymphatic drainage of the left chambers, anterior view.

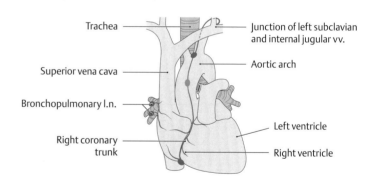

B Lymphatic drainage of the right chambers, anterior view.

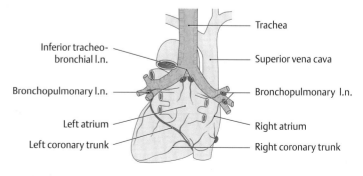

C Posterior view.

The paraesophageal nodes drain the esophagus. Lymphatic drainage of the cervical part of the esophagus is primarily cranial, to the deep cervical lymph nodes and then to the jugular trunk. The thoracic part of the esophagus drains to the bronchomediastinal trunks in two parts: the upper half drains cranially, and the lower half drains inferiorly via the superior phrenic lymph nodes. The bronchopulmonary and paratracheal nodes drain lymph from the lungs, bronchi, and trachea into the bronchomediastinal trunk (see p. 118).

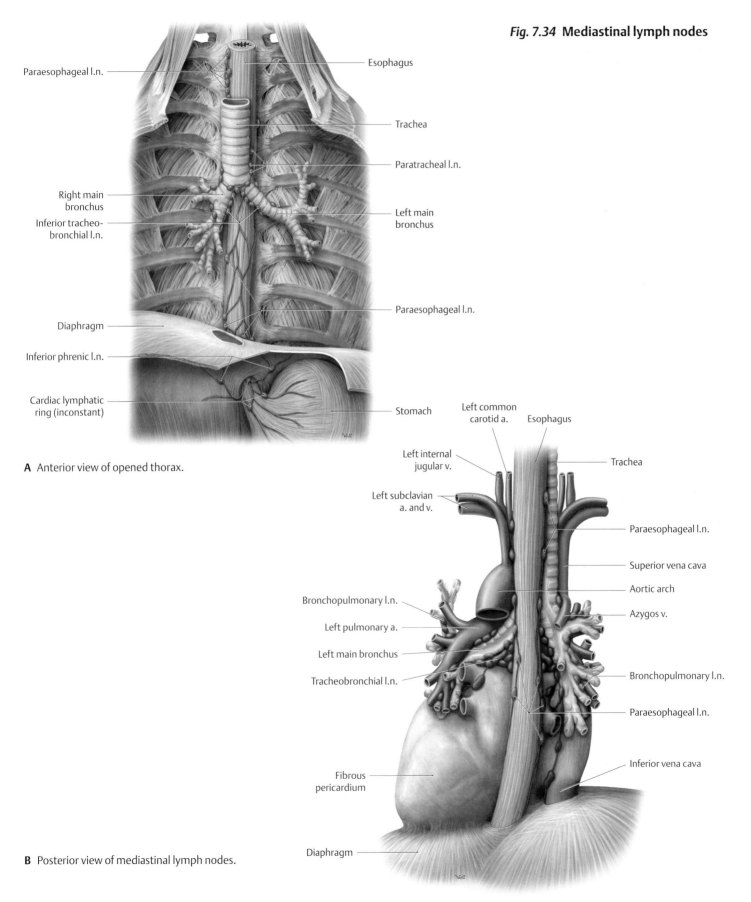

***Fig. 7.34* Mediastinal lymph nodes**

A Anterior view of opened thorax.

B Posterior view of mediastinal lymph nodes.

Pleural Cavity

 The paired pleural cavities contain the left and right lungs. They are completely separated from each other by the mediastinum and are under negative atmospheric pressure (see respiratory mechanics, pp. 112–113).

Fig. 8.1 Pleural cavity

Pleural cavities and lungs projected onto thoracic skeleton.

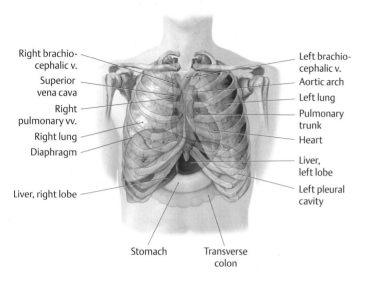

A Anterior view.

B Posterior view.

Fig. 8.2 Boundaries of the pleural cavities and lungs

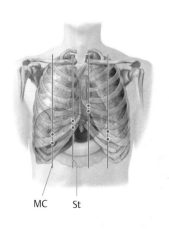

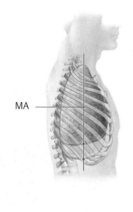

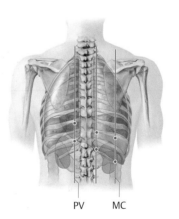

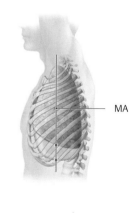

A Anterior view.   **B** Right lateral view.   **C** Posterior view.   **D** Left lateral view.

Table 8.1	Pleural cavity boundaries and reference points			
Reference line	**Right parietal pleura**	**Right lung**	**Left lung**	**Left parietal pleura**
Sternal line (St)	7th rib	6th rib	4th rib	4th rib
Midclavicular line (MC)	8th costal cartilage	6th rib	6th rib	8th rib
Midaxillary line (MA)	10th rib	8th rib	8th rib	10th rib
Paravertebral line (PV)	T12 vertebra	10th rib	10th rib	T12 vertebra

Fig. 8.3 Parietal pleura

The pleural cavity is bounded by two serous layers. The visceral (pulmonary) pleura covers the lungs, and the parietal pleura lines the inner surface of the thoracic cavity. The four parts of the parietal pleura (costal, diaphragmatic, mediastinal, and cervical) are continuous.

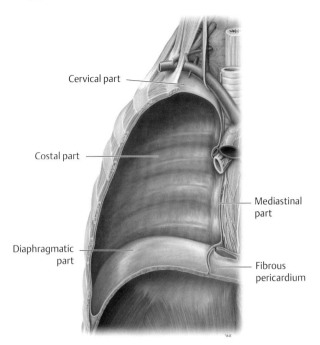

A Parts of the parietal pleura. *Opened:* Right pleural cavity, anterior view.

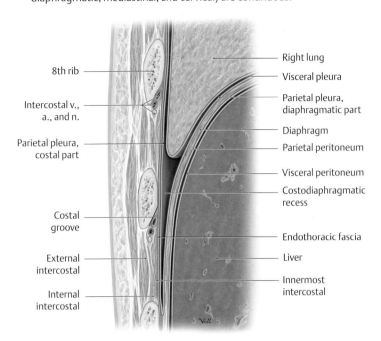

B Costodiaphragmatic recess, coronal section, anterior view. Reflection of the diaphragmatic pleura onto the inner thoracic wall (becoming the costal pleura) forms the costodiaphragmatic recess.

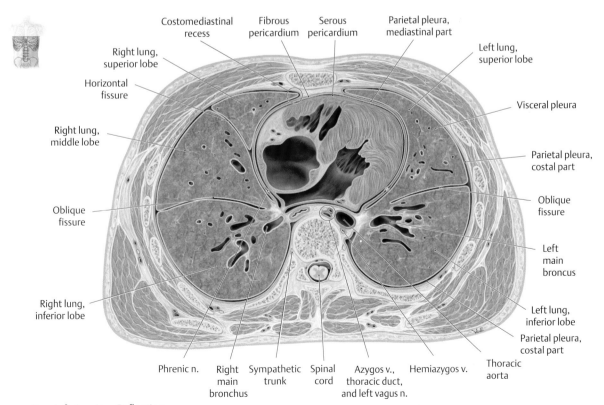

C Transverse section, inferior view. Reflection of the costal pleura onto the pericardium forms the costomediastinal recess.

Lungs in Situ

Fig. 8.4 Lungs in situ
The left and right lungs occupy the full volume of the pleural cavity. Note that the left lung is slightly smaller than the right due to the asymmetrical position of the heart.

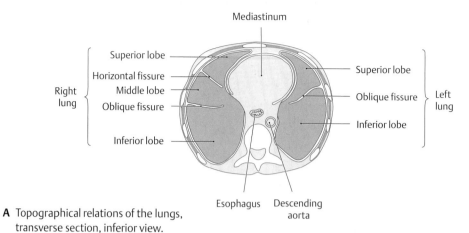

A Topographical relations of the lungs, transverse section, inferior view.

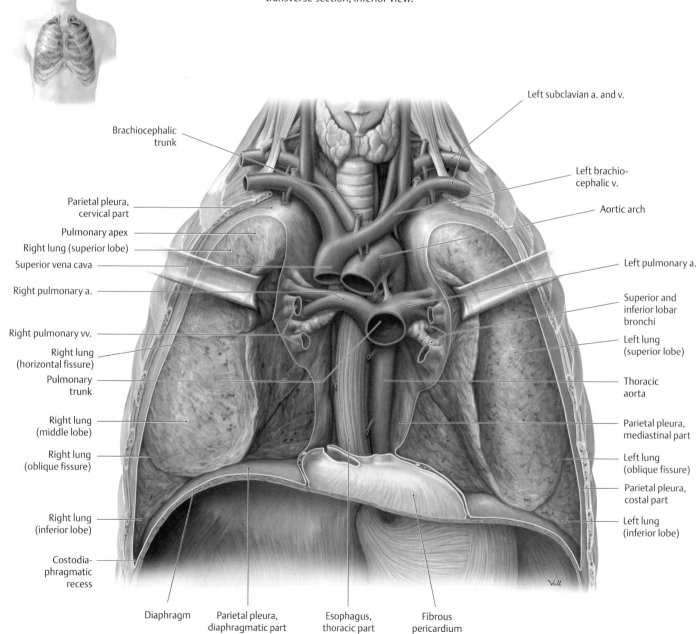

B Anterior view with lungs retracted.

The oblique and horizontal fissures divide the right lung into three lobes: superior, middle, and inferior. The oblique fissure divides the left lung into two lobes: superior and inferior. The apex of each lung extends into the root of the neck. The hilum is the location at which the bronchi and neurovascular structures connect to the lung.

Fig. 8.5 Gross anatomy of the lungs

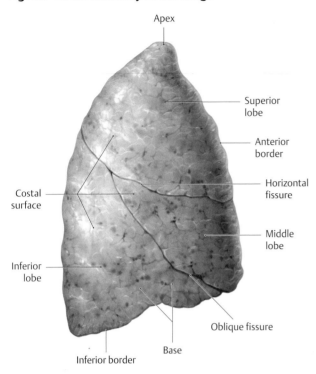

A Right lung, lateral view.

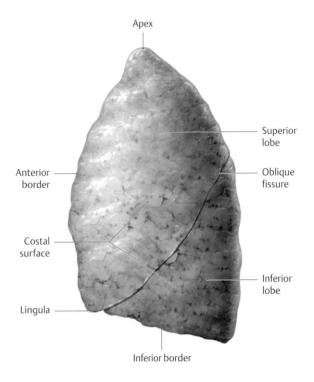

B Left lung, lateral view.

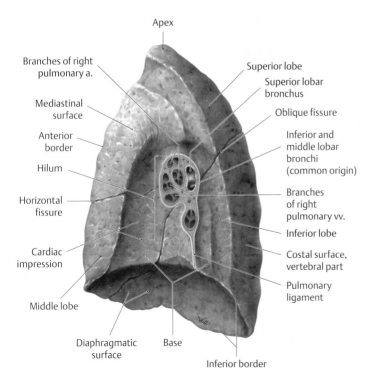

C Right lung, medial view.

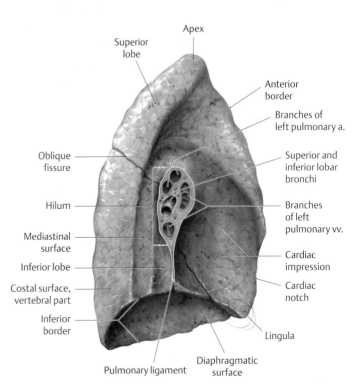

D Left lung, medial view.

Lung: Radiology

The regions of the lungs show varying degrees of lucency in chest radiographs. The perihilar region where the main bronchi and vessels enter and exit the lung is less radiolucent than the peripheral region, which contains small-caliber vascular branches and segmental bronchi. The perihilar lung region is also covered by the heart. These "shadows" appear as white or bright areas on the radiograph (radiographs are negatives: areas that are impermeable to light will appear bright).

Fig. 8.6 Radiographic appearance of the lungs

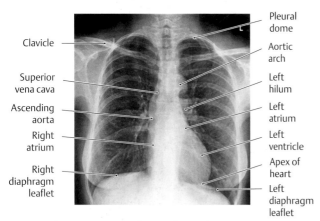

Clavicle
Superior vena cava
Ascending aorta
Right atrium
Right diaphragm leaflet

Pleural dome
Aortic arch
Left hilum
Left atrium
Left ventricle
Apex of heart
Left diaphragm leaflet

A Normal anteroposterior chest radiograph.

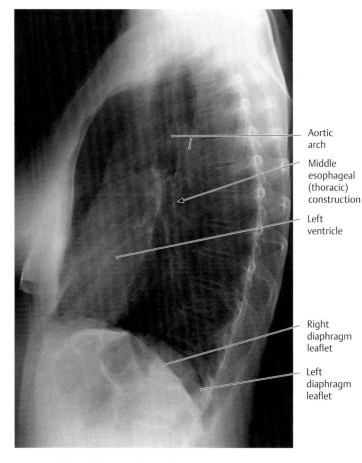

Aortic arch
Middle esophageal (thoracic) construction
Left ventricle
Right diaphragm leaflet
Left diaphragm leaflet

B Normal lateral chest radiograph.

Fig. 8.7 Opacity in lung diseases

Lateral and anterior views of the right and left lungs. Opacity (decreased radiolucency) may be observed in diseased lung areas. Increased opacity may be due to fluid infiltration (inflammation) or tissue proliferation (neoplasia). These opacities are easier to detect in the peripheral part of the lung, which is inherently more radiolucent. *Note:* Opacities that conform to segmental lung boundaries are almost invariably due to pulmonary inflammation.

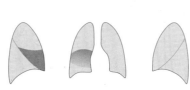

A Apical segment opacity.

B Upper lobe opacity.

C Middle lobe opacity.
   Note: The left lung has no middle lobe.

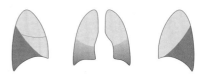

D Lower lobe opacity.

Diseases of the lung

Increased opacity in the lungs does not necessarly correspond to segmental boundaries. Fluid accumulation in the lungs also creates characteristic "shadows" in pulmonary radiographs.

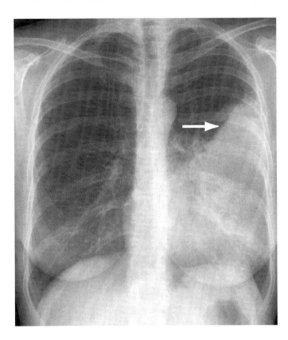

A Lingular pneumonia. The horizontal fissure can be seen (arrow). *Note*: The heart is much more difficult to visualize here due to increased opacity of segments IV and V.

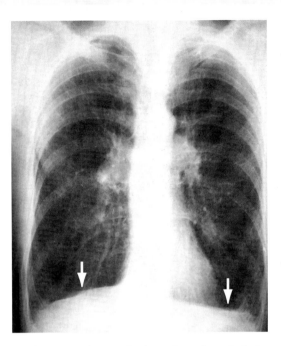

B Pulmonary emphysema. The chest radiograph reveals diaphragmatic depression (flattening of the domes of the diaphragm, arrows) with corresponding changes in the orientation of the cardiac shadow. The heart assumes a vertical orientation due to the low diaphragm (a lateral radiograph would reveal an increased retrosternal space). The central pulmonary arteries are dilated but taper dramatically at the segmental level.

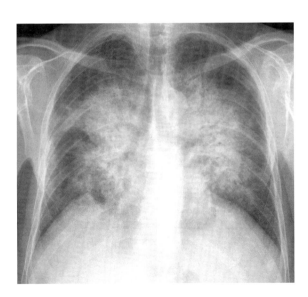

C Pulmonary edema complicating acute myocardial infarction. Dilation of vessels increases the number of visible vascular structures. This image shows a butterfly pattern of edema and bilateral pleural effusion.

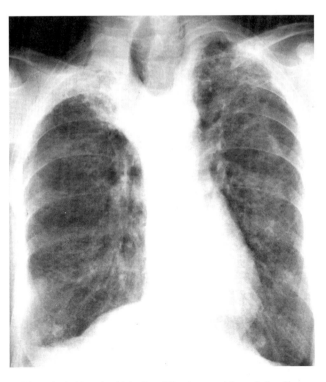

D Tuberculosis. Note the thickening of the pleura and the radiating fibrous bands. This image does not contain the small pulmonary nodules (tuberculomas) often found in the upper zones of the lung.

Bronchopulmonary Segments of the Lungs

 The lung lobes are subdivided into bronchopulmonary segments, each supplied by a tertiary (segmental) bronchus. *Note:* These subdivisions are not defined by surface boundaries but by origin.

Fig. 8.8 Segmentation of the lung
Anterior view. See pp. 110–111 for details of the trachea and bronchial tree.

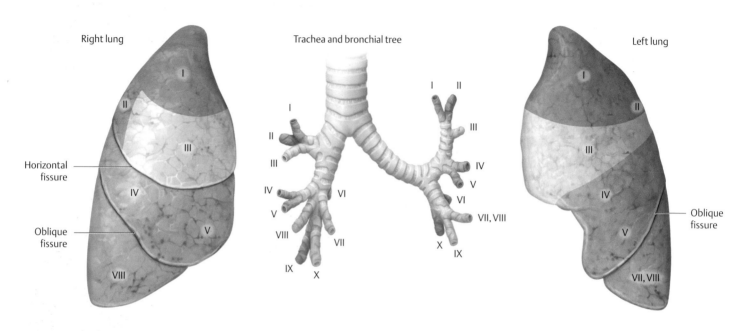

Right lung

Horizontal fissure

Oblique fissure

Trachea and bronchial tree

Left lung

Oblique fissure

Fig. 8.9 Posteroanterior bronchogram
Anterior view of right lung.

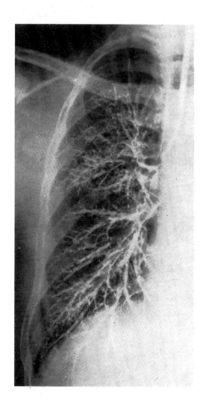

Table 8.2	Segmental architecture of the lungs		
Each segment is supplied by a segmental bronchus of the same name (e.g., the apical segmental bronchus supplies the apical segment). See pp. 110–111 for details of the trachea and bronchial tree.			
	Right lung		**Left lung**
	Superior lobe		
I	Apical segment	Apicoposterior segment	I
II	Posterior segment		II
III	Anterior segment		III
	Middle lobe	**Lingula**	
IV	Lateral segment	Superior lingular segment	IV
V	Medial segment	Inferior lingular segment	V
	Inferior lobe		
VI	Superior segment		VI
VII	Medial basal segment		VII
VIII	Anterior basal segment		VIII
IX	Lateral basal segment		IX
X	Posterior basal segment		X

Fig. 8.10 Right lung: Bronchopulmonary segments

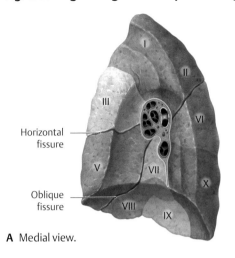

Horizontal fissure

Oblique fissure

A Medial view.

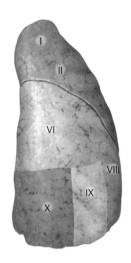

B Posterior view.

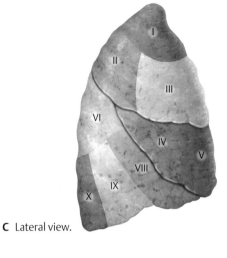

C Lateral view.

Fig. 8.11 Left lung: Bronchopulmonary segments

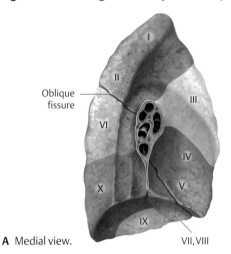

Oblique fissure

A Medial view.

VII, VIII

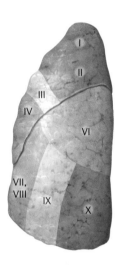

B Posterior view.

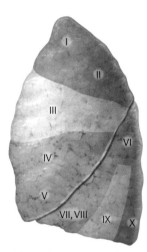

C Lateral view.

✳ Clinical

Lung resections

Lung cancer, emphysema, or tuberculosis may necessitate the surgical removal of damaged portions of the lung. Surgeons exploit the anatomical subdivision of the lungs into lobes and segments when excising damaged tissue.

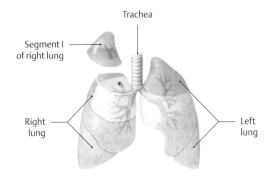

Trachea

Segment I of right lung

Right lung

Left lung

A Segmentectomy (wedge resection): Removal of one or more segments.

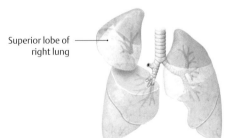

Superior lobe of right lung

B Lobectomy: Removal of lobe.

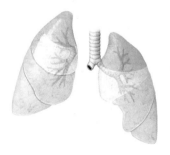

C Pneumonectomy: Removal of entire lung.

Trachea & Bronchial Tree

 At or near the level of the sternal angle, the lowest tracheal cartilage extends anteroposteriorly, forming the carina. The trachea bifurcates at the carina into the right and left main bronchi. Each bronchus gives off lobar branches to the corresponding lung.

Fig. 8.12 **Trachea**
See p. 574 for the structures of the thyroid.

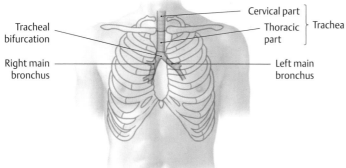

A Projection of trachea onto chest.

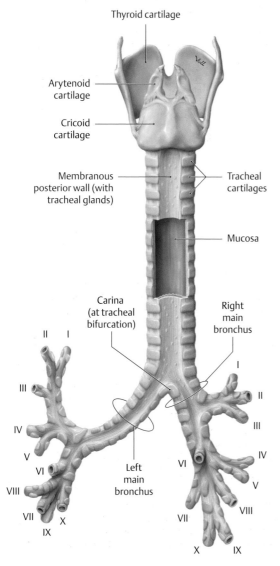

C Posterior view with opened posterior wall.

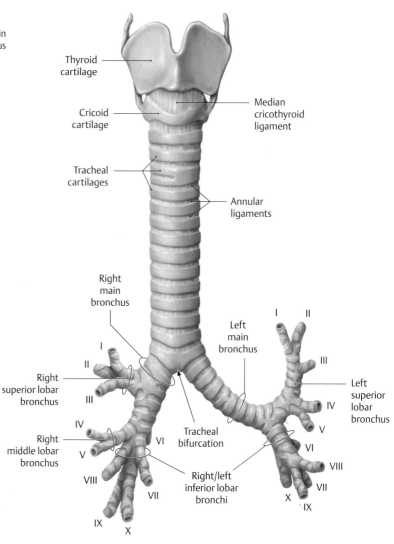

B Anterior view.

✳ Clinical

Foreign body aspiration
Toddlers are at particularly high risk of potentially fatal aspiration of foreign bodies. In general, foreign bodies are more likely to become lodged in the right main bronchus than the left: the left bronchus diverges more sharply at the tracheal bifurcation, while the right bronchus is relatively straight.

The conducting portion of the bronchial tree extends from the tracheal bifurcation to the terminal bronchiole, inclusive. The respiratory portion consists of the respiratory bronchiole, alveolar ducts, alveolar sacs, and alveoli.

Fig. 8.13 **Bronchial tree**

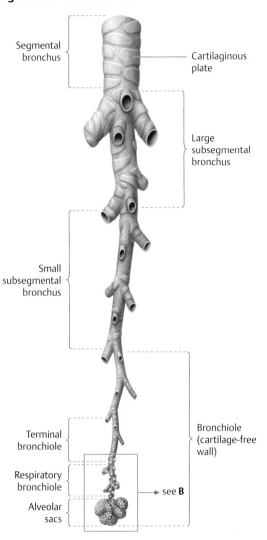

Segmental bronchus

Cartilaginous plate

Large subsegmental bronchus

Small subsegmental bronchus

Terminal bronchiole

Respiratory bronchiole

Alveolar sacs

Bronchiole (cartilage-free wall)

→ see **B**

A Divisions of the bronchial tree.

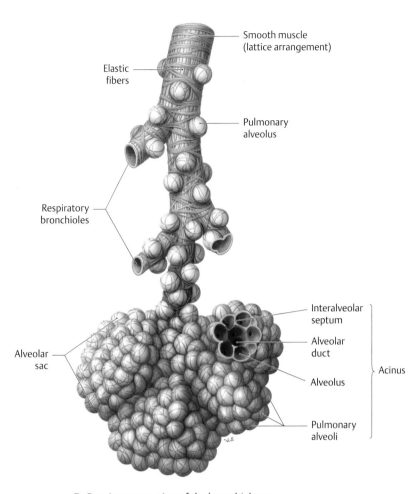

Smooth muscle (lattice arrangement)

Elastic fibers

Pulmonary alveolus

Respiratory bronchioles

Alveolar sac

Interalveolar septum

Alveolar duct

Alveolus

Pulmonary alveoli

Acinus

B Respiratory portion of the bronchial tree.

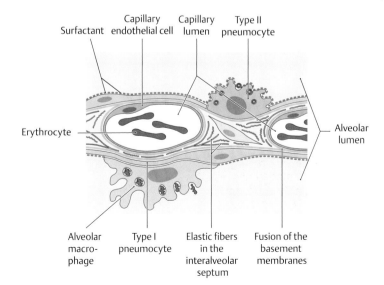

Surfactant

Capillary endothelial cell

Capillary lumen

Type II pneumocyte

Erythrocyte

Alveolar lumen

Alveolar macrophage

Type I pneumocyte

Elastic fibers in the interalveolar septum

Fusion of the basement membranes

C Epithelial lining of the alveoli.

Clinical

Respiratory compromise

The most common cause of respiratory compromise at the bronchial level is asthma. Compromise at the alveolar level may result from increased diffusion distance, decreased aeration (emphysema), or fluid infiltration (e.g., pneumonia).

Diffusion distance: Gaseous exchange takes place between the alveolar and capillary lumens in the alveoli (see Fig. 8.13C). At these sites, the basement membranes of capillary endothelial cells are fused with those of type I alveolar epithelial cells, lowering the exchange distance to 0.5 μm. Diseases that increase this diffusion distance (e.g., edematous fluid collection or inflammation) result in compromised respiration.

Condition of alveoli: In diseases like emphysema, which occurs in chronic obstructive pulmonary disease (COPD), alveoli are destroyed or damaged. This reduces the surface area available for gaseous exchange.

Production of surfactant: Surfactant is a protein-phospholipid film that lowers the surface tension of the alveoli, making it easier for the lung to expand. The immature lungs of a preterm infant often fail to produce sufficient surfactant, leading to respiratory problems. Surfactant is produced and absorbed by alveolar epithelial cells (pneumocytes). Type I alveolar epithelial cells absorb surfactant; type II produce and distribute it.

Respiratory Mechanics

 The mechanics of respiration are based on a rhythmic increase and decrease in thoracic volume, with an associated expansion and contraction of the lungs. *Inspiration* (red): Contraction of the diaphragm leaflets lowers the diaphragm into the inspiratory position, increasing the volume of the pleural cavity along the vertical axis. Contraction of the thoracic muscles (external intercostals with the scalene, intercartilaginous, and posterior serratus muscles) elevates the ribs, expanding the pleural cavity along the sagittal and transverse axes (Fig. 8.15A,B). Surface tension in the pleural space causes the visceral and parietal pleura to adhere; thus, changes in thoracic volume alter the volume of the lungs. This is particularly evident in the pleural recesses: at functional residual capacity (resting position between inspiration and expiration), the lung does not fully occupy the pleural cavity. As the pleural cavity expands, a negative intrapleural pressure is generated. The air pressure differential results in an influx of air (inspiration). *Expiration* (blue): During passive expiration, the muscles of the thoracic cage relax and the diaphragm returns to its expiratory position. Contraction of the lungs increases the pulmonary pressure and expels air from the lungs. For forcible expiration, the internal intercostal muscles (with the transverse thoracic and subcostal mucosa) can actively lower the rib cage more rapidly and to a greater extent than through passive elastic recoil.

Fig. 8.14 Respiratory changes in thoracic volume
Inspiratory position (red); expiratory position (blue).

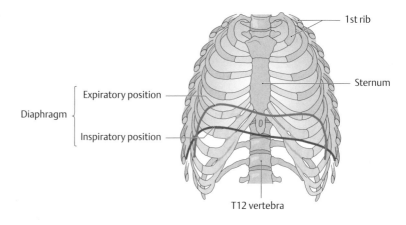

Fig. 8.15 Inspiration: Pleural cavity expansion

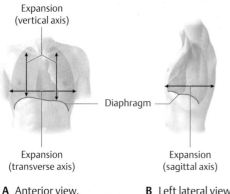

A Anterior view.   **B** Left lateral view.   **C** Anterolateral view.

Fig. 8.16 Expiration: Pleural cavity contraction

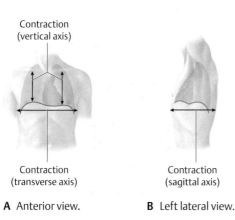

A Anterior view.   **B** Left lateral view.   **C** Anterolateral view.

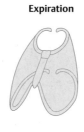

Fig. 8.17 Respiratory changes in lung volume

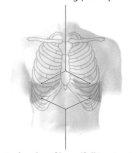

Fig. 8.18 Inspiration: Lung expansion

Right lung (full inspiration)

Diaphragm

Costodiaphragmatic recess

Fig. 8.19 Expiration: Lung contraction

Right lung (full expiration)

Pleural space

Diaphragm

Costodiaphragmatic recess

Fig. 8.20 Movements of the lung and bronchial tree

As the volume of the lung changes with the thoracic cavity, the entire bronchial tree moves within the lung. These structural movements are more pronounced in portions of the bronchial tree distant from the pulmonary hilum.

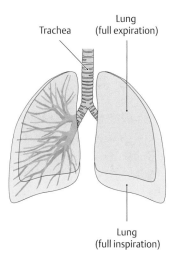

Trachea

Lung (full expiration)

Lung (full inspiration)

✳ Clinical

Pneumothorax

The pleural space is normally sealed from the outside environment. Injury to the parietal pleura, visceral pleura, or lung allows air to enter the pleural cavity (pneumothorax). The lung collapses due to its inherent elasticity, and the patient's ability to breathe is compromised. The uninjured lung continues to function under normal pressure variations, resulting in "mediastinal flutter": the mediastinum shifts toward the normal side during inspiration and returns to the midline during expiration. Tension (valve) pneumothorax occurs when traumatically detached and displaced tissuere covers the defect in the thoracic wall from the inside. This mobile flap allows air to enter, but not escape, the pleural cavity, causing a pressure buildup. The mediastinum shifts to the normal side, which may cause kinking of the great vessels and prevent the return of venous blood to the heart. Without treatment, tension pneumothorax is invariably fatal.

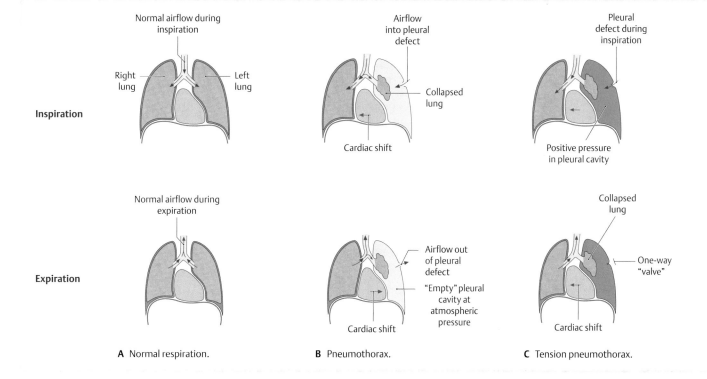

Normal airflow during inspiration

Right lung

Left lung

Inspiration

Normal airflow during expiration

Expiration

A Normal respiration.

Airflow into pleural defect

Collapsed lung

Cardiac shift

Airflow out of pleural defect

"Empty" pleural cavity at atmospheric pressure

Cardiac shift

B Pneumothorax.

Pleural defect during inspiration

Positive pressure in pleural cavity

Collapsed lung

One-way "valve"

Cardiac shift

C Tension pneumothorax.

Pulmonary Arteries & Veins

Thorax

 The pulmonary trunk arises from the right ventricle and divides into a left and right pulmonary artery for each lung. The paired pulmonary veins open into the left atrium on each side. The pulmonary arteries accompany and follow the branching of the bronchial tree, whereas the pulmonary veins do not, being located at the margins of the pulmonary lobules.

Fig. 8.21 **Pulmonary arteries and veins**
Anterior view.

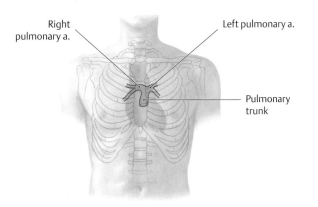

A Projection of pulmonary arteries on chest wall.

B Projection of pulmonary veins on chest wall.

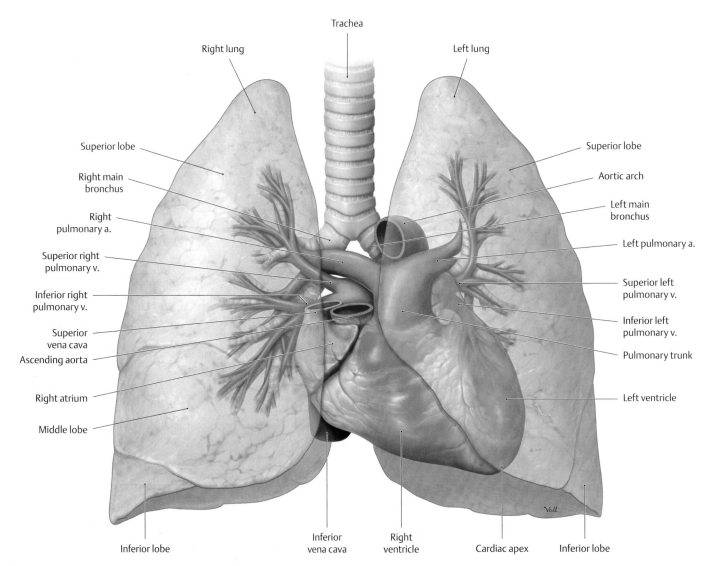

C Distribution of the pulmonary arteries and veins, anterior view.

114

Fig. 8.22 Pulmonary arteries

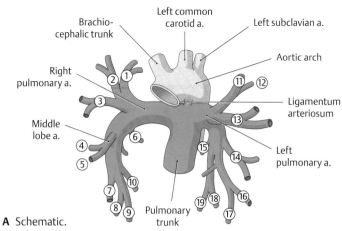

A Schematic.

Table 8.3 · Pulmonary arteries and their branches

	Right pulmonary artery		Left pulmonary artery
Superior lobe arteries			
①	Apical segmental a.		⑪
②	Posterior segmental a.		⑫
③	Anterior segmental a.		⑬
Middle lobe arteries			
④	Lateral segmental a.	Lingular a.	⑭
⑤	Medial segmental a.		
Inferior lobe arteries			
⑥	Superior segmental a.		⑮
⑦	Anterior basal segmental a.		⑯
⑧	Lateral basal segmental a.		⑰
⑨	Posterior basal segmental a.		⑱
⑩	Medial basal segmental a.		⑲

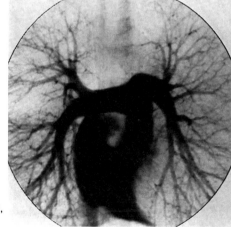

B Pulmonary arteriogram, arterial phase, anterior view.

Fig. 8.23 Pulmonary veins

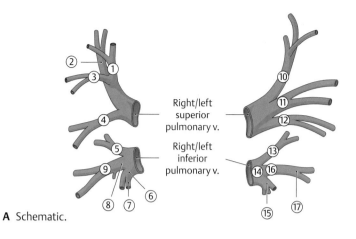

A Schematic.

Table 8.4 · Pulmonary veins and their tributaries

	Right pulmonary vein	Left pulmonary vein	
Superior pulmonary veins			
①	Apical v.	Apicoposterior v.	⑩
②	Posterior v.		
③	Anterior v.	Anterior v.	⑪
④	Middle lobe v.	Lingular v.	⑫
Inferior pulmonary veins			
⑤	Superior v.		⑬
⑥	Common basal v.		⑭
⑦	Inferior basal v.		⑮
⑧	Superior basal v.		⑯
⑨	Anterior basal v.		⑰

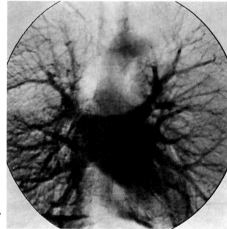

B Pulmonary arteriogram, venous phase, anterior view.

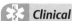 **Clinical**

Pulmonary embolism

Potentially life-threatening pulmonary embolism occurs when blood clots migrate through the venous system and become lodged in one of the arteries supplying the lungs. Symptoms include dyspnea (difficulty breathing) and tachycardia (increased heart rate). Most pulmonary emboli originate from stagnant blood in the veins of the lower limb and pelvis (venous thromboemboli). Causes include immobilization, disordered blood coagulation, and trauma. *Note:* A thromboembolus is a thrombus (blood clot) that has migrated (embolised).

Neurovasculature of the Tracheobronchial Tree

Fig. 8.24 Pulmonary vasculature

The pulmonary system is responsible for gaseous exchange within the lung. Pulmonary arteries (shown in blue) carry *deoxygenated* blood and follow the bronchial tree. The pulmonary vein (red) is the only vein in the body carrying *oxygenated* blood, which it receives from the alveolar capillaries at the periphery of the lobule.

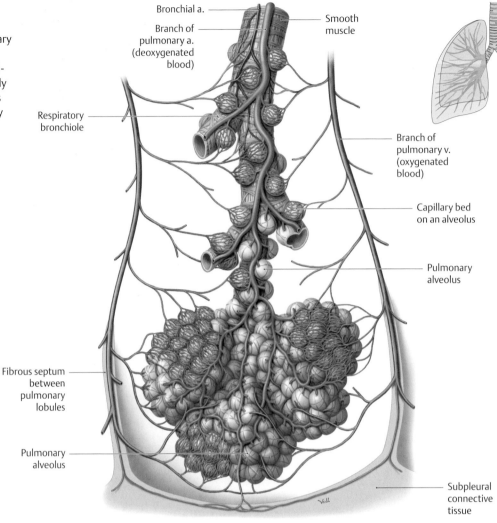

Fig. 8.25 Arteries of the tracheobronchial tree

The bronchial tree receives its nutrients via the bronchial arteries, found in the adventitia of the airways. Typically, there are one to three bronchial arteries arising directly from the aorta. Origin from a posterior intercostal artery may also occur.

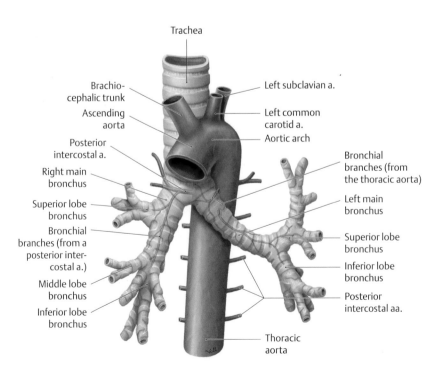

Fig. 8.26 Veins of the tracheobronchial tree

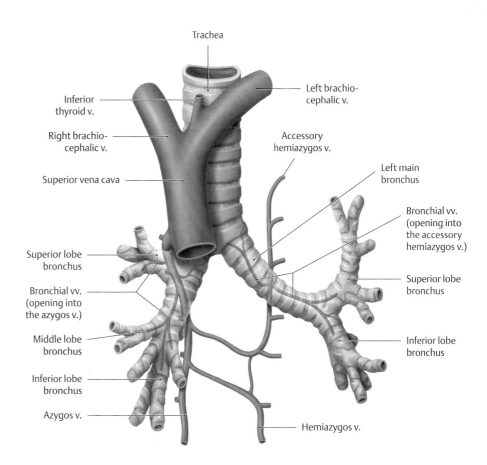

Trachea
Inferior thyroid v.
Left brachiocephalic v.
Right brachiocephalic v.
Accessory hemiazygos v.
Superior vena cava
Left main bronchus
Bronchial vv. (opening into the accessory hemiazygos v.)
Superior lobe bronchus
Superior lobe bronchus
Bronchial vv. (opening into the azygos v.)
Middle lobe bronchus
Inferior lobe bronchus
Inferior lobe bronchus
Azygos v.
Hemiazygos v.

Fig. 8.27 Autonomic innervation of the tracheobronchial tree

Sympathetic innervation (red); parasympathetic innervation (blue).

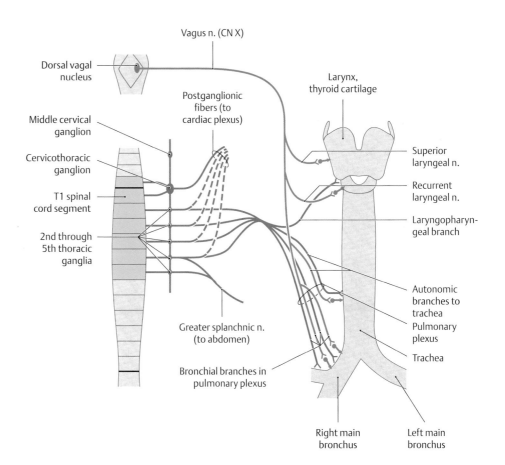

Vagus n. (CN X)
Dorsal vagal nucleus
Postganglionic fibers (to cardiac plexus)
Larynx, thyroid cartilage
Middle cervical ganglion
Cervicothoracic ganglion
Superior laryngeal n.
T1 spinal cord segment
Recurrent laryngeal n.
Laryngopharyngeal branch
2nd through 5th thoracic ganglia
Autonomic branches to trachea
Pulmonary plexus
Greater splanchnic n. (to abdomen)
Trachea
Bronchial branches in pulmonary plexus
Right main bronchus
Left main bronchus

Lymphatics of the Pleural Cavity

 The lungs and bronchi are drained by two lymphatic drainage systems. The peribronchial network follows the bronchial tree, draining lymph from the bronchi and most of the lungs. The subpleural network collects lymph from the peripheral lung and visceral pleura.

Fig. 8.28 Lymphatic drainage of the pleural cavity
Transverse section, inferior view.

A Peribronchial network, coronal section. (Intra)pulmonary nodes along the bronchial tree drain lymph from the lungs into the bronchopulmonary (hilar) nodes. Lymph then passes sequentially through the inferior and superior tracheobronchial nodes, paratracheal nodes, bronchomediastinal trunk, and finally to the right lymphatic or thoracic duct. *Note:* Significant amounts of lymph from the left lower lobe drain to the right superior tracheobronchial nodes.

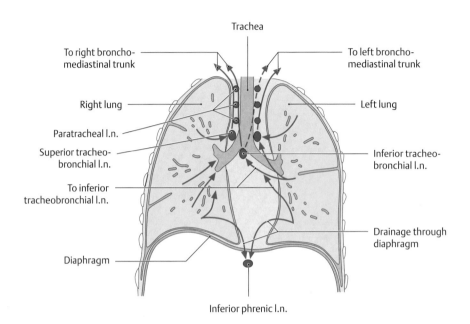

B Subpleural network, transverse section, superior view.

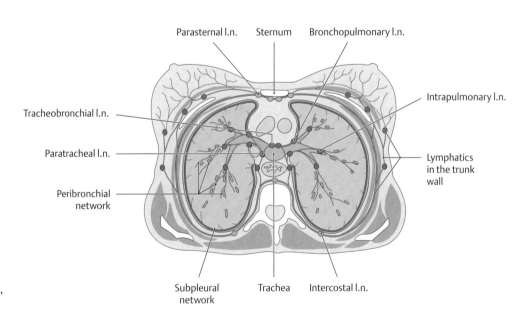

Fig. 8.29 **Lymph nodes of the pleural cavity**
Anterior view of pulmonary nodes.

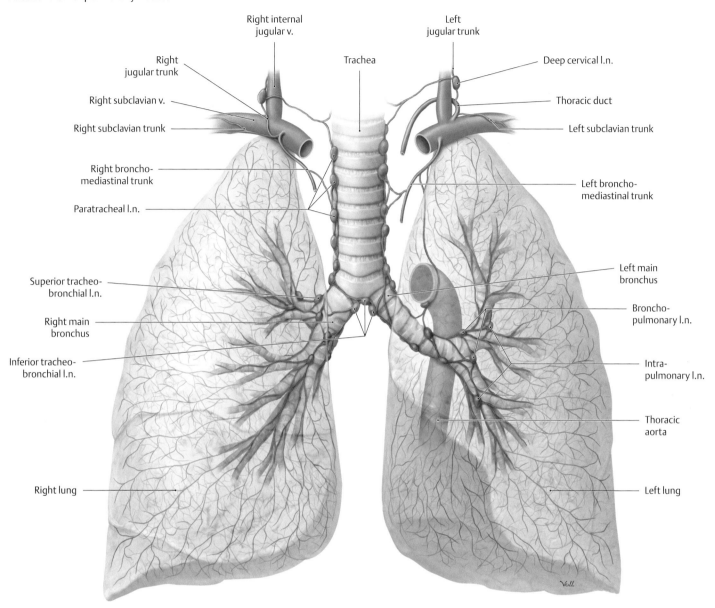

Right internal
jugular v.

Left
jugular trunk

Trachea

Right
jugular trunk

Deep cervical l.n.

Right subclavian v.

Thoracic duct

Right subclavian trunk

Left subclavian trunk

Right broncho-
mediastinal trunk

Left broncho-
mediastinal trunk

Paratracheal l.n.

Left main
bronchus

Superior tracheo-
bronchial l.n.

Broncho-
pulmonary l.n.

Right main
bronchus

Inferior tracheo-
bronchial l.n.

Intra-
pulmonary l.n.

Thoracic
aorta

Right lung

Left lung

Surface Anatomy

Fig. 9.1 Palpable structures in the thorax

Anterior view. See pp. 40–41 for structures of the back.

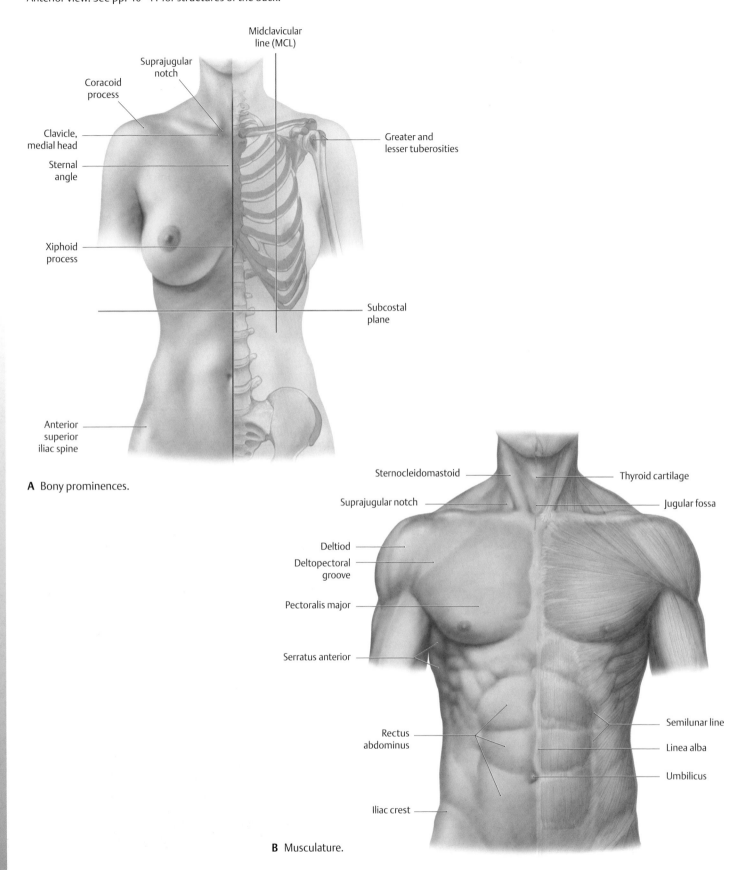

Midclavicular
line (MCL)

Suprajugular
notch

Coracoid
process

Clavicle,
medial head

Sternal
angle

Xiphoid
process

Greater and
lesser tuberosities

Subcostal
plane

Anterior
superior
iliac spine

A Bony prominences.

Sternocleidomastoid

Suprajugular notch

Thyroid cartilage

Jugular fossa

Deltiod

Deltopectoral
groove

Pectoralis major

Serratus anterior

Rectus
abdominus

Semilunar line

Linea alba

Umbilicus

Iliac crest

B Musculature.

Fig. 9.2 **Surface anatomy of the thorax**

Anterior view. See pp. 40–41 for structures of the back.

Q1: A female patient has given a history of detecting a "lump" during a self-examination. How would you proceed? Where would you palpate for lymph nodes?

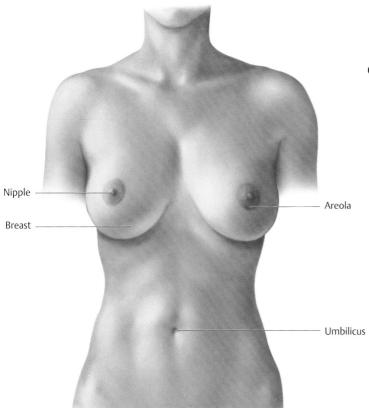

Nipple

Breast

Areola

Umbilicus

A Female thorax.

Q2: You are presented with the anterior chest of your first hospital patient. How would you formulate a plan to optimally examine the four valves of the heart?

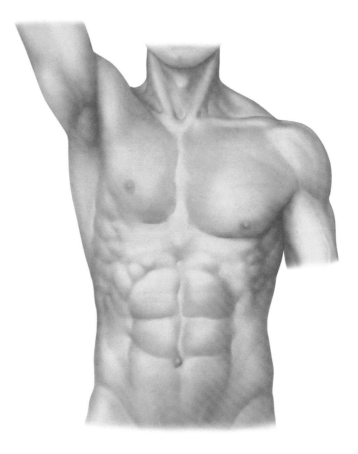

See answers beginning on p. 626.

B Male thorax.

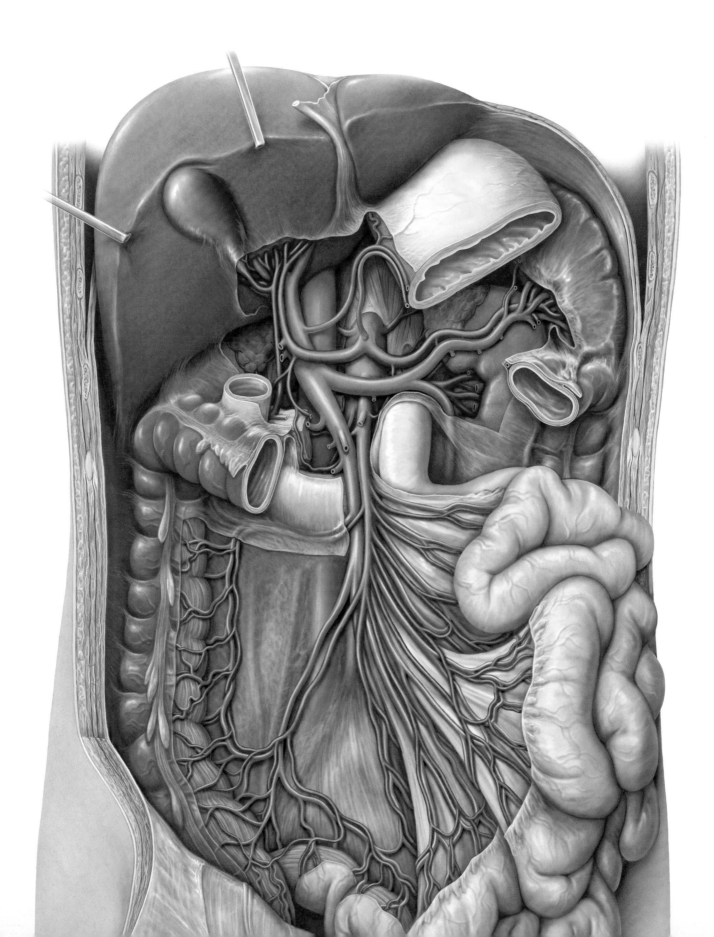

Abdomen & Pelvis

Pelvic Girdle

(see p. 358).

Fig. 10.1 Pelvic girdle

Anterosuperior view. The pelvic girdle consists of the two hip bones and the sacrum (see p. 358).

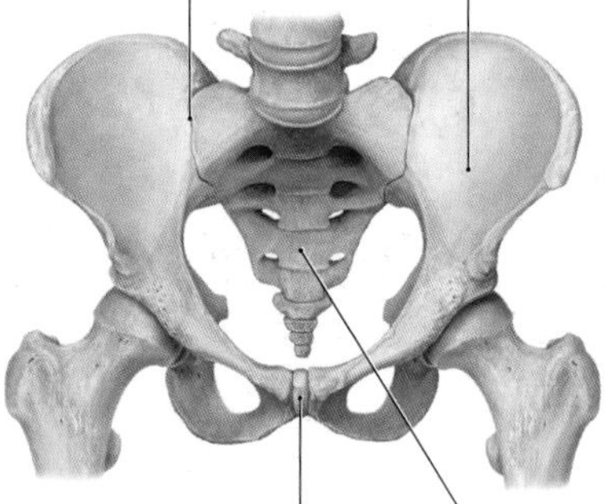

Sacroiliac joint

Hip bone

Pubic symphysis

Sacrum

Fig. 10.2 Hip bone

Right hip bone (male).

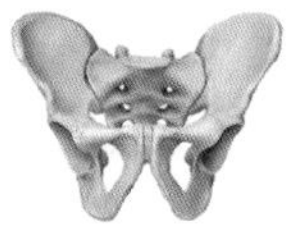

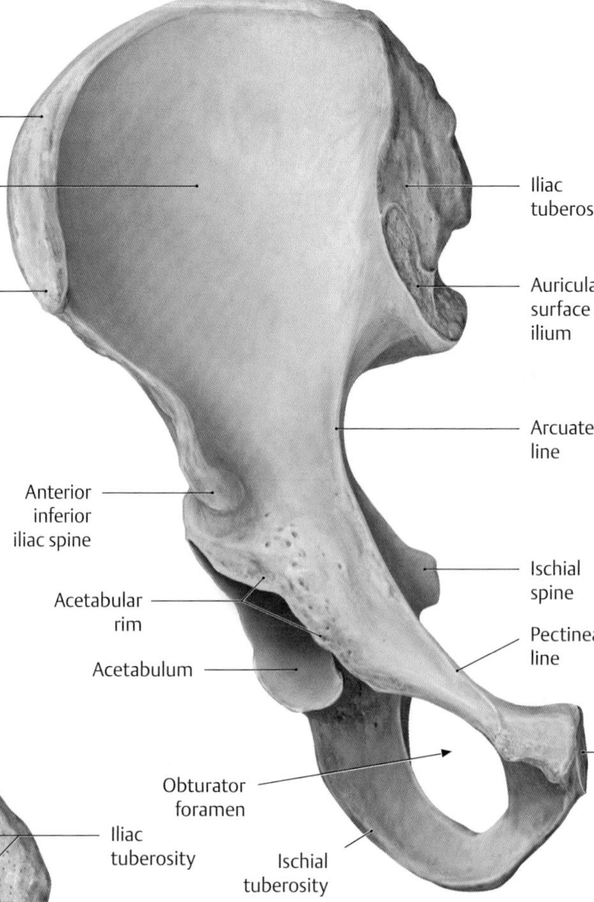

Iliac crest

Iliac fossa

Anterior superior iliac spine

Anterior inferior iliac spine

Acetabular rim

Acetabulum

Obturator foramen

Iliac tuberosity

Auricular surface of ilium

Arcuate line

Ischial spine

Pectineal line

Symphyseal surface

Ischial tuberosity

A Anterior view.

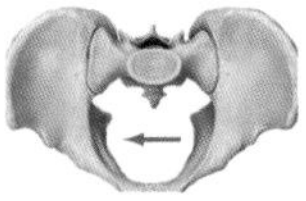

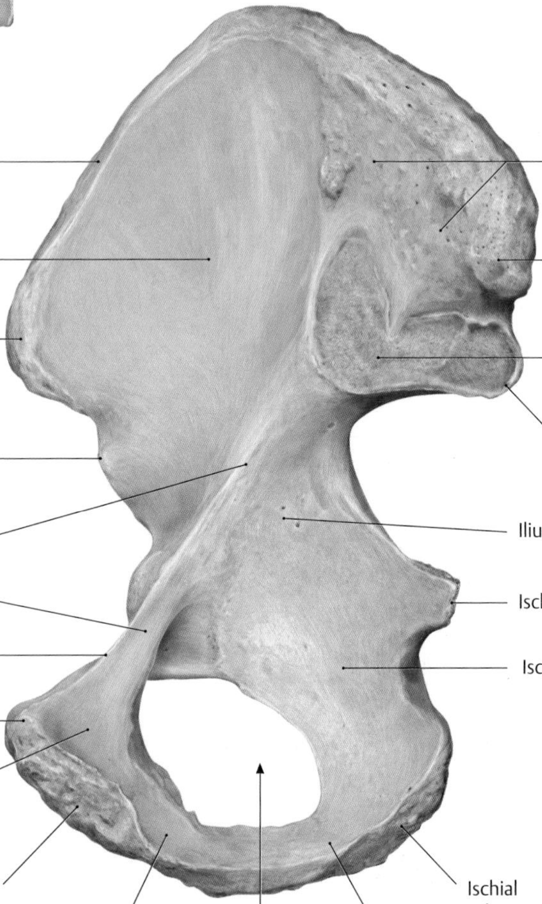

Iliac crest

Iliac fossa

Anterior superior iliac spine

Anterior inferior iliac spine

Arcuate line

Superior pubic ramus

Pectineal line

Pubic tubercle

Pubis (body)

Symphyseal surface

Inferior pubic ramus

Obturator foramen

Ischial ramus

Ischial tuberosity

Ischium (body)

Ischial spine

Ilium (body)

Posterior inferior iliac spine

Auricular surface of ilium

Posterior superior iliac spine

Iliac tuberosity

B Medial view.

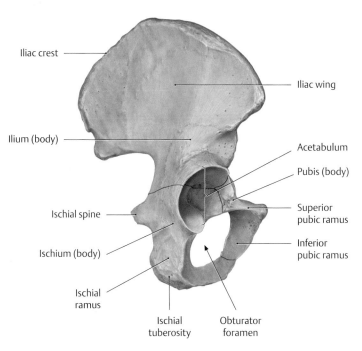

Iliac crest

Iliac wing

Ilium (body)

Acetabulum

Pubis (body)

Ischial spine

Superior pubic ramus

Ischium (body)

Inferior pubic ramus

Ischial ramus

Ischial tuberosity

Obturator foramen

A Junction of the triradiate cartilage.

Fig. 10.3 Triradiate cartilage of the hip bone
Right hip bone, lateral view. The hip bone consists of the ilium, ischium, and pubis.

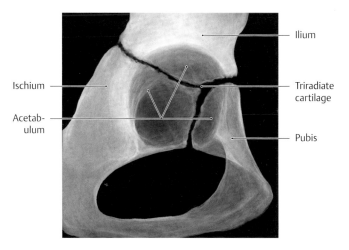

Ilium

Ischium

Triradiate cartilage

Acetab-ulum

Pubis

B Radiograph of a child's acetabulum. Right hip bone, lateral view.

Fig. 10.4 Hip bone: Lateral view
Right hip bone (male).

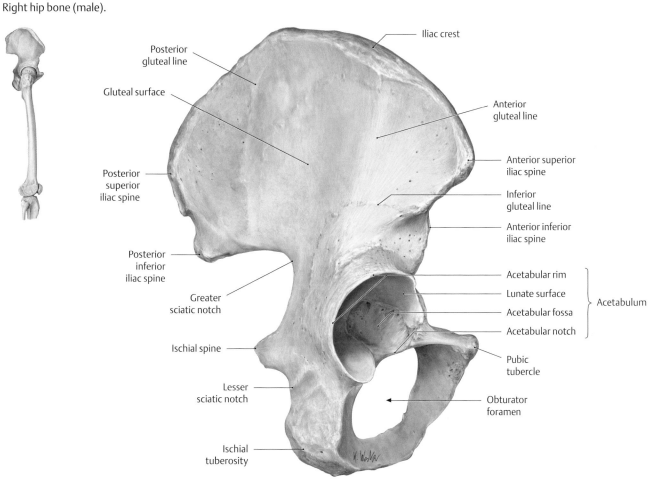

Iliac crest

Posterior gluteal line

Gluteal surface

Anterior gluteal line

Posterior superior iliac spine

Anterior superior iliac spine

Inferior gluteal line

Anterior inferior iliac spine

Posterior inferior iliac spine

Acetabular rim

Lunate surface

Acetabular fossa

Acetabulum

Greater sciatic notch

Acetabular notch

Ischial spine

Pubic tubercle

Lesser sciatic notch

Obturator foramen

Ischial tuberosity

125

Male & Female Pelvis

Fig. 10.5 **Female pelvis**

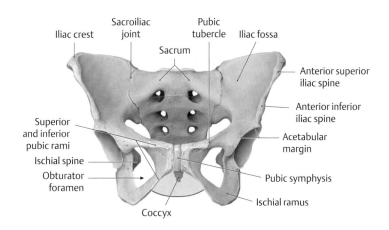

Iliac crest
Sacroiliac joint
Pubic tubercle
Iliac fossa
Sacrum
Iliac crest
Anterior superior iliac spine
Anterior inferior iliac spine
Superior and inferior pubic rami
Acetabular margin
Ischial spine
Obturator foramen
Pubic symphysis
Coccyx
Ischial ramus

A Anterior view.

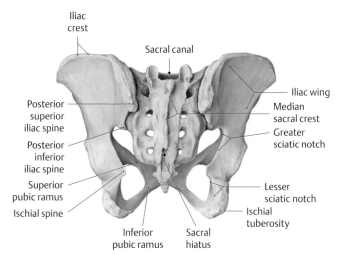

Iliac crest
Sacral canal
Posterior superior iliac spine
Iliac wing
Median sacral crest
Posterior inferior iliac spine
Greater sciatic notch
Superior pubic ramus
Ischial spine
Lesser sciatic notch
Ischial tuberosity
Inferior pubic ramus
Sacral hiatus

B Posterior view.

Fig. 10.6 **Male pelvis**

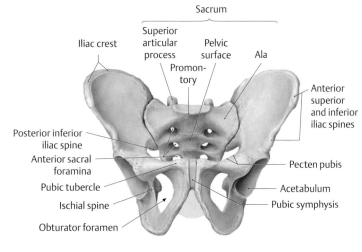

Sacrum
Superior articular process
Pelvic surface
Ala
Promontory
Iliac crest
Anterior superior and inferior iliac spines
Posterior inferior iliac spine
Anterior sacral foramina
Pubic tubercle
Pecten pubis
Ischial spine
Acetabulum
Obturator foramen
Pubic symphysis

A Anterior view.

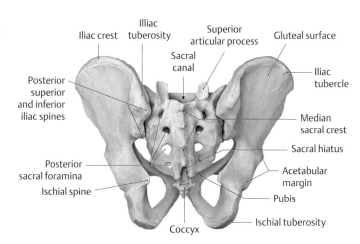

Iliac crest
Iliac tuberosity
Superior articular process
Gluteal surface
Sacral canal
Iliac tubercle
Posterior superior and inferior iliac spines
Median sacral crest
Posterior sacral foramina
Sacral hiatus
Ischial spine
Acetabular margin
Pubis
Coccyx
Ischial tuberosity

B Posterior view.

Fig. 10.7 Female pelvis: Superior view

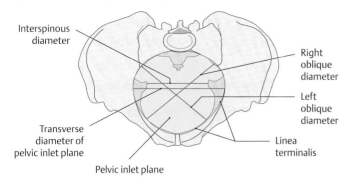

A Pelvic measurements.

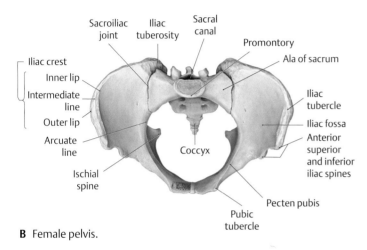

B Female pelvis.

Fig. 10.8 Male pelvis: Superior view

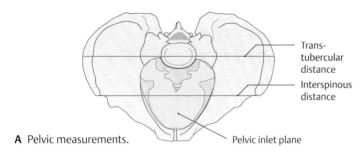

A Pelvic measurements.

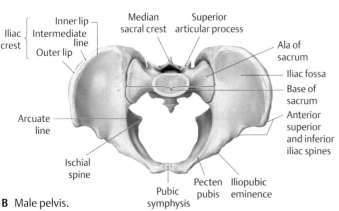

B Male pelvis.

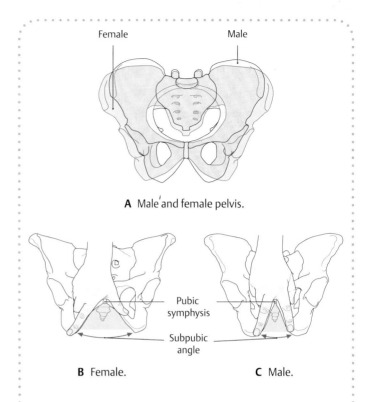

A Male and female pelvis.

B Female.

C Male.

Table 10.1	Gender-specific features of the pelvis	
Structure	**♀**	**♂**
False pelvis	Wide and shallow	Narrow and deep
Pelvic inlet	Transversely oval	Heart-shaped
Pelvic outlet	Roomy and round	Narrow and oblong
Ischial tuberosities	Everted	Inverted
Pelvic cavity	Roomy and shallow	Narrow and deep
Sacrum	Short, wide, and flat	Long, narrow, and convex
Subpubic angle	90–100 degrees	70 degrees

✴ Clinical

Childbirth

A non-optimal relation between the maternal pelvis and the fetal head may lead to complications during childbirth, potentially necessitating a caesarean section. Maternal causes include earlier pelvic trauma and innate malformations. Fetal causes include hydrocephalus (disturbed circulation of cerebrospinal fluid, leading to brain dilation and cranial expansion).

Pelvic Ligaments

***Fig. 10.9* Ligaments of the pelvis**
Male pelvis.

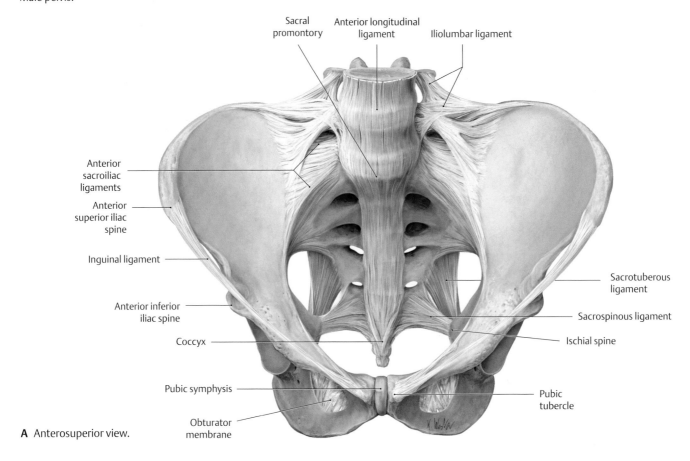

Sacral promontory
Anterior longitudinal ligament
Iliolumbar ligament
Anterior sacroiliac ligaments
Anterior superior iliac spine
Inguinal ligament
Anterior inferior iliac spine
Coccyx
Pubic symphysis
Obturator membrane
Sacrotuberous ligament
Sacrospinous ligament
Ischial spine
Pubic tubercle

A Anterosuperior view.

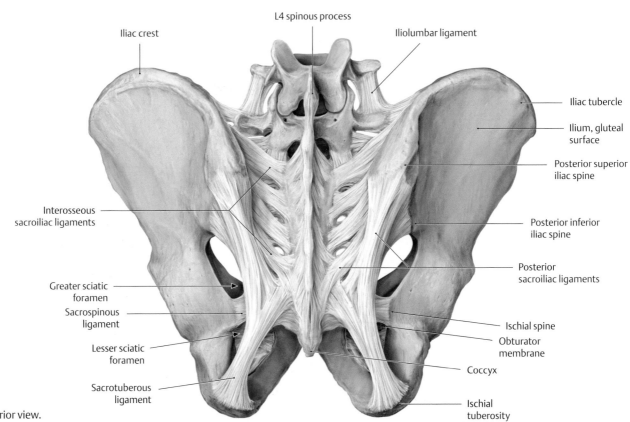

Iliac crest
L4 spinous process
Iliolumbar ligament
Iliac tubercle
Ilium, gluteal surface
Posterior superior iliac spine
Interosseous sacroiliac ligaments
Posterior inferior iliac spine
Posterior sacroiliac ligaments
Greater sciatic foramen
Sacrospinous ligament
Ischial spine
Obturator membrane
Lesser sciatic foramen
Coccyx
Sacrotuberous ligament
Ischial tuberosity

B Posterior view.

Fig. 10.10 Ligaments of the sacroiliac joint
Male pelvis.

Fig. 10.11 Pelvic measurements
Right half of female pelvis, medial view.
See Table 10.1.

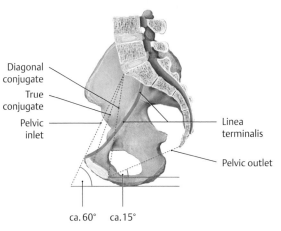

Diagonal conjugate
True conjugate
Pelvic inlet
Linea terminalis
Pelvic outlet

ca. 60° ca. 15°

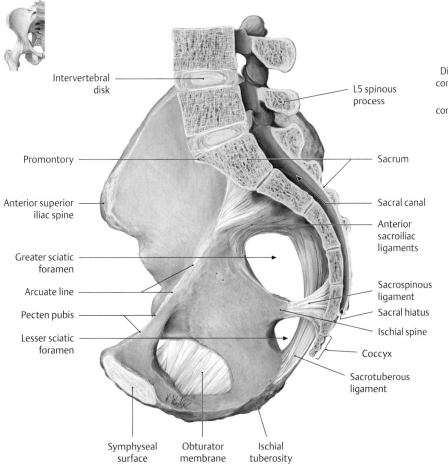

Intervertebral disk
L5 spinous process
Promontory
Sacrum
Anterior superior iliac spine
Sacral canal
Anterior sacroiliac ligaments
Greater sciatic foramen
Arcuate line
Sacrospinous ligament
Pecten pubis
Sacral hiatus
Ischial spine
Lesser sciatic foramen
Coccyx
Sacrotuberous ligament
Symphyseal surface
Obturator membrane
Ischial tuberosity

A Right half of pelvis, medial view.

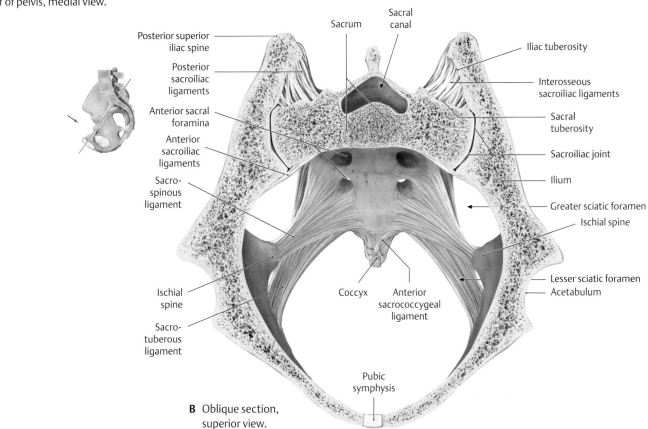

Sacrum
Sacral canal
Posterior superior iliac spine
Iliac tuberosity
Posterior sacroiliac ligaments
Interosseous sacroiliac ligaments
Anterior sacral foramina
Sacral tuberosity
Anterior sacroiliac ligaments
Sacroiliac joint
Sacrospinous ligament
Ilium
Greater sciatic foramen
Ischial spine
Ischial spine
Lesser sciatic foramen
Acetabulum
Coccyx
Anterior sacrococcygeal ligament
Sacrotuberous ligament
Pubic symphysis

B Oblique section, superior view.

Muscles of the Abdominal Wall

 The oblique muscles of the abdominal wall consist of the external and internal obliques and the transversus abdominis. The poste-rior or deep abdominal wall muscles (notably the psoas major) are functionally hip muscles (see p. 138).

Fig. 11.1 **Muscles of the abdominal wall**
Right side, anterior view.

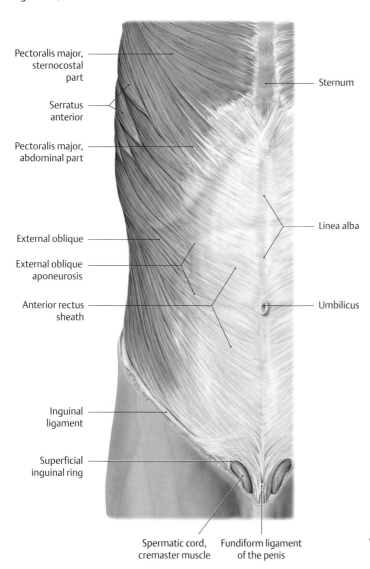

Pectoralis major, sternocostal part

Serratus anterior

Pectoralis major, abdominal part

External oblique

External oblique aponeurosis

Anterior rectus sheath

Inguinal ligament

Superficial inguinal ring

Spermatic cord, cremaster muscle

Fundiform ligament of the penis

Sternum

Linea alba

Umbilicus

A Superficial abdominal wall muscles.

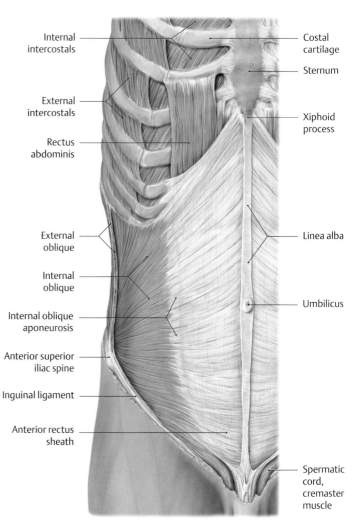

Internal intercostals

External intercostals

Rectus abdominis

External oblique

Internal oblique

Internal oblique aponeurosis

Anterior superior iliac spine

Inguinal ligament

Anterior rectus sheath

Costal cartilage

Sternum

Xiphoid process

Linea alba

Umbilicus

Spermatic cord, cremaster muscle

B *Removed:* External oblique, pectoralis major, and serratus anterior.

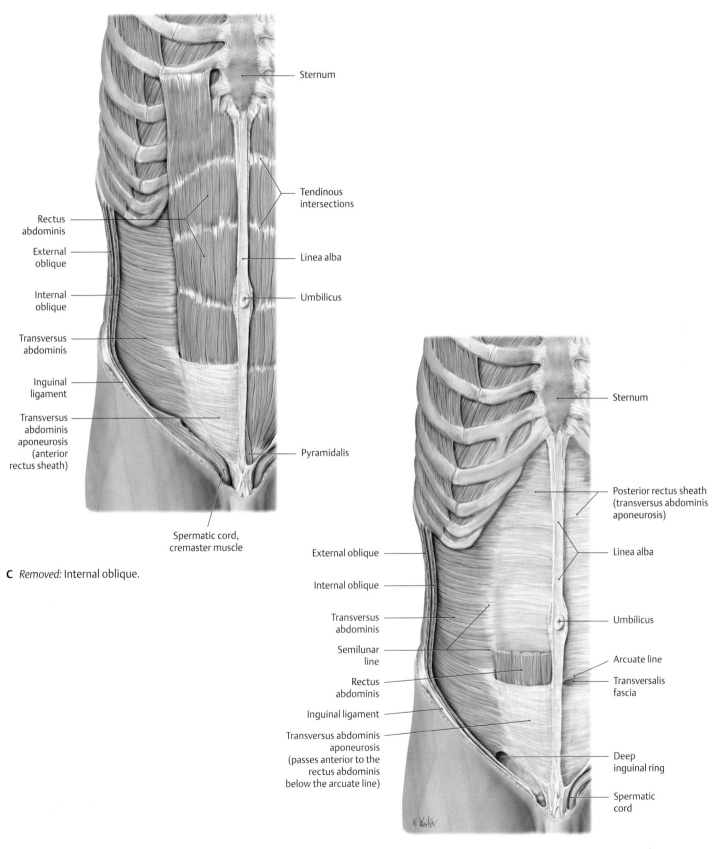

C *Removed:* Internal oblique.

Sternum

Tendinous
intersections

Rectus
abdominis

External
oblique

Internal
oblique

Linea alba

Transversus
abdominis

Umbilicus

Inguinal
ligament

Transversus
abdominis
aponeurosis
(anterior
rectus sheath)

Pyramidalis

Spermatic cord,
cremaster muscle

Sternum

Posterior rectus sheath
(transversus abdominis
aponeurosis)

External oblique

Internal oblique

Linea alba

Transversus
abdominis

Semilunar
line

Umbilicus

Rectus
abdominis

Arcuate line

Transversalis
fascia

Inguinal ligament

Transversus abdominis
aponeurosis
(passes anterior to the
rectus abdominis
below the arcuate line)

Deep
inguinal ring

Spermatic
cord

D *Removed:* Rectus abdominis.

Inguinal Region & Canal

 The inguinal region is the junction of the anterior abdominal wall and the anterior thigh. The inguinal canal is an important site for the passage of structures into and out of the abdominal cavity (e.g., components of the spermatic cord).

***Fig. 11.2* Inguinal region**
Right side, anterior view.

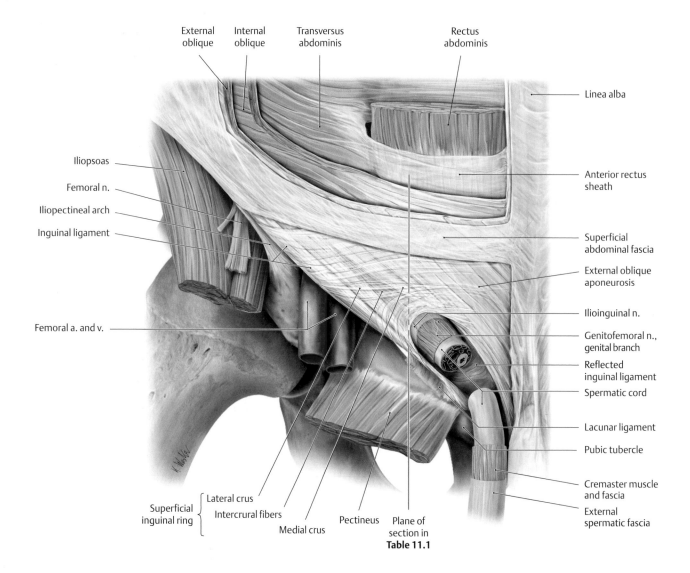

Table 11.1	Structures of the inguinal canal		
Structures			**Formed by**
Wall	Anterior wall	①	External oblique aponeurosis
	Roof	②	Internal oblique muscles
		③	Transversus abdominis
	Posterior wall	④	Transversalis fascia
		⑤	Parietal peritoneum
	Floor	⑥	Inguinal ligament (densely interwoven fibers of the lower external oblique aponeurosis and adjacent fascia lata of thigh)
Openings	Superficial inguinal ring		Opening in external oblique aponeurosis; bounded by medial and lateral crus, intercrural fibers, and reflected inguinal ligament
	Deep inguinal ring		Outpouching of the transversalis fascia lateral to the lateral umbilical fold (inferior epigastric vessels)
Sagittal section through plane in Fig. 11.2.			

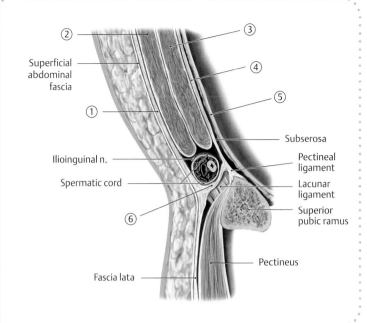

Fig. 11.3 Dissection of the inguinal region
Right side, anterior view.

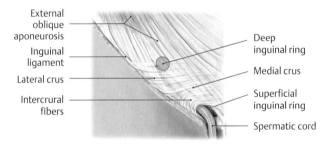

A Superficial layer.

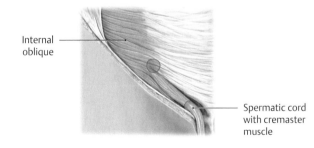

B *Removed:* External oblique aponeurosis.

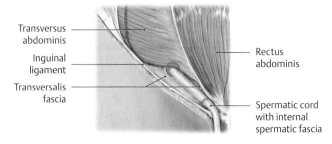

C *Removed:* Internal oblique.

Fig. 11.4 Opening of the inguinal canal
Right side, anterior view.

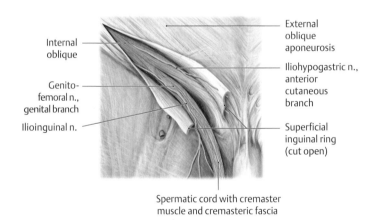

A *Divided:* External oblique aponeurosis.

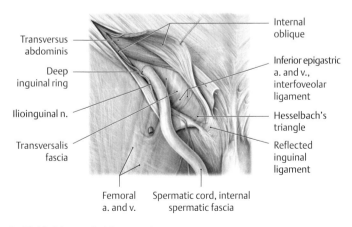

B *Divided:* Internal oblique and cremaster.

Abdominal Wall & Inguinal Hernias

 The rectus sheath is created by fusion of the aponeuroses of the transversus abdominis and abdominal oblique muscles. The inferior edge of the posterior rectus sheath is called the arcuate line.

Fig. 11.5 Abdominal wall and rectus sheath

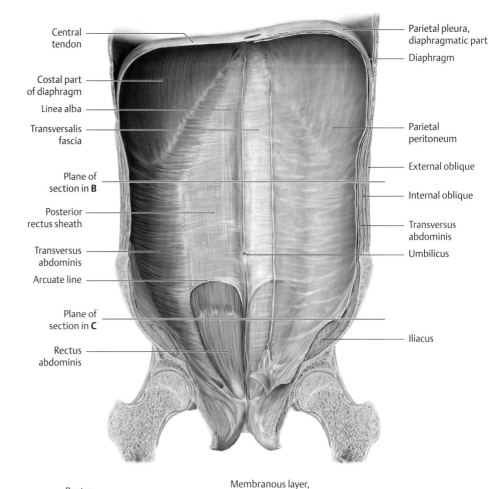

Central tendon

Costal part of diaphragm

Linea alba

Transversalis fascia

Plane of section in **B**

Posterior rectus sheath

Transversus abdominis

Arcuate line

Plane of section in **C**

Rectus abdominis

Parietal pleura, diaphragmatic part

Diaphragm

Parietal peritoneum

External oblique

Internal oblique

Transversus abdominis

Umbilicus

Iliacus

A Posterior (internal) view of the anterior abdominal wall.

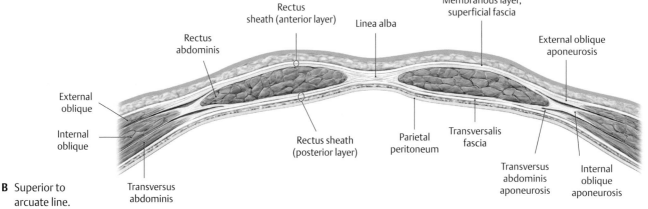

Rectus abdominis

Rectus sheath (anterior layer)

Linea alba

Membranous layer, superficial fascia

External oblique aponeurosis

External oblique

Internal oblique

Transversus abdominis

Rectus sheath (posterior layer)

Parietal peritoneum

Transversalis fascia

Transversus abdominis aponeurosis

Internal oblique aponeurosis

B Superior to arcuate line.

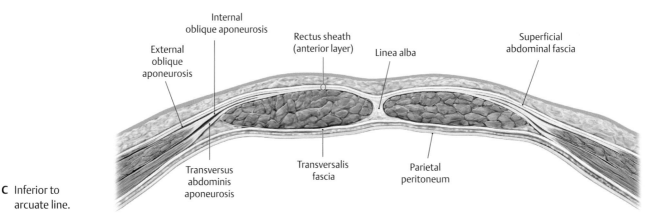

Internal oblique aponeurosis

External oblique aponeurosis

Rectus sheath (anterior layer)

Linea alba

Superficial abdominal fascia

Transversus abdominis aponeurosis

Transversalis fascia

Parietal peritoneum

C Inferior to arcuate line.

Fig. 11.6 Abdominal wall: Internal surface anatomy

Coronal section, posterior view. The three fossae of the anterior abdominal wall (*circled*) are sites of potential herniation.

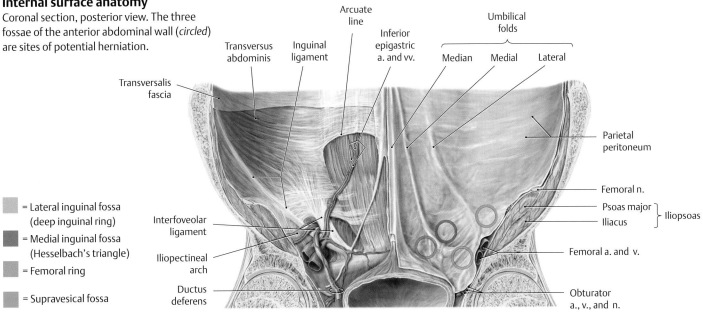

= Lateral inguinal fossa (deep inguinal ring)

= Medial inguinal fossa (Hesselbach's triangle)

= Femoral ring

= Supravesical fossa

Clinical

Inguinal and femoral hernias

Indirect inguinal hernias occur in younger males and may be congenital or acquired; direct inguinal hernias are always acquired. Femoral hernias are acquired and more common in females.

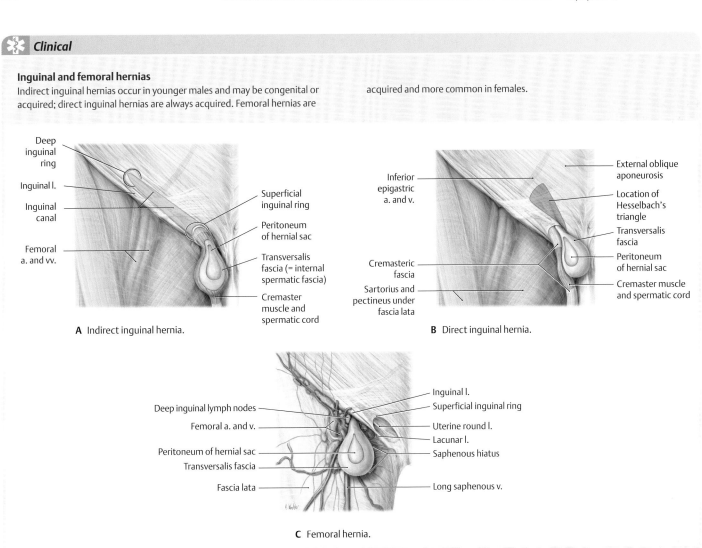

A Indirect inguinal hernia.

B Direct inguinal hernia.

C Femoral hernia.

Perineal Region

***Fig. 11.7* Perineum and pelvic floor: Female**
Lithotomy position, caudal (inferior) view. See p. 192
for the external genitalia.

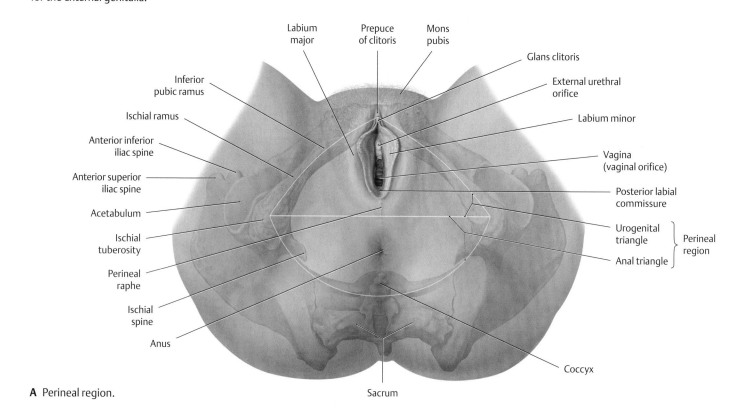

A Perineal region.

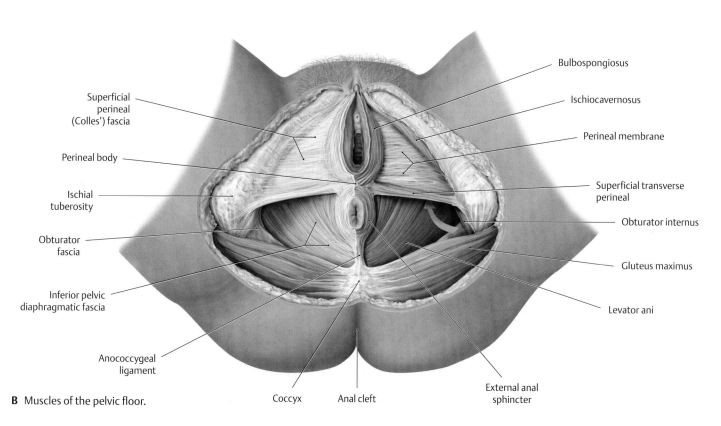

B Muscles of the pelvic floor.

The bilateral boundaries of the perineum in both sexes are the pubic symphysis, ischiopubic ramus, ischial tuberosity, sacro- tuberous ligament, and the coccyx. The green arrows indicate the anterior recess of the ischioanal fossa, superior to the urogenital muscles.

Fig. 11.8 **Perineum and pelvic floor: Male**
Lithotomy position, caudal (inferior) view. See p. 196 for the genitalia.

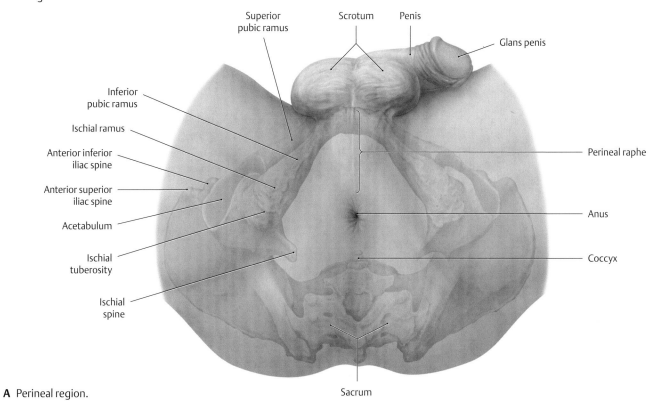

Superior pubic ramus — Scrotum — Penis — Glans penis — Inferior pubic ramus — Ischial ramus — Anterior inferior iliac spine — Anterior superior iliac spine — Acetabulum — Ischial tuberosity — Ischial spine — Perineal raphe — Anus — Coccyx — Sacrum

A Perineal region.

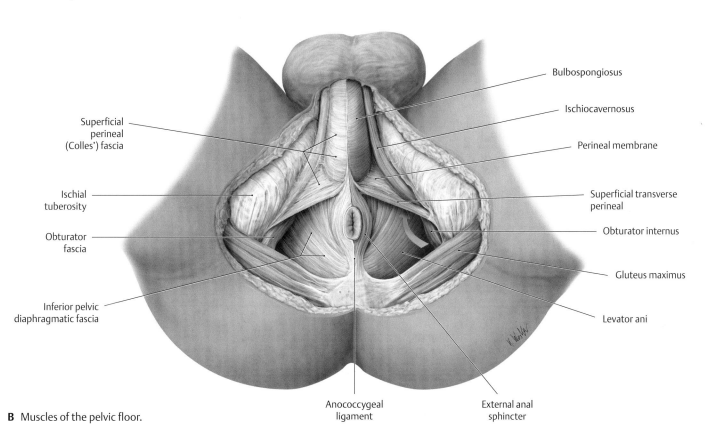

Bulbospongiosus — Ischiocavernosus — Perineal membrane — Superficial transverse perineal — Obturator internus — Gluteus maximus — Levator ani — Superficial perineal (Colles') fascia — Ischial tuberosity — Obturator fascia — Inferior pelvic diaphragmatic fascia — Anococcygeal ligament — External anal sphincter

B Muscles of the pelvic floor.

Abdominal Wall Muscle Facts

Fig. 11.9 Anterior muscles
Anterior view.

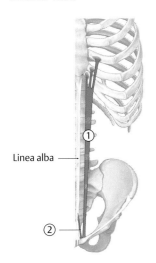

Linea alba —

Fig. 11.10 Anterolateral muscles
Anterior view.

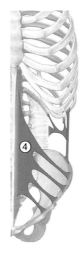

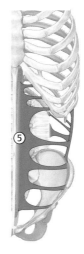

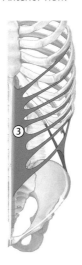

A External oblique.

B Internal oblique.

C Transversus abdominis.

Fig. 11.11 Posterior muscles
Anterior view. The psoas major and iliacus are together known as the iliopsoas.

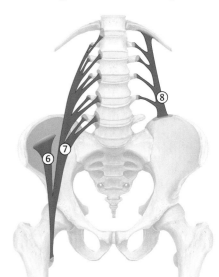

Table 11.2	Abdominal wall muscles				
Muscle	**Origin**	**Insertion**	**Innervation**	**Action**
Anterior abdominal wall muscles				
① Rectus abdominis	Pubis (between pubic tubercle and symphysis)	Cartilages of 5th to 7th ribs, xiphoid process of sternum	Intercostal nn. (T5–T12)	Flexes trunk, compresses abdomen, stabilizes pelvis
② Pyramidalis	Pubis (anterior to rectus abdominis)	Linea alba (runs within the rectus sheath)	Subcostal n. (12th intercostal n.)	Tenses linea alba
Anterolateral abdominal wall muscles				
③ External oblique	5th to 12th ribs (outer surface)	Linea alba, pubic tubercle, anterior iliac crest	Intercostal nn. (T7–T12)	*Unilateral:* Bends trunk to same side, rotates trunk to opposite side
④ Internal oblique	Thoracolumbar fascia (deep layer), iliac crest (intermediate line), anterior superior iliac spine, iliopsoas fascia	10th to 12th ribs (lower borders), linea alba (anterior and posterior layers)	Intercostal nn. (T7–T12), iliohypogastric n., ilioinguinal n.	*Bilateral:* Flexes trunk, compresses abdomen, stabilizes pelvis
⑤ Transversus abdominis	7th to 12th costal cartilages (inner surfaces), thoracolumbar fascia (deep layer), iliac crest, anterior superior iliac spine (inner lip), iliopsoas fascia	Linea alba, pubic crest		*Unilateral:* Rotates trunk to same side *Bilateral:* Compresses abdomen
Posterior abdominal wall muscles				
⑥ Psoas major — Superficial layer	T12–L4 vertebral bodies and associated intervertebral disks (lateral surfaces)	Femur (lesser trochanter), joint insertion as iliopsoas muscle	Direct branches from lumbar plexus (L2–L4)	Hip joint: Flexion and external rotation Lumbar spine (with femur fixed): *Unilateral:* Contraction bends trunk laterally
⑥ Psoas major — Deep layer	L1–L5 (costal processes)			
⑦ Iliacus	Iliac fossa		Femoral n. (L2–L4)	*Bilateral:* Contraction raises trunk from supine position
⑧ Quadratus lumborum	Iliac crest and iliolumbar ligament (not shown)	12th rib, L1–L4 vertebrae (transverse processes)	T12, L1–L4 spinal nn.	*Unilateral:* Bends trunk to same side *Bilateral:* Bearing down and expiration, stabilizes 12th rib

Fig. 11.12 Anterior and posterior abdominal wall muscles
Anterior view.

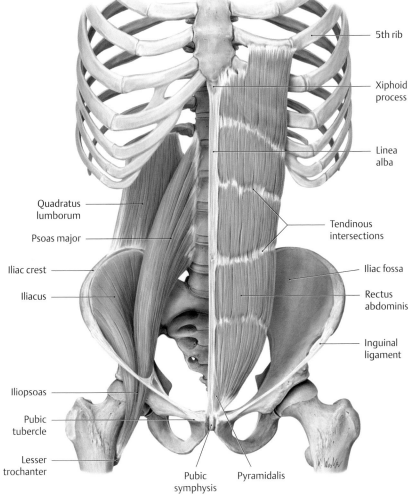

5th rib

Xiphoid process

Linea alba

Tendinous intersections

Quadratus lumborum

Psoas major

Iliac crest

Iliacus

Iliac fossa

Rectus abdominis

Inguinal ligament

Iliopsoas

Pubic tubercle

Lesser trochanter

Pubic symphysis

Pyramidalis

A Anterior and posterior muscles.

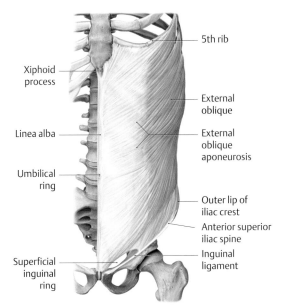

Xiphoid process

5th rib

Linea alba

External oblique

External oblique aponeurosis

Umbilical ring

Outer lip of iliac crest

Anterior superior iliac spine

Superficial inguinal ring

Inguinal ligament

B External oblique.

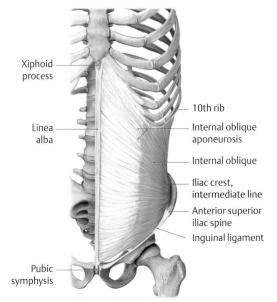

Xiphoid process

10th rib

Internal oblique aponeurosis

Linea alba

Internal oblique

Iliac crest, intermediate line

Anterior superior iliac spine

Inguinal ligament

Pubic symphysis

C Internal oblique.

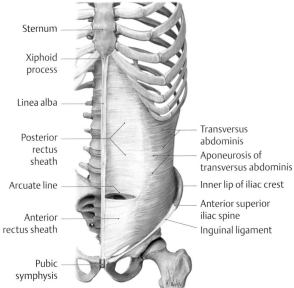

Sternum

Xiphoid process

Linea alba

Transversus abdominis

Posterior rectus sheath

Aponeurosis of transversus abdominis

Inner lip of iliac crest

Arcuate line

Anterior superior iliac spine

Anterior rectus sheath

Inguinal ligament

Pubic symphysis

D Transversus abdominis.

139

Pelvic Floor Muscle Facts

Fig. 11.13 Muscles of the pelvic floor
Superior view.

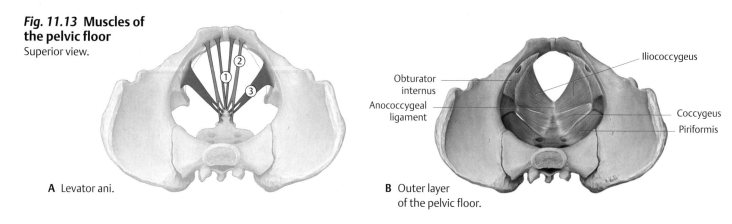

A Levator ani.

B Outer layer of the pelvic floor.

Table 11.3		Muscles of the pelvic floor			
Muscle		**Origin**	**Insertion**	**Innervation**	**Action**
Muscles of the pelvic diaphragm					
Levator ani	① Puborectalis	Superior pubic ramus (both sides of pubic symphysis)	Anococcygeal ligament	Direct branches of sacral plexus (S4), inferior anal n.	Pelvic diaphragm: Supports pelvic viscera
	② Pubococcygeus	Pubis (lateral to origin of puborectalis)	Anococcygeal ligament, coccyx		
	③ Iliococcygeus	Internal obturator fascia of levator ani (tendinous arch)			
Coccygeus		Sacrum (inferior end)	Ischial spine	Direct branches from sacral plexus (S4–S5)	Supports pelvic viscera, flexes coccyx
Muscles of the pelvic wall (parietal muscles)					
Piriformis*		Sacrum (pelvic surface)	Femur (apex of greater trochanter)	Direct branches from sacral plexus (S1–S2)	Hip joint: External rotation, stabilization, and abduction of flexed hip
Obturator internus*		Obturator membrane and bony boundaries (inner surface)	Femur (greater trochanter, medial surface)	Direct branches from sacral plexus (L5–S1)	Hip joint: External rotation and abduction of flexed hip
Sphincter and erector muscles					
④ External anal sphincter		Encircles anus (runs posteriorly from perineal body to anococcygeal ligament)		Pudendal n. (S2–S4)	Closes anus
⑤ External urethral sphincter		Encircles urethra (division of deep transverse perineal muscle)			Closes urethra
⑥ Bulbospongiosus		Runs anteriorly from perineal body to clitoris (females) or penile raphe (males)			Females: Compresses greater vestibular gland Males: Assists in erection
⑦ Ischiocavernosus		Ischial ramus	Crus of clitoris or penis		Maintains erection by squeezing blood into corpus cavernosum of clitoris or penis

*The piriformis and obturator internus are considered muscles of the hip (see p. 374).
The female and male external genitalia are shown on pp. 194, 203.

Fig. 11.14 Sphincter and erector muscles of the pelvic floor
Inferior view. See pp. 194, 203.

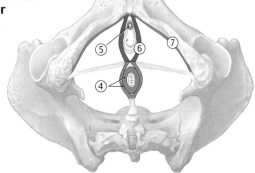

Fig. 11.15 Pelvic floor

Female pelvis.

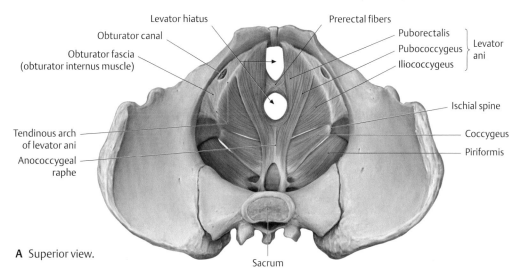

Levator hiatus

Obturator canal

Obturator fascia
(obturator internus muscle)

Prerectal fibers

Puborectalis ⎱
Pubococcygeus ⎰ Levator
Iliococcygeus ⎰ ani

Ischial spine

Tendinous arch
of levator ani

Coccygeus

Anococcygeal
raphe

Piriformis

Sacrum

A Superior view.

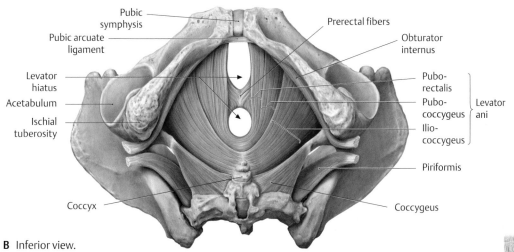

Pubic
symphysis

Pubic arcuate
ligament

Levator
hiatus

Acetabulum

Ischial
tuberosity

Coccyx

Prerectal fibers

Obturator
internus

Pubo-
rectalis

Pubo-
coccygeus

Ilio-
coccygeus

Levator
ani

Piriformis

Coccygeus

B Inferior view.

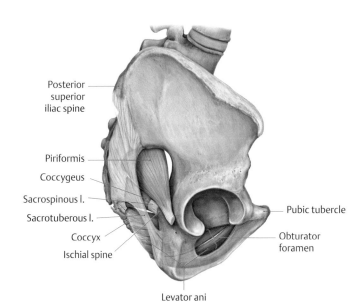

Posterior
superior
iliac spine

Piriformis

Coccygeus

Sacrospinous l.

Sacrotuberous l.

Coccyx

Ischial spine

Pubic tubercle

Obturator
foramen

Levator ani

D Right lateral view.

Anterior sacroiliac ll.

Arcuate line

Obturator
internus fascia

Tendinous arch
of levator ani

Pubic symphysis

Deep transverse
perineal

Piriformis

Coccygeus

Ischial spine

Anococcygeal l.

Iliococcygeus ⎱
Pubococcygeus ⎰ Levator
Puborectalis ⎰ ani

C Medial view of right hemipelvis.

Divisions of the Abdominopelvic Cavity

Fig. 12.1 **Organ layers and quadrants**

Anterior view. The organs of the abdomen and pelvis can be classified by layer, by quadrant (using the umbilicus at L4), by level (upper and lower abdomen, and pelvis), or with respect to the presence of a mesentery (Table 12.1).

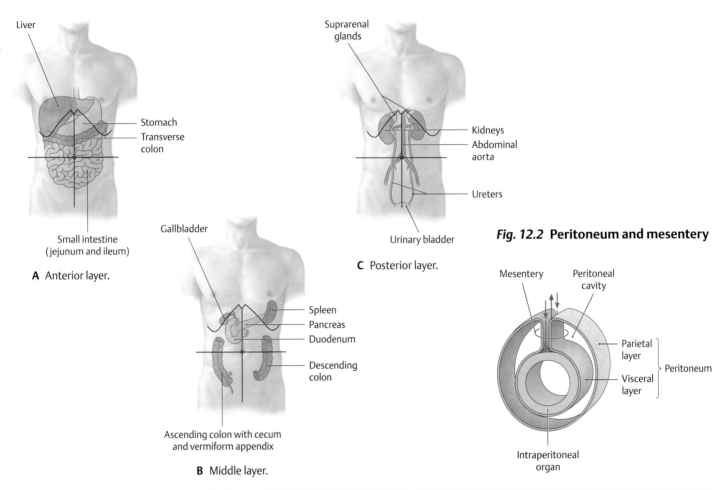

Liver

Stomach
Transverse colon

Small intestine (jejunum and ileum)

A Anterior layer.

Gallbladder

Spleen
Pancreas
Duodenum

Descending colon

Ascending colon with cecum and vermiform appendix

B Middle layer.

Suprarenal glands

Kidneys
Abdominal aorta

Ureters

Urinary bladder

C Posterior layer.

Fig. 12.2 **Peritoneum and mesentery**

Mesentery
Peritoneal cavity

Parietal layer
Visceral layer
Peritoneum

Intraperitoneal organ

Table 12.1	Organs of the abdomen and pelvis		
Location	**Organs**		
Intraperitoneal organs: These organs have a mesentery and are completely covered by the peritoneum.			
Abdominal peritoneal cavity	• Stomach • Small intestine (jejunum, ileum, some of the superior part of the duodenum) • Spleen • Liver	• Gallbladder • Cecum with vermiform appendix (portions of variable size may be retroperitoneal) • Large intestine (transverse and sigmoid colons)	
Pelvic peritoneal cavity	• Uterus (fundus and body)	• Ovaries	• Uterine tubes
Extraperitoneal organs: These organs either have no mesentery or lost it during development.			
Retroperitoneal	Primarily	• Kidneys	• Suprarenal glands	• Uterine cervix
	Secondarily	• Duodenum (descending, horizontal, and ascending) • Pancreas	• Ascending and descending colon • Rectum (upper 2/3)	
Infraperitoneal/subperitoneal		• Urinary bladder • Distal ureters • Prostate	• Seminal vesicle • Uterine cervix	• Vagina • Rectum (lower 1/3)

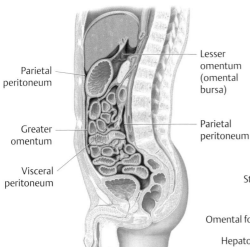

Parietal peritoneum

Lesser omentum (omental bursa)

Greater omentum

Parietal peritoneum

Visceral peritoneum

A Peritoneal cavity. The peritoneum is shown in red.

Fig. 12.3 **Peritoneal relationships**
Midsagittal section through male pelvis, viewed from the left side.

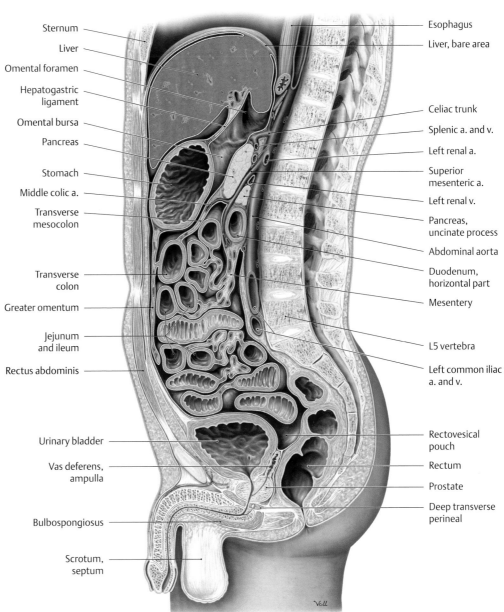

Sternum

Liver

Omental foramen

Hepatogastric ligament

Omental bursa

Pancreas

Stomach

Middle colic a.

Transverse mesocolon

Transverse colon

Greater omentum

Jejunum and ileum

Rectus abdominis

Urinary bladder

Vas deferens, ampulla

Bulbospongiosus

Scrotum, septum

Esophagus

Liver, bare area

Celiac trunk

Splenic a. and v.

Left renal a.

Superior mesenteric a.

Left renal v.

Pancreas, uncinate process

Abdominal aorta

Duodenum, horizontal part

Mesentery

L5 vertebra

Left common iliac a. and v.

Rectovesical pouch

Rectum

Prostate

Deep transverse perineal

B Organs of the abdomen and pelvis.

 Clinical

Acute abdominal pain

Acute abdominal pain ("acute abdomen") may be so severe that the abdominal wall becomes extremely sensitive to touch ("guarding") and the intestines stop functioning. Causes include organ inflammation such as appendicitis, perforation due to a gastric ulcer (see p. 159), or organ blockage by a stone, tumor, etc. In women, gynecological processes or ectopic pregnancies may produce severe abdominal pain.

Peritoneal Cavity & Greater Sac

 The largest part of the peritoneal cavity is the greater sac. The greater omentum is an apron-like fold of peritoneum suspended from the greater curvature of the stomach and covering the anterior surface of the transverse colon. The transverse colon divides the peritoneal cavity into a supracolic compartment (liver, gallbladder, and stomach) and an infracolic compartment (intestines).

***Fig. 12.4* Dissection of the peritoneal cavity**
Anterior view.

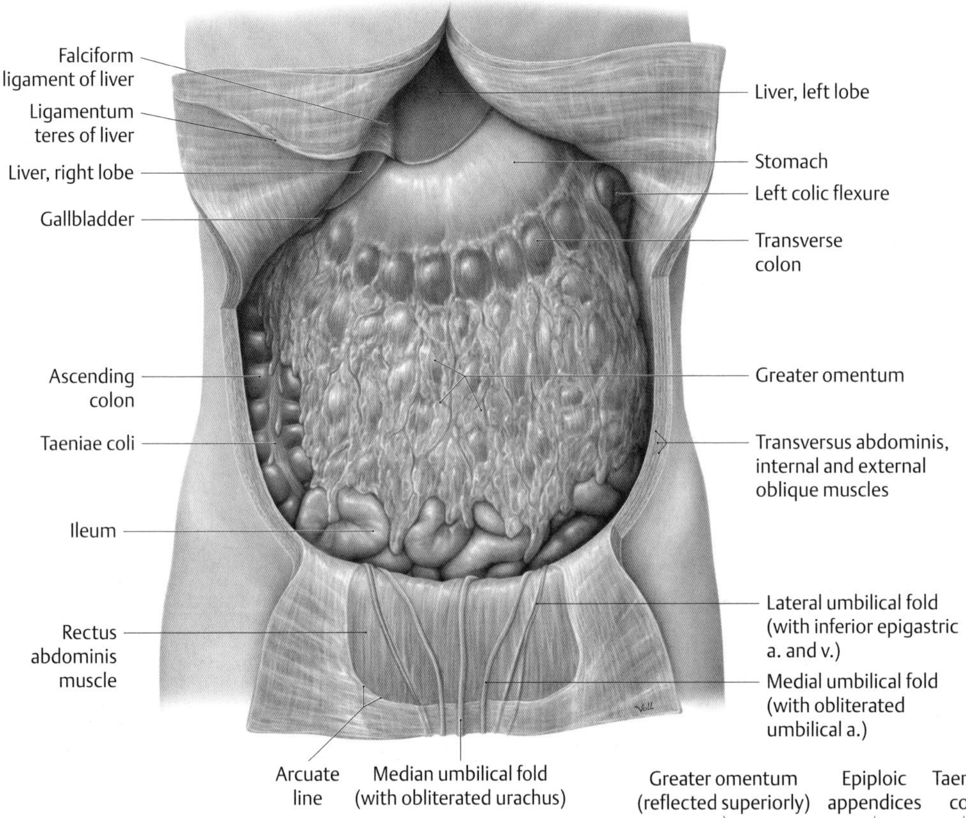

Falciform ligament of liver
Ligamentum teres of liver
Liver, right lobe
Gallbladder
Ascending colon
Taeniae coli
Ileum
Rectus abdominis muscle
Arcuate line
Median umbilical fold (with obliterated urachus)

Liver, left lobe
Stomach
Left colic flexure
Transverse colon
Greater omentum
Transversus abdominis, internal and external oblique muscles
Lateral umbilical fold (with inferior epigastric a. and v.)
Medial umbilical fold (with obliterated umbilical a.)

A Greater sac. *Retracted:* Abdominal wall.

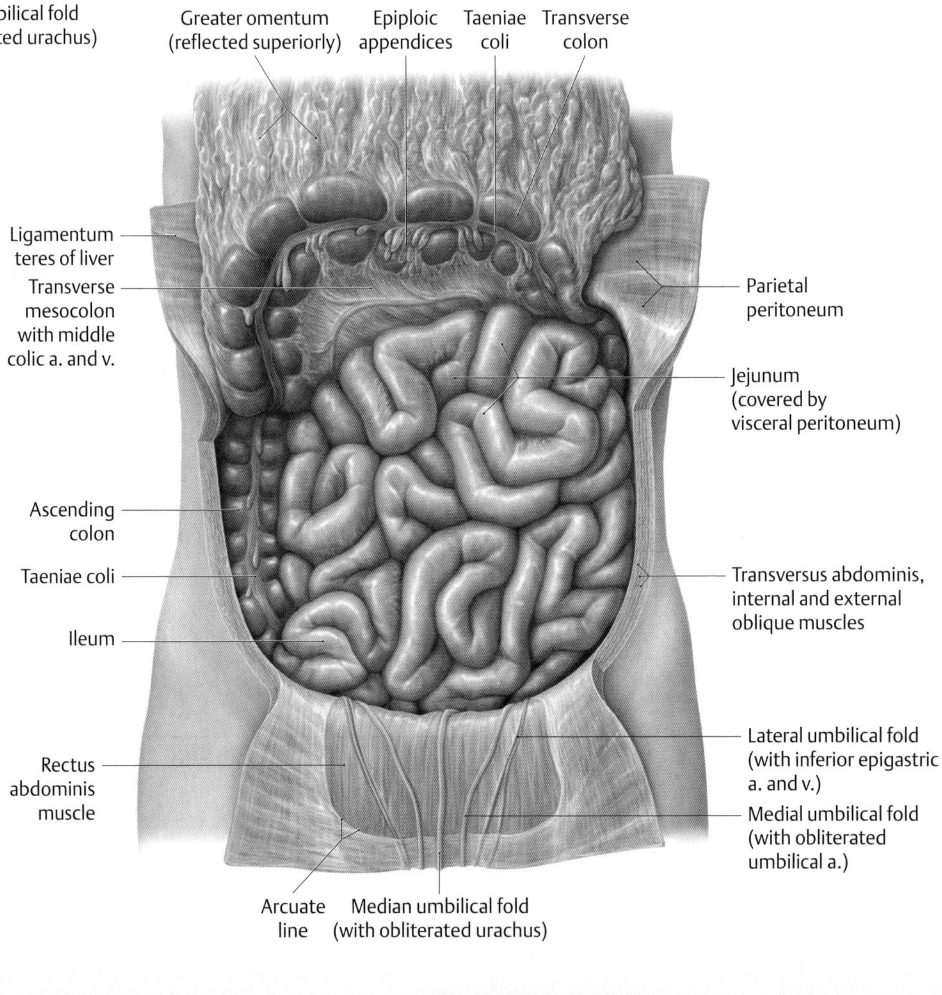

Greater omentum (reflected superiorly)
Epiploic appendices
Taeniae coli
Transverse colon

Ligamentum teres of liver
Transverse mesocolon with middle colic a. and v.
Ascending colon
Taeniae coli
Ileum
Rectus abdominis muscle

Parietal peritoneum
Jejunum (covered by visceral peritoneum)
Transversus abdominis, internal and external oblique muscles
Lateral umbilical fold (with inferior epigastric a. and v.)
Medial umbilical fold (with obliterated umbilical a.)

Arcuate line
Median umbilical fold (with obliterated urachus)

B Infracolic compartment. *Reflected:* Greater omentum and transverse colon.

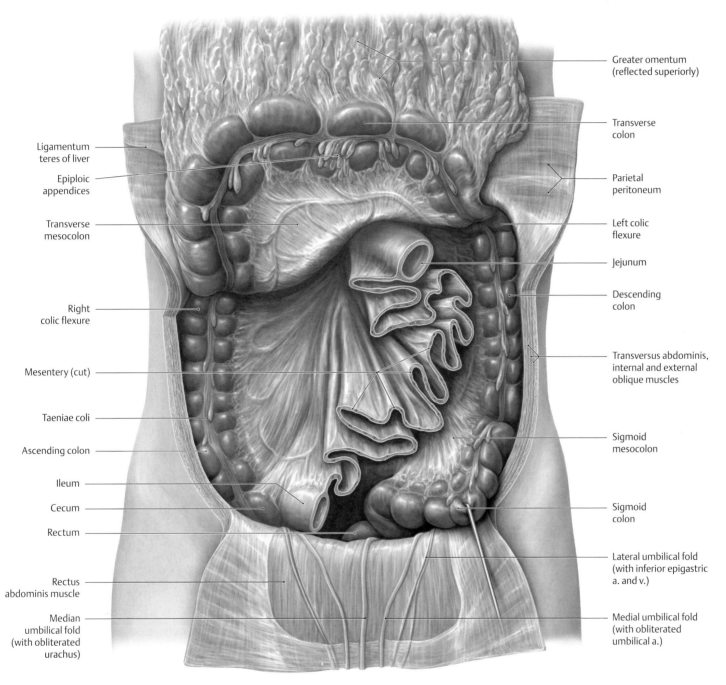

Greater omentum
(reflected superiorly)

Transverse
colon

Ligamentum
teres of liver

Epiploic
appendices

Parietal
peritoneum

Transverse
mesocolon

Left colic
flexure

Jejunum

Right
colic flexure

Descending
colon

Transversus abdominis,
internal and external
oblique muscles

Mesentery (cut)

Taeniae coli

Ascending colon

Sigmoid
mesocolon

Ileum

Cecum

Sigmoid
colon

Rectum

Rectus
abdominis muscle

Lateral umbilical fold
(with inferior epigastric
a. and v.)

Median
umbilical fold
(with obliterated
urachus)

Medial umbilical fold
(with obliterated
umbilical a.)

C Mesenteries. *Reflected:* Greater omentum and transverse
colon. *Removed:* Intraperitoneal small intestines.

Lesser Sac

Fig. 12.5 Lesser sac (Omental bursa)

Anterior view. The lesser sac (omental bursa) is the portion of the peritoneal cavity located behind the lesser omentum and stomach.

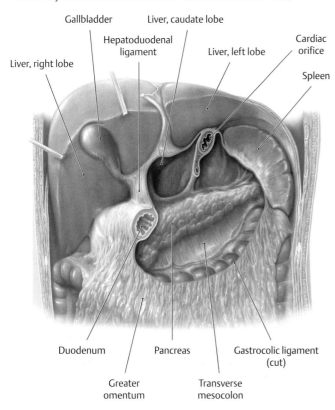

A Boundaries of the lesser sac (omental bursa).

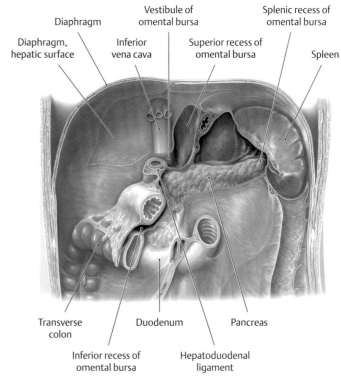

B Posterior wall of the lesser sac (omental bursa).

Fig. 12.6 Location of the lesser sac

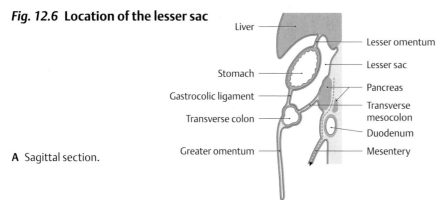

A Sagittal section.

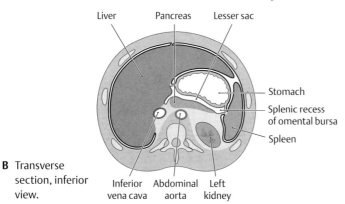

B Transverse section, inferior view.

Table 12.2	Boundaries of the lesser sac (omental bursa)	
Direction	**Boundary**	**Recess**
Anterior	Lesser omentum, gastrocolic ligament	—
Inferior	Transverse mesocolon	Inferior recess
Superior	Liver (with caudate lobe)	Superior recess
Posterior	Pancreas, aorta (abdominal part), celiac trunk, splenic a. and v., gastrosplenic fold, left suprarenal gland, left kidney (superior pole)	—
Right	Liver, duodenal bulb	—
Left	Spleen, gastrosplenic ligament	Splenic recess

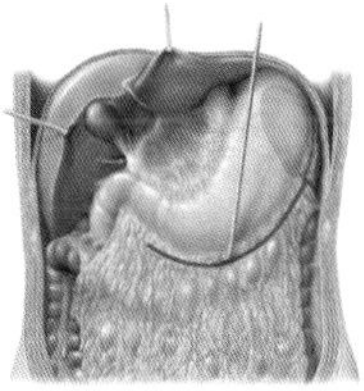

Fig. 12.7 Omental bursa in situ

Anterior view. *Divided:* Gastrocolic ligament. *Retracted:* Liver.
Reflected: Stomach.

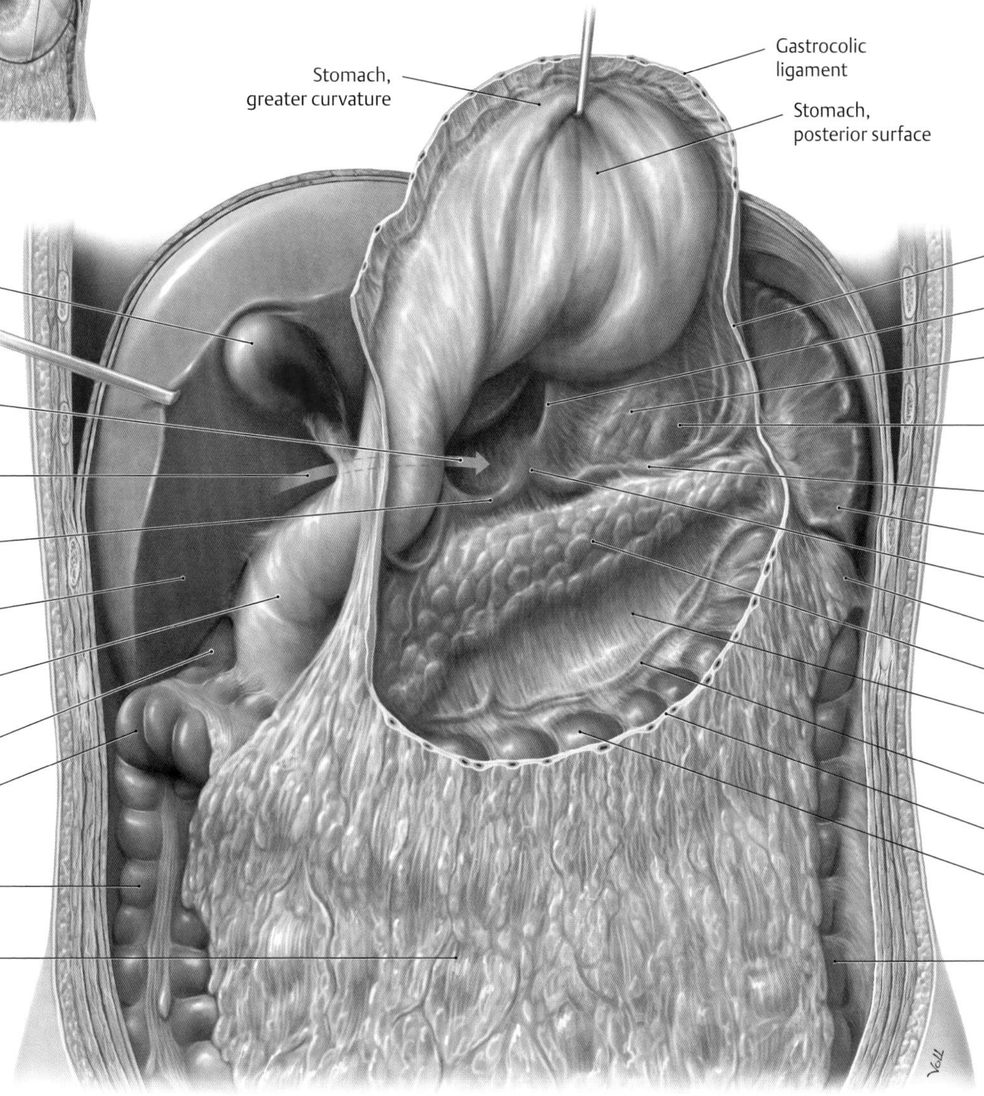

Stomach, greater curvature

Gastrocolic ligament

Stomach, posterior surface

Gallbladder

Vestibule of omental bursa

Omental foramen

Common hepatic a.

Liver, right lobe

Duodenum, descending part

Right kidney

Right colic flexure

Ascending colon

Greater omentum

Gastrosplenic ligament

Left gastric a.

Left suprarenal gland

Left kidney, superior pole

Splenic a.

Spleen

Celiac trunk

Phrenicocolic ligament

Pancreas

Transverse mesocolon

Middle colic a. and v.

Gastrocolic ligament

Transverse colon

Descending colon

Table 12.3	**Boundaries of the omental foramen**

The communication between the greater and lesser sacs is the omental (epiploic) foramen (see arrow in Fig. 12.7).

Direction	Boundary
Anterior	Hepatoduodenal ligament with the portal v., proper hepatic a., and bile duct
Inferior	Duodenum (superior part)
Posterior	Inferior vena cava, diaphragm (right crus)
Superior	Liver (caudate lobe)

Mesenteries & Posterior Wall

Fig. 12.8 Mesenteries and organs of the peritoneal cavity
Anterior view. *Removed:* Stomach, jejunum, and ileum. *Reflected:* Liver.

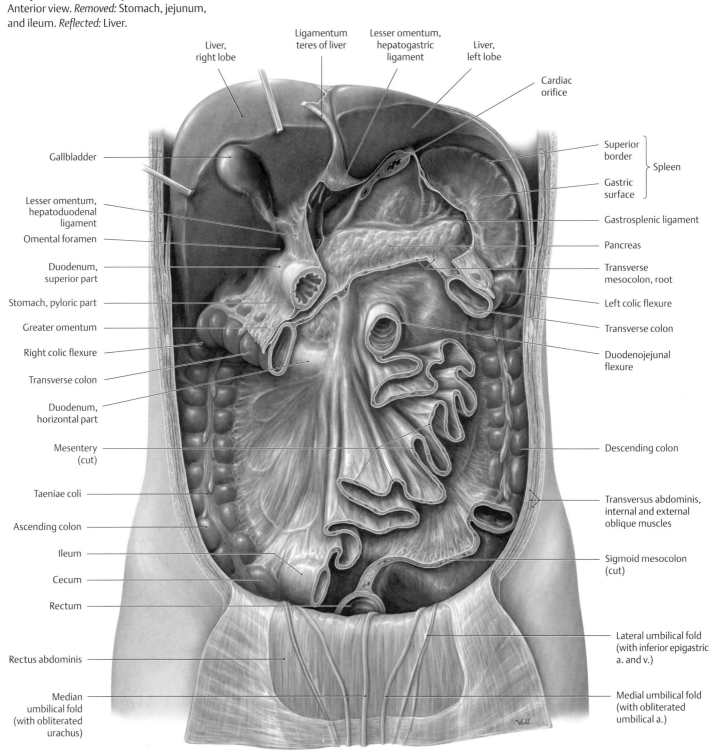

Liver, right lobe
Ligamentum teres of liver
Lesser omentum, hepatogastric ligament
Liver, left lobe
Cardiac orifice
Gallbladder
Superior border
Spleen
Gastric surface
Lesser omentum, hepatoduodenal ligament
Gastrosplenic ligament
Omental foramen
Pancreas
Duodenum, superior part
Transverse mesocolon, root
Stomach, pyloric part
Left colic flexure
Greater omentum
Transverse colon
Right colic flexure
Duodenojejunal flexure
Transverse colon
Duodenum, horizontal part
Mesentery (cut)
Descending colon
Taeniae coli
Transversus abdominis, internal and external oblique muscles
Ascending colon
Ileum
Sigmoid mesocolon (cut)
Cecum
Rectum
Lateral umbilical fold (with inferior epigastric a. and v.)
Rectus abdominis
Medial umbilical fold (with obliterated umbilical a.)
Median umbilical fold (with obliterated urachus)

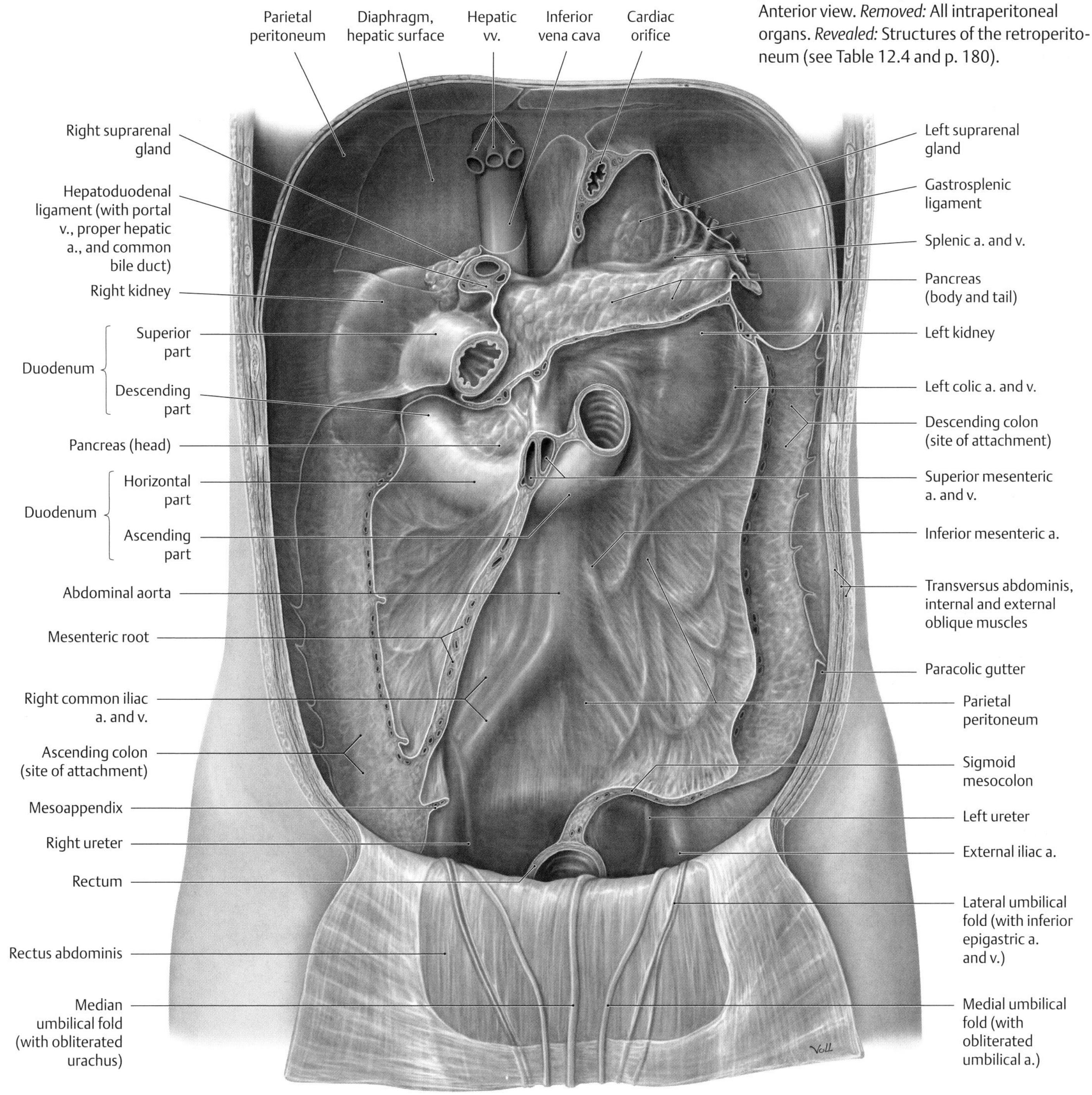
Parietal peritoneum
Diaphragm, hepatic surface
Hepatic vv.
Inferior vena cava
Cardiac orifice
Right suprarenal gland
Hepatoduodenal ligament (with portal v., proper hepatic a., and common bile duct)
Right kidney
Duodenum
Superior part
Descending part
Pancreas (head)
Duodenum
Horizontal part
Ascending part
Abdominal aorta
Mesenteric root
Right common iliac a. and v.
Ascending colon (site of attachment)
Mesoappendix
Right ureter
Rectum
Rectus abdominis
Median umbilical fold (with obliterated urachus)
Left suprarenal gland
Gastrosplenic ligament
Splenic a. and v.
Pancreas (body and tail)
Left kidney
Left colic a. and v.
Descending colon (site of attachment)
Superior mesenteric a. and v.
Inferior mesenteric a.
Transversus abdominis, internal and external oblique muscles
Paracolic gutter
Parietal peritoneum
Sigmoid mesocolon
Left ureter
External iliac a.
Lateral umbilical fold (with inferior epigastric a. and v.)
Medial umbilical fold (with obliterated umbilical a.)

Fig. 12.9 **Posterior wall of the peritoneal cavity**
Anterior view. *Removed:* All intraperitoneal organs. *Revealed:* Structures of the retroperitoneum (see Table 12.4 and p. 180).

Table 12.4 **Structures of the retroperitoneum**

See pp. 216, 228, 239 for neurovascular structures of the retroperitoneum.

Classification	Organs	Vessels	Nerves
Primarily retroperitoneal (Retroperitoneal when formed)	• Kidneys • Suprarenal glands • Ureters	• Aorta (abdominal part) • Inferior vena cava and tributaries • Ascending lumbar vv. • Portal v. and tributaries • Lumbar, sacral, and iliac lymph nodes • Lumbar trunks and cisterna chyli	• Lumbar plexus branches ∘ Iliohypogastric n. ∘ Ilioinguinal n. ∘ Genitofemoral n. ∘ Lateral femoral cutaneous n. ∘ Femoral n. ∘ Obturator n. • Sympathetic trunk • Autonomic ganglia and plexuses
Secondarily retroperitoneal (Mesentery lost during development)	• Pancreas • Duodenum (descending and horizontal parts; some of ascending part) • Ascending and descending colon • Cecum (portions; variable) • Rectum (upper 2/3)		

Contents of the Pelvis

Fig. 12.10 **Male pelvis**

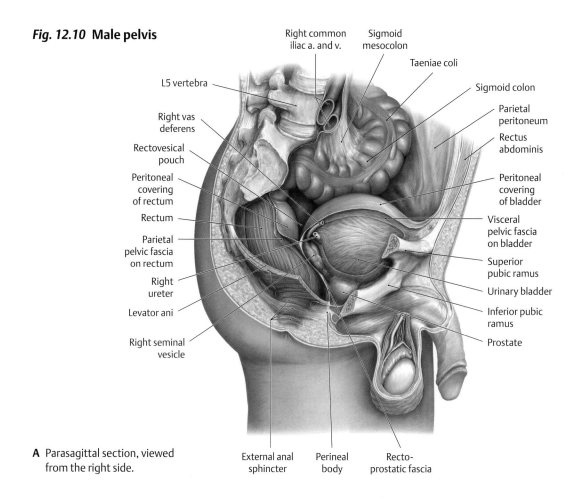

A Parasagittal section, viewed from the right side.

Labels (clockwise): Right common iliac a. and v. — Sigmoid mesocolon — Taeniae coli — Sigmoid colon — Parietal peritoneum — Rectus abdominis — Peritoneal covering of bladder — Visceral pelvic fascia on bladder — Superior pubic ramus — Urinary bladder — Inferior pubic ramus — Prostate — Recto-prostatic fascia — Perineal body — External anal sphincter — Right seminal vesicle — Levator ani — Right ureter — Parietal pelvic fascia on rectum — Rectum — Peritoneal covering of rectum — Rectovesical pouch — Right vas deferens — L5 vertebra

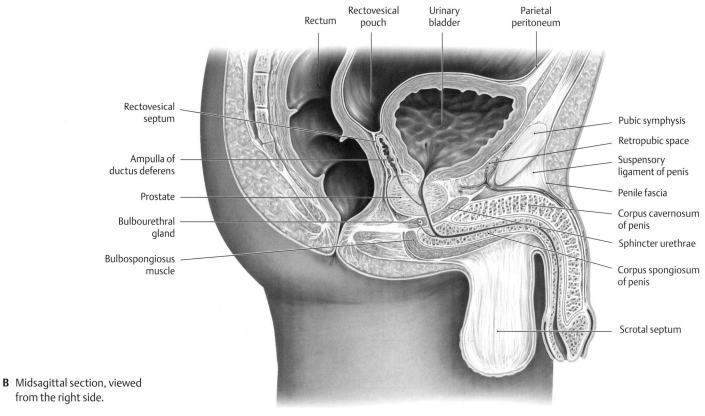

B Midsagittal section, viewed from the right side.

Labels: Rectum — Rectovesical pouch — Urinary bladder — Parietal peritoneum — Rectovesical septum — Ampulla of ductus deferens — Prostate — Bulbourethral gland — Bulbospongiosus muscle — Pubic symphysis — Retropubic space — Suspensory ligament of penis — Penile fascia — Corpus cavernosum of penis — Sphincter urethrae — Corpus spongiosum of penis — Scrotal septum

150

Fig. 12.11 Female pelvis

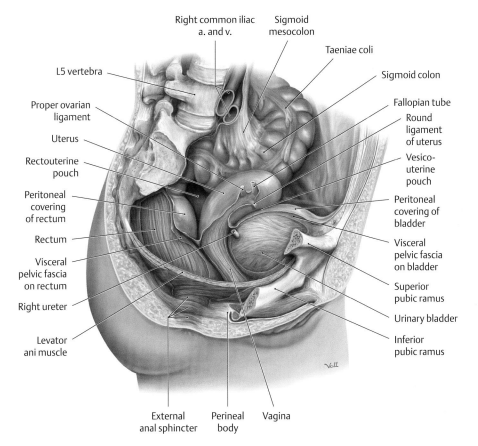

Right common iliac a. and v.

Sigmoid mesocolon

Taeniae coli

Sigmoid colon

Fallopian tube

Round ligament of uterus

Vesico-uterine pouch

Peritoneal covering of bladder

Visceral pelvic fascia on bladder

Superior pubic ramus

Urinary bladder

Inferior pubic ramus

L5 vertebra

Proper ovarian ligament

Uterus

Rectouterine pouch

Peritoneal covering of rectum

Rectum

Visceral pelvic fascia on rectum

Right ureter

Levator ani muscle

External anal sphincter

Perineal body

Vagina

A Parasagittal section, viewed from the right side.

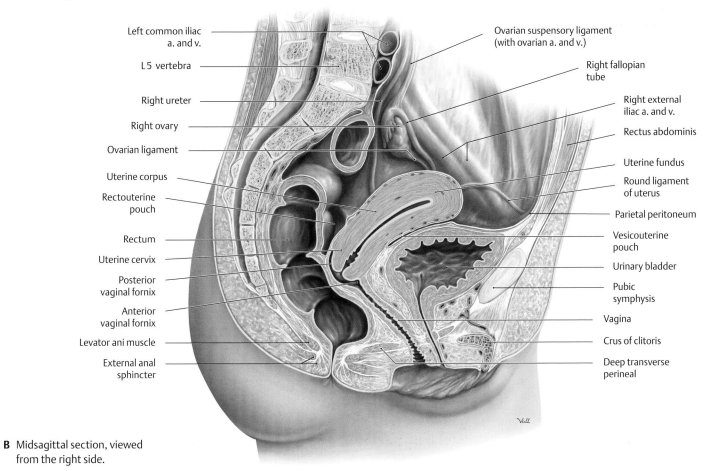

Left common iliac a. and v.

L5 vertebra

Right ureter

Right ovary

Ovarian ligament

Uterine corpus

Rectouterine pouch

Rectum

Uterine cervix

Posterior vaginal fornix

Anterior vaginal fornix

Levator ani muscle

External anal sphincter

Ovarian suspensory ligament (with ovarian a. and v.)

Right fallopian tube

Right external iliac a. and v.

Rectus abdominis

Uterine fundus

Round ligament of uterus

Parietal peritoneum

Vesicouterine pouch

Urinary bladder

Pubic symphysis

Vagina

Crus of clitoris

Deep transverse perineal

B Midsagittal section, viewed from the right side.

Peritoneal Relationships

Fig. 12.12 **Peritoneal relationships in the pelvis: Female**

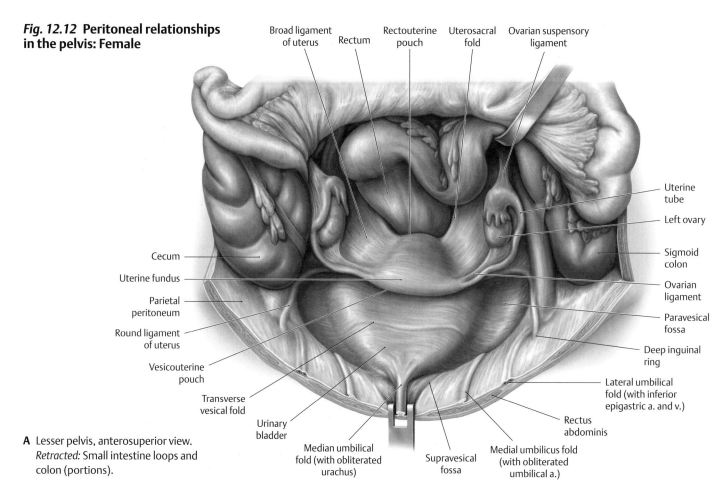

A Lesser pelvis, anterosuperior view. *Retracted:* Small intestine loops and colon (portions).

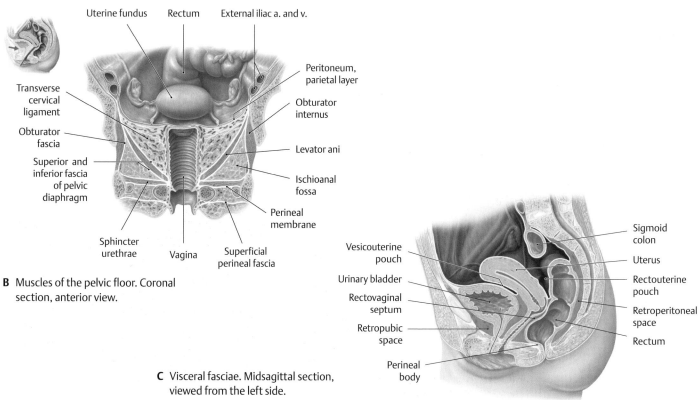

B Muscles of the pelvic floor. Coronal section, anterior view.

C Visceral fasciae. Midsagittal section, viewed from the left side.

Fig. 12.13 Peritoneal relationships in the pelvis: Male

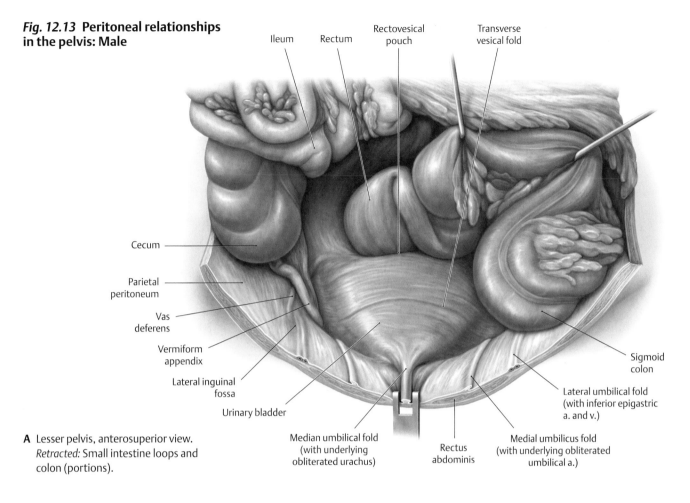

Ileum

Rectum

Rectovesical pouch

Transverse vesical fold

Cecum

Parietal peritoneum

Vas deferens

Vermiform appendix

Lateral inguinal fossa

Urinary bladder

Median umbilical fold (with underlying obliterated urachus)

Rectus abdominis

Medial umbilicus fold (with underlying obliterated umbilical a.)

Lateral umbilical fold (with inferior epigastric a. and v.)

Sigmoid colon

A Lesser pelvis, anterosuperior view. *Retracted:* Small intestine loops and colon (portions).

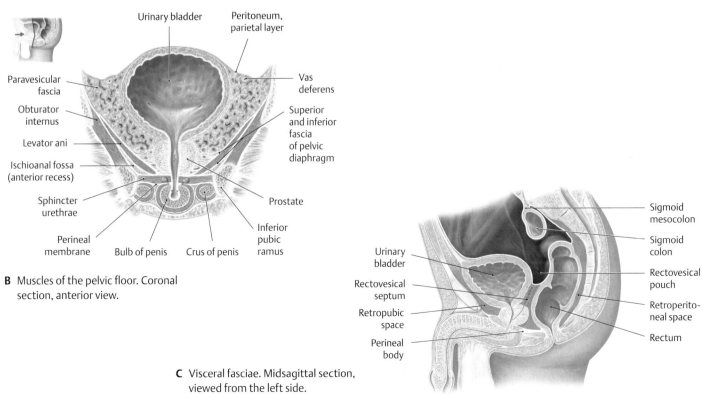

Urinary bladder

Peritoneum, parietal layer

Paravesicular fascia

Obturator internus

Levator ani

Ischioanal fossa (anterior recess)

Sphincter urethrae

Perineal membrane

Bulb of penis

Crus of penis

Vas deferens

Superior and inferior fascia of pelvic diaphragm

Prostate

Inferior pubic ramus

B Muscles of the pelvic floor. Coronal section, anterior view.

Urinary bladder

Rectovesical septum

Retropubic space

Perineal body

Sigmoid mesocolon

Sigmoid colon

Rectovesical pouch

Retroperitoneal space

Rectum

C Visceral fasciae. Midsagittal section, viewed from the left side.

Pelvis & Perineum

Table 12.5	Divisions of the pelvis and perineum

The levels of the pelvis are determined by bony landmarks (iliac crest and pelvis inlet, see p. 126). The contents of the perineum are separated by the pelvic diaphragm and two fascial layers.

Iliac crest			
Pelvis	**False pelvis**	• Ileum (coils)	
		• Cecum and appendix	
		• Sigmoid colon	
		• Common and external iliac aa. and vv.	
		• Lumbar plexus (branches)	
	Pelvic inlet		
	Pelvis proper	• Distal ureters	
		• Urinary bladder	
		• Rectum	
		♀: Vagina, uterus, uterine tubes, and ovaries	
		♂: Ductus deferens, seminal vesicle, and prostate	
		• Internal iliac a. and v. and branches	
		• Sacral plexus	
		• Inferior hypogastric plexus	

Pelvic diaphragm (Levator ani with superficial and inferior pelvic diaphragmatic fascia)

Perineum	**Deep pouch**	• Sphincter urethrae and deep transverse perineal mm.
		• Urethra (membranous)
		• Vagina
		• Rectum
		• Bulbourethral gland
		• Ischioanal fossa
		• Internal pudendal a. and v., pudendal n. and branches
	Perineal membrane	
	Superficial pouch	• Ischiocavernosus, bulbocavernosus, and superficial transverse perineal mm.
		• Urethra (penile)
		• Clitoris and penis
		• Internal pudendal a. and v., pudendal n. and branches
	Superficial perineal (Colles') fascia	
	Subcutaneous perineal space	• Fat

Skin

Fig. 12.14 Pelvis and urogenital triangle
Coronal section, anterior view.

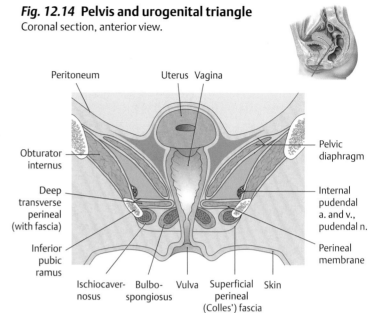

A Female.

Labels: Peritoneum, Uterus, Vagina, Obturator internus, Deep transverse perineal (with fascia), Inferior pubic ramus, Ischiocavernosus, Bulbospongiosus, Vulva, Superficial perineal (Colles') fascia, Skin, Pelvic diaphragm, Internal pudendal a. and v., pudendal n., Perineal membrane

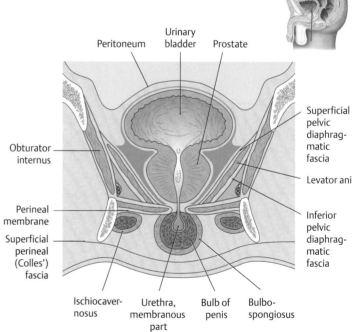

B Male.

Labels: Peritoneum, Urinary bladder, Prostate, Obturator internus, Perineal membrane, Superficial perineal (Colles') fascia, Ischiocavernosus, Urethra, membranous part, Bulb of penis, Bulbospongiosus, Superficial pelvic diaphragmatic fascia, Levator ani, Inferior pelvic diaphragmatic fascia

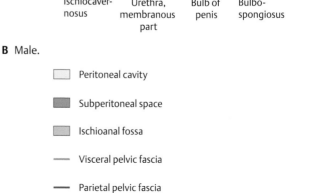

- Peritoneal cavity
- Subperitoneal space
- Ischioanal fossa
- Visceral pelvic fascia
- Parietal pelvic fascia

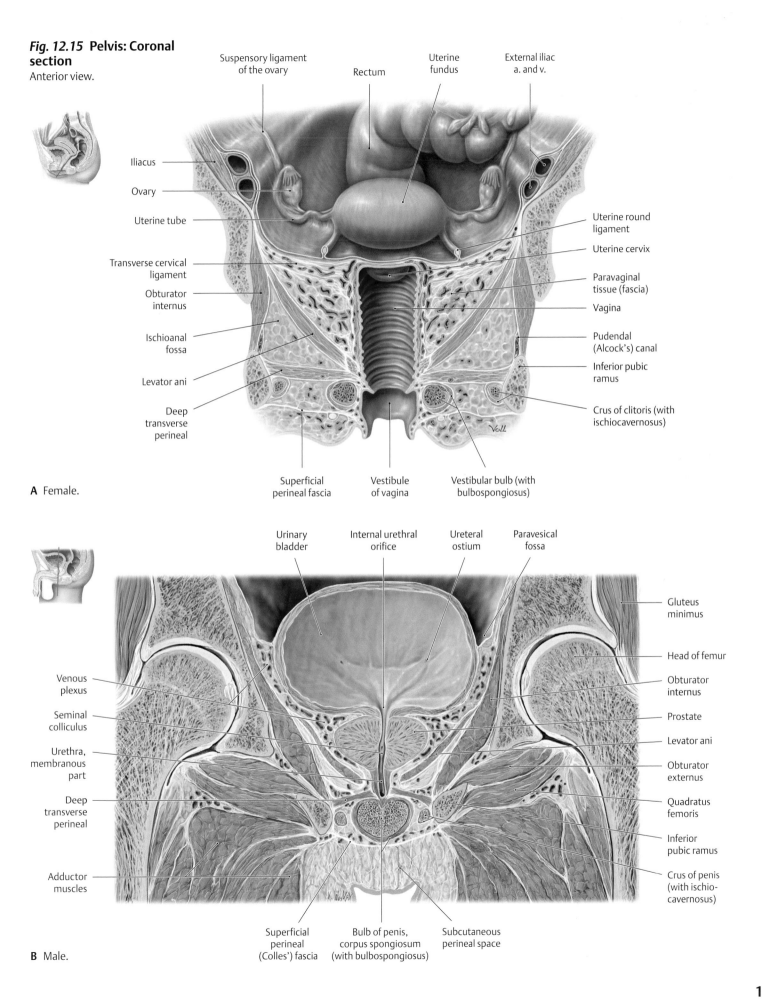

Fig. 12.15 **Pelvis: Coronal section**
Anterior view.

Suspensory ligament of the ovary

Rectum

Uterine fundus

External iliac a. and v.

Iliacus

Ovary

Uterine tube

Transverse cervical ligament

Obturator internus

Ischioanal fossa

Levator ani

Deep transverse perineal

Uterine round ligament

Uterine cervix

Paravaginal tissue (fascia)

Vagina

Pudendal (Alcock's) canal

Inferior pubic ramus

Crus of clitoris (with ischiocavernosus)

Superficial perineal fascia

Vestibule of vagina

Vestibular bulb (with bulbospongiosus)

A Female.

Urinary bladder

Internal urethral orifice

Ureteral ostium

Paravesical fossa

Venous plexus

Seminal colliculus

Urethra, membranous part

Deep transverse perineal

Adductor muscles

Gluteus minimus

Head of femur

Obturator internus

Prostate

Levator ani

Obturator externus

Quadratus femoris

Inferior pubic ramus

Crus of penis (with ischiocavernosus)

Superficial perineal (Colles') fascia

Bulb of penis, corpus spongiosum (with bulbospongiosus)

Subcutaneous perineal space

B Male.

Transverse Sections

Fig. 12.16 **Abdomen: Transverse section**
Inferior view.

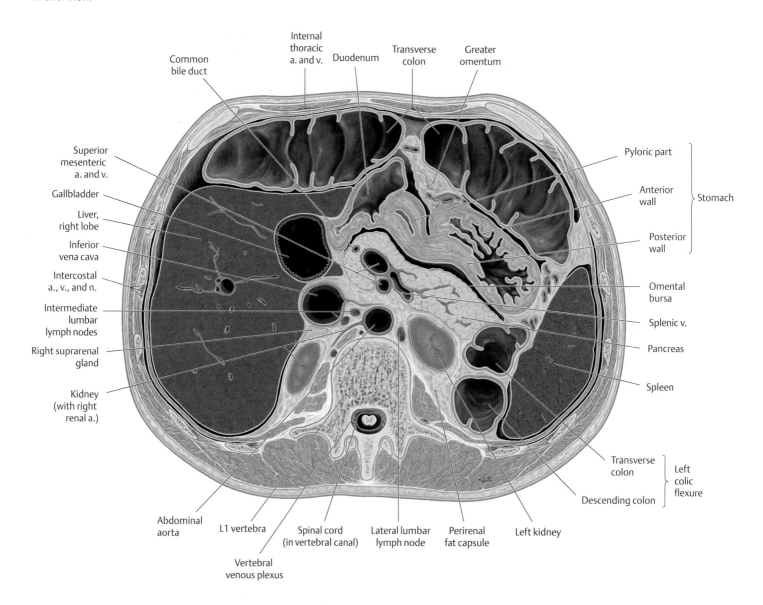

Common bile duct

Internal thoracic a. and v.

Duodenum

Transverse colon

Greater omentum

Pyloric part

Anterior wall

Stomach

Posterior wall

Superior mesenteric a. and v.

Gallbladder

Liver, right lobe

Inferior vena cava

Intercostal a., v., and n.

Intermediate lumbar lymph nodes

Right suprarenal gland

Kidney (with right renal a.)

Omental bursa

Splenic v.

Pancreas

Spleen

Transverse colon

Descending colon

Left colic flexure

Abdominal aorta

L1 vertebra

Spinal cord (in vertebral canal)

Lateral lumbar lymph node

Perirenal fat capsule

Left kidney

Vertebral venous plexus

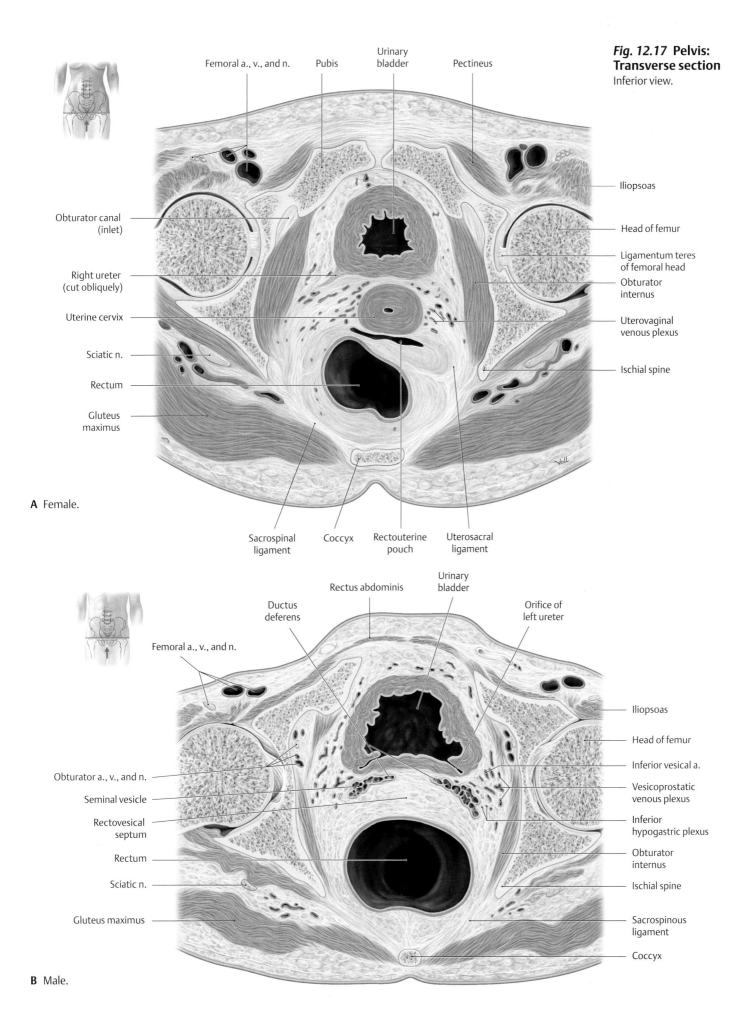

Fig. 12.17 **Pelvis: Transverse section**
Inferior view.

Femoral a., v., and n. **Pubis** **Urinary bladder** **Pectineus**

Obturator canal (inlet)

Right ureter (cut obliquely)

Uterine cervix

Sciatic n.

Rectum

Gluteus maximus

Iliopsoas

Head of femur

Ligamentum teres of femoral head

Obturator internus

Uterovaginal venous plexus

Ischial spine

A Female.

Sacrospinal ligament   Coccyx   Rectouterine pouch   Uterosacral ligament

Rectus abdominis   Urinary bladder

Ductus deferens

Orifice of left ureter

Femoral a., v., and n.

Obturator a., v., and n.

Seminal vesicle

Rectovesical septum

Rectum

Sciatic n.

Gluteus maximus

Iliopsoas

Head of femur

Inferior vesical a.

Vesicoprostatic venous plexus

Inferior hypogastric plexus

Obturator internus

Ischial spine

Sacrospinous ligament

Coccyx

B Male.

Stomach

Fig. 13.1 Stomach: Location

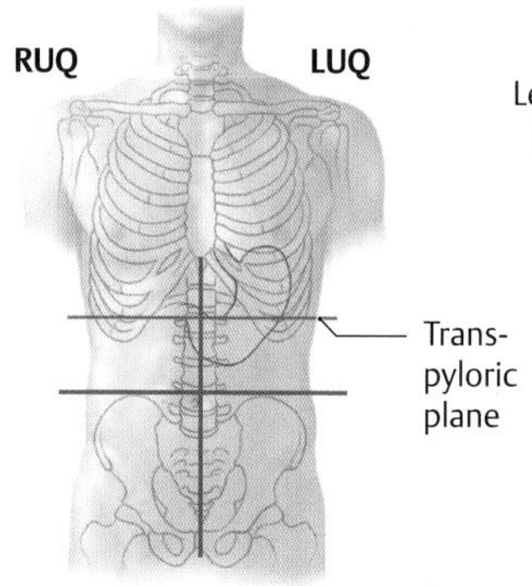

RUQ LUQ

Transpyloric plane

A Anterior view.

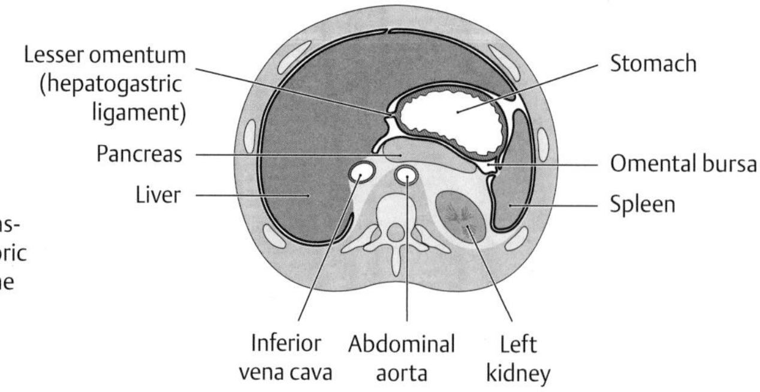

Lesser omentum (hepatogastric ligament)

Pancreas

Liver

Stomach

Omental bursa

Spleen

Inferior vena cava

Abdominal aorta

Left kidney

B Transverse section, inferior view.

Fig. 13.2 Surfaces of the stomach

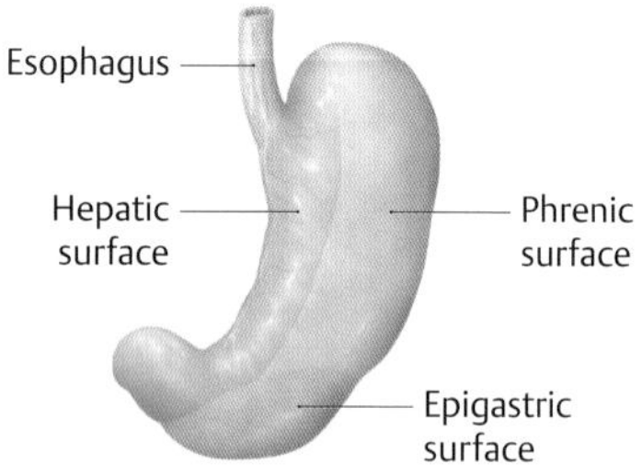

Esophagus

Hepatic surface

Phrenic surface

Epigastric surface

A Anterior view.

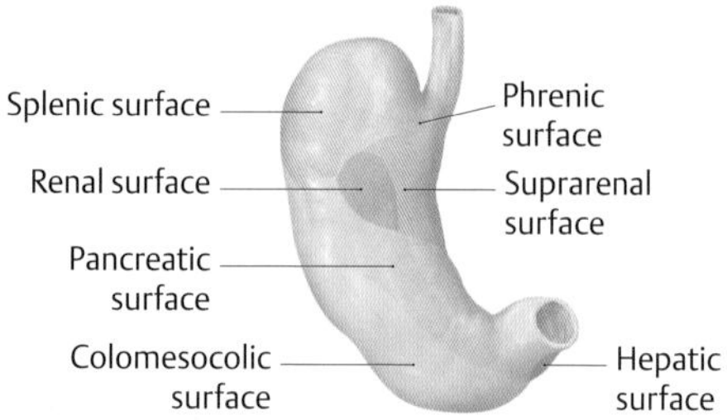

Splenic surface

Renal surface

Pancreatic surface

Colomesocolic surface

Phrenic surface

Suprarenal surface

Hepatic surface

B Posterior view.

Fig. 13.3 Stomach

Anterior view.

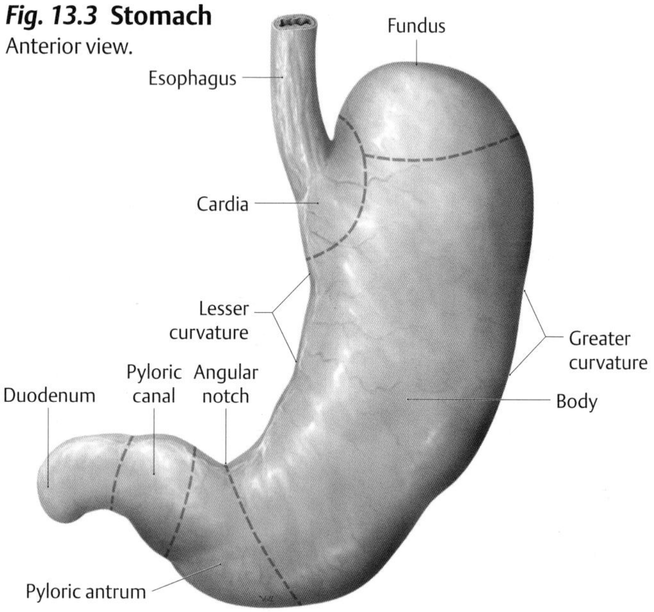

Esophagus

Fundus

Cardia

Lesser curvature

Pyloric canal

Angular notch

Duodenum

Greater curvature

Body

Pyloric antrum

A Anterior wall.

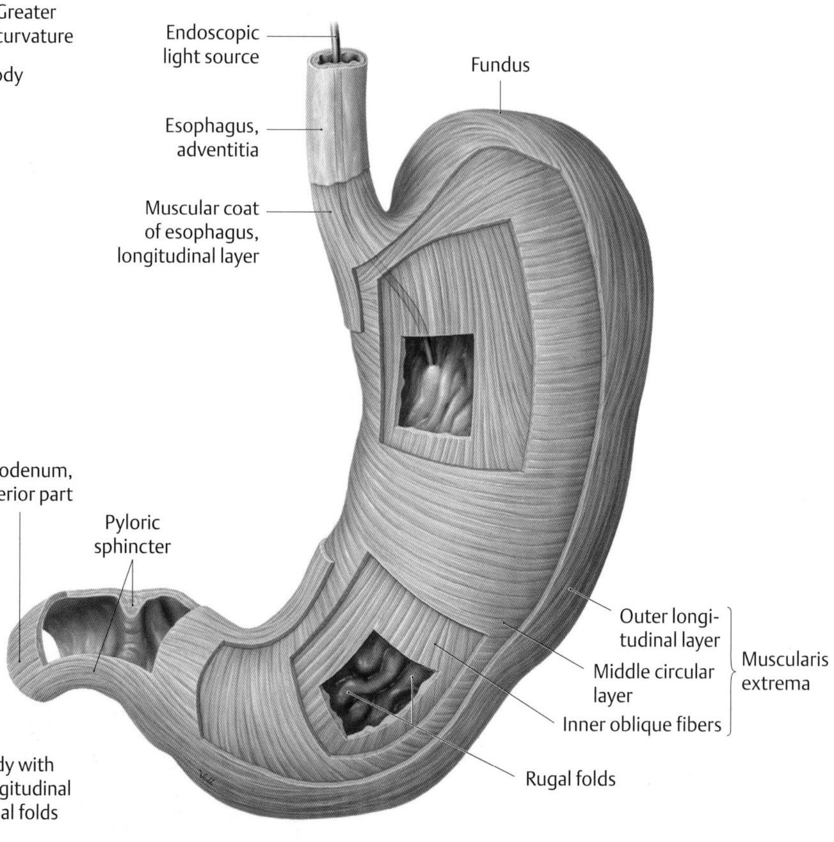

Esophagus

Cardia

Duodenum

Pyloric sphincter

Angular notch

Duodenum, superior part

Pyloric sphincter

Body with longitudinal rugal folds

Pyloric orifice

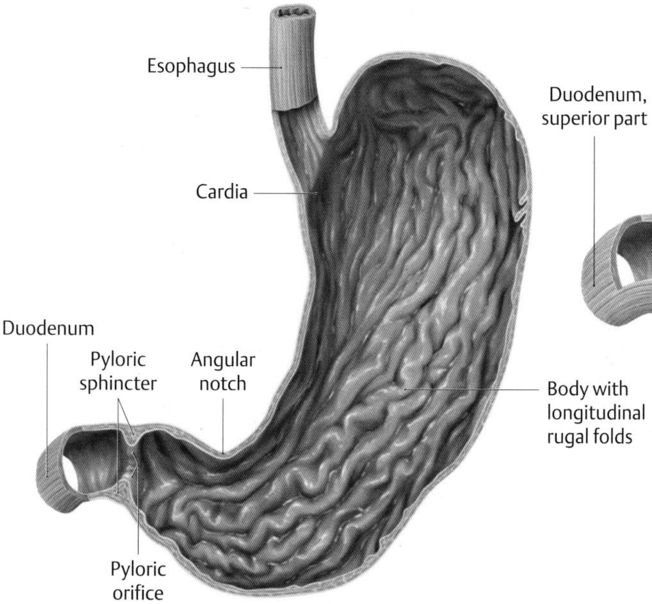

C Interior. *Removed:* Anterior wall.

Endoscopic light source

Esophagus, adventitia

Muscular coat of esophagus, longitudinal layer

Fundus

Outer longitudinal layer

Middle circular layer

Inner oblique fibers

Muscularis extrema

Rugal folds

B Muscular layers. *Removed:* Serosa and subserosa. *Windowed:* Muscular coat.

The stomach is found in the right and left upper quadrants. It is intraperitoneal, its mesenteries being the lesser and greater omenta.

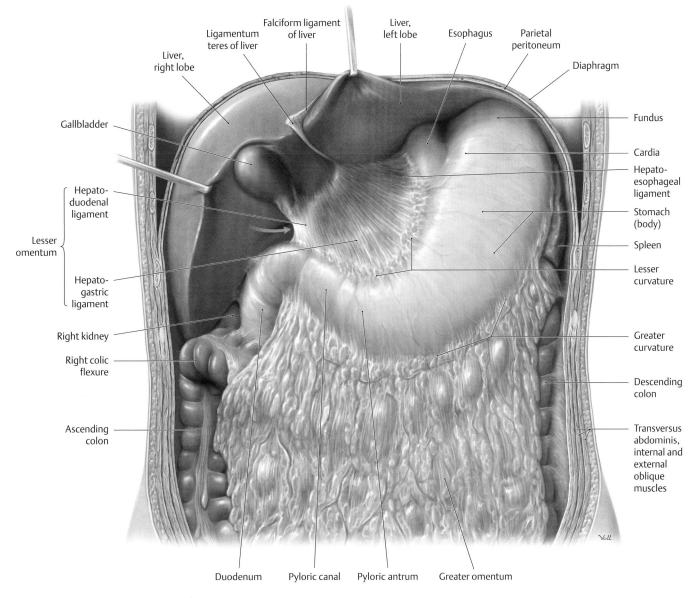

- Liver, right lobe
- Ligamentum teres of liver
- Falciform ligament of liver
- Liver, left lobe
- Esophagus
- Parietal peritoneum
- Diaphragm
- Gallbladder
- Fundus
- Cardia
- Hepato-esophageal ligament
- Hepato-duodenal ligament
- Lesser omentum
- Hepato-gastric ligament
- Stomach (body)
- Spleen
- Lesser curvature
- Right kidney
- Right colic flexure
- Ascending colon
- Greater curvature
- Descending colon
- Transversus abdominis, internal and external oblique muscles
- Duodenum
- Pyloric canal
- Pyloric antrum
- Greater omentum

 Clinical

Gastritis and gastric ulcers

Gastritis and gastric ulcers, the two most common diseases of the stomach, are associated with increased acid production and are caused by alcohol, drugs such as aspirin, and the bacterium *Helicobacter pylori*. Symptoms include lessened appetite, pain, and even bleeding, which manifests as black stool or dark brown material in vomit. Gastritis is limited to the inner surface of the stomach, while gastric ulcers extend into the stomach wall. The gastric ulcer in **C** is covered with fibrin and shows hematin spots.

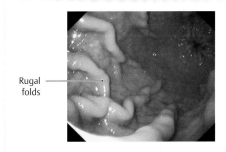

Rugal folds

A Body of normal stomach.

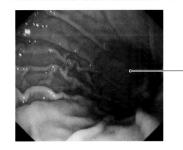

Gastric antrum

B Normal pyloric antrum.

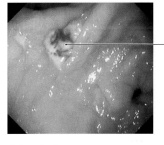

Gastric ulcer

C Gastric ulcer.

Duodenum

 The small intestine consists of the duodenum, jejunum, and ileum (see p. 162). The duodenum is primarily retroperitoneal and divided into four parts: superior, descending, horizontal, and ascending.

Fig. 13.5 **Duodenum: Location**
Anterior view.

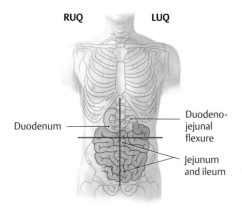

Fig. 13.6 **Parts of the duodenum**
Anterior view.

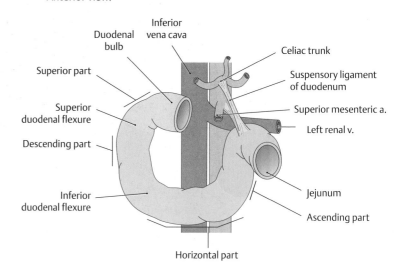

Fig. 13.7 **Duodenum**
Anterior view with the anterior wall opened.

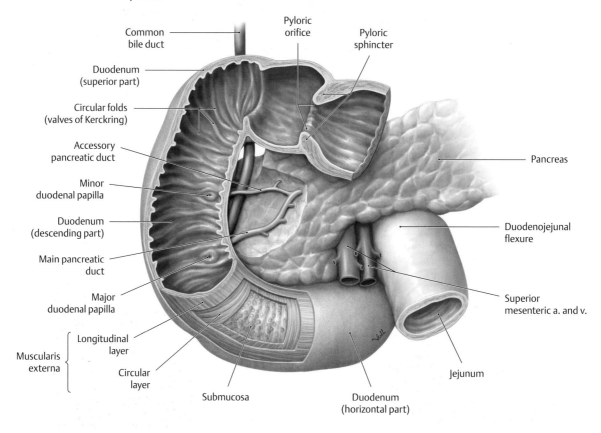

Fig. 13.8 Duodenum in situ

Anterior view. *Removed:* Stomach, liver, small intestine, and large portions of the transverse colon. *Thinned:* Retroperitoneal fat and connective tissue.

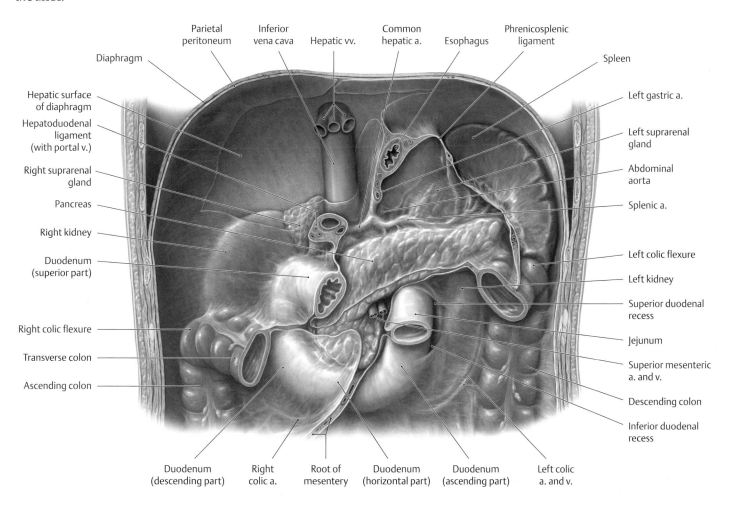

Clinical

Endoscopy of the papillary region

Two important ducts end in the papillary region of the duodenum: the common bile duct and the pancreatic duct (see Fig. 13.7). These ducts may be examined by X-ray through endoscopic retrograde cholangiopancreatography (ERCP), in which dye is injected endoscopically into the duodenal papilla. Duodenal diverticula (generally harmless outpouchings) may complicate the procedure.

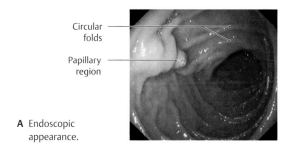

A Endoscopic appearance.

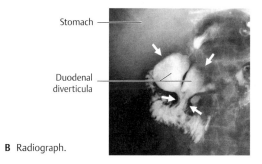

B Radiograph.

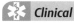

Jejunum & Ileum

Fig. 13.9 **Jejunum and ileum: Location**

Anterior view. The intraperitoneal jejunum and ileum are enclosed by the mesentery proper.

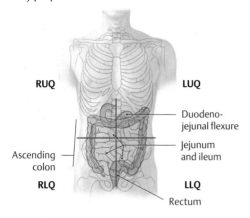

RUQ

LUQ

Duodeno-
jejunal flexure

Jejunum
and ileum

Ascending
colon

RLQ

LLQ

Rectum

Fig. 13.10 **Wall structure of the small intestine**

Macroscopic views of the longitudinally opened small intestine.

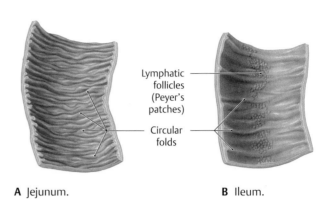

Lymphatic
follicles
(Peyer's
patches)

Circular
folds

A Jejunum.

B Ileum.

Fig. 13.11 **Jejunum and ileum in situ**

Anterior view. *Reflected:* Transverse colon.

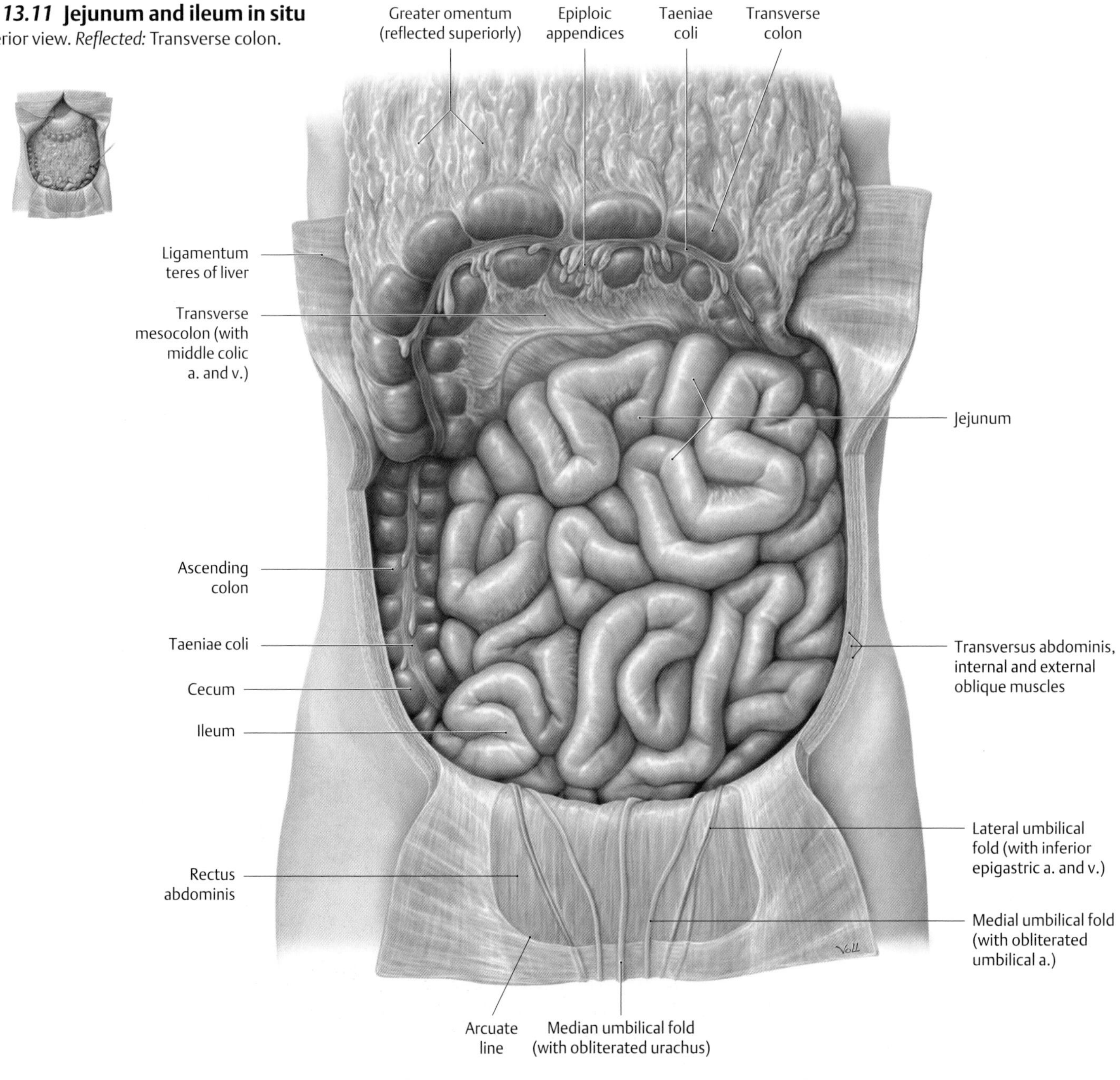

Greater omentum
(reflected superiorly)

Epiploic
appendices

Taeniae
coli

Transverse
colon

Ligamentum
teres of liver

Transverse
mesocolon (with
middle colic
a. and v.)

Jejunum

Ascending
colon

Taeniae coli

Cecum

Ileum

Transversus abdominis,
internal and external
oblique muscles

Lateral umbilical
fold (with inferior
epigastric a. and v.)

Rectus
abdominis

Medial umbilical fold
(with obliterated
umbilical a.)

Arcuate
line

Median umbilical fold
(with obliterated urachus)

Crohn's disease

Crohn's disease, a chronic inflammation of the digestive tract, occurs most often in the terminal ileum (30% of cases). Patients are generally young and suffer from abdominal pain, nausea, elevated body temperature, and diarrhea. Initially, these symptoms can be confused with appendicitis. Complications of Crohn's disease often include anal fistulae (**B**).

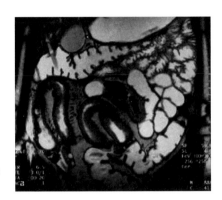

A MRI showing thickened wall of terminal ileum.

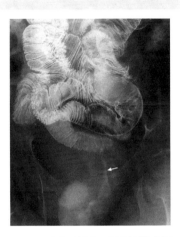

B Double-contrast radiograph. Arrow indicates fistula.

Fig. 13.12 **Mesentery of the small intestine**

Anterior view. *Removed:* Stomach, jejunum, and ileum. *Reflected:* Liver.

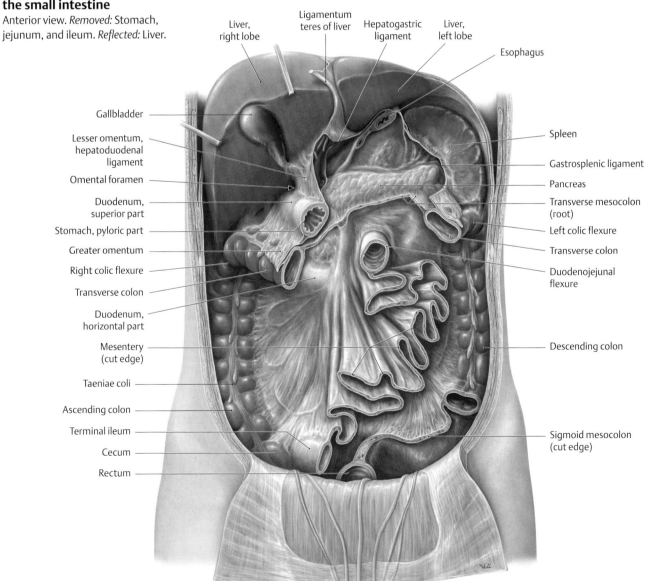

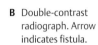

Liver, right lobe — Ligamentum teres of liver — Hepatogastric ligament — Liver, left lobe — Esophagus

Gallbladder

Lesser omentum, hepatoduodenal ligament

Omental foramen

Duodenum, superior part

Stomach, pyloric part

Greater omentum

Right colic flexure

Transverse colon

Duodenum, horizontal part

Mesentery (cut edge)

Taeniae coli

Ascending colon

Terminal ileum

Cecum

Rectum

Spleen

Gastrosplenic ligament

Pancreas

Transverse mesocolon (root)

Left colic flexure

Transverse colon

Duodenojejunal flexure

Descending colon

Sigmoid mesocolon (cut edge)

Cecum, Appendix & Colon

 The large intestine consists of the cecum, appendix, colon, and rectum (see p. 166). The colon is divided into four parts: ascending, transverse, descending, and sigmoid. The appendix, trans- verse colon, and sigmoid colon are intraperitoneal (suspended by the mesoappendix, transverse mesocolon, and sigmoid mesocolon, respectively).

Fig. 13.13 **Large intestine: Location**
Anterior view.

RUQ

LUQ

Right colic flexure

Ascending colon

Cecum

Left colic flexure

Transverse colon

Descending colon

Sigmoid colon

RLQ

LLQ

Rectum

Fig. 13.14 **Ileocecal orifice**
Anterior view of longitudinal coronal section.

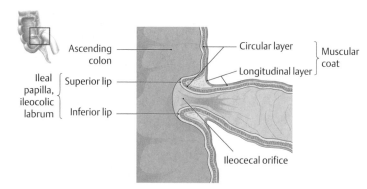

Ascending colon

Ileal papilla, ileocolic labrum

Superior lip

Inferior lip

Circular layer

Longitudinal layer

Muscular coat

Ileocecal orifice

Fig. 13.15 **Large intestine**
Anterior view.

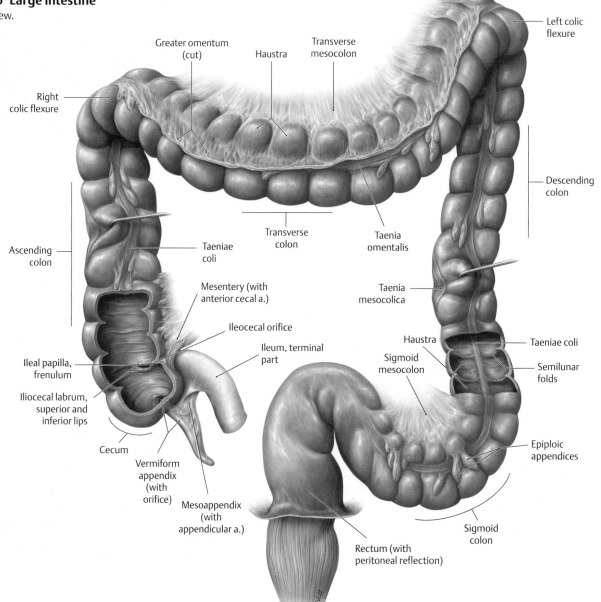

Right colic flexure

Greater omentum (cut)

Haustra

Transverse mesocolon

Left colic flexure

Ascending colon

Taeniae coli

Transverse colon

Taenia omentalis

Descending colon

Mesentery (with anterior cecal a.)

Ileocecal orifice

Ileum, terminal part

Taenia mesocolica

Ileal papilla, frenulum

Iliocecal labrum, superior and inferior lips

Cecum

Vermiform appendix (with orifice)

Mesoappendix (with appendicular a.)

Rectum (with peritoneal reflection)

Sigmoid mesocolon

Haustra

Sigmoid colon

Taeniae coli

Semilunar folds

Epiploic appendices

Fig. 13.16 Large intestine in situ

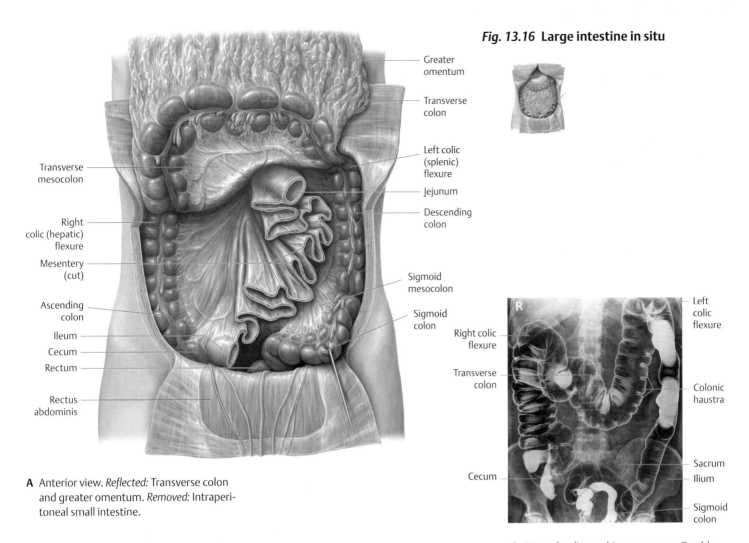

Greater omentum

Transverse colon

Left colic (splenic) flexure

Jejunum

Descending colon

Transverse mesocolon

Right colic (hepatic) flexure

Mesentery (cut)

Ascending colon

Ileum

Cecum

Rectum

Rectus abdominis

Sigmoid mesocolon

Sigmoid colon

A Anterior view. *Reflected:* Transverse colon and greater omentum. *Removed:* Intraperitoneal small intestine.

Right colic flexure

Transverse colon

Cecum

Left colic flexure

Colonic haustra

Sacrum

Ilium

Sigmoid colon

B Normal radiographic appearance. Double-contrast radiograph, anterior view.

Clinical

Colitis

Ulcerative colitis is a chronic inflammation of the large intestine, often starting in the rectum. Typical symptoms include diarrhea (sometimes with blood), pain, weight loss, and inflammation of other organs. Patients are also at higher risk for colorectal carcinomas.

Colon carcinoma

Malignant tumors of the colon and rectum are among the most frequent solid tumors. More than 90% occur in patients over the age of 50. In early stages, the tumor may be asymptomatic; later symptoms include loss of appetite, changes in bowel movements, and weight loss. Blood in the stools is particularly incriminating, necessitating a thorough examination. Hemorrhoids are not a sufficient explanation for blood in stools unless all other tests (including a colonoscopy) are negative.

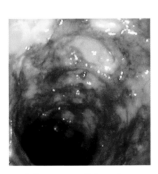

A Colonoscopy of ulcerative colitis.

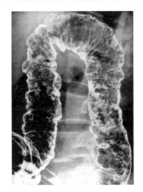

B Early-phase colitis. Residual normal mucosa appears as pseudopolyps.

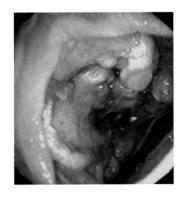

C Colonoscopy of colon carcinoma. The tumor partially blocks the lumen of the colon.

Rectum & Anal Canal

Fig. 13.17 **Rectum: Location**

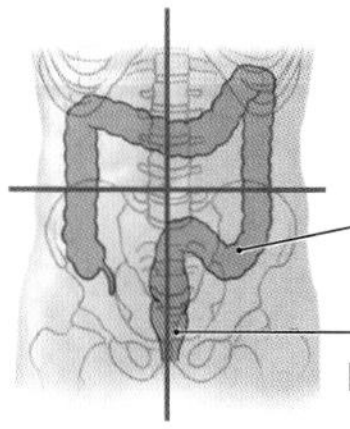

A Anterior view.

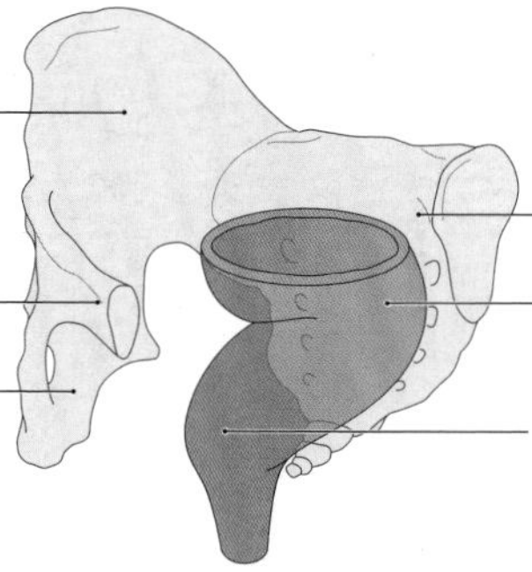

Sigmoid colon

Rectum

RLQ   LLQ

Ilium

Pubis

Ischium

Sacrum

Sacral flexure

Perineal flexure

Rectum

B Left anterolateral view.

Fig. 13.18 **Closure of the rectum**

Left lateral view. The puborectalis acts as a muscular sling that kinks the anorectal junction. It functions in the maintenance of fecal continence.

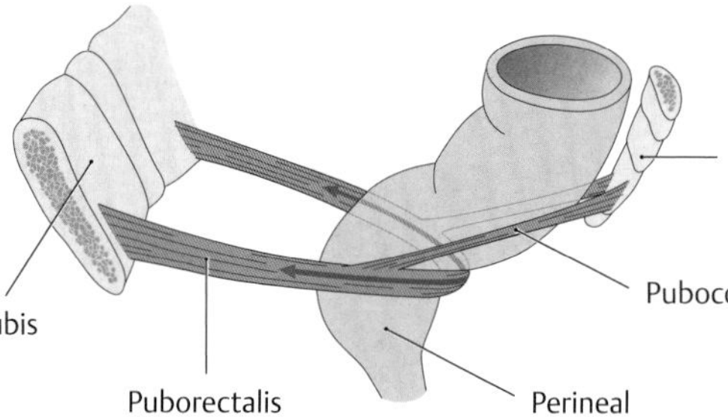

Coccyx

Pubococcygeus

Pubis

Puborectalis

Perineal flexure

Fig. 13.19 **Rectum in situ**

Coronal section, anterior view of the female pelvis. The upper third of the rectum is covered with visceral peritoneum on its anterior and lateral sides. The middle third is covered only anteriorly and the lower third is inferior to the parietal peritoneum.

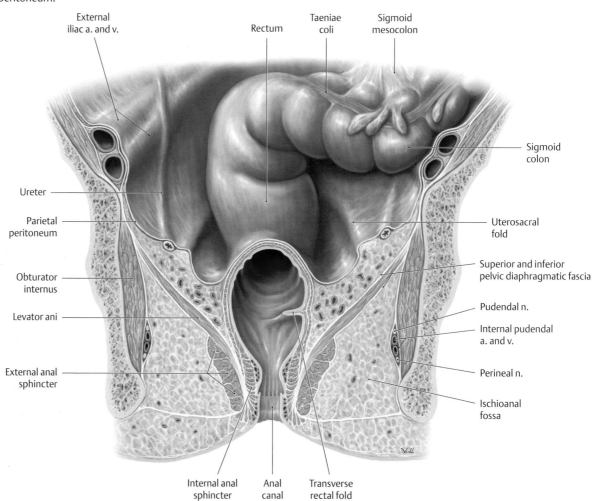

External iliac a. and v.

Rectum

Taeniae coli

Sigmoid mesocolon

Sigmoid colon

Ureter

Parietal peritoneum

Obturator internus

Levator ani

External anal sphincter

Uterosacral fold

Superior and inferior pelvic diaphragmatic fascia

Pudendal n.

Internal pudendal a. and v.

Perineal n.

Ischioanal fossa

Internal anal sphincter

Anal canal

Transverse rectal fold

Fig. 13.20 Rectum and anal canal

Coronal section, anterior view with the anterior wall removed.

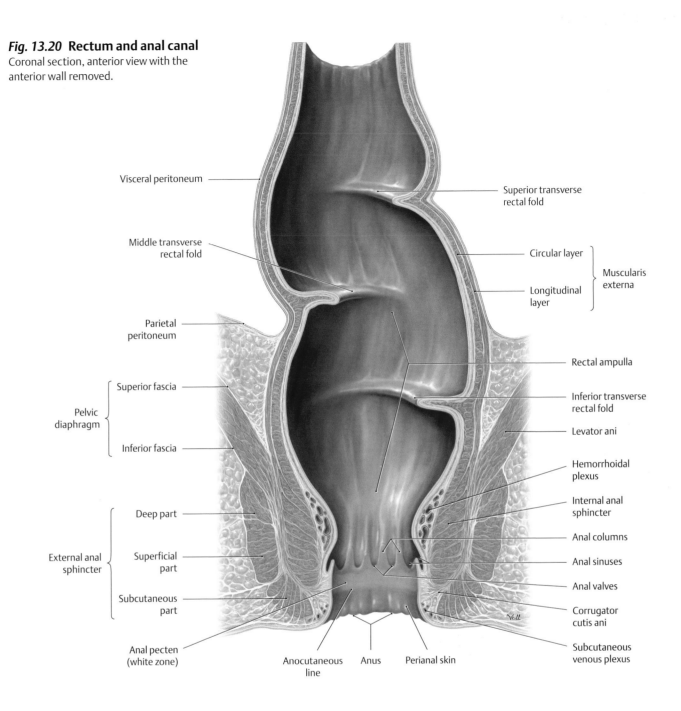

Visceral peritoneum

Middle transverse rectal fold

Parietal peritoneum

Pelvic diaphragm
- Superior fascia
- Inferior fascia

External anal sphincter
- Deep part
- Superficial part
- Subcutaneous part

Anal pecten (white zone)

Anocutaneous line

Anus

Perianal skin

Superior transverse rectal fold

Circular layer — Muscularis externa

Longitudinal layer

Rectal ampulla

Inferior transverse rectal fold

Levator ani

Hemorrhoidal plexus

Internal anal sphincter

Anal columns

Anal sinuses

Anal valves

Corrugator cutis ani

Subcutaneous venous plexus

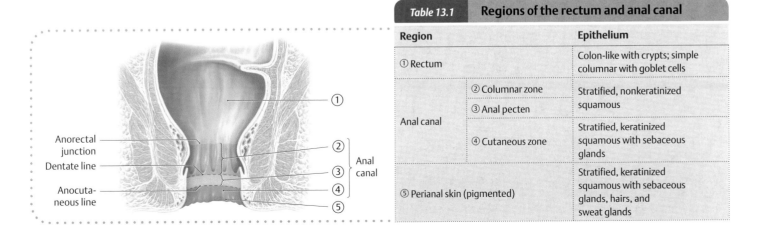

Anorectal junction

Dentate line

Anocutaneous line

① ② ③ ④ ⑤ — Anal canal

Table 13.1		Regions of the rectum and anal canal
Region		**Epithelium**
① Rectum		Colon-like with crypts; simple columnar with goblet cells
Anal canal	② Columnar zone	Stratified, nonkeratinized squamous
	③ Anal pecten	
	④ Cutaneous zone	Stratified, keratinized squamous with sebaceous glands
⑤ Perianal skin (pigmented)		Stratified, keratinized squamous with sebaceous glands, hairs, and sweat glands

167

Liver: Overview

Fig. 13.21 **Liver: Location**

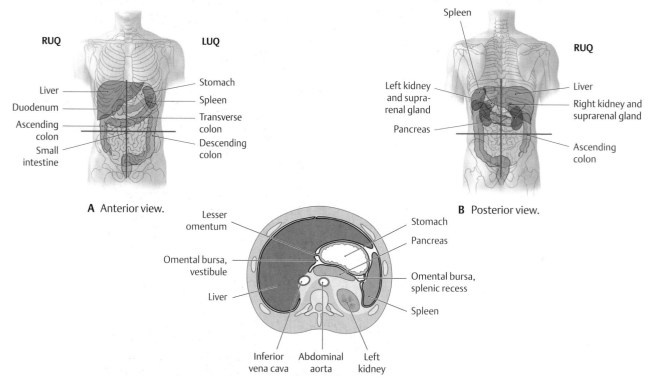

A Anterior view.

B Posterior view.

C Transverse section, inferior view.

Fig. 13.22 **Liver in situ**

Anterior view with liver retracted. *Removed:* Stomach, jejunum, and ileum. The liver is intraperitoneal except for its "bare area" (see Fig. 13.26); its mesenteries include the falciform, coronary, and triangular ligaments (see Fig. 13.27).

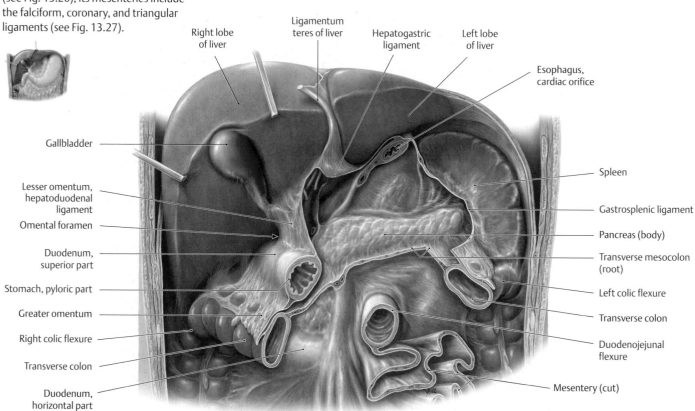

Fig. 13.23 Abdominal MRI

Inferior view.

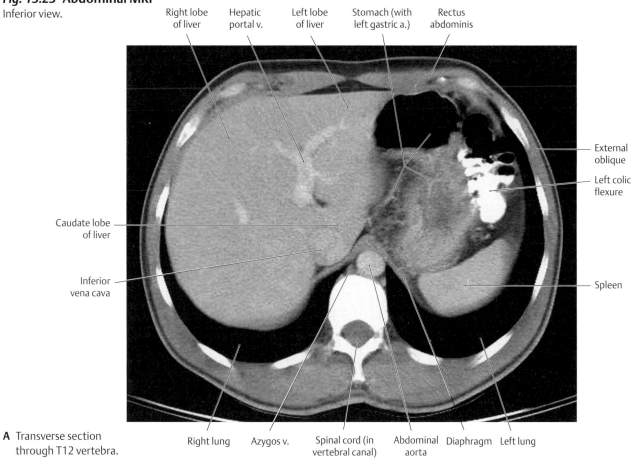

Right lobe of liver — Hepatic portal v. — Left lobe of liver — Stomach (with left gastric a.) — Rectus abdominis

Caudate lobe of liver

Inferior vena cava

External oblique

Left colic flexure

Spleen

A Transverse section through T12 vertebra.

Right lung — Azygos v. — Spinal cord (in vertebral canal) — Abdominal aorta — Diaphragm — Left lung

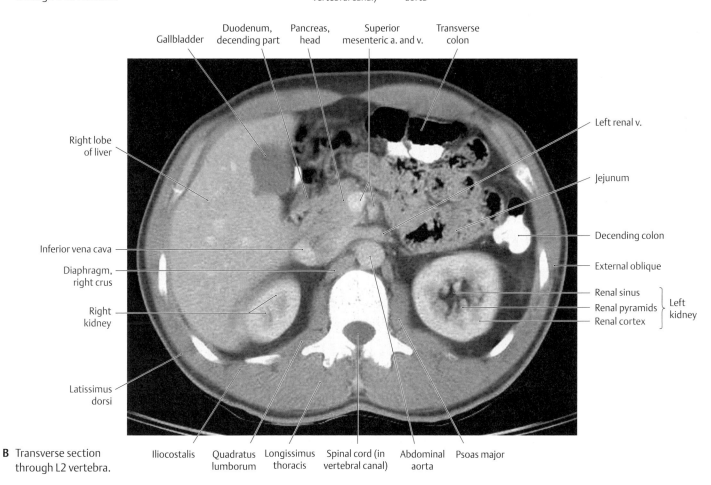

Gallbladder — Duodenum, decending part — Pancreas, head — Superior mesenteric a. and v. — Transverse colon

Right lobe of liver

Inferior vena cava

Diaphragm, right crus

Right kidney

Latissimus dorsi

Left renal v.

Jejunum

Decending colon

External oblique

Renal sinus
Renal pyramids } Left kidney
Renal cortex

B Transverse section through L2 vertebra.

Iliocostalis — Quadratus lumborum — Longissimus thoracis — Spinal cord (in vertebral canal) — Abdominal aorta — Psoas major

Liver: Segments & Lobes

Fig. 13.24 Segmentation of the liver

Anterior view. The components portal triad (hepatic artery, portal vein, and hepatic duct, see pp. 172, 219) divides the liver into hepatic segments (see Table 13.2).

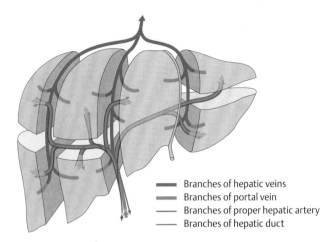

Branches of hepatic veins
Branches of portal vein
Branches of proper hepatic artery
Branches of hepatic duct

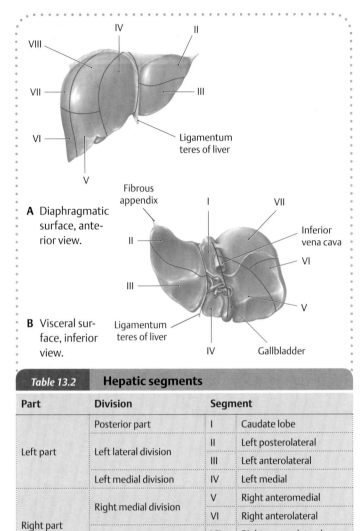

A Diaphragmatic surface, anterior view.

B Visceral surface, inferior view.

Fig. 13.25 Liver: Areas of organ contact

Visceral surface, inferior view.

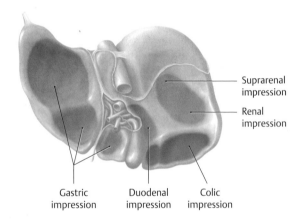

Suprarenal impression
Renal impression
Gastric impression
Duodenal impression
Colic impression

Table 13.2	Hepatic segments		
Part	**Division**	**Segment**	
Left part	Posterior part	I	Caudate lobe
	Left lateral division	II	Left posterolateral
		III	Left anterolateral
	Left medial division	IV	Left medial
Right part	Right medial division	V	Right anteromedial
		VI	Right anterolateral
	Right lateral division	VII	Right posterolateral
		VIII	Right posteromedial

Fig. 13.26 Attachment of liver to diaphragm

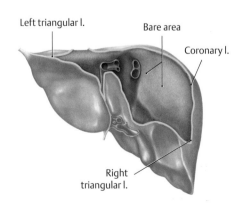

Left triangular l.
Bare area
Coronary l.
Right triangular l.

A Diaphragmatic surface of the liver, posterior view.

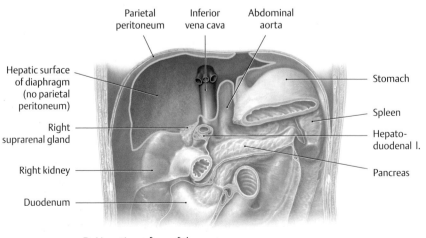

Parietal peritoneum
Inferior vena cava
Abdominal aorta
Hepatic surface of diaphragm (no parietal peritoneum)
Right suprarenal gland
Right kidney
Duodenum
Stomach
Spleen
Hepato-duodenal l.
Pancreas

B Hepatic surface of the diaphragm, anterior view.

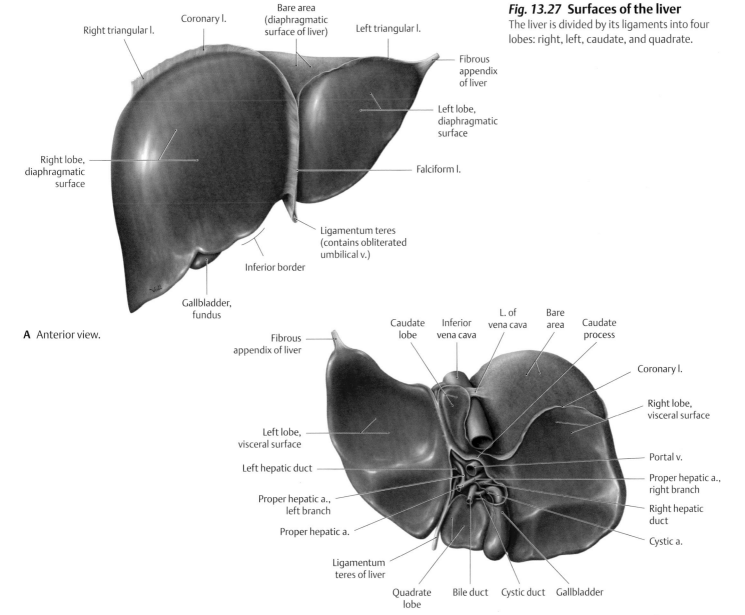

Right triangular l.

Coronary l.

Bare area (diaphragmatic surface of liver)

Left triangular l.

Fibrous appendix of liver

Left lobe, diaphragmatic surface

Fig. 13.27 **Surfaces of the liver**
The liver is divided by its ligaments into four lobes: right, left, caudate, and quadrate.

Right lobe, diaphragmatic surface

Falciform l.

Ligamentum teres (contains obliterated umbilical v.)

Inferior border

Gallbladder, fundus

A Anterior view.

Fibrous appendix of liver

Caudate lobe

Inferior vena cava

L. of vena cava

Bare area

Caudate process

Coronary l.

Right lobe, visceral surface

Left lobe, visceral surface

Left hepatic duct

Portal v.

Proper hepatic a., right branch

Proper hepatic a., left branch

Right hepatic duct

Proper hepatic a.

Cystic a.

Ligamentum teres of liver

Quadrate lobe

Bile duct

Cystic duct

Gallbladder

B Inferior view.

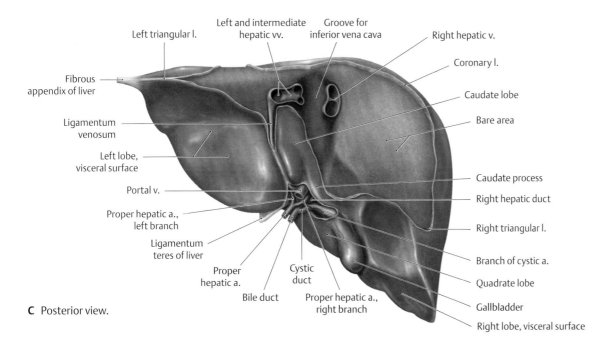

Left triangular l.

Left and intermediate hepatic vv.

Groove for inferior vena cava

Right hepatic v.

Coronary l.

Fibrous appendix of liver

Caudate lobe

Bare area

Ligamentum venosum

Caudate process

Left lobe, visceral surface

Right hepatic duct

Portal v.

Right triangular l.

Proper hepatic a., left branch

Ligamentum teres of liver

Branch of cystic a.

Proper hepatic a.

Quadrate lobe

Bile duct

Cystic duct

Proper hepatic a., right branch

Gallbladder

Right lobe, visceral surface

C Posterior view.

171

Gallbladder & Bile Ducts

Fig. 13.28 **Gallbladder: Location**

RUQ

Right hepatic duct

Cystic duct

Gallbladder

Left hepatic duct

Common hepatic duct

Bile duct

A Anterior view.

Fig. 13.29 **Hepatic bile ducts: Location**
Projection onto surface of the liver, anterior view.

Right duct of caudate lobe

Left duct of caudate lobe

Right hepatic duct

Common hepatic duct

Cystic duct

Liver, right lobe

Liver, left lobe

Left hepatic duct

Bile duct

Gallbladder

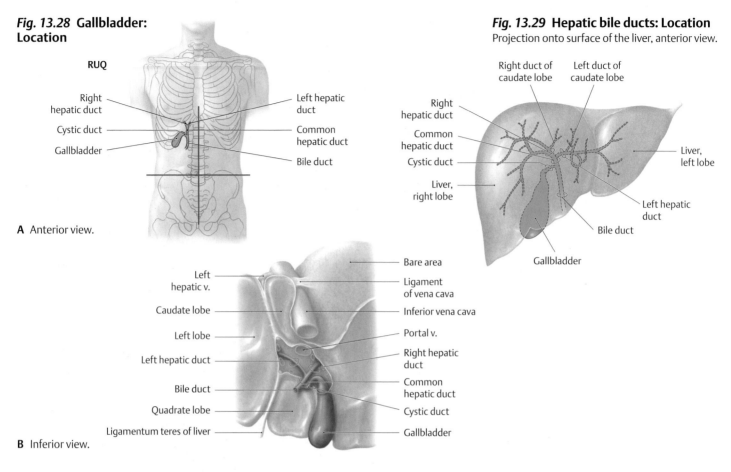

Bare area

Left hepatic v.

Caudate lobe

Left lobe

Left hepatic duct

Bile duct

Quadrate lobe

Ligamentum teres of liver

Ligament of vena cava

Inferior vena cava

Portal v.

Right hepatic duct

Common hepatic duct

Cystic duct

Gallbladder

B Inferior view.

Fig. 13.30 **Biliary sphincter system**

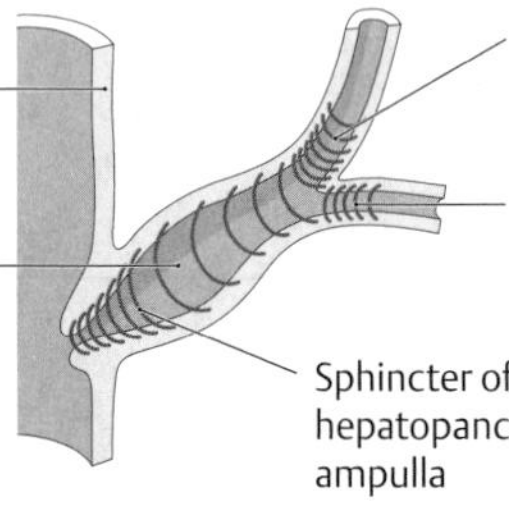

Duodenum (wall)

Hepato-pancreatic ampulla

Sphincter of bile duct

Sphincter of pancreatic duct

Sphincter of hepatopancreatic ampulla

A Sphincters of the pancreatic and bile ducts.

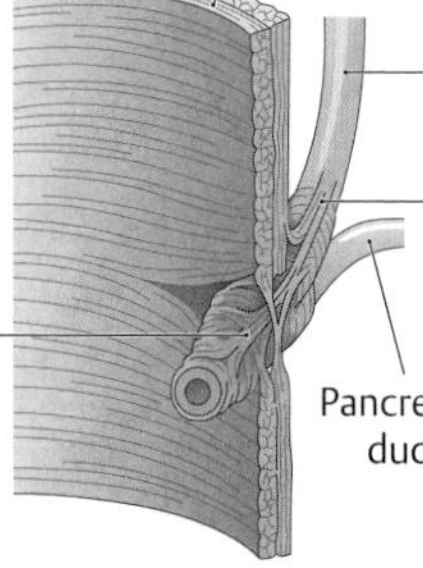

Duodenum, muscularis externa

Longitudinal layer

Circular layer

Bile duct

Longitudinal slips of duodenal muscle on bile duct

Sphincter of hepato-pancreatic ampulla

Pancreatic duct

B Sphincter system in the duodenal wall.

Fig. 13.31 **Extrahepatic bile ducts**
Anterior view. *Opened:* Gallbladder and duodenum.

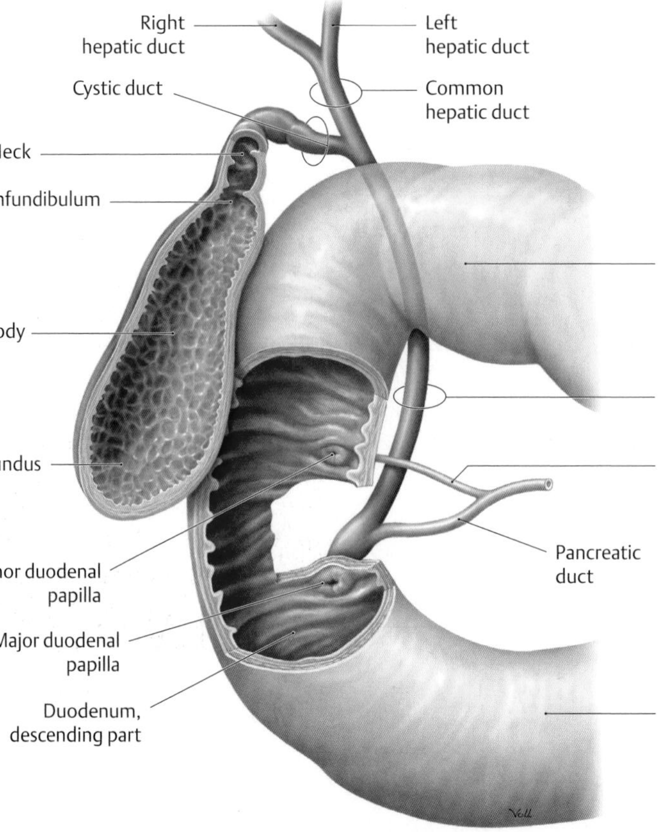

Right hepatic duct

Cystic duct

Neck

Infundibulum

Gall-bladder

Body

Fundus

Minor duodenal papilla

Major duodenal papilla

Duodenum, descending part

Left hepatic duct

Common hepatic duct

Duodenum, superior part

Bile duct

Accessory pancreatic duct

Pancreatic duct

Duodenum, horizontal part

Fig. 13.32 **Biliary tract in situ**

Anterior view. *Removed:* Stomach, small intestine, transverse colon, and large portions of the liver. The gallbladder is intraperitoneal, covered by visceral peritoneum where it is not attached to the liver.

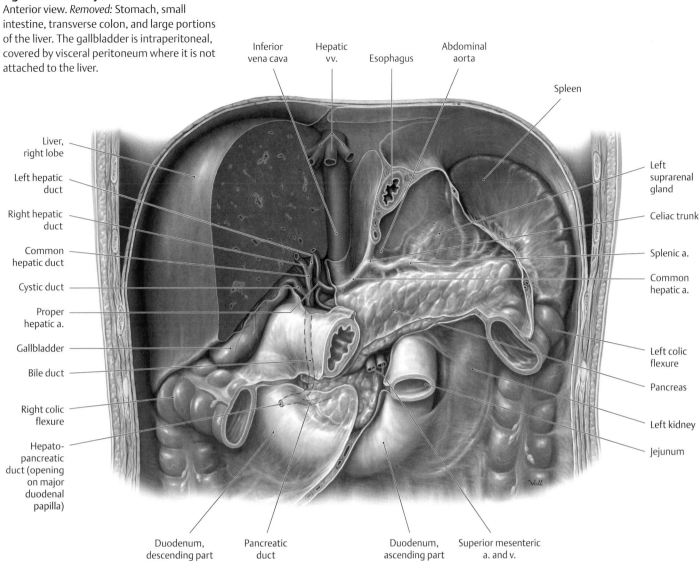

Liver, right lobe
Left hepatic duct
Right hepatic duct
Common hepatic duct
Cystic duct
Proper hepatic a.
Gallbladder
Bile duct
Right colic flexure
Hepato-pancreatic duct (opening on major duodenal papilla)

Inferior vena cava
Hepatic vv.
Esophagus
Abdominal aorta
Spleen
Left suprarenal gland
Celiac trunk
Splenic a.
Common hepatic a.
Left colic flexure
Pancreas
Left kidney
Jejunum

Duodenum, descending part
Pancreatic duct
Duodenum, ascending part
Superior mesenteric a. and v.

Clinical

Obstruction of the bile duct

As bile is stored and concentrated in the gallbladder, certain substances, such as cholesterol, may crystallize, resulting in the formation of gallstones. Migration of gallstones into the bile duct causes severe pain (colic). Gallstones may also block the pancreatic duct in the papillary regions, causing highly acute or even life-threatening pancreatitis.

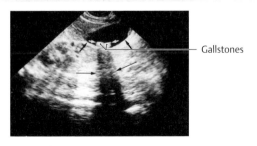

Gallstones

Ultrasound appearance of two gallstones. Black arrows mark the echo-free area behind the stones.

Pancreas & Spleen

Fig. 13.33 Pancreas and spleen: Location

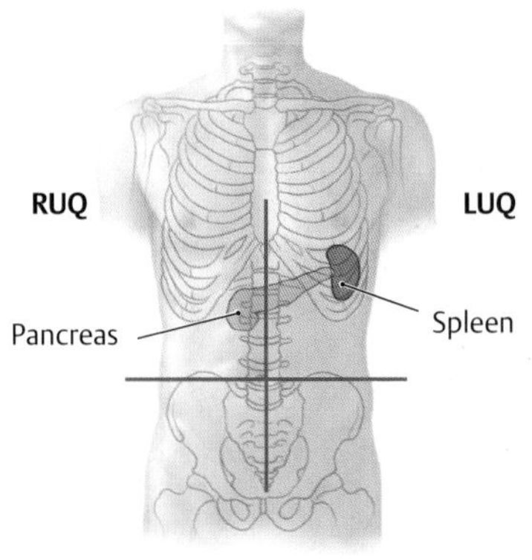

RUQ   LUQ

Pancreas   Spleen

A Anterior view.

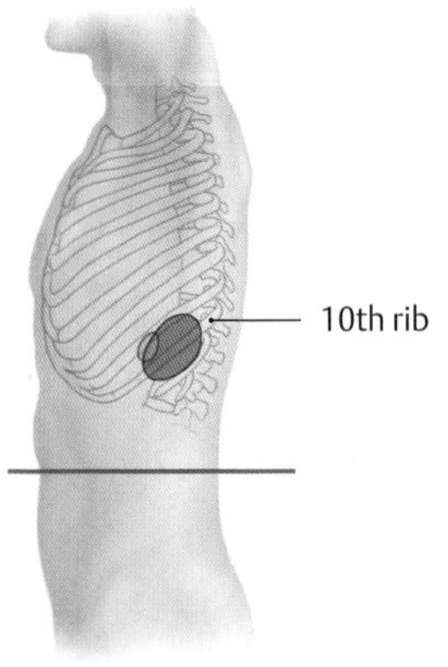

10th rib

B Left lateral view.

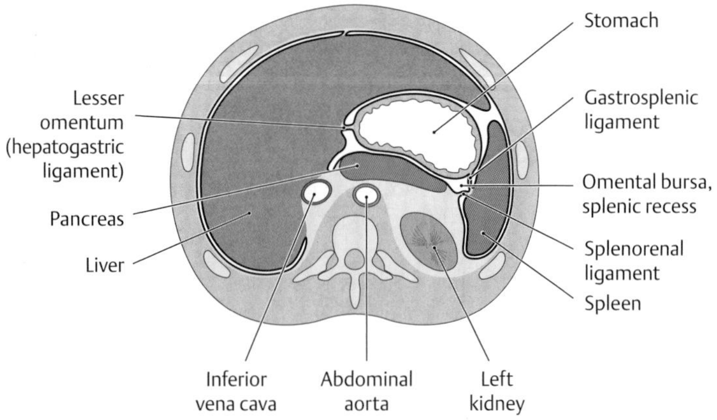

Lesser omentum (hepatogastric ligament)

Pancreas

Liver

Stomach

Gastrosplenic ligament

Omental bursa, splenic recess

Splenorenal ligament

Spleen

Inferior vena cava   Abdominal aorta   Left kidney

C Transverse section, inferior view.

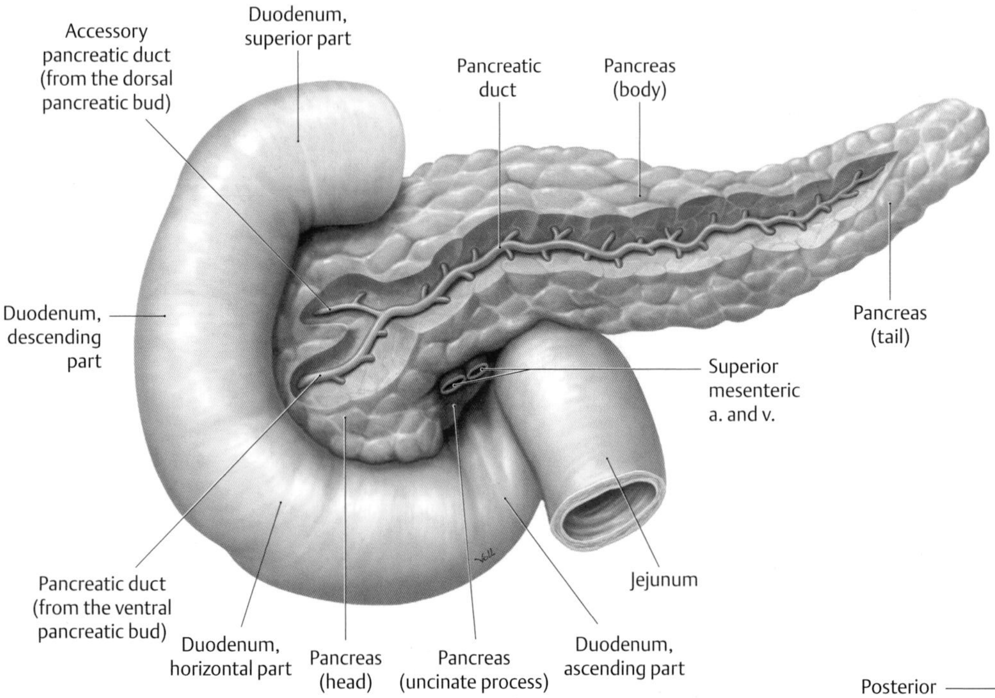

Accessory pancreatic duct (from the dorsal pancreatic bud)

Duodenum, superior part

Pancreatic duct

Pancreas (body)

Duodenum, descending part

Pancreas (tail)

Superior mesenteric a. and v.

Pancreatic duct (from the ventral pancreatic bud)

Duodenum, horizontal part

Pancreas (head)

Pancreas (uncinate process)

Duodenum, ascending part

Jejunum

Fig. 13.34 Pancreas

Anterior view with dissection of the pancreatic duct.

Fig. 13.35 Spleen

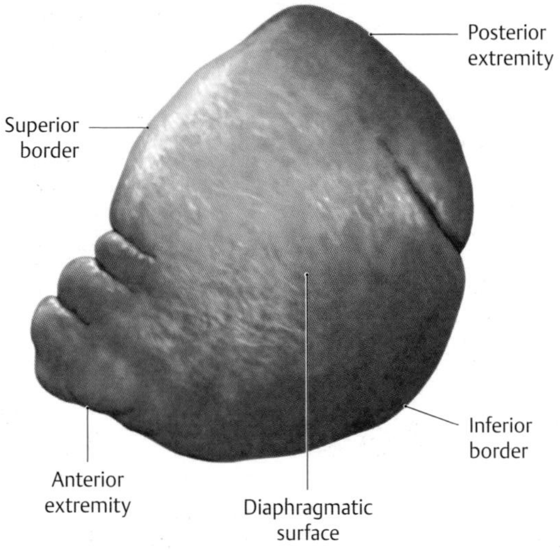

Posterior extremity

Superior border

Anterior extremity

Diaphragmatic surface

Inferior border

A Costal surface.

Posterior extremity

Splenic a.

Splenic v.

Renal surface

Inferior border

Colic surface

Superior border

Gastric surface

Hilum

Anterior extremity

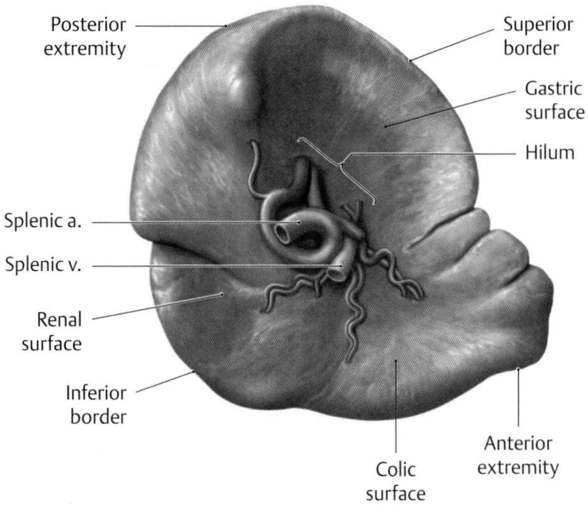

B Visceral surface.

Fig. 13.36 Pancreas and spleen in situ

Anterior view. *Removed:* Liver, stomach, small intestine, and large intestine. The pancreas is retroperitoneal, while the spleen is intraperitoneal.

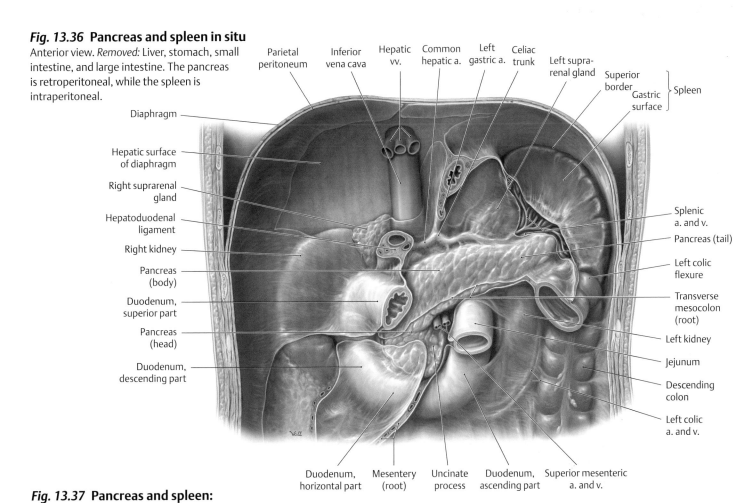

Labels (clockwise from top): Parietal peritoneum · Inferior vena cava · Hepatic vv. · Common hepatic a. · Left gastric a. · Celiac trunk · Left supra-renal gland · Superior border · Gastric surface · Spleen · Splenic a. and v. · Pancreas (tail) · Left colic flexure · Transverse mesocolon (root) · Left kidney · Jejunum · Descending colon · Left colic a. and v. · Superior mesenteric a. and v. · Duodenum, ascending part · Uncinate process · Mesentery (root) · Duodenum, horizontal part · Duodenum, descending part · Pancreas (head) · Duodenum, superior part · Pancreas (body) · Right kidney · Hepatoduodenal ligament · Right suprarenal gland · Hepatic surface of diaphragm · Diaphragm

Fig. 13.37 Pancreas and spleen: Transverse section

Inferior view. Section through L1 vertebra.

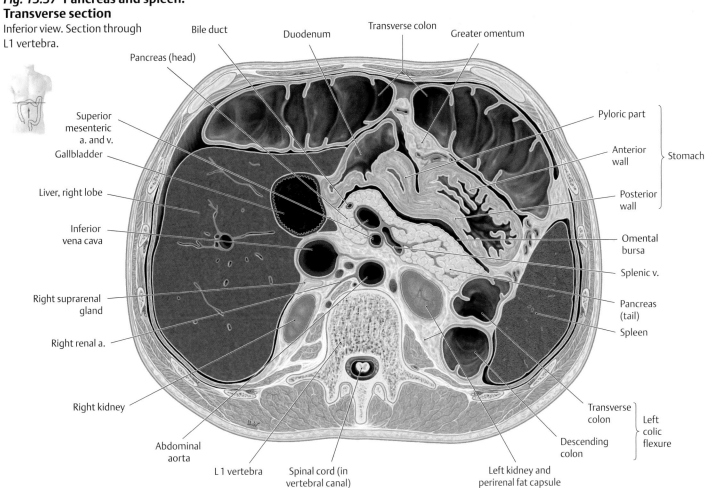

Labels: Bile duct · Duodenum · Transverse colon · Greater omentum · Pancreas (head) · Superior mesenteric a. and v. · Gallbladder · Liver, right lobe · Inferior vena cava · Right suprarenal gland · Right renal a. · Right kidney · Abdominal aorta · L1 vertebra · Spinal cord (in vertebral canal) · Left kidney and perirenal fat capsule · Descending colon · Transverse colon · Left colic flexure · Spleen · Pancreas (tail) · Splenic v. · Omental bursa · Posterior wall · Anterior wall · Pyloric part · Stomach

Kidneys & Suprarenal Glands: Overview

Fig. 13.38 **Kidneys and suprarenal glands: Location**

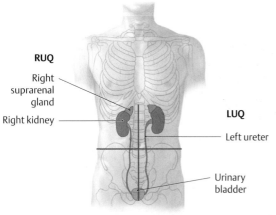

RUQ

Right suprarenal gland

Right kidney

LUQ

Left ureter

Urinary bladder

A Anterior view.

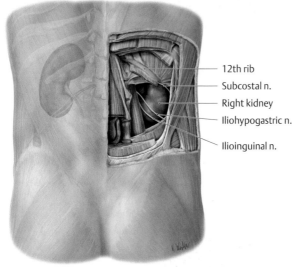

12th rib

Subcostal n.

Right kidney

Iliohypogastric n.

Ilioinguinal n.

B Posterior view with the trunk wall opened.

Fig. 13.39 **Kidneys: Areas of organ contact**
Anterior view.

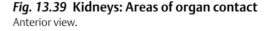
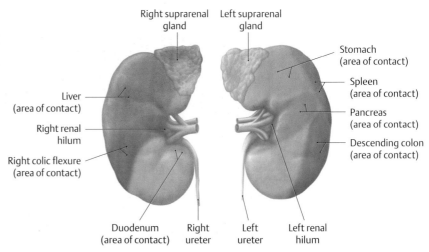

Right suprarenal gland

Left suprarenal gland

Stomach (area of contact)

Spleen (area of contact)

Pancreas (area of contact)

Descending colon (area of contact)

Liver (area of contact)

Right renal hilum

Right colic flexure (area of contact)

Duodenum (area of contact)

Right ureter

Left ureter

Left renal hilum

Fig. 13.40 **Right kidney in the renal bed**
Sagittal section through the right renal bed.

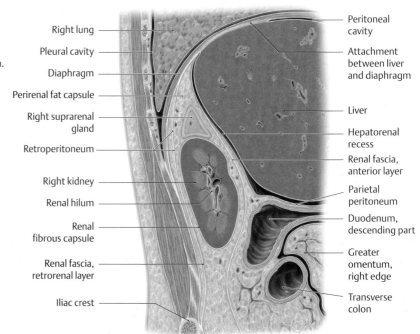

Right lung

Pleural cavity

Diaphragm

Perirenal fat capsule

Right suprarenal gland

Retroperitoneum

Right kidney

Renal hilum

Renal fibrous capsule

Renal fascia, retrorenal layer

Iliac crest

Peritoneal cavity

Attachment between liver and diaphragm

Liver

Hepatorenal recess

Renal fascia, anterior layer

Parietal peritoneum

Duodenum, descending part

Greater omentum, right edge

Transverse colon

Fig. 13.41 **Suprarenal gland**
Anterior view.

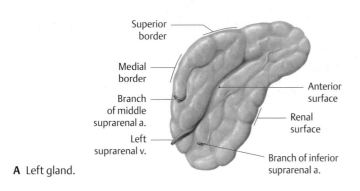

Superior border

Medial border

Branch of middle suprarenal a.

Left suprarenal v.

Anterior surface

Renal surface

Branch of inferior suprarenal a.

A Left gland.

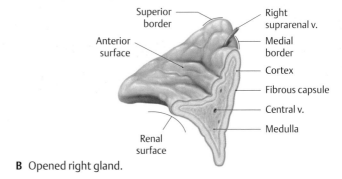

Superior border

Anterior surface

Renal surface

Right suprarenal v.

Medial border

Cortex

Fibrous capsule

Central v.

Medulla

B Opened right gland.

Fig. 13.42 **Kidneys and suprarenal glands in the retroperitoneum**

Anterior view. Both the kidneys and suprarenal glands are retroperitoneal.

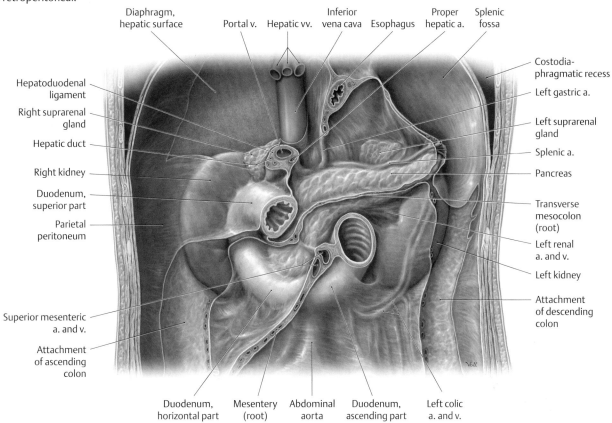

Diaphragm, hepatic surface — Portal v. — Hepatic vv. — Inferior vena cava — Esophagus — Proper hepatic a. — Splenic fossa

Hepatoduodenal ligament

Right suprarenal gland

Hepatic duct

Right kidney

Duodenum, superior part

Parietal peritoneum

Superior mesenteric a. and v.

Attachment of ascending colon

Costodia- phragmatic recess

Left gastric a.

Left suprarenal gland

Splenic a.

Pancreas

Transverse mesocolon (root)

Left renal a. and v.

Left kidney

Attachment of descending colon

Duodenum, horizontal part — Mesentery (root) — Abdominal aorta — Duodenum, ascending part — Left colic a. and v.

A *Removed:* Intraperitoneal organs, along with portions of the ascending and descending colon.

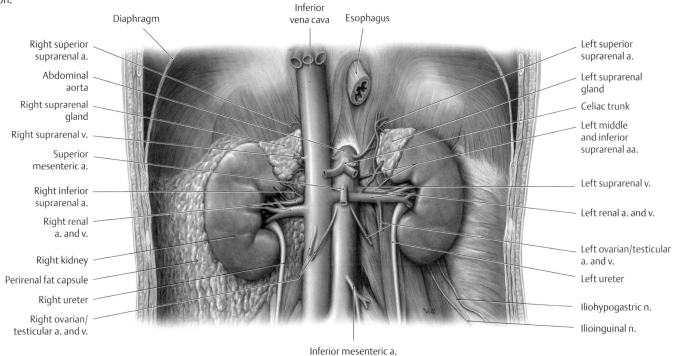

Diaphragm — Inferior vena cava — Esophagus

Right superior suprarenal a.

Abdominal aorta

Right suprarenal gland

Right suprarenal v.

Superior mesenteric a.

Right inferior suprarenal a.

Right renal a. and v.

Right kidney

Perirenal fat capsule

Right ureter

Right ovarian/ testicular a. and v.

Left superior suprarenal a.

Left suprarenal gland

Celiac trunk

Left middle and inferior suprarenal aa.

Left suprarenal v.

Left renal a. and v.

Left ovarian/testicular a. and v.

Left ureter

Iliohypogastric n.

Ilioinguinal n.

Inferior mesenteric a.

B *Removed:* Peritoneum, spleen, and gastro- intestinal organs, along with fat capsule (left side). *Retracted:* Esophagus.

Kidneys & Suprarenal Glands: Features

Fig. 13.43 Right kidney and suprarenal gland
Anterior view. *Removed:* Perirenal fat capsule.
Retracted: Inferior vena cava.

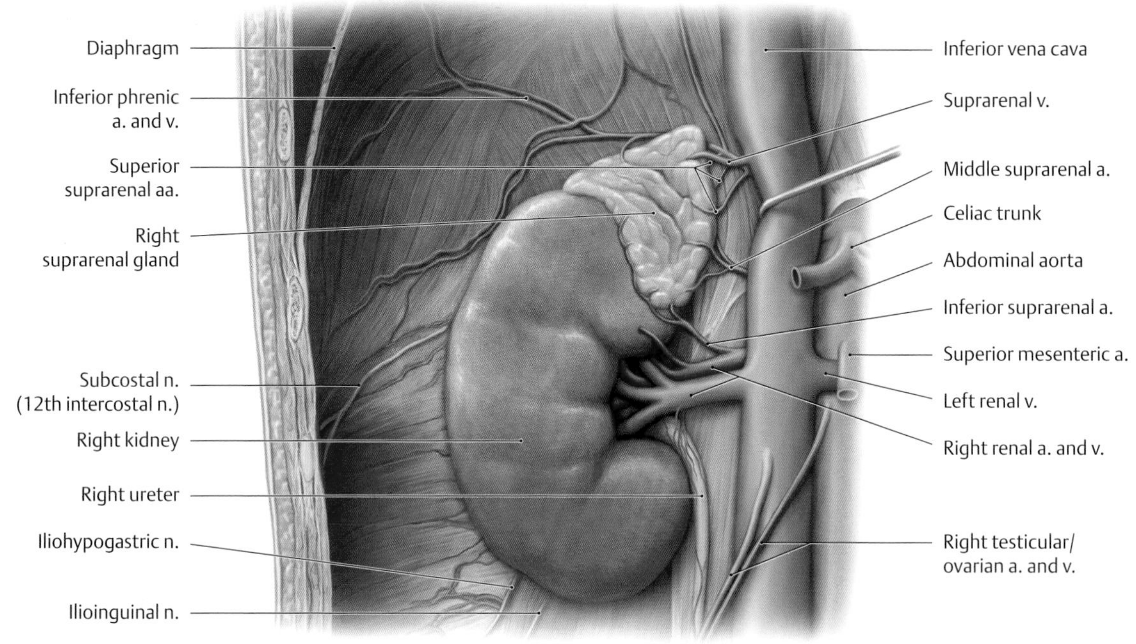

Diaphragm
Inferior phrenic a. and v.
Superior suprarenal aa.
Right suprarenal gland
Subcostal n. (12th intercostal n.)
Right kidney
Right ureter
Iliohypogastric n.
Ilioinguinal n.
Inferior vena cava
Suprarenal v.
Middle suprarenal a.
Celiac trunk
Abdominal aorta
Inferior suprarenal a.
Superior mesenteric a.
Left renal v.
Right renal a. and v.
Right testicular/ ovarian a. and v.

Fig. 13.45 Kidney: Structure
Right kidney with suprarenal gland.

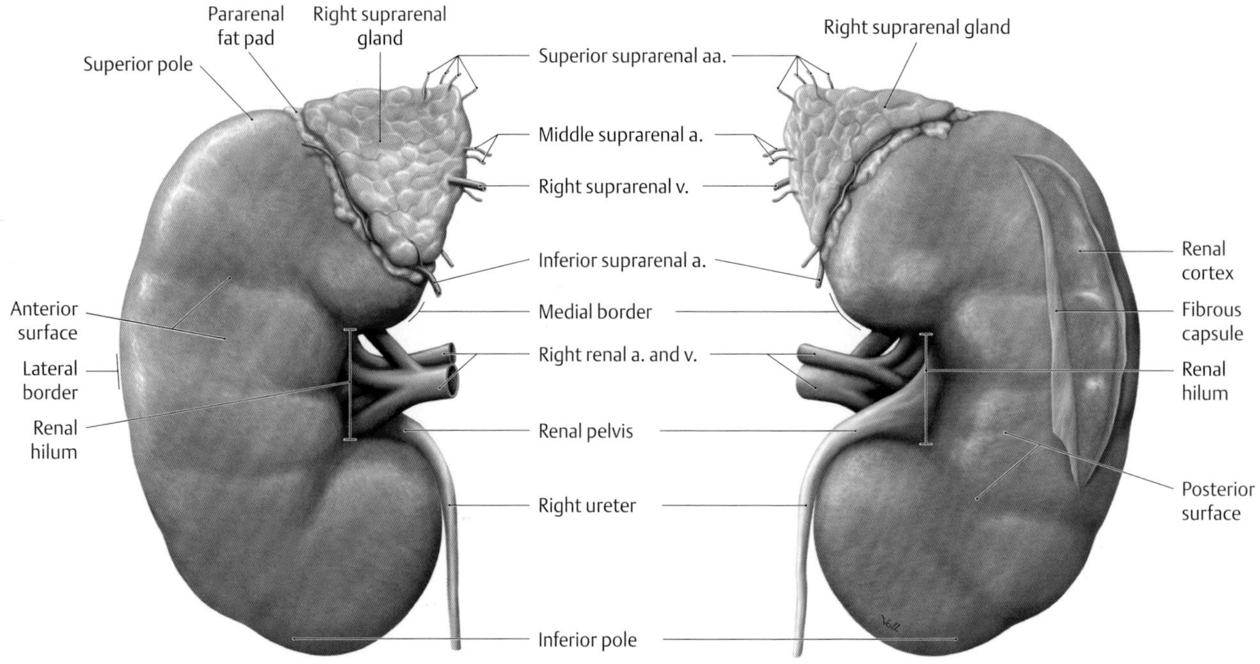

Pararenal fat pad
Right suprarenal gland
Superior pole
Superior suprarenal aa.
Middle suprarenal a.
Right suprarenal v.
Inferior suprarenal a.
Medial border
Right renal a. and v.
Renal pelvis
Right ureter
Inferior pole
Anterior surface
Lateral border
Renal hilum
Right suprarenal gland
Renal cortex
Fibrous capsule
Renal hilum
Posterior surface

A Anterior view.

B Posterior view.

Fig. 13.44 Left kidney and suprarenal gland

Anterior view. *Removed:* Perirenal fat capsule.
Retracted: Pancreas.

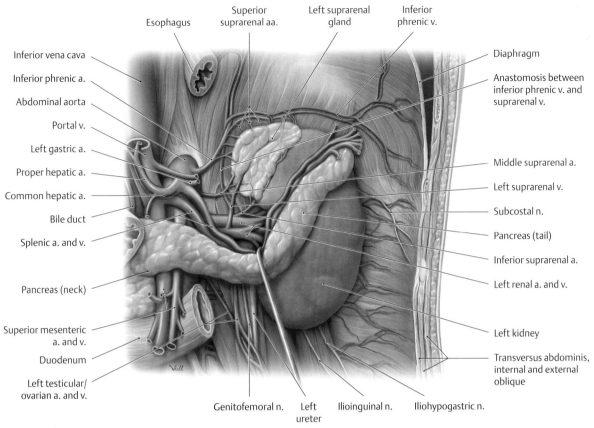

C Posterior view with upper half partially removed.

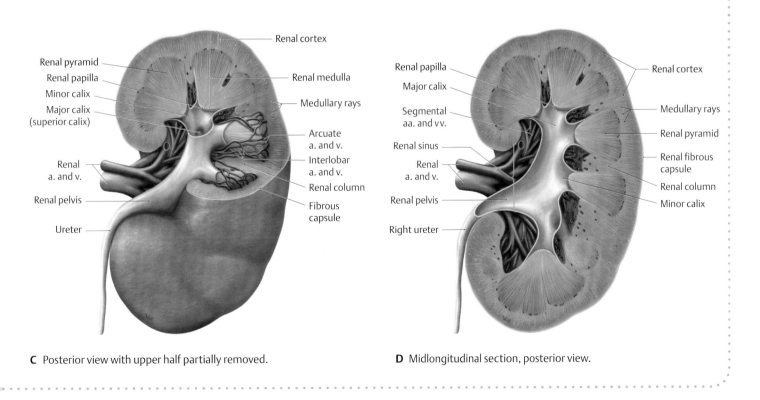

D Midlongitudinal section, posterior view.

Ureter

Fig. 13.46 Ureters: Location
Anterior view.

The ureters cross the common iliac artery at its bifurcation into the external and internal iliac arteries.

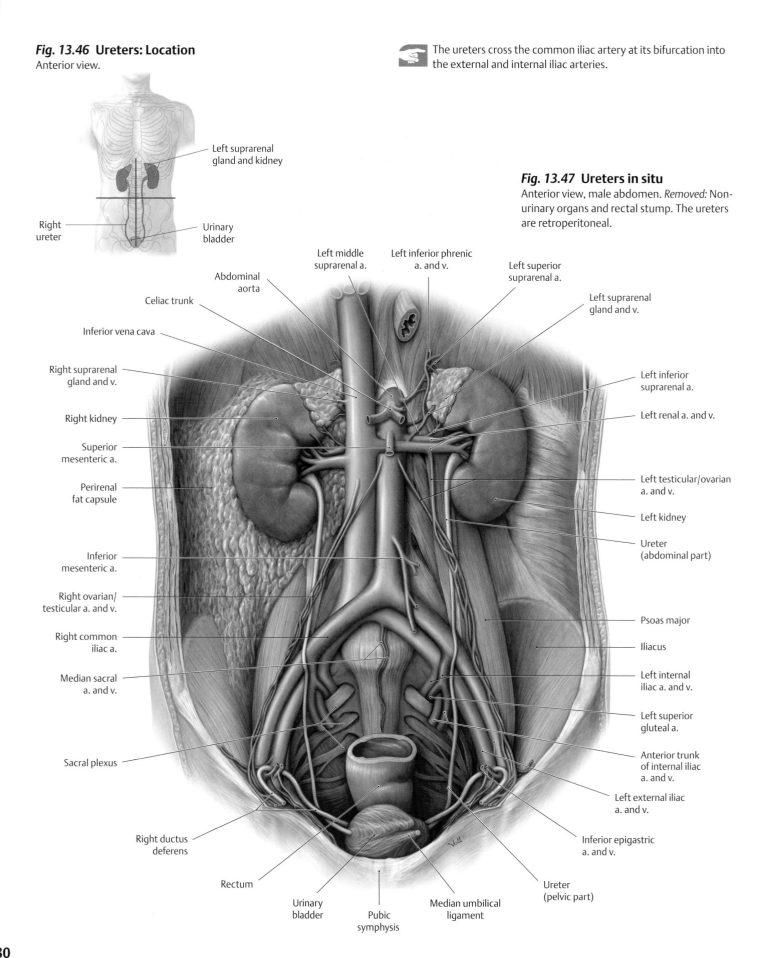

Fig. 13.47 Ureters in situ
Anterior view, male abdomen. *Removed:* Non-urinary organs and rectal stump. The ureters are retroperitoneal.

Left suprarenal gland and kidney

Right ureter

Urinary bladder

Left middle suprarenal a.

Abdominal aorta

Celiac trunk

Inferior vena cava

Right suprarenal gland and v.

Right kidney

Superior mesenteric a.

Perirenal fat capsule

Inferior mesenteric a.

Right ovarian/ testicular a. and v.

Right common iliac a.

Median sacral a. and v.

Sacral plexus

Right ductus deferens

Rectum

Urinary bladder

Pubic symphysis

Left inferior phrenic a. and v.

Left superior suprarenal a.

Left suprarenal gland and v.

Left inferior suprarenal a.

Left renal a. and v.

Left testicular/ovarian a. and v.

Left kidney

Ureter (abdominal part)

Psoas major

Iliacus

Left internal iliac a. and v.

Left superior gluteal a.

Anterior trunk of internal iliac a. and v.

Left external iliac a. and v.

Inferior epigastric a. and v.

Ureter (pelvic part)

Median umbilical ligament

Fig. 13.48 **Ureter in the male pelvis**
Superior view.

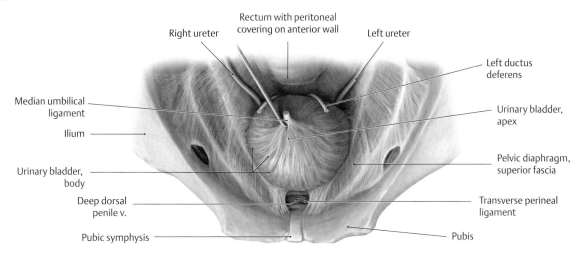

Right ureter

Rectum with peritoneal covering on anterior wall

Left ureter

Left ductus deferens

Median umbilical ligament

Ilium

Urinary bladder, body

Deep dorsal penile v.

Pubic symphysis

Urinary bladder, apex

Pelvic diaphragm, superior fascia

Transverse perineal ligament

Pubis

Fig. 13.49 **Ureter in the female pelvis**
Superior view.

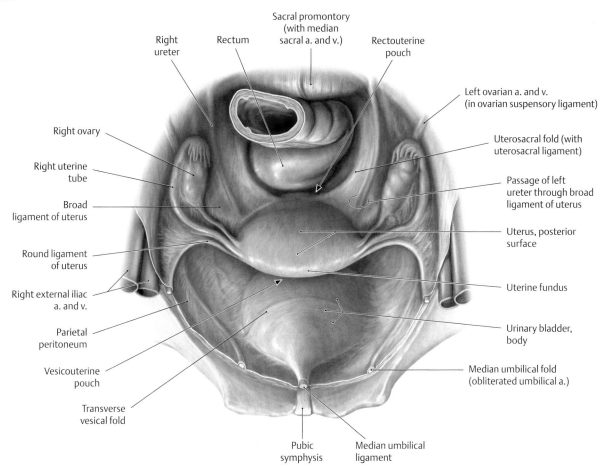

Right ureter

Rectum

Sacral promontory (with median sacral a. and v.)

Rectouterine pouch

Left ovarian a. and v. (in ovarian suspensory ligament)

Right ovary

Right uterine tube

Broad ligament of uterus

Round ligament of uterus

Right external iliac a. and v.

Parietal peritoneum

Vesicouterine pouch

Transverse vesical fold

Pubic symphysis

Median umbilical ligament

Uterosacral fold (with uterosacral ligament)

Passage of left ureter through broad ligament of uterus

Uterus, posterior surface

Uterine fundus

Urinary bladder, body

Median umbilical fold (obliterated umbilical a.)

181

Urinary Bladder

Fig. 13.50 Male urinary bladder

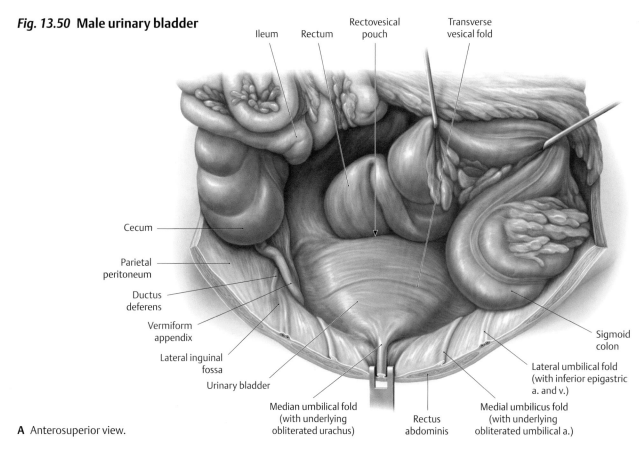

Ileum

Rectum

Rectovesical pouch

Transverse vesical fold

Cecum

Parietal peritoneum

Ductus deferens

Vermiform appendix

Lateral inguinal fossa

Urinary bladder

Median umbilical fold (with underlying obliterated urachus)

Rectus abdominis

Medial umbilicus fold (with underlying obliterated umbilical a.)

Lateral umbilical fold (with inferior epigastric a. and v.)

Sigmoid colon

A Anterosuperior view.

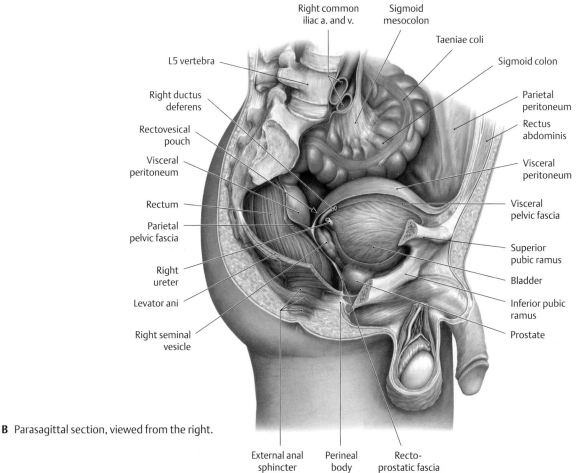

Right common iliac a. and v.

Sigmoid mesocolon

Taeniae coli

Sigmoid colon

L5 vertebra

Right ductus deferens

Rectovesical pouch

Visceral peritoneum

Rectum

Parietal pelvic fascia

Right ureter

Levator ani

Right seminal vesicle

Parietal peritoneum

Rectus abdominis

Visceral peritoneum

Visceral pelvic fascia

Superior pubic ramus

Bladder

Inferior pubic ramus

Prostate

External anal sphincter

Perineal body

Recto-prostatic fascia

B Parasagittal section, viewed from the right.

The urinary bladder is retropubic and retroperitoneal in location.

Fig. 13.51 Female urinary bladder

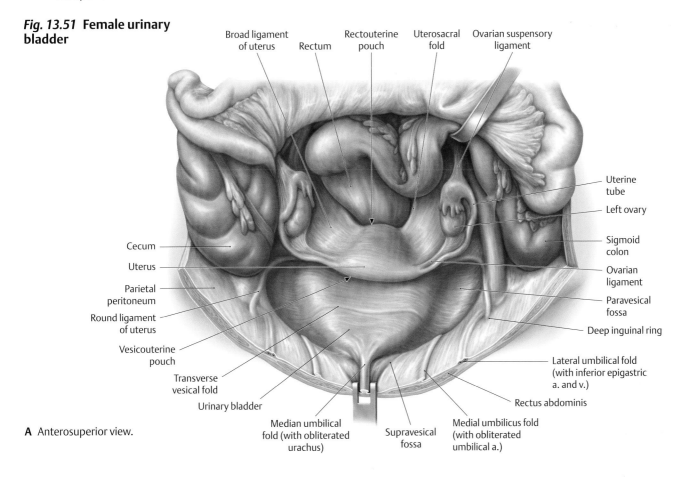

Broad ligament of uterus · Rectum · Rectouterine pouch · Uterosacral fold · Ovarian suspensory ligament

Uterine tube
Left ovary
Sigmoid colon
Ovarian ligament
Paravesical fossa
Deep inguinal ring
Lateral umbilical fold (with inferior epigastric a. and v.)
Rectus abdominis
Medial umbilicus fold (with obliterated umbilical a.)

Cecum
Uterus
Parietal peritoneum
Round ligament of uterus
Vesicouterine pouch
Transverse vesical fold
Urinary bladder
Median umbilical fold (with obliterated urachus)
Supravesical fossa

A Anterosuperior view.

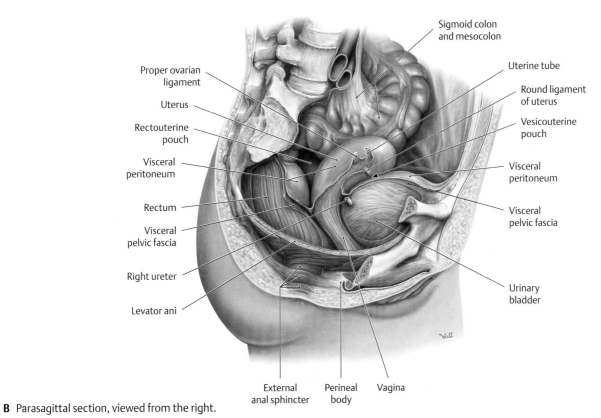

Sigmoid colon and mesocolon
Uterine tube
Round ligament of uterus
Vesicouterine pouch
Visceral peritoneum
Visceral pelvic fascia
Urinary bladder

Proper ovarian ligament
Uterus
Rectouterine pouch
Visceral peritoneum
Rectum
Visceral pelvic fascia
Right ureter
Levator ani

External anal sphincter
Perineal body
Vagina

B Parasagittal section, viewed from the right.

183

Urinary Bladder & Urethra

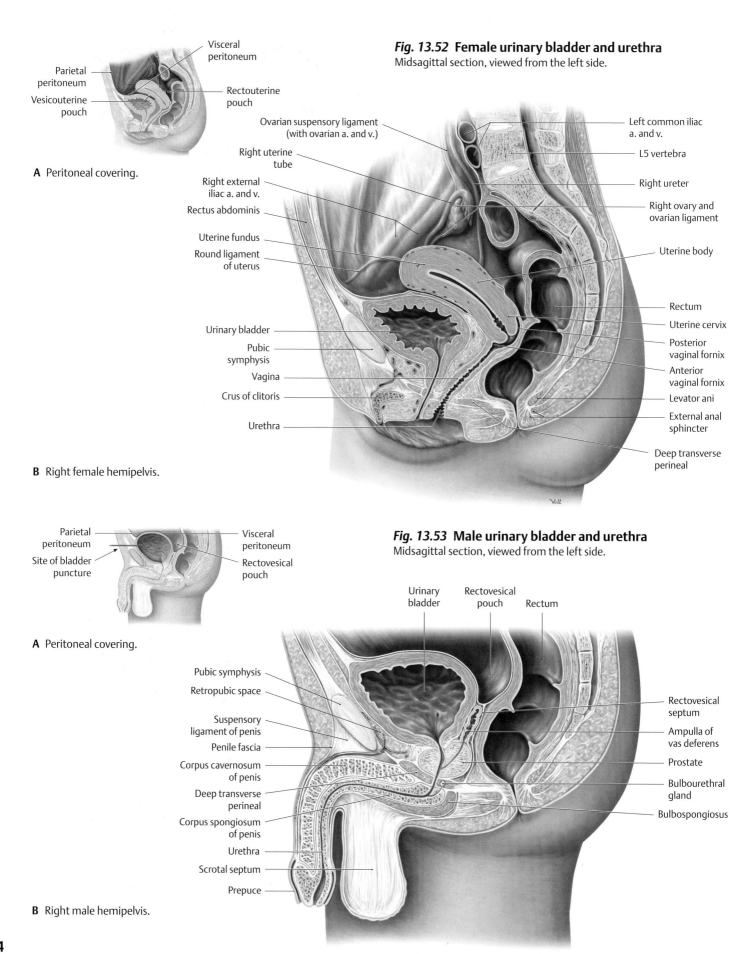

Visceral peritoneum

Parietal peritoneum

Vesicouterine pouch

Rectouterine pouch

A Peritoneal covering.

B Right female hemipelvis.

Fig. 13.52 Female urinary bladder and urethra
Midsagittal section, viewed from the left side.

Ovarian suspensory ligament (with ovarian a. and v.)

Right uterine tube

Right external iliac a. and v.

Rectus abdominis

Uterine fundus

Round ligament of uterus

Urinary bladder

Pubic symphysis

Vagina

Crus of clitoris

Urethra

Left common iliac a. and v.

L5 vertebra

Right ureter

Right ovary and ovarian ligament

Uterine body

Rectum

Uterine cervix

Posterior vaginal fornix

Anterior vaginal fornix

Levator ani

External anal sphincter

Deep transverse perineal

Parietal peritoneum

Site of bladder puncture

Visceral peritoneum

Rectovesical pouch

A Peritoneal covering.

B Right male hemipelvis.

Fig. 13.53 Male urinary bladder and urethra
Midsagittal section, viewed from the left side.

Urinary bladder

Rectovesical pouch

Rectum

Pubic symphysis

Retropubic space

Suspensory ligament of penis

Penile fascia

Corpus cavernosum of penis

Deep transverse perineal

Corpus spongiosum of penis

Urethra

Scrotal septum

Prepuce

Rectovesical septum

Ampulla of vas deferens

Prostate

Bulbourethral gland

Bulbospongiosus

Fig. 13.54 Wall structure
Anterior view of coronal section.

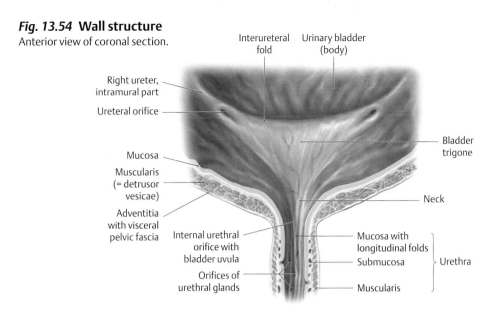

Labels (clockwise):
- Interureteral fold
- Urinary bladder (body)
- Right ureter, intramural part
- Ureteral orifice
- Mucosa
- Muscularis (= detrusor vesicae)
- Adventitia with visceral pelvic fascia
- Internal urethral orifice with bladder uvula
- Orifices of urethral glands
- Bladder trigone
- Neck
- Mucosa with longitudinal folds
- Submucosa
- Muscularis
- Urethra

Fig. 13.55 Urinary bladder and urethra
Anterior view.

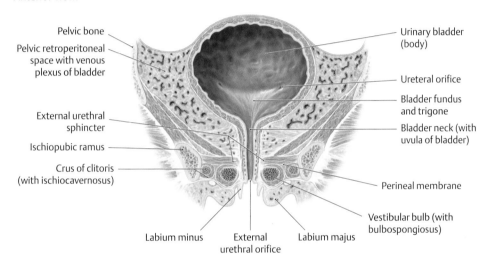

Labels:
- Pelvic bone
- Pelvic retroperitoneal space with venous plexus of bladder
- External urethral sphincter
- Ischiopubic ramus
- Crus of clitoris (with ischiocavernosus)
- Labium minus
- External urethral orifice
- Labium majus
- Urinary bladder (body)
- Ureteral orifice
- Bladder fundus and trigone
- Bladder neck (with uvula of bladder)
- Perineal membrane
- Vestibular bulb (with bulbospongiosus)

A Female pelvis in coronal section.

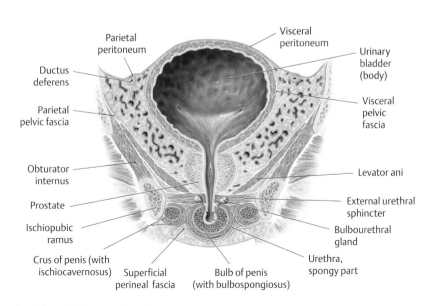

Labels:
- Parietal peritoneum
- Ductus deferens
- Parietal pelvic fascia
- Obturator internus
- Prostate
- Ischiopubic ramus
- Crus of penis (with ischiocavernosus)
- Superficial perineal fascia
- Bulb of penis (with bulbospongiosus)
- Visceral peritoneum
- Urinary bladder (body)
- Visceral pelvic fascia
- Levator ani
- External urethral sphincter
- Bulbourethral gland
- Urethra, spongy part

B Male pelvis in coronal section.

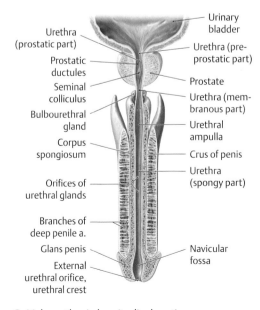

Labels:
- Urethra (prostatic part)
- Prostatic ductules
- Seminal colliculus
- Bulbourethral gland
- Corpus spongiosum
- Orifices of urethral glands
- Branches of deep penile a.
- Glans penis
- External urethral orifice, urethral crest
- Urinary bladder
- Urethra (pre-prostatic part)
- Prostate
- Urethra (membranous part)
- Urethral ampulla
- Crus of penis
- Urethra (spongy part)
- Navicular fossa

C Male urethra in longitudinal section.

Overview of the Genital Organs

 The genital organs can be classified topographically (external versus internal), functionally (Tables 14.1 and 14.2), or ontogenetically (see p. 204).

Table 14.1		Female genital organs	
Organ			**Function**
Internal genitalia	Ovary		Germ cell and hormone production
	Uterine (fallopian) tube		Site of conception and transport organ for zygote
	Uterus		Organ of incubation and parturition
	Vagina (upper portion)		Organ of copulation and parturition
External genitalia	Vulva	Vagina (vestibule)	
		Labia majora and minora	Copulatory organ
		Clitoris	
		Greater and lesser vestibular glands	Production of secretions
		Mons pubis	Protection of the pubic bone

Fig. 14.1 **Female genital organs**

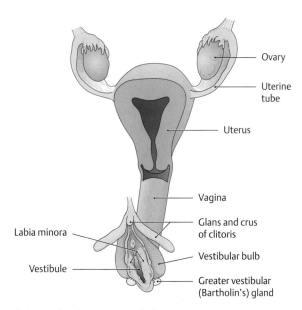

A Internal and external genitalia.

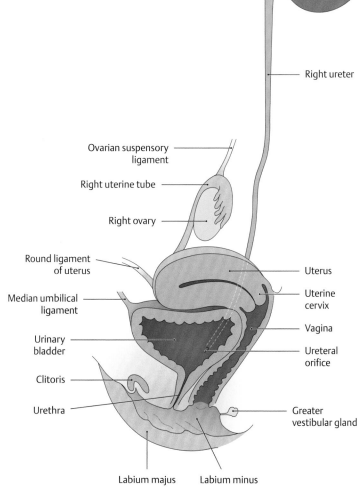

B Urogenital system. *Note:* The female urinary and genital tracts are functionally separate, though topographically close.

Table 14.2 Male genital organs

	Organ		Function
Internal genitalia	Testis		Germ cell and hormone production
	Epididymis		Reservoir for sperm
	Ductus deferens		Transport organ for sperm
	Accessory sex glands	Prostate	Production of secretions (semen)
		Seminal vesicles	
		Bulbourethral gland	
External genitalia	Penis		Copulatory and urinary organ
	Urethra		Urinary organ and transport organ for sperm
	Scrotum		Protection of testis
	Coverings of the testis		

Fig. 14.2 Male genital organs

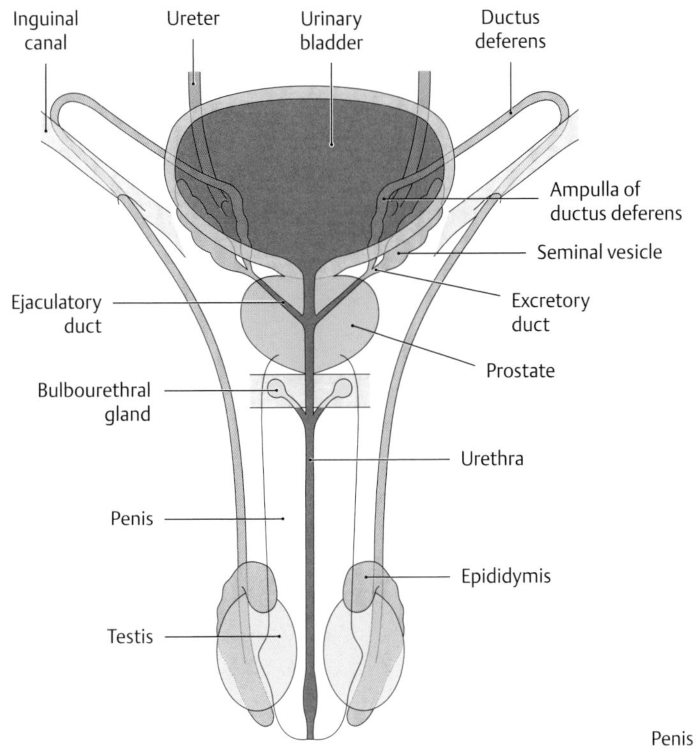

A Seminiferous structures.

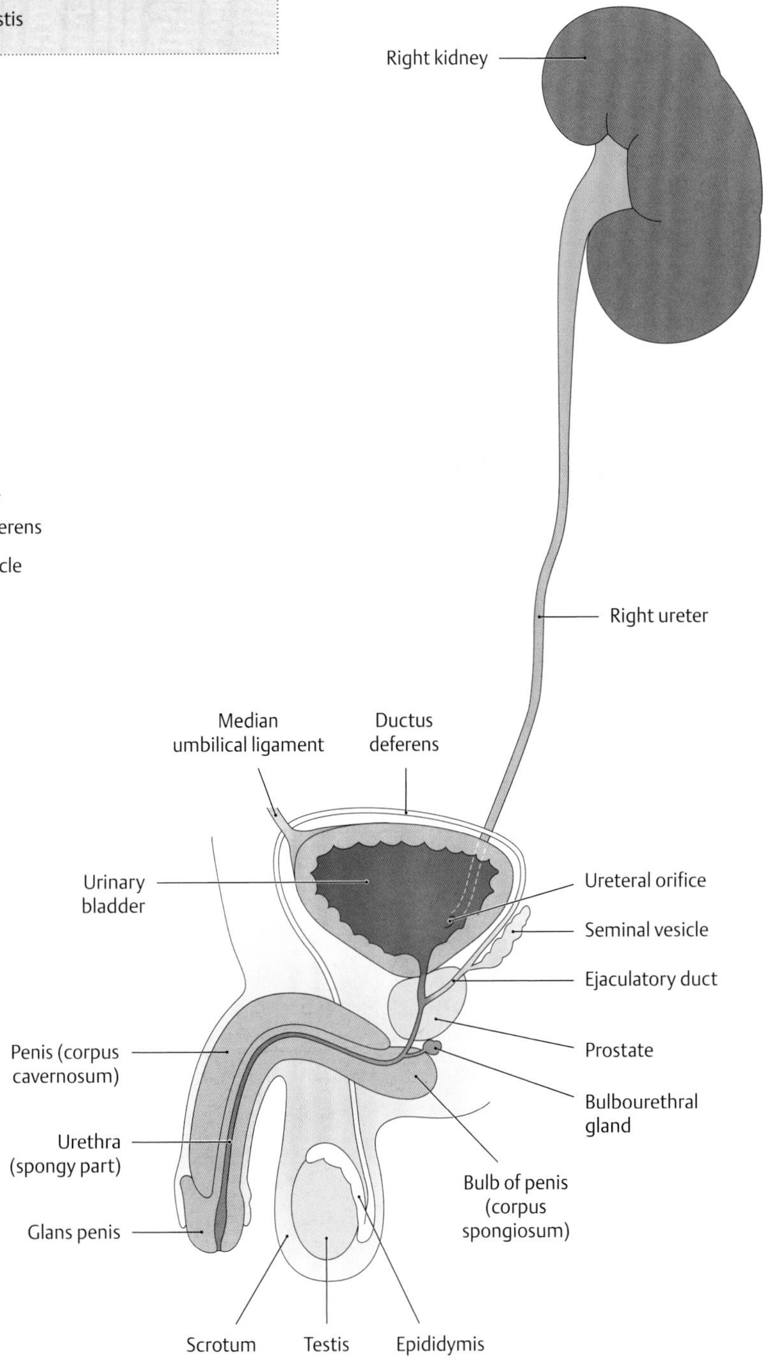

B Urogenital system. *Note:* The male urethra serves as a common urinary and genital passage.

Uterus & Ovaries

Fig. 14.3 Female internal genitalia

The uterus and ovaries are suspended by the mesovarium and mesometrium (portions of the broad ligament).

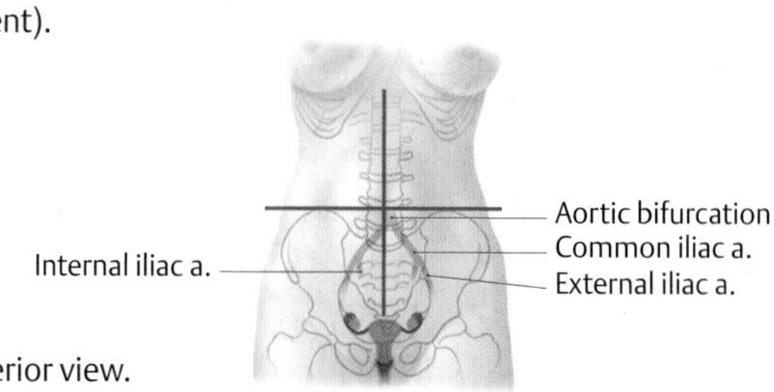

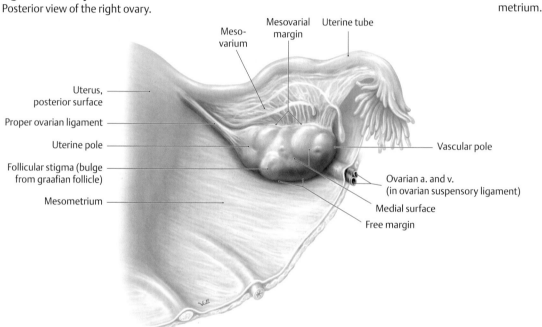

A Location. Anterior view.

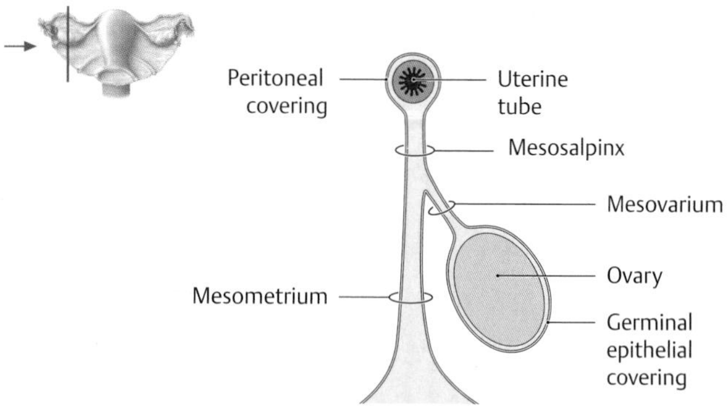

Internal iliac a.
Aortic bifurcation
Common iliac a.
External iliac a.

Peritoneal covering
Uterine tube
Mesosalpinx
Mesovarium
Ovary
Mesometrium
Germinal epithelial covering

B Mesenteries. Sagittal section. The broad ligament of the uterus is a combination of the mesosalpinx, mesovarium, amd mesometrium.

Fig. 14.4 Ovary

Posterior view of the right ovary.

Meso-varium
Mesovarial margin
Uterine tube
Uterus, posterior surface
Proper ovarian ligament
Uterine pole
Follicular stigma (bulge from graafian follicle)
Mesometrium
Vascular pole
Ovarian a. and v. (in ovarian suspensory ligament)
Medial surface
Free margin

Fig. 14.5 Curvature of the uterus

Midsagittal section, left lateral view. The position of the uterus can be described in terms of flexion (①) and version (②).

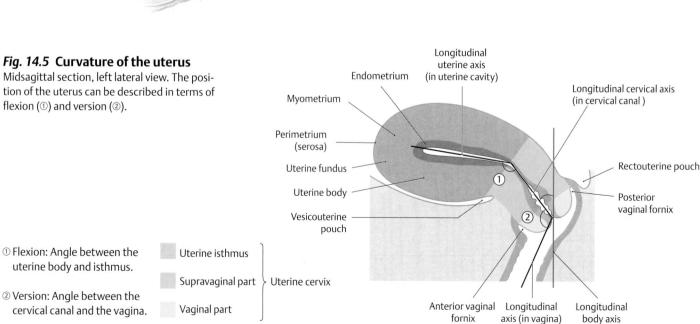

Longitudinal uterine axis (in uterine cavity)
Endometrium
Myometrium
Perimetrium (serosa)
Uterine fundus
Uterine body
Vesicouterine pouch
Longitudinal cervical axis (in cervical canal)
Rectouterine pouch
Posterior vaginal fornix
Anterior vaginal fornix
Longitudinal axis (in vagina)
Longitudinal body axis

① Flexion: Angle between the uterine body and isthmus.

② Version: Angle between the cervical canal and the vagina.

Uterine isthmus
Supravaginal part } Uterine cervix
Vaginal part

Fig. 14.6 **Uterus and uterine tube**

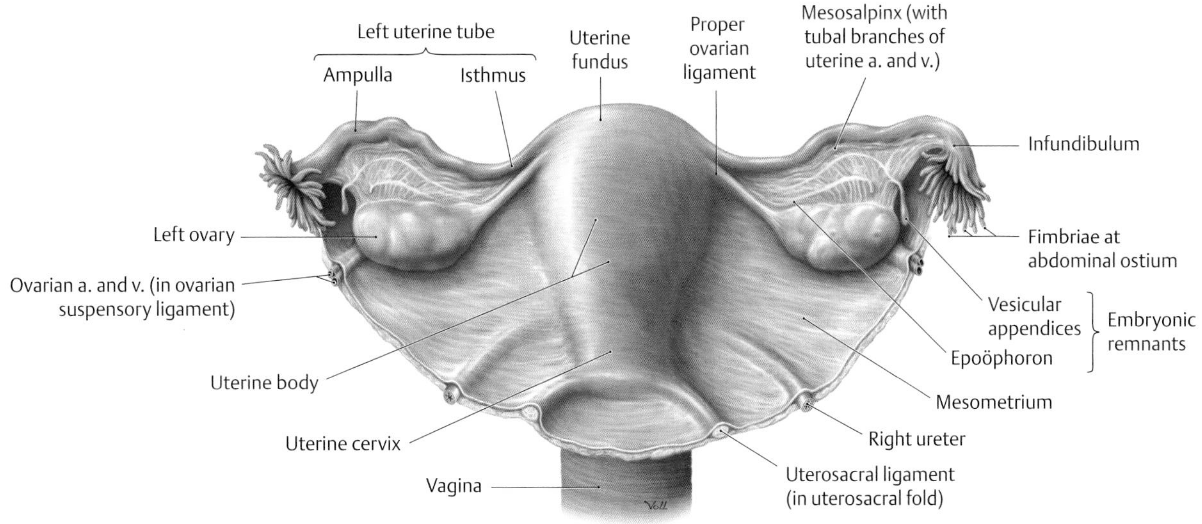

A Posterosuperior view.

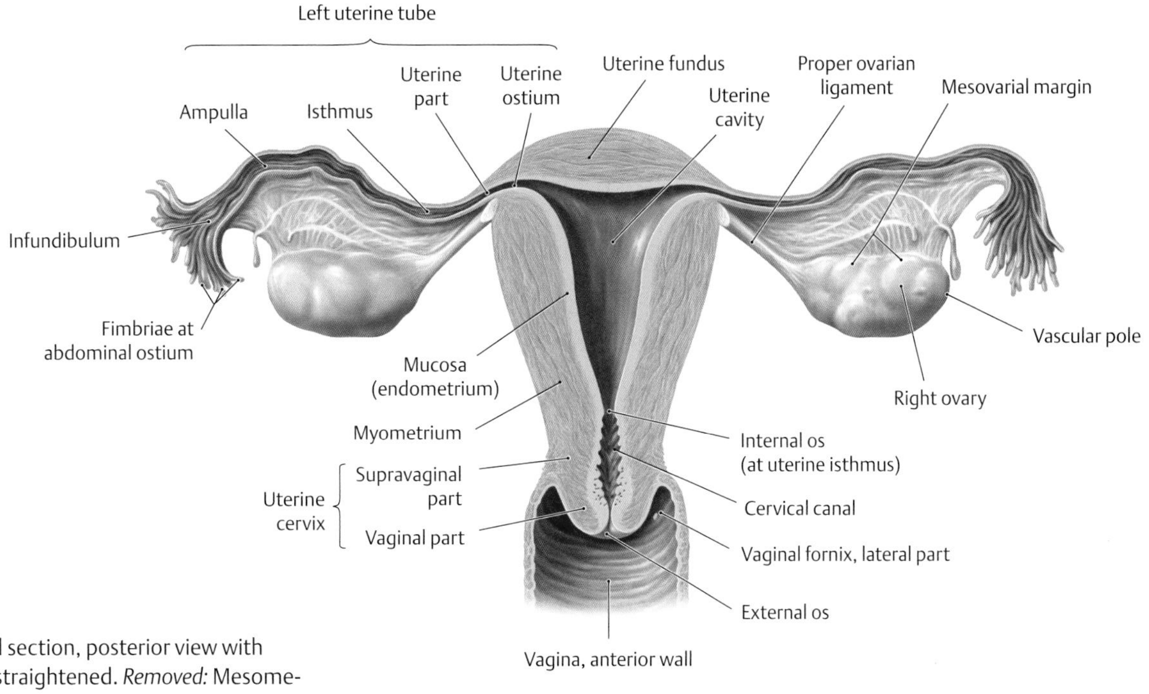

B Coronal section, posterior view with uterus straightened. *Removed:* Mesometrium.

Clinical

Ectopic pregnancy

After fertilization, the ovum usually implants in the wall of the uterine cavity. However, it may become implanted at other sites (e.g., the uterine tube or even the peritoneal cavity). Tubal pregnancies, the most common type of ectopic pregnancy, pose the risk of tubal wall rupture and potentially life-threatening bleeding into the peritoneal cavity. Tubal pregnancies are promoted by adhesion of the tubal mucosa, mostly due to inflammation.

Vagina

Fig. 14.7 Location
Midsagittal section, left lateral view.

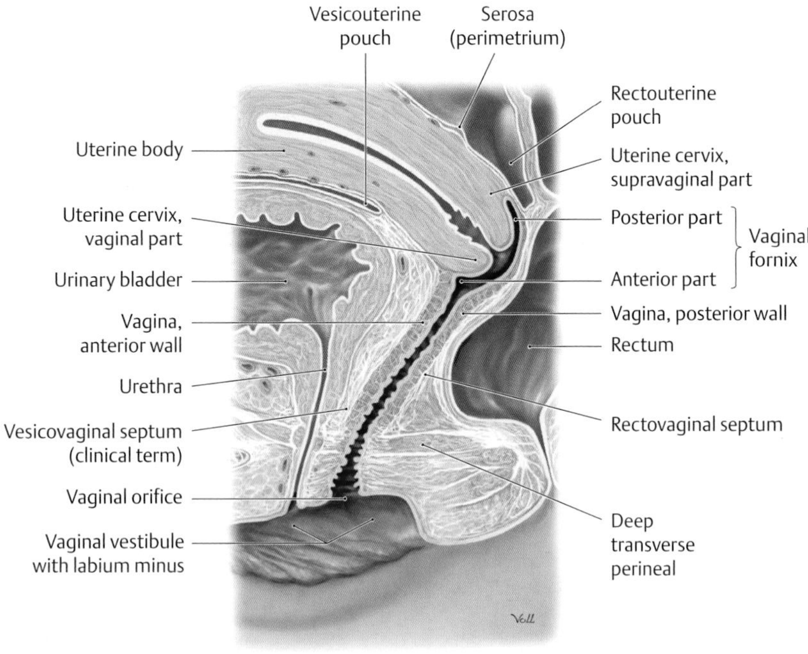

Vesicouterine pouch

Serosa (perimetrium)

Rectouterine pouch

Uterine cervix, supravaginal part

Uterine body

Posterior part ⎫
Anterior part ⎬ Vaginal fornix

Uterine cervix, vaginal part

Urinary bladder

Vagina, posterior wall

Vagina, anterior wall

Rectum

Urethra

Rectovaginal septum

Vesicovaginal septum (clinical term)

Vaginal orifice

Deep transverse perineal

Vaginal vestibule with labium minus

Fig. 14.8 Structure
Posteriorly angled coronal section, posterior view.

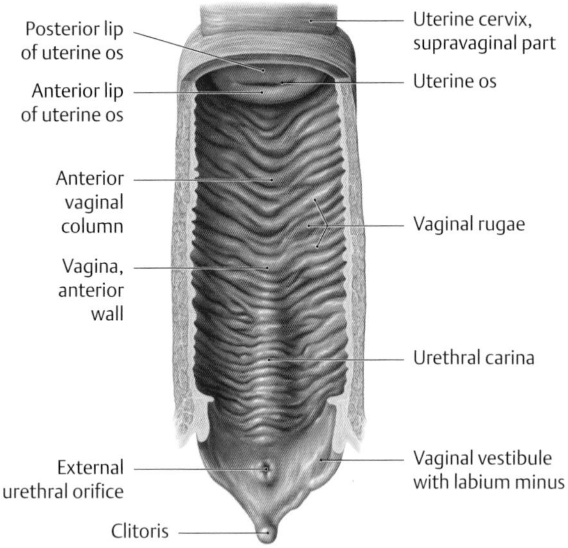

Posterior lip of uterine os

Uterine cervix, supravaginal part

Anterior lip of uterine os

Uterine os

Anterior vaginal column

Vaginal rugae

Vagina, anterior wall

Urethral carina

External urethral orifice

Vaginal vestibule with labium minus

Clitoris

Fig. 14.9 Uterine cervix: Transverse section
Inferior view.

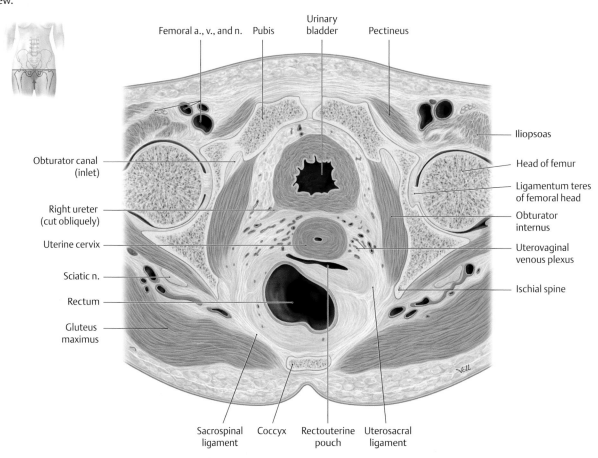

Femoral a., v., and n.   Pubis   Urinary bladder   Pectineus

Obturator canal (inlet)

Iliopsoas

Head of femur

Ligamentum teres of femoral head

Right ureter (cut obliquely)

Obturator internus

Uterine cervix

Uterovaginal venous plexus

Sciatic n.

Ischial spine

Rectum

Gluteus maximus

Sacrospinal ligament   Coccyx   Rectouterine pouch   Uterosacral ligament

Fig. 14.10 Female genital organs: Coronal section

Anterior view. The vagina is both pelvic and perineal in location. It is also retroperitoneal.

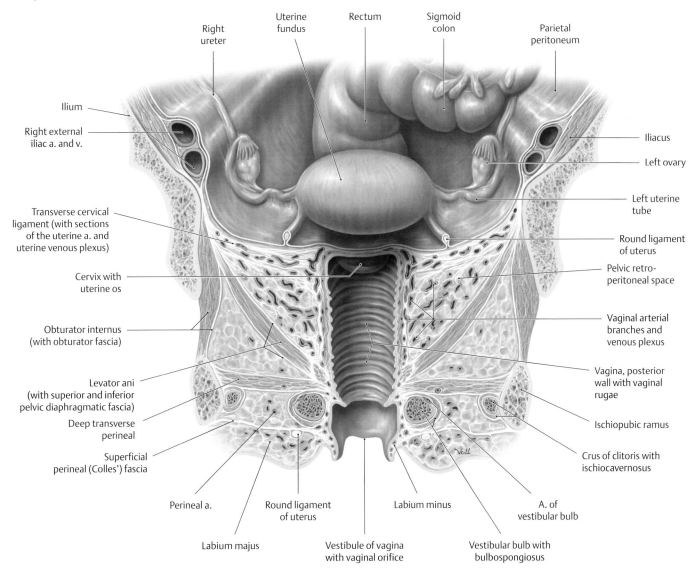

Fig. 14.11 Vagina: Location in the pelvic floor

Inferior view.

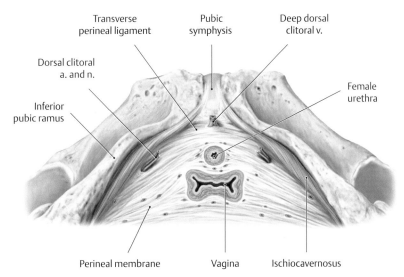

Female External Genitalia

Fig. 14.12 Female external genitalia
Lithotomy position with labia minora separated.

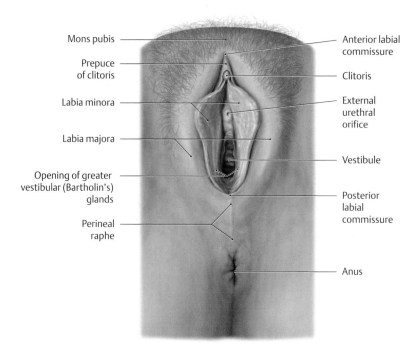

Mons pubis

Prepuce
of clitoris

Labia minora

Labia majora

Opening of greater
vestibular (Bartholin's)
glands

Perineal
raphe

Anterior labial
commissure

Clitoris

External
urethral
orifice

Vestibule

Posterior
labial
commissure

Anus

Fig. 14.13 Vestibule and vestibular glands
Lithotomy position with labia separated.

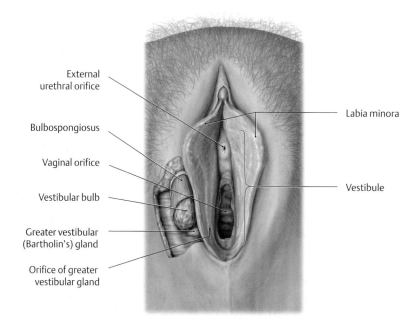

External
urethral orifice

Bulbospongiosus

Vaginal orifice

Vestibular bulb

Greater vestibular
(Bartholin's) gland

Orifice of greater
vestibular gland

Labia minora

Vestibule

Fig. 14.14 **Erectile muscles and tissue: Female**

Lithotomy position. *Removed:* Labia, skin, and perineal membrane; erectile muscles (left side).

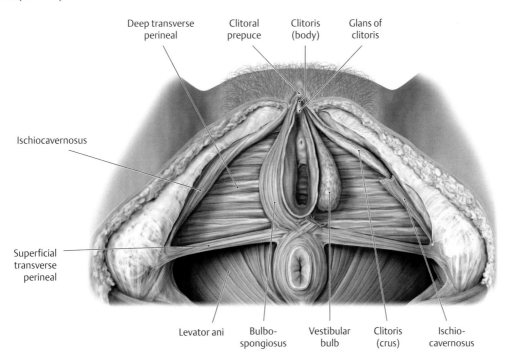

Episiotomy

Episiotomy is a common obstetric procedure used to enlarge the birth canal during the expulsive stage of labor. The procedure is generally used to expedite the delivery of a baby at risk for hypoxia during the expulsive stage. Alternately, if the perineal skin turns white (indicating diminished blood flow), there is imminent danger of perineal laceration, and an episiotomy is often performed. More lateral incisions gain more room, but they are more difficult to repair.

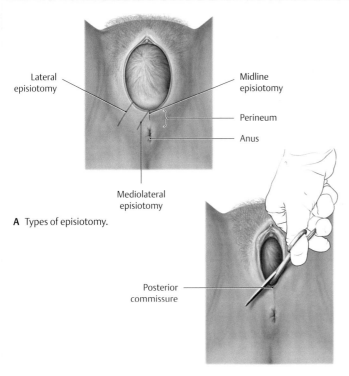

A Types of episiotomy.

B Mediolateral episiotomy at height of contraction.

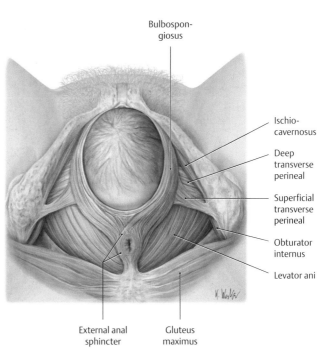

C Pelvic floor with crowning of fetal head.

Neurovasculature of the Female Genitalia

Fig. 14.15 **Nerves of the female perineum and genitalia**

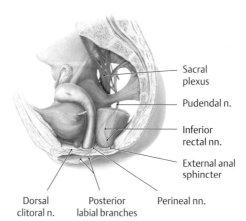

A Nerve supply to the female external genitalia. Lesser pelvis, left lateral view.

Sacral plexus

Pudendal n.

Inferior rectal nn.

External anal sphincter

Dorsal clitoral n.

Posterior labial branches

Perineal nn.

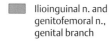
Ilioinguinal n. and genitofemoral n., genital branch

Pudendal n.

Posterior femoral cutaneous n.

Middle cluneal nn.

Superior cluneal nn.

Inferior cluneal nn.

Anococcygeal nn.

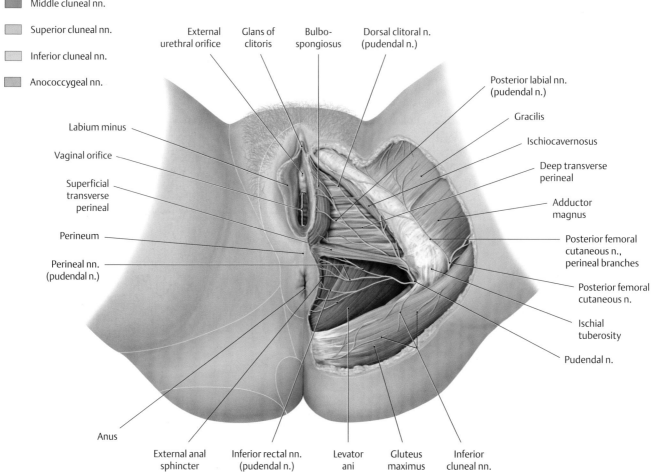

External urethral orifice

Glans of clitoris

Bulbo-spongiosus

Dorsal clitoral n. (pudendal n.)

Posterior labial nn. (pudendal n.)

Gracilis

Ischiocavernosus

Deep transverse perineal

Adductor magnus

Labium minus

Vaginal orifice

Superficial transverse perineal

Perineum

Perineal nn. (pudendal n.)

Posterior femoral cutaneous n., perineal branches

Posterior femoral cutaneous n.

Ischial tuberosity

Pudendal n.

Anus

External anal sphincter

Inferior rectal nn. (pudendal n.)

Levator ani

Gluteus maximus

Inferior cluneal nn.

B Sensory innervation of the female perineum. Lithotomy position.

Fig. 14.16 Blood vessels of the female external genitalia

Inferior view.

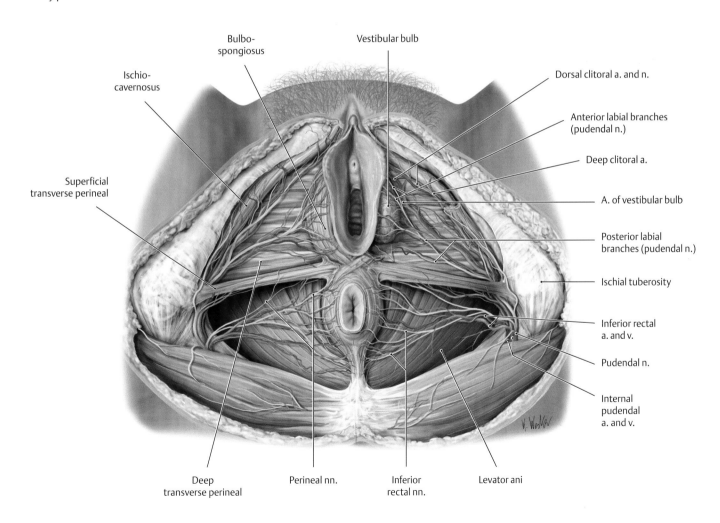

Dorsal clitoral a.

Deep clitoral a.

A. of vestibular bulb

Posterior labial branches

Internal pudendal a.

Vestibular bulb

Superficial transverse perineal

Perineal a.

Inferior rectal a.

A Arterial supply.

Crus of clitoris

Deep clitoral vv.

V. of vestibular bulb

Perineal vv.

Inferior rectal vv.

Deep dorsal clitoral v.

Venous plexus of vestibular bulb

Posterior labial vv.

Internal pudendal v.

B Venous drainage.

Fig. 14.17 Neurovasculature of the female perineum

Lithotomy position.

Bulbo-spongiosus

Ischio-cavernosus

Superficial transverse perineal

Vestibular bulb

Dorsal clitoral a. and n.

Anterior labial branches (pudendal n.)

Deep clitoral a.

A. of vestibular bulb

Posterior labial branches (pudendal n.)

Ischial tuberosity

Inferior rectal a. and v.

Pudendal n.

Internal pudendal a. and v.

Deep transverse perineal

Perineal nn.

Inferior rectal nn.

Levator ani

Penis, Scrotum & Spermatic Cord

Fig. 14.18 Penis, scrotum, and spermatic cord
Anterior view. *Removed:* Skin over the scrotum and spermatic cord.

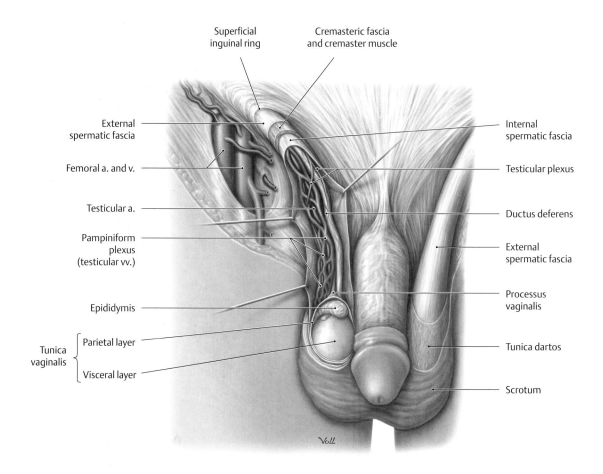

Superficial inguinal ring

Cremasteric fascia and cremaster muscle

External spermatic fascia

Femoral a. and v.

Testicular a.

Pampiniform plexus (testicular vv.)

Epididymis

Tunica vaginalis { Parietal layer / Visceral layer }

Internal spermatic fascia

Testicular plexus

Ductus deferens

External spermatic fascia

Processus vaginalis

Tunica dartos

Scrotum

Fig. 14.19 Spermatic cord: Contents
Cross section.

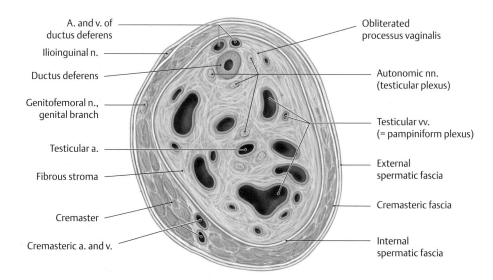

A. and v. of ductus deferens

Ilioinguinal n.

Ductus deferens

Genitofemoral n., genital branch

Testicular a.

Fibrous stroma

Cremaster

Cremasteric a. and v.

Obliterated processus vaginalis

Autonomic nn. (testicular plexus)

Testicular vv. (= pampiniform plexus)

External spermatic fascia

Cremasteric fascia

Internal spermatic fascia

Fig. 14.20 Penis

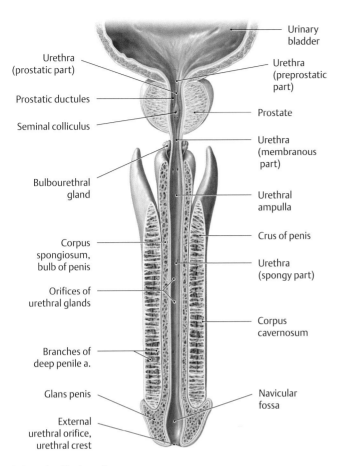

Urinary bladder

Urethra (prostatic part)

Prostatic ductules

Seminal colliculus

Urethra (preprostatic part)

Prostate

Urethra (membranous part)

Bulbourethral gland

Urethral ampulla

Crus of penis

Corpus spongiosum, bulb of penis

Urethra (spongy part)

Orifices of urethral glands

Corpus cavernosum

Branches of deep penile a.

Glans penis

Navicular fossa

External urethral orifice, urethral crest

A Longitudinal section.

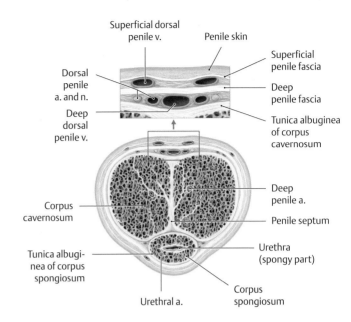

Superficial dorsal penile v.

Penile skin

Dorsal penile a. and n.

Superficial penile fascia

Deep dorsal penile v.

Deep penile fascia

Tunica albuginea of corpus cavernosum

Corpus cavernosum

Deep penile a.

Penile septum

Tunica albuginea of corpus spongiosum

Urethra (spongy part)

Urethral a.

Corpus spongiosum

B Cross section through the shaft of the penis.

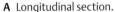

Pubic symphysis

Dorsal penile a. and n.

Deep dorsal penile v.

Corpus cavernosum

Deep penile a.

Urethra (spongy part)

Bulb of penis, corpus spongiosum

Bulbo-spongiosus

Urethral a.

C Cross section through the root of the penis.

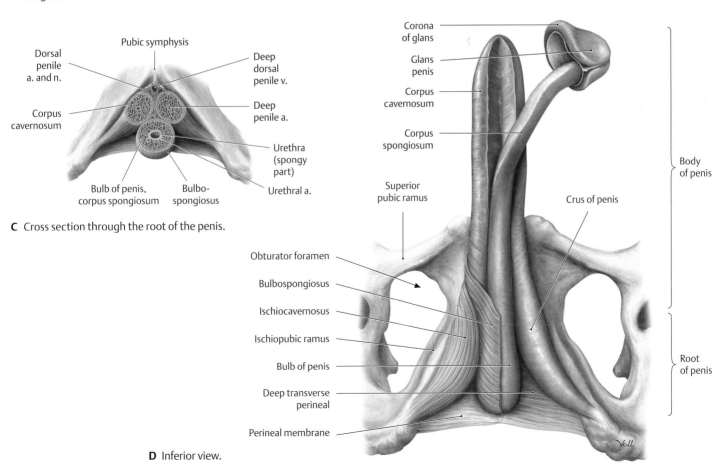

Corona of glans

Glans penis

Corpus cavernosum

Corpus spongiosum

Superior pubic ramus

Crus of penis

Body of penis

Obturator foramen

Bulbospongiosus

Ischiocavernosus

Ischiopubic ramus

Bulb of penis

Deep transverse perineal

Perineal membrane

Root of penis

D Inferior view.

197

Testis & Epididymis

***Fig. 14.21* Testis and epididymis**
Left lateral view.

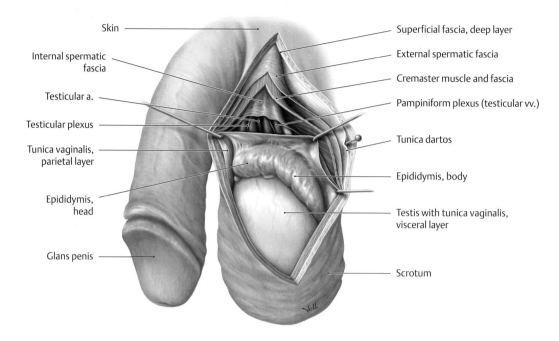

A Testis and epididymis in situ.

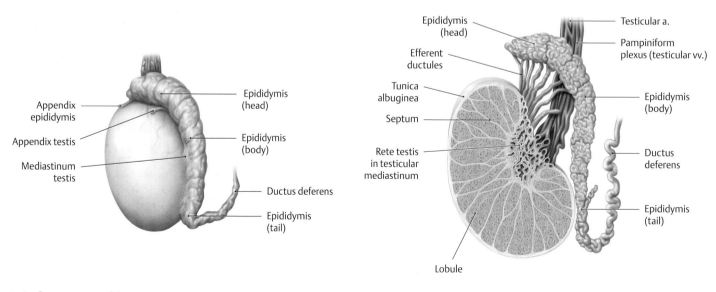

B Surface anatomy of the
testis and epididymis.

C Sagittal section.

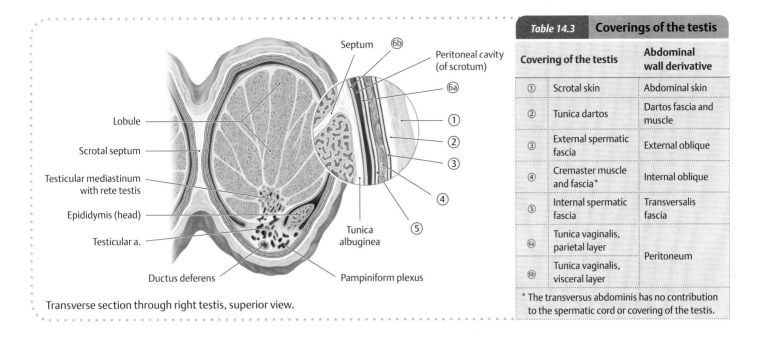

Transverse section through right testis, superior view.

Table 14.3	**Coverings of the testis**	
Covering of the testis		**Abdominal wall derivative**
①	Scrotal skin	Abdominal skin
②	Tunica dartos	Dartos fascia and muscle
③	External spermatic fascia	External oblique
④	Cremaster muscle and fascia*	Internal oblique
⑤	Internal spermatic fascia	Transversalis fascia
⑥a	Tunica vaginalis, parietal layer	Peritoneum
⑥b	Tunica vaginalis, visceral layer	

* The transversus abdominis has no contribution to the spermatic cord or covering of the testis.

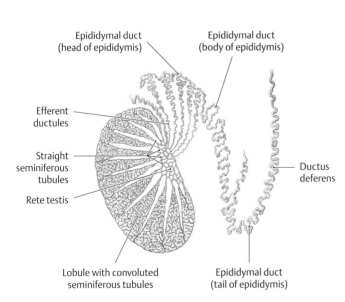

D Seminiferous tubules.

Fig. 14.22 **Blood vessels of the testis**
Left lateral view.

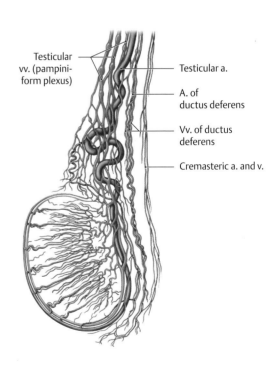

Male Accessory Sex Glands

Fig. 14.23 Accessory sex glands

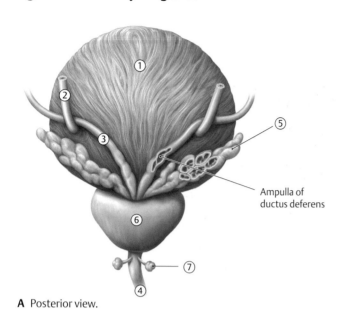

① Urinary bladder	⑤ Seminal vesicle
② Ureter (spongy part)	⑥ Prostate
③ Ductus deferens	⑦ Bulbourethral gland
④ Urethra	

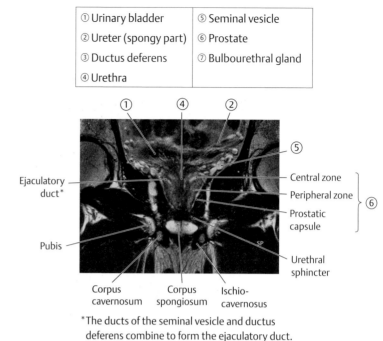

Ejaculatory duct*

Pubis

Central zone

Peripheral zone

Prostatic capsule

⑥

Urethral sphincter

Corpus cavernosum

Corpus spongiosum

Ischio-cavernosus

*The ducts of the seminal vesicle and ductus deferens combine to form the ejaculatory duct.

Ampulla of ductus deferens

A Posterior view.

B MRI. Coronal section, anterior view.

Fig. 14.24 Prostate
The prostate may be divided anatomically (top row) or clinically (bottom row).

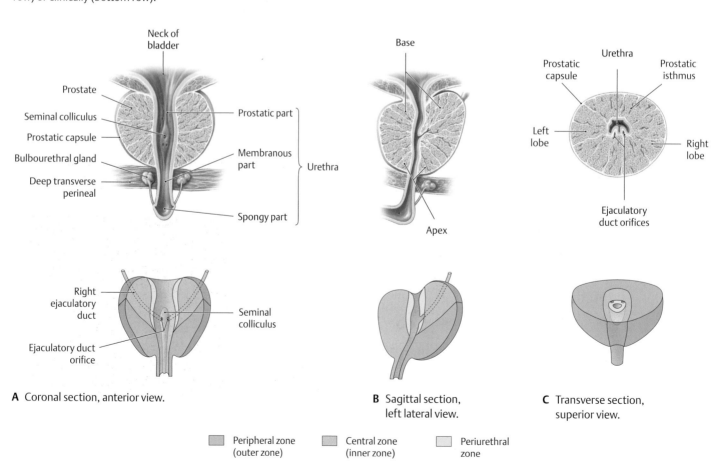

Neck of bladder

Prostate

Seminal colliculus

Prostatic capsule

Bulbourethral gland

Deep transverse perineal

Prostatic part

Membranous part

Spongy part

Urethra

Base

Apex

Urethra

Prostatic capsule

Prostatic isthmus

Left lobe

Right lobe

Ejaculatory duct orifices

Right ejaculatory duct

Ejaculatory duct orifice

Seminal colliculus

A Coronal section, anterior view.

B Sagittal section, left lateral view.

C Transverse section, superior view.

Peripheral zone (outer zone)

Central zone (inner zone)

Periurethral zone

Fig. 14.25 **Prostate in situ**
Sagittal section through the male pelvis, left lateral view.

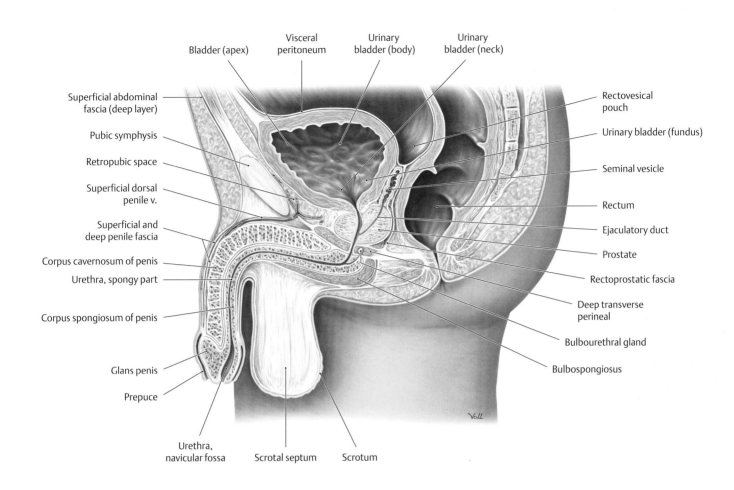

Superficial abdominal fascia (deep layer)

Pubic symphysis

Retropubic space

Superficial dorsal penile v.

Superficial and deep penile fascia

Corpus cavernosum of penis

Urethra, spongy part

Corpus spongiosum of penis

Glans penis

Prepuce

Bladder (apex)

Visceral peritoneum

Urinary bladder (body)

Urinary bladder (neck)

Rectovesical pouch

Urinary bladder (fundus)

Seminal vesicle

Rectum

Ejaculatory duct

Prostate

Rectoprostatic fascia

Deep transverse perineal

Bulbourethral gland

Bulbospongiosus

Urethra, navicular fossa

Scrotal septum

Scrotum

 Clinical

Prostatic carcinoma and hypertrophy

Prostatic carcinoma is one of the most common malignant tumors in older men, often growing at a subcapsular location in the peripheral zone of the prostate. Unlike benign prostatic hyperplasia, which begins in the central part of the gland, prostatic carcinoma does not cause urinary outflow obstruction in its early stages. Being in the peripheral zone, the tumor is palpable as a firm mass through the anterior wall of the rectum during rectal examination.

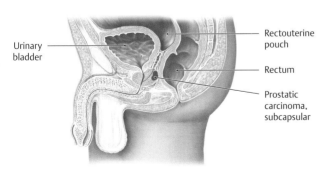

Urinary bladder

Rectouterine pouch

Rectum

Prostatic carcinoma, subcapsular

A Common site of prostatic carcinoma.

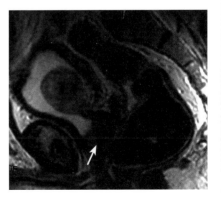

B Prostatic carcinoma (arrow) with bladder infiltration.

In certain prostate diseases, especially cancer, increased amounts of a protein, prostate-specific antigen or PSA, appear in the blood. This protein can be measured by a simple blood test.

201

Neurovasculature of the Male Genitalia

Fig. 14.26 Neurovasculature of the male genitalia
Left lateral view.

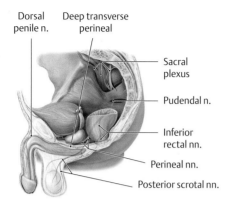

A Nerve supply.

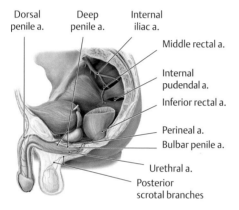

B Arterial supply.

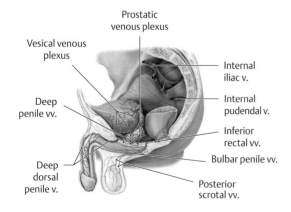

C Venous drainage.

Fig. 14.27 Neurovasculature of the penis and scrotum

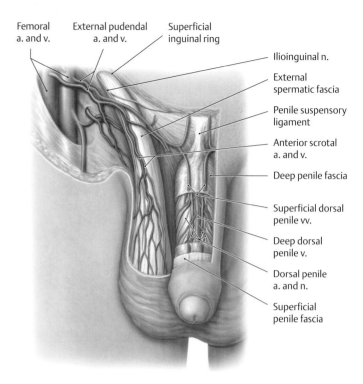

A Anterior view. *Partially removed:* Skin and fascia.

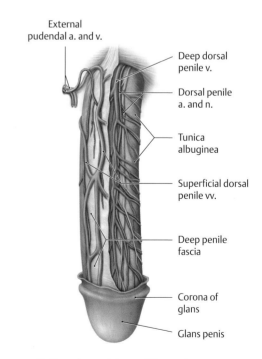

B Dorsal vasculature of the penis.

Fig. 14.28 Nerves of the male perineum and genitalia

Lithotomy position.

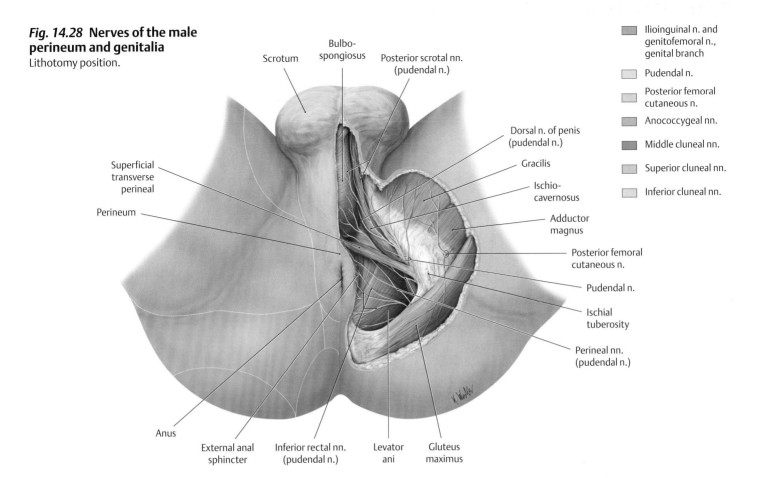

Scrotum

Bulbo-spongiosus

Posterior scrotal nn. (pudendal n.)

Superficial transverse perineal

Perineum

Anus

External anal sphincter

Inferior rectal nn. (pudendal n.)

Levator ani

Gluteus maximus

Dorsal n. of penis (pudendal n.)

Gracilis

Ischio-cavernosus

Adductor magnus

Posterior femoral cutaneous n.

Pudendal n.

Ischial tuberosity

Perineal nn. (pudendal n.)

Ilioinguinal n. and genitofemoral n., genital branch

Pudendal n.

Posterior femoral cutaneous n.

Anococcygeal nn.

Middle cluneal nn.

Superior cluneal nn.

Inferior cluneal nn.

Fig. 14.29 Neurovasculature of the male perineum

Lithotomy position.

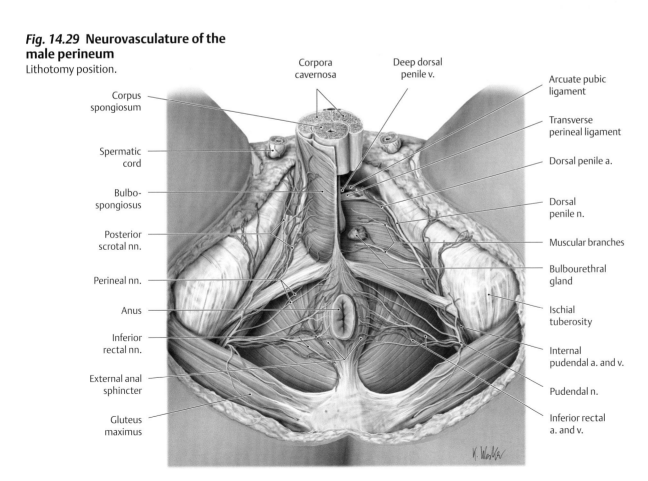

Corpora cavernosa

Deep dorsal penile v.

Corpus spongiosum

Spermatic cord

Bulbo-spongiosus

Posterior scrotal nn.

Perineal nn.

Anus

Inferior rectal nn.

External anal sphincter

Gluteus maximus

Arcuate pubic ligament

Transverse perineal ligament

Dorsal penile a.

Dorsal penile n.

Muscular branches

Bulbourethral gland

Ischial tuberosity

Internal pudendal a. and v.

Pudendal n.

Inferior rectal a. and v.

Development of the Genitalia

 The male and female genitalia are derived from a common gonadal primordium.

Fig. 14.30 **Development of the external genitalia**

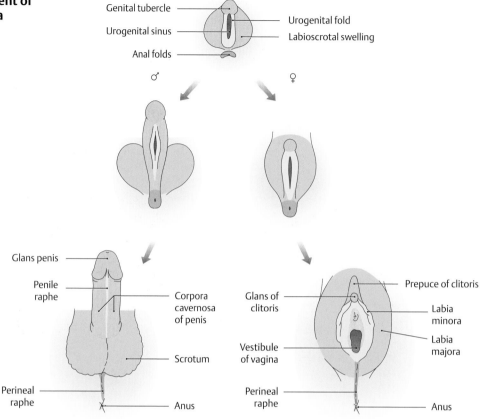

Fig. 14.31 **Descent of the testis**
Left lateral view.

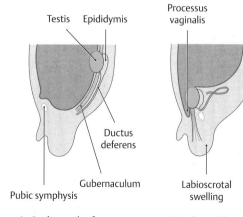

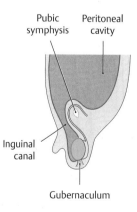

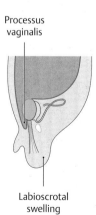

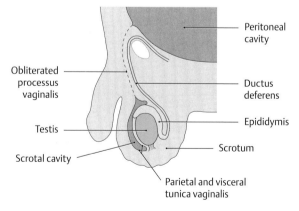

A 2nd month of development.

B 3rd month.

C Birth.

D After obliteration of the processus vaginalis of the peritoneum.

Fig. 14.32 Development of the internal genitalia

Anterior view.

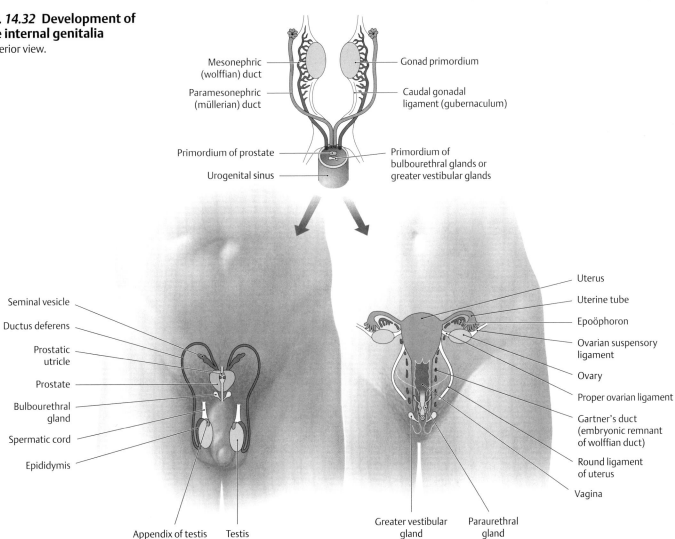

Mesonephric (wolffian) duct
Paramesonephric (müllerian) duct
Primordium of prostate
Urogenital sinus
Gonad primordium
Caudal gonadal ligament (gubernaculum)
Primordium of bulbourethral glands or greater vestibular glands

Seminal vesicle
Ductus deferens
Prostatic utricle
Prostate
Bulbourethral gland
Spermatic cord
Epididymis
Appendix of testis
Testis

Uterus
Uterine tube
Epoöphoron
Ovarian suspensory ligament
Ovary
Proper ovarian ligament
Gartner's duct (embryonic remnant of wolffian duct)
Round ligament of uterus
Vagina
Greater vestibular gland
Paraurethral gland

A Genetically male embryo (testicular primordium).

B Genetically female embryo (ovarian primordium).

Table 14.4	Derivatives of embryonic urogenital structures	
Nonfunctioning remnants in italics. Structures common to both sexes in bold.		
Rudiment	**Male structure**	**Female structure**
Undifferentiated gonad	Testis	Ovary
Cortex	Seminiferous tubules	Follicle
Medulla	Rete testis	Ovarian stroma
Mesonephric ductule	Efferent ductules of testis, *paradidymis*	*Epo- and paroöphoron*
Mesonephric (wolffian) duct	**Ureter, renal pelvis and calices, collecting ducts**	
	Epididymal duct, ductus deferens, ejaculatory duct, seminal vesicle	—
Paramesonephric (müllerian) duct	*Appendix of testis*	Uterine tube, uterus, vagina (superior portion), *Morgagni's hydatids*
Urogenital sinus	**Bladder, urethra**	
	Prostate, bulbourethral gland, *prostatic utricle*	Vagina (inferior portion), greater and lesser vestibular glands
Phallus (genital tubercle)	Corpus cavernosum of penis	Clitoris, glans of clitoris
Genital folds	Glans of penis, *penile raphe*	Labia minora, vestibular bulb
Labioscrotal swellings	Scrotum	Labia majora
Gubernaculum	*Gubernaculum of testis*	Proper ovarian ligament, round ligament of uterus
Genital tubercle (of Müller)	*Seminal colliculus*	*Hymen*

Arteries of the Abdomen

Fig. 15.1 Abdominal aorta and major branches

Anterior view. The abdominal aorta enters the abdomen at the T12 level through the aortic aperture of the diaphragm (see p. 54). Before bifurcating at L4 into its terminal branches, the common iliac arteries, the abdominal aorta gives off the renal arteries (see p. 209) and three major trunks that supply the organs of the alimentary canal:

Celiac trunk: Supplies the structures of the foregut, the anterior portion of the alimentary canal. The foregut consists of the esophagus (distal half), stomach, duodenum (proximal half), liver, gallbladder, and pancreas (superior portion).

Superior mesenteric artery: Supplies the structures of the midgut: the duodenum (distal half), jejunum and ileum, cecum and appendix, ascending and transverse colons, and right colic (hepatic) flexure.

Inferior mesenteric artery: Supplies the structures of the hindgut: the transverse colon (distal third), left colic (splenic) flexure, descending and sigmoid colons, rectum, and anal canal (upper part).

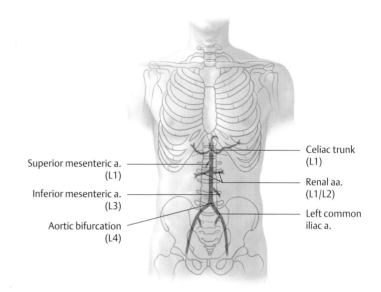

Superior mesenteric a. (L1)
Inferior mesenteric a. (L3)
Aortic bifurcation (L4)
Celiac trunk (L1)
Renal aa. (L1/L2)
Left common iliac a.

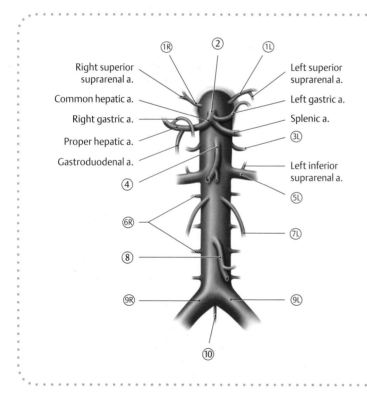

Right superior suprarenal a.
Common hepatic a.
Right gastric a.
Proper hepatic a.
Gastroduodenal a.
④
⑥R
⑧
⑨R

Left superior suprarenal a.
Left gastric a.
Splenic a.
③L
Left inferior suprarenal a.
⑤L
⑦L
⑨L
⑩
①R ② ①L

Table 15.1		Branches of the abdominal aorta		

The abdominal aorta gives rise to three major unpaired trunks (bold) and the unpaired median sacral artery, as well as six paired branches.

Branch from abdominal aorta			Branches		
①R	①L	Inferior phrenic aa. (paired)	Superior suprarenal aa.		
②		**Celiac trunk**	Left gastric a.		
			Splenic a.		
			Common hepatic a.	Proper hepatic a.	
				Right gastric a.	
				Gastroduodenal a.	
③R	③L	Middle suprarenal aa. (paired)			
④		**Superior mesenteric a.**			
⑤R	⑤L	Renal aa. (paired)	Inferior suprarenal aa.		
⑥R	⑥L	Lumbar aa. (1st through 4th, paired)			
⑦R	⑦L	Testicular/ovarian aa. (paired)			
⑧		**Inferior mesenteric a.**			
⑨R	⑨L	Common iliac aa. (paired)	External iliac a.		
			Internal iliac a.		
⑩		Median sacral a.			

Fig. 15.2 Celiac trunk

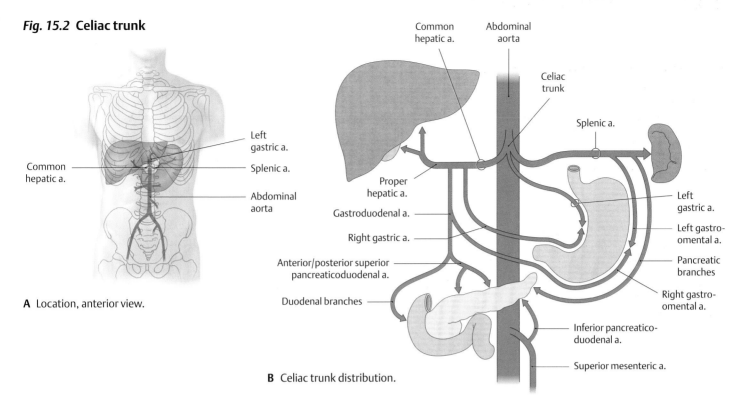

A Location, anterior view.

B Celiac trunk distribution.

Fig. 15.3 Superior mesenteric artery
Anterior view.

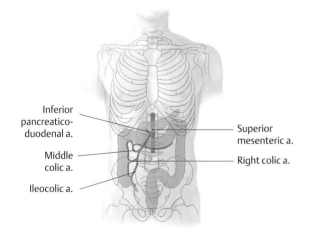

Fig. 15.4 Inferior mesenteric artery
Anterior view.

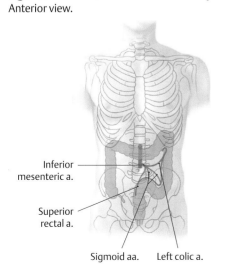

Fig. 15.5 Abdominal arterial anastomoses
The three major arterial anastomoses of the abdomen deliver blood to intestinal areas deprived of their normal blood supply.

① Celiac trunk
(supplies the foregut):
- Esophagus
- Stomach
- Liver
- Gallbladder
- Pancreas
- Duodenum

② Superior mesenteric a.
(supplies the midgut):
- Jejunum and ileum
- Cecum and appendix
- Ascending colon
- Hepatic (right colic) flexure
- Transverse colon

③ Inferior mesenteric a.
(supplies the hindgut):
- Splenic (left colic) flexure
- Descending and sigmoid colons
- Rectum
- Anal canal (upper part)

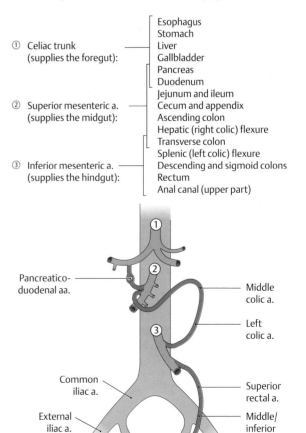

Abdominal Aorta & Renal Arteries

Fig. 15.6 Abdominal aorta

Anterior view of the female abdomen. *Removed:* Abdominal organs and peritoneum. The abdominal aorta is the distal continuation of the thoracic aorta (see p. 68). It enters the abdomen at the T12 level and bifurcates into the common iliac arteries at L4.

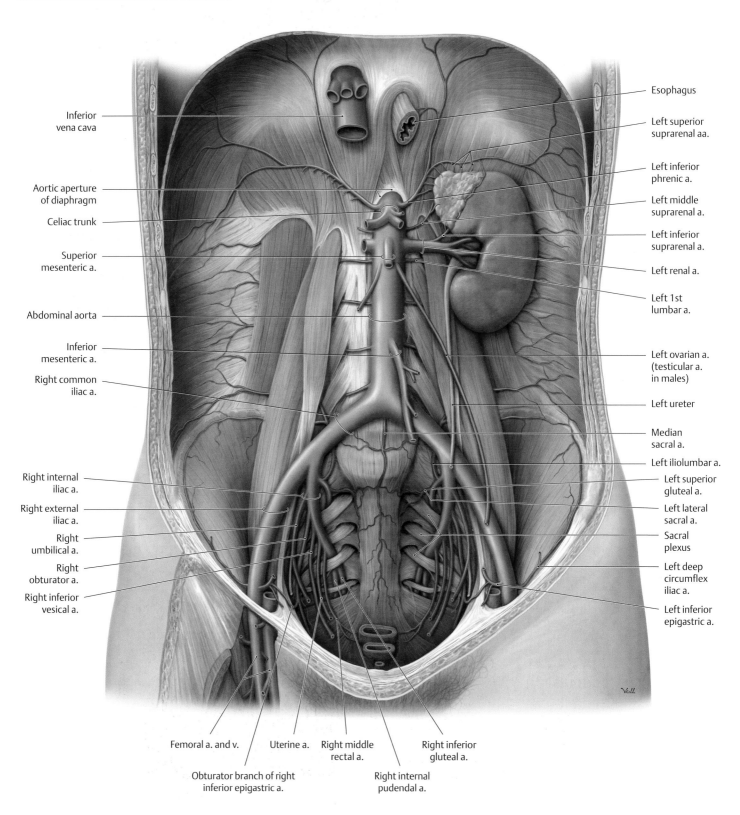

Inferior vena cava

Aortic aperture of diaphragm

Celiac trunk

Superior mesenteric a.

Abdominal aorta

Inferior mesenteric a.

Right common iliac a.

Right internal iliac a.

Right external iliac a.

Right umbilical a.

Right obturator a.

Right inferior vesical a.

Esophagus

Left superior suprarenal aa.

Left inferior phrenic a.

Left middle suprarenal a.

Left inferior suprarenal a.

Left renal a.

Left 1st lumbar a.

Left ovarian a. (testicular a. in males)

Left ureter

Median sacral a.

Left iliolumbar a.

Left superior gluteal a.

Left lateral sacral a.

Sacral plexus

Left deep circumflex iliac a.

Left inferior epigastric a.

Femoral a. and v.

Uterine a.

Right middle rectal a.

Right inferior gluteal a.

Obturator branch of right inferior epigastric a.

Right internal pudendal a.

Fig. 15.7 Renal arteries

Left kidney, anterior view. The renal arteries arise at approximately the level of L2. Each renal artery divides into an anterior and a posterior branch. The anterior branch further divides into four segmental arteries (circled).

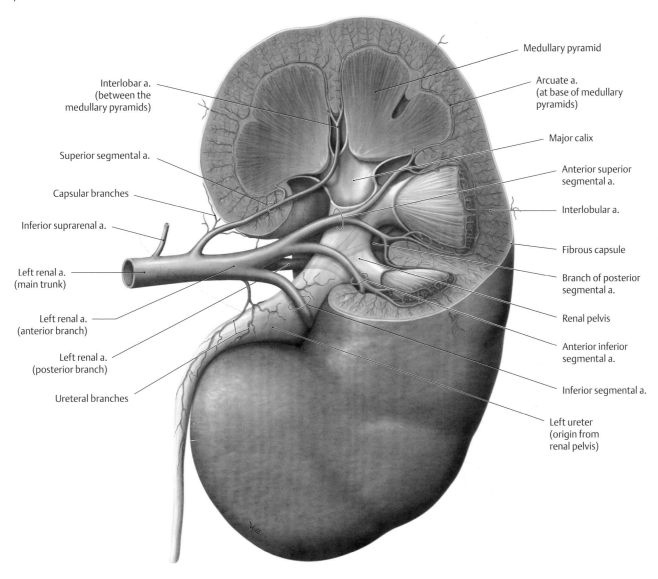

Clinical

Renal hypertension

The kidney is an important blood pressure sensor and regulator. Stenosis of the renal artery reduces blood flow through the kidney and stimulates increased production of renin, a hormone that cleaves angiotensinogen to form angiotensin I. Subsequent cleavage yields angiotensin II, which induces vasoconstriction and an increase in blood pressure. Renal hypertension must be excluded (or confirmed) when diagnosing high blood pressure.

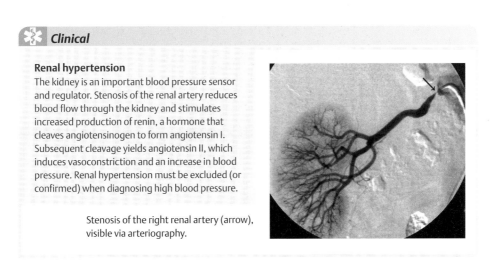

Stenosis of the right renal artery (arrow), visible via arteriography.

Celiac Trunk

 The distribution of the celiac trunk is shown on p. 207.

Fig. 15.8 **Celiac trunk: Stomach, liver, and gallbladder**
Anterior view. *Opened:* Lesser omentum. *Incised:* Greater omentum. The celiac trunk arises from the abdominal aorta at about the level of L1.

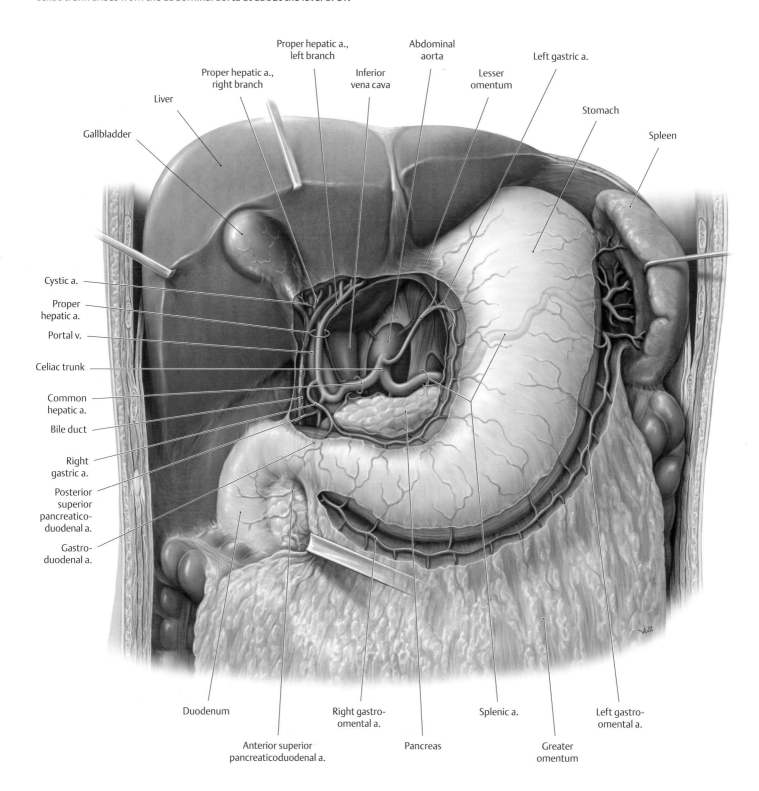

Fig. 15.9 Celiac trunk: Pancreas, duodenum, and spleen

Anterior view. *Removed:* Stomach (body) and lesser omentum.

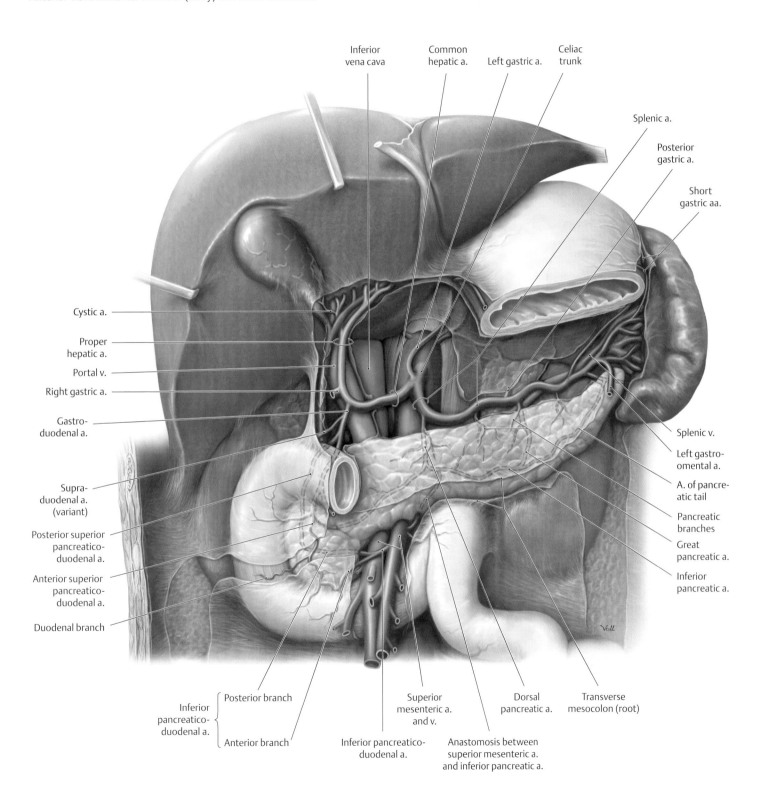

Inferior vena cava

Common hepatic a.

Left gastric a.

Celiac trunk

Splenic a.

Posterior gastric a.

Short gastric aa.

Cystic a.

Proper hepatic a.

Portal v.

Right gastric a.

Gastro-duodenal a.

Supra-duodenal a. (variant)

Posterior superior pancreatico-duodenal a.

Anterior superior pancreatico-duodenal a.

Duodenal branch

Splenic v.

Left gastro-omental a.

A. of pancreatic tail

Pancreatic branches

Great pancreatic a.

Inferior pancreatic a.

Inferior pancreatico-duodenal a. {
Posterior branch

Anterior branch
}

Superior mesenteric a. and v.

Inferior pancreatico-duodenal a.

Dorsal pancreatic a.

Anastomosis between superior mesenteric a. and inferior pancreatic a.

Transverse mesocolon (root)

211

Superior & Inferior Mesenteric Arteries

Fig. 15.10 Superior mesenteric artery

Anterior view. *Partially removed:* Stomach and peritoneum.
Note: The middle colic artery has been truncated (see Fig. 15.11). The superior and inferior mesenteric arteries arise from the aorta opposite L2 and L3, respectively.

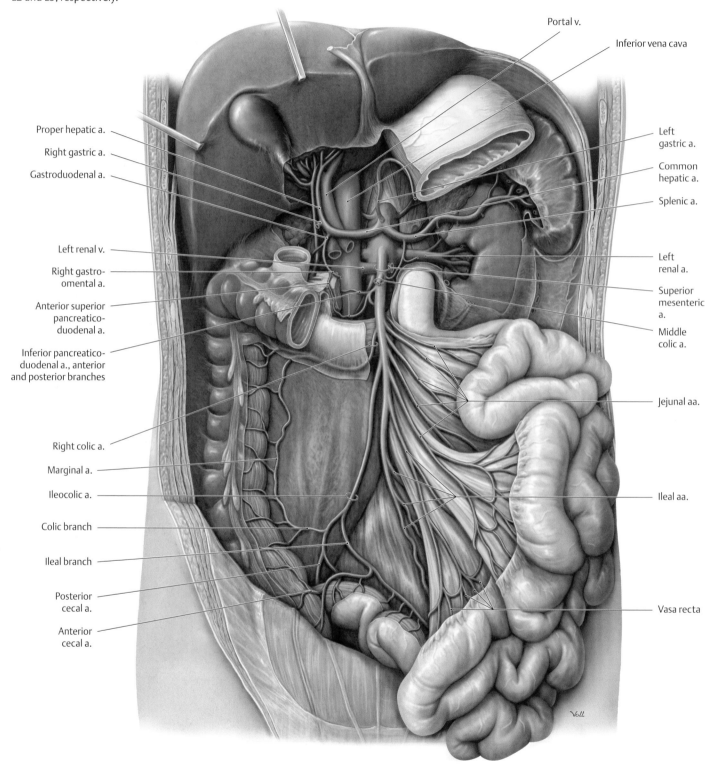

Proper hepatic a.
Right gastric a.
Gastroduodenal a.
Left renal v.
Right gastro-omental a.
Anterior superior pancreatico-duodenal a.
Inferior pancreatico-duodenal a., anterior and posterior branches
Right colic a.
Marginal a.
Ileocolic a.
Colic branch
Ileal branch
Posterior cecal a.
Anterior cecal a.

Portal v.
Inferior vena cava
Left gastric a.
Common hepatic a.
Splenic a.
Left renal a.
Superior mesenteric a.
Middle colic a.
Jejunal aa.
Ileal aa.
Vasa recta

Fig. 15.11 **Inferior mesenteric artery**
Anterior view. *Removed:* Jejunum and ileum. *Reflected:* Transverse colon.

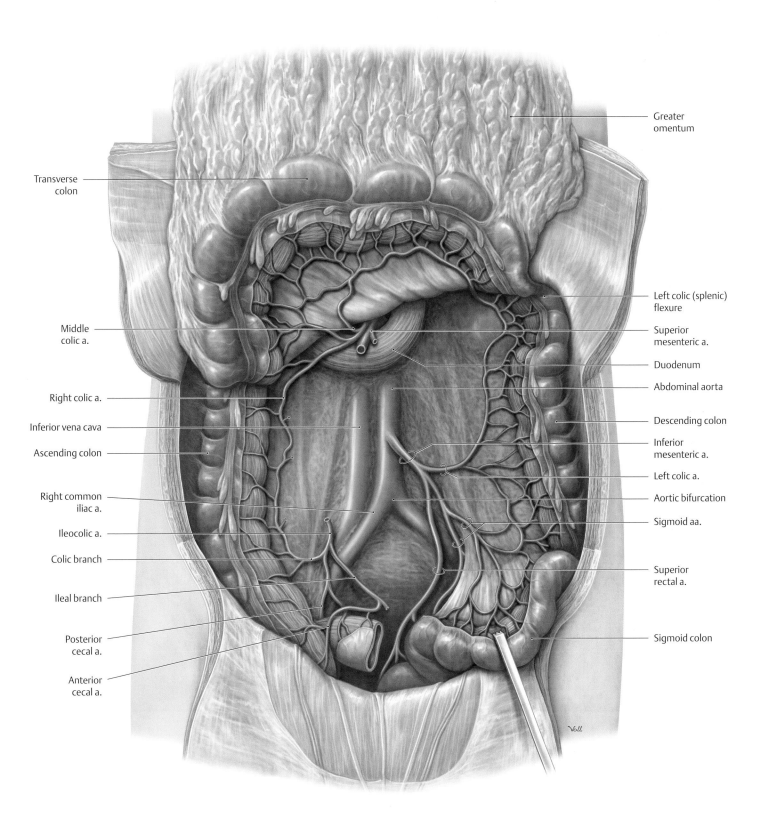

Greater omentum

Transverse colon

Left colic (splenic) flexure

Middle colic a.

Superior mesenteric a.

Duodenum

Right colic a.

Abdominal aorta

Inferior vena cava

Descending colon

Ascending colon

Inferior mesenteric a.

Left colic a.

Right common iliac a.

Aortic bifurcation

Ileocolic a.

Sigmoid aa.

Colic branch

Superior rectal a.

Ileal branch

Posterior cecal a.

Sigmoid colon

Anterior cecal a.

Veins of the Abdomen

Fig. 15.12 Inferior vena cava: Location
Anterior view.

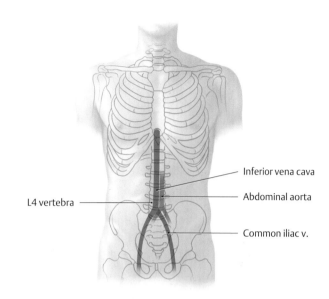

- Inferior vena cava
- Abdominal aorta
- L4 vertebra
- Common iliac v.

Fig. 15.13 Tributaries of the renal veins
Anterior view.

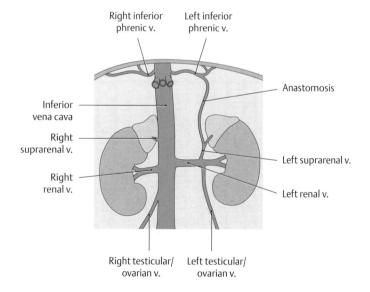

- Right inferior phrenic v.
- Left inferior phrenic v.
- Anastomosis
- Inferior vena cava
- Right suprarenal v.
- Left suprarenal v.
- Right renal v.
- Left renal v.
- Right testicular/ovarian v.
- Left testicular/ovarian v.

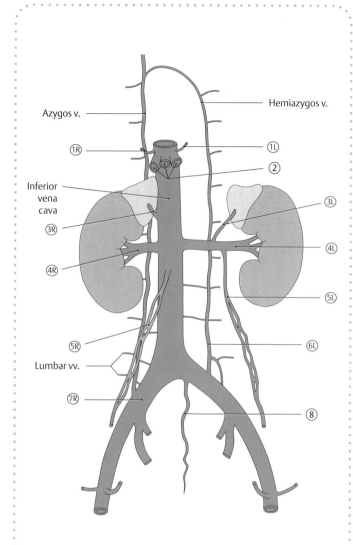

- Azygos v.
- Hemiazygos v.
- ①R
- ①L
- ②
- Inferior vena cava
- ③L
- ③R
- ④L
- ④R
- ⑤L
- ⑤R
- ⑥L
- Lumbar vv.
- ⑦R
- ⑧

Table 15.2		Tributaries of the inferior vena cava
①R	①L	Inferior phrenic vv. (paired)
	②	Hepatic vv. (3)
③R	③L	Suprarenal vv. (the right vein is a direct tributary)
④R	④L	Renal vv. (paired)
⑤R	⑤L	Testicular/ovarian vv. (the right vein is a direct tributary)
⑥R	⑥L	Ascending lumbar vv. (paired)
⑦R	⑦L	Common iliac vv. (paired)
	⑧	Median sacral v.

Fig. 15.14 Portal vein

The portal vein (see p. 218) drains venous blood from the abdominopelvic organs supplied by the celiac trunk and superior and inferior mesenteric arteries.

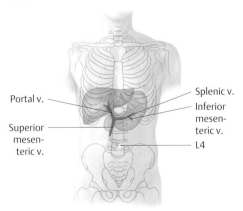

A Location, anterior view.

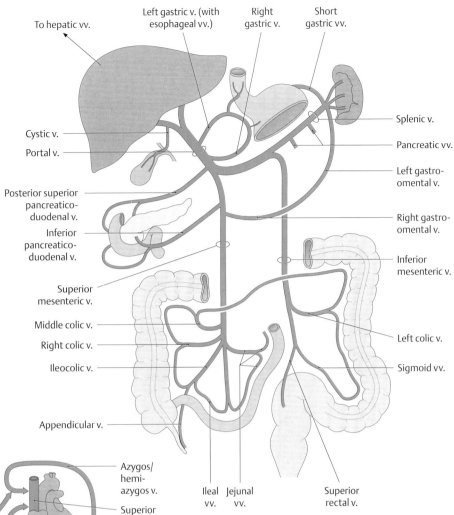

B Portal vein distribution.

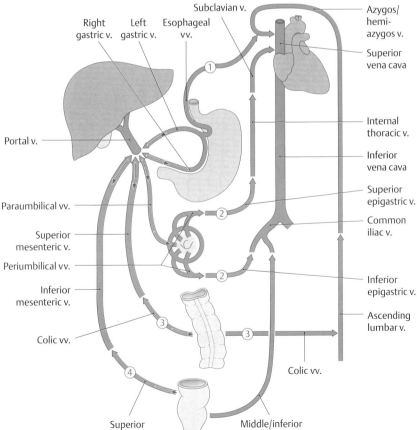
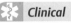

C Collateral pathways (portosystemic collaterals). When the portal system is compromised, nutrient-laden blood may be transported to the heart via the venae cavae without passing through the liver. Red arrows indicate flow reversal.

✴ Clinical

Cancer metastases

Tumors in the region drained by the superior rectal vein may spread through the portal venous system to the capillary bed of the liver (hepatic metastasis). Tumors drained by the middle or inferior rectal veins may metastasize to the capillary bed of the lung (pulmonary metastasis) via the inferior vena cava and right heart.

Inferior Vena Cava & Renal Veins

Fig. 15.15 Inferior vena cava
Anterior view of the female abdomen. *Removed:* All organs (except the left kidney and suprarenal gland).

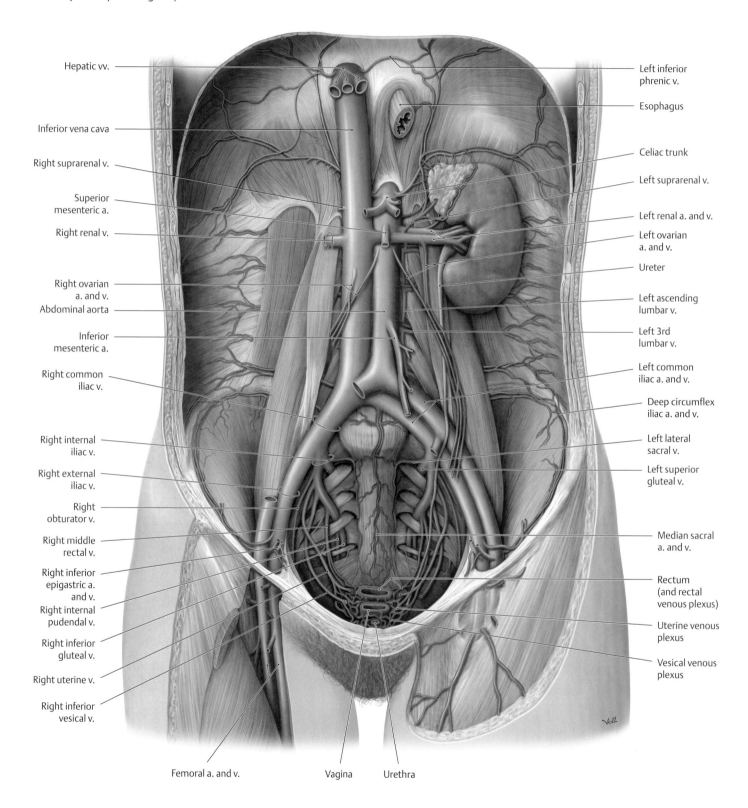

Hepatic vv.

Inferior vena cava

Right suprarenal v.

Superior mesenteric a.

Right renal v.

Right ovarian a. and v.

Abdominal aorta

Inferior mesenteric a.

Right common iliac v.

Right internal iliac v.

Right external iliac v.

Right obturator v.

Right middle rectal v.

Right inferior epigastric a. and v.

Right internal pudendal v.

Right inferior gluteal v.

Right uterine v.

Right inferior vesical v.

Left inferior phrenic v.

Esophagus

Celiac trunk

Left suprarenal v.

Left renal a. and v.

Left ovarian a. and v.

Ureter

Left ascending lumbar v.

Left 3rd lumbar v.

Left common iliac a. and v.

Deep circumflex iliac a. and v.

Left lateral sacral v.

Left superior gluteal v.

Median sacral a. and v.

Rectum (and rectal venous plexus)

Uterine venous plexus

Vesical venous plexus

Femoral a. and v.

Vagina

Urethra

Fig. 15.16 **Renal veins**

Anterior view. See p. 209 for the renal arteries in isolation.

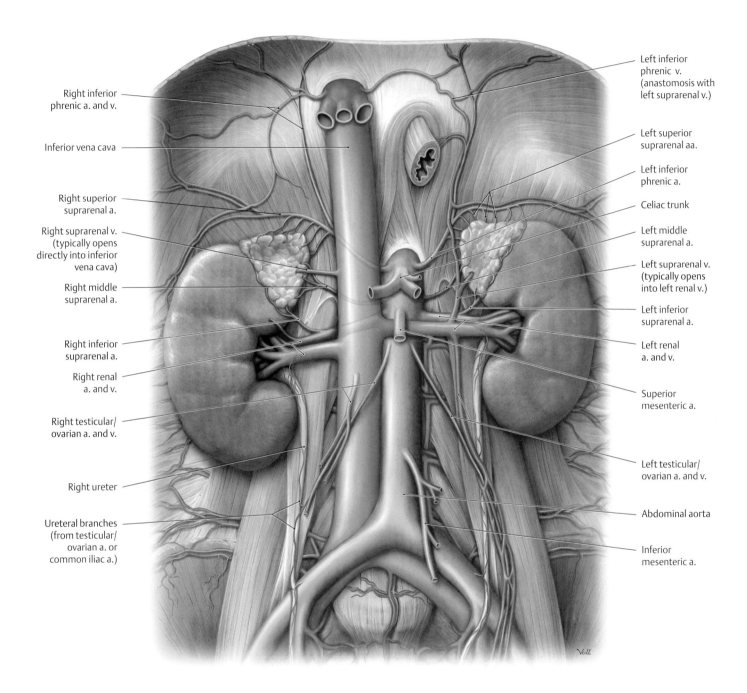

Right inferior phrenic a. and v.

Inferior vena cava

Right superior suprarenal a.

Right suprarenal v. (typically opens directly into inferior vena cava)

Right middle suprarenal a.

Right inferior suprarenal a.

Right renal a. and v.

Right testicular/ovarian a. and v.

Right ureter

Ureteral branches (from testicular/ovarian a. or common iliac a.)

Left inferior phrenic v. (anastomosis with left suprarenal v.)

Left superior suprarenal aa.

Left inferior phrenic a.

Celiac trunk

Left middle suprarenal a.

Left suprarenal v. (typically opens into left renal v.)

Left inferior suprarenal a.

Left renal a. and v.

Superior mesenteric a.

Left testicular/ovarian a. and v.

Abdominal aorta

Inferior mesenteric a.

Portal Vein

 The portal vein is typically formed by the union of the superior mesenteric and the splenic veins posterior to the neck of the pancreas. The distribution of the portal vein is shown on p. 215.

Fig. 15.17 **Portal vein: Stomach and duodenum**
Anterior view. *Removed:* Liver, lesser omentum, and peritoneum.
Opened: Greater omentum.

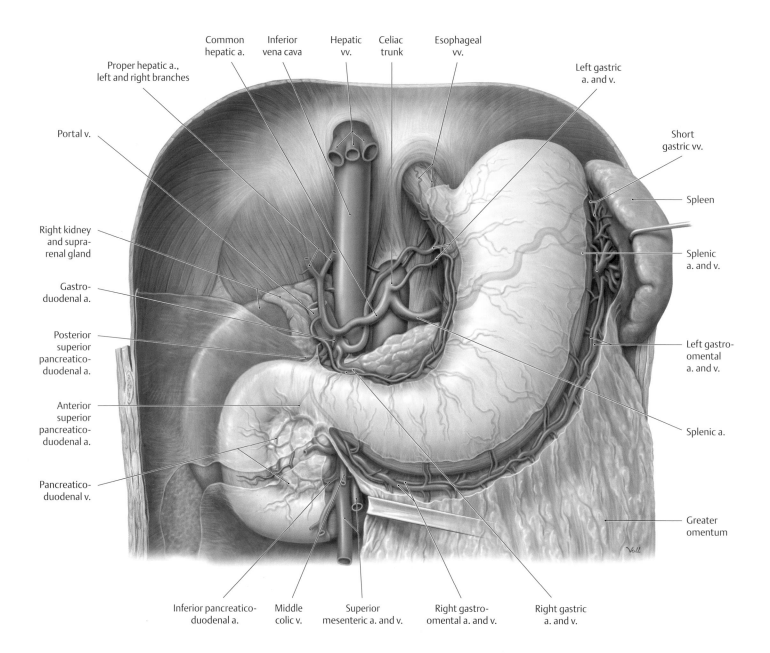

Fig. 15.18 Portal vein: Pancreas and spleen

Anterior view. *Partially removed:* Stomach, pancreas, and peritoneum.

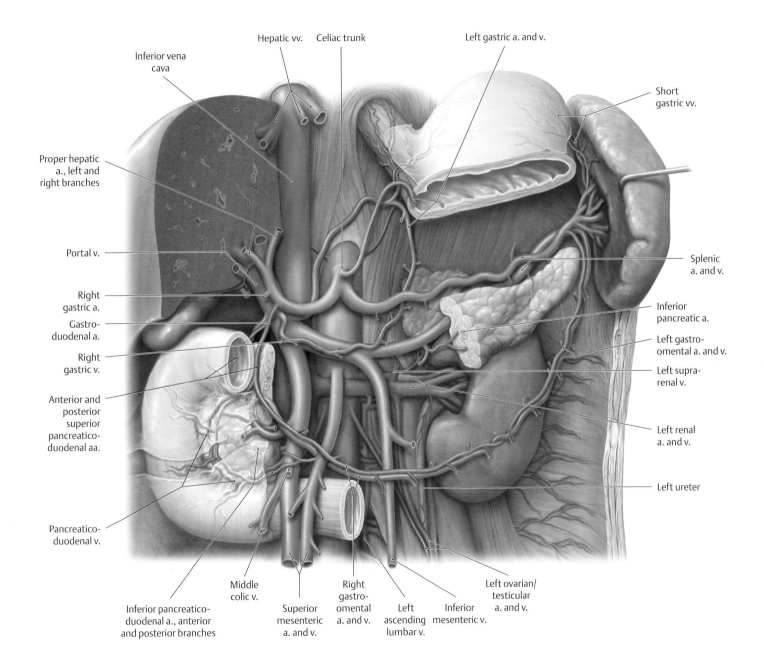

Superior & Inferior Mesenteric Veins

Fig. 15.19 Superior mesenteric vein

Anterior view. *Partially removed:* Stomach, pancreas, peritoneum, mesentery, and transverse colon. *Displaced:* Small intestine.

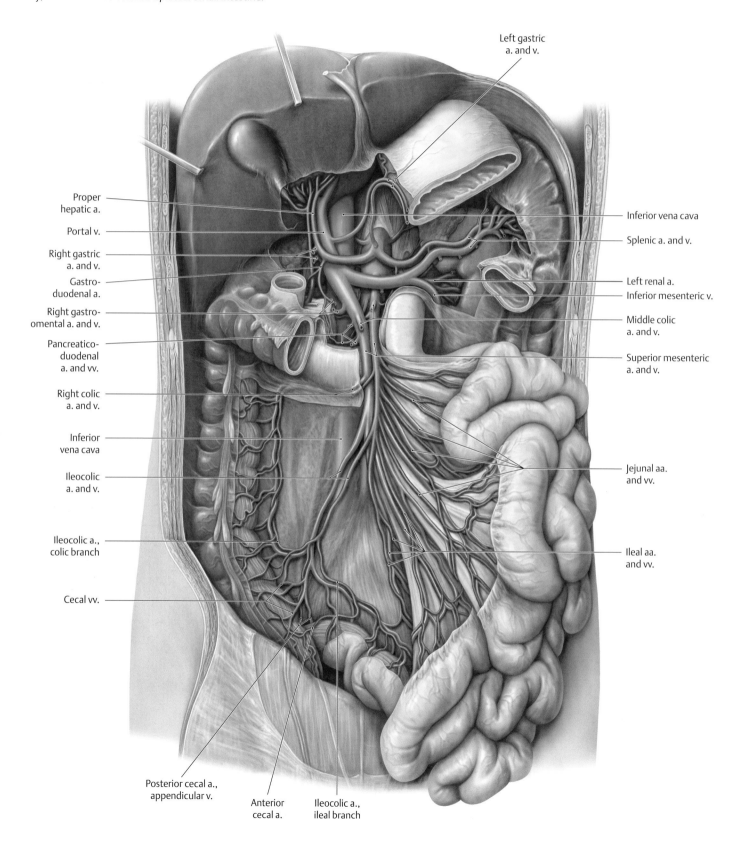

Left gastric a. and v.

Proper hepatic a.

Portal v.

Right gastric a. and v.

Gastro-duodenal a.

Right gastro-omental a. and v.

Pancreatico-duodenal a. and vv.

Right colic a. and v.

Inferior vena cava

Ileocolic a. and v.

Ileocolic a., colic branch

Cecal vv.

Posterior cecal a., appendicular v.

Anterior cecal a.

Ileocolic a., ileal branch

Inferior vena cava

Splenic a. and v.

Left renal a.

Inferior mesenteric v.

Middle colic a. and v.

Superior mesenteric a. and v.

Jejunal aa. and vv.

Ileal aa. and vv.

Fig. 15.20 **Inferior mesenteric vein**

Anterior view. *Removed:* Stomach, pancreas, small intestine, and peritoneum.

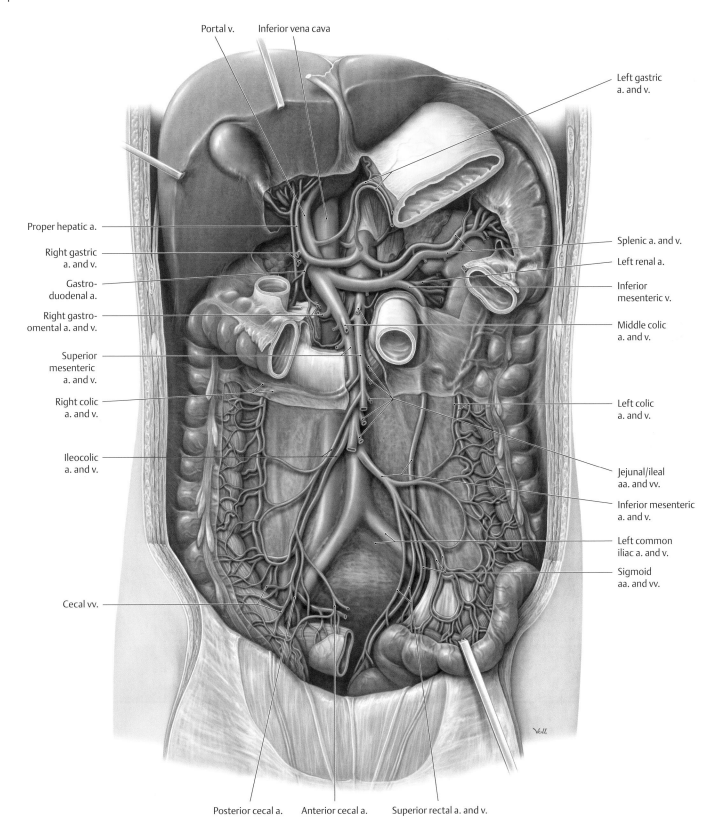

Portal v.

Inferior vena cava

Left gastric a. and v.

Proper hepatic a.

Right gastric a. and v.

Gastro-duodenal a.

Right gastro-omental a. and v.

Superior mesenteric a. and v.

Right colic a. and v.

Ileocolic a. and v.

Cecal vv.

Splenic a. and v.

Left renal a.

Inferior mesenteric v.

Middle colic a. and v.

Left colic a. and v.

Jejunal/ileal aa. and vv.

Inferior mesenteric a. and v.

Left common iliac a. and v.

Sigmoid aa. and vv.

Posterior cecal a.

Anterior cecal a.

Superior rectal a. and v.

Arteries & Veins of the Pelvis

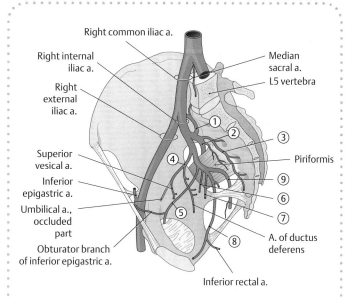

A Male pelvis.

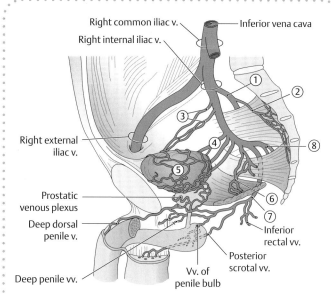

A Male pelvis.

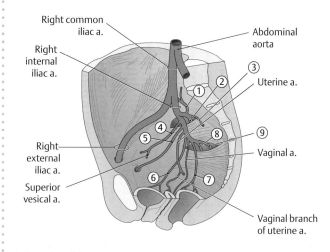

B Female pelvis.

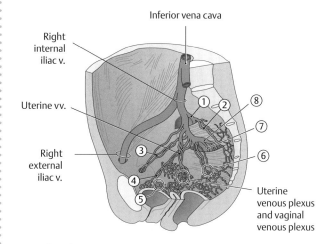

B Female pelvis.

Table 15.3	Branches of the internal iliac artery	

The internal iliac artery gives off five parietal (pelvic wall) and four visceral (pelvic organs) branches.* Parietal branches are shown in italics.

Branches		
①	*Iiolumbar a.*	
②	*Superior gluteal a.*	
③	*Lateral sacral a.*	
④	Umbilical a.	A. of ductus deferens
		Superior vesical a.
⑤	*Obturator a.*	
⑥	Inferior vesical a.	
⑦	Middle rectal a.	
⑧	Internal pudendal a.	Inferior rectal a.
⑨	*Inferior gluteal a.*	

* In the female pelvis, the uterine and vaginal arteries may arise directly from the internal iliac artery.

Table 15.4	Venous drainage of the pelvis

Tributaries	
①	Superior gluteal v.
②	Lateral sacral v.
③	Obturator vv.
④	Vesical vv.
⑤	Vesical venous plexus
⑥	Middle rectal vv. (rectal venous plexus) (also superior and inferior rectal vv., not shown)
⑦	Internal pudendal v.
⑧	Inferior gluteal vv.

The male pelvis also contains a prostatic venous plexus and veins draining the penis and scrotum. The female pelvis contains the uterine and vaginal venous plexus.

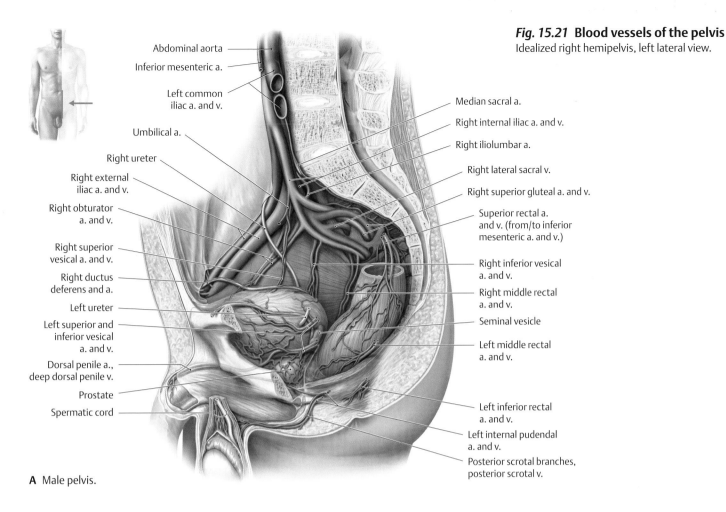

***Fig. 15.21* Blood vessels of the pelvis**
Idealized right hemipelvis, left lateral view.

Abdominal aorta

Inferior mesenteric a.

Left common iliac a. and v.

Umbilical a.

Right ureter

Right external iliac a. and v.

Right obturator a. and v.

Right superior vesical a. and v.

Right ductus deferens and a.

Left ureter

Left superior and inferior vesical a. and v.

Dorsal penile a., deep dorsal penile v.

Prostate

Spermatic cord

Median sacral a.

Right internal iliac a. and v.

Right iliolumbar a.

Right lateral sacral v.

Right superior gluteal a. and v.

Superior rectal a. and v. (from/to inferior mesenteric a. and v.)

Right inferior vesical a. and v.

Right middle rectal a. and v.

Seminal vesicle

Left middle rectal a. and v.

Left inferior rectal a. and v.

Left internal pudendal a. and v.

Posterior scrotal branches, posterior scrotal v.

A Male pelvis.

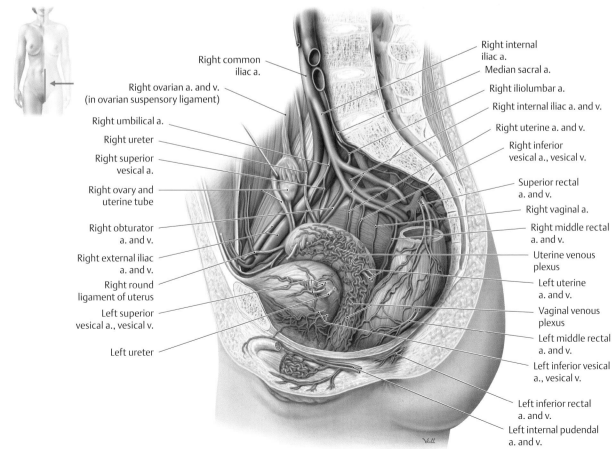

Right common iliac a.

Right ovarian a. and v. (in ovarian suspensory ligament)

Right umbilical a.

Right ureter

Right superior vesical a.

Right ovary and uterine tube

Right obturator a. and v.

Right external iliac a. and v.

Right round ligament of uterus

Left superior vesical a., vesical v.

Left ureter

Right internal iliac a.

Median sacral a.

Right iliolumbar a.

Right internal iliac a. and v.

Right uterine a. and v.

Right inferior vesical a., vesical v.

Superior rectal a. and v.

Right vaginal a.

Right middle rectal a. and v.

Uterine venous plexus

Left uterine a. and v.

Vaginal venous plexus

Left middle rectal a. and v.

Left inferior vesical a., vesical v.

Left inferior rectal a. and v.

Left internal pudendal a. and v.

B Female pelvis.

Arteries & Veins of the Rectum & Genitalia

Fig. 15.22 **Blood vessels of the rectum**

Posterior view. The main blood supply to the rectum is from the superior rectal arteries; the middle rectal arteries serve as an anastomosis between the superior and inferior rectal arteries.

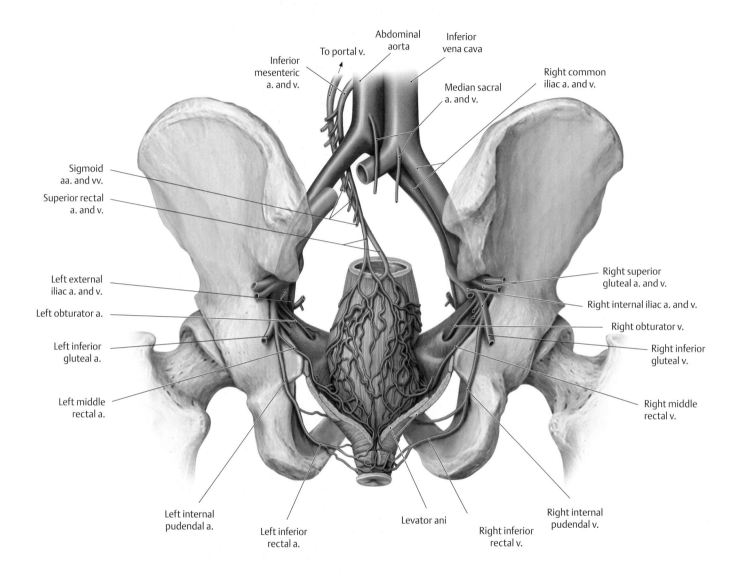

Fig. 15.23 Blood vessels of the genitalia

Anterior view.

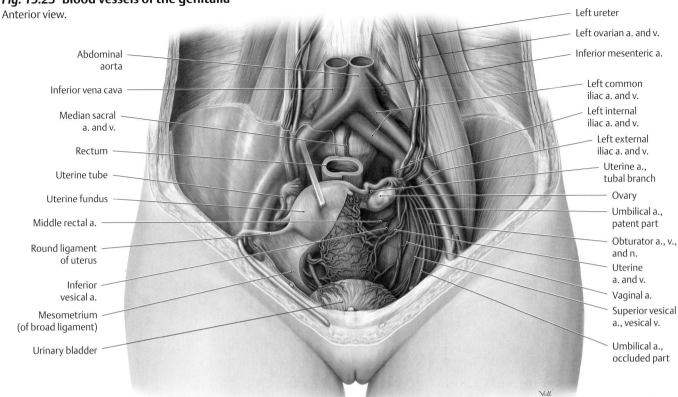

Abdominal aorta

Inferior vena cava

Median sacral a. and v.

Rectum

Uterine tube

Uterine fundus

Middle rectal a.

Round ligament of uterus

Inferior vesical a.

Mesometrium (of broad ligament)

Urinary bladder

Left ureter

Left ovarian a. and v.

Inferior mesenteric a.

Left common iliac a. and v.

Left internal iliac a. and v.

Left external iliac a. and v.

Uterine a., tubal branch

Ovary

Umbilical a., patent part

Obturator a., v., and n.

Uterine a. and v.

Vaginal a.

Superior vesical a., vesical v.

Umbilical a., occluded part

A Female pelvis. *Removed:* Peritoneum (left side). *Displaced:* Uterus.

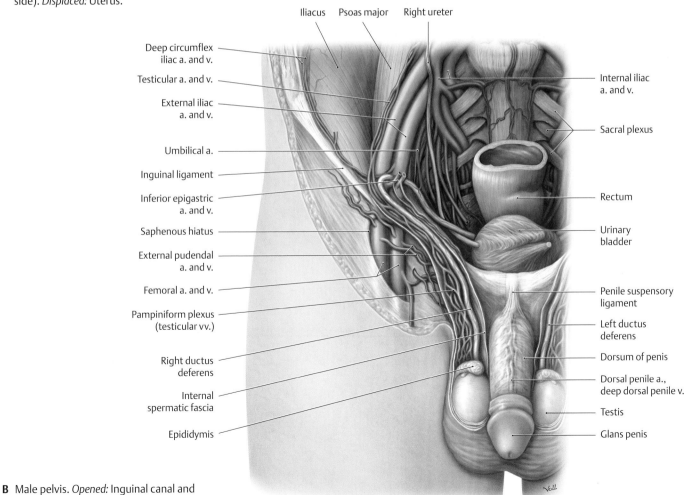

Iliacus Psoas major Right ureter

Deep circumflex iliac a. and v.

Testicular a. and v.

External iliac a. and v.

Umbilical a.

Inguinal ligament

Inferior epigastric a. and v.

Saphenous hiatus

External pudendal a. and v.

Femoral a. and v.

Pampiniform plexus (testicular vv.)

Right ductus deferens

Internal spermatic fascia

Epididymis

Internal iliac a. and v.

Sacral plexus

Rectum

Urinary bladder

Penile suspensory ligament

Left ductus deferens

Dorsum of penis

Dorsal penile a., deep dorsal penile v.

Testis

Glans penis

B Male pelvis. *Opened:* Inguinal canal and coverings of the spermatic cord.

Lymph Nodes of the Abdomen & Pelvis

Fig. 16.1 Lymphatic drainage of the internal organs

See Table 16.1 for numbering. Lymph drainage from the abdomen, pelvis, and lower limb ultimately passes through the lumbar lymph nodes (clinically: aortic nodes). The lumbar lymph nodes consist of the right (caval) and left lateral aortic nodes, the preaortic nodes, and the retroaortic nodes. Efferent lymph vessels from the lumbar and preaortic nodes form the lumbar and intestinal trunks, respectively. The lumbar and intestinal trunks terminate into the cisterna chyli.

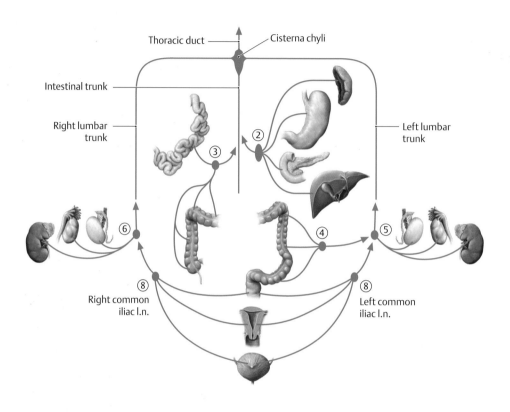

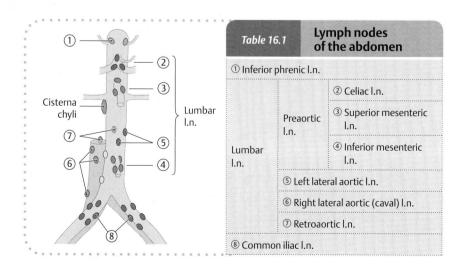

Table 16.1	Lymph nodes of the abdomen		
① Inferior phrenic l.n.			
Lumbar l.n.	Preaortic l.n.	② Celiac l.n.	
		③ Superior mesenteric l.n.	
		④ Inferior mesenteric l.n.	
	⑤ Left lateral aortic l.n.		
	⑥ Right lateral aortic (caval) l.n.		
	⑦ Retroaortic l.n.		
⑧ Common iliac l.n.			

Fig. 16.2 Lymphatic drainage of the rectum
Anterior view.

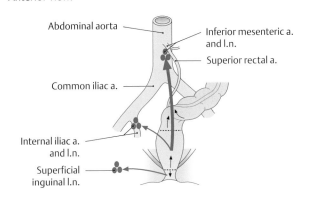

Fig. 16.3 Lymphatic drainage of the bladder and urethra
Anterior view.

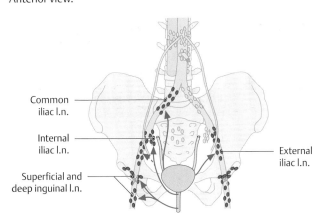

Fig. 16.4 Lymphatic drainage of the male genitalia
Anterior view.

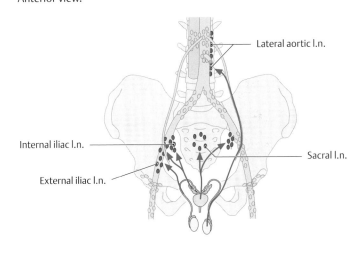

Fig. 16.5 Lymphatic drainage of the female genitalia
Anterior view.

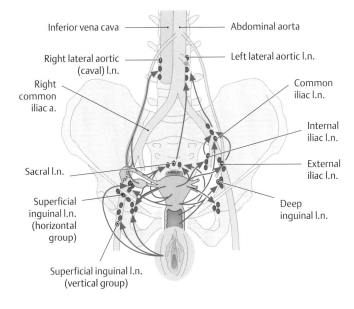

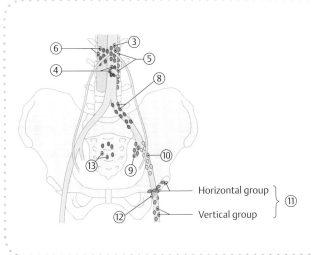

Table 16.2	Lymph nodes of the pelvis	
Numbers continued from Table 16.1.		
Preaortic l.n.	③ Superior mesenteric l.n.	
	④ Inferior mesenteric l.n.	
⑤ Left lateral aortic l.n.		
⑥ Right lateral aortic (caval) l.n.		
⑧ Common iliac l.n.		
⑨ Internal iliac l.n.		
⑩ External iliac l.n.		
⑪ Superficial inguinal l.n.	Horizontal group	
	Vertical group	
⑫ Deep inguinal l.n.		
⑬ Sacral l.n.		

Lymph Nodes of the Posterior Abdominal Wall

 Lymph nodes in the abdomen and pelvis may be classified as either parietal or visceral. The majority of the parietal lymph nodes are located on the posterior abdominal wall.

Fig. 16.6 Parietal lymph nodes in the abdomen and pelvis
Anterior view. *Removed:* All visceral structures (except vessels).

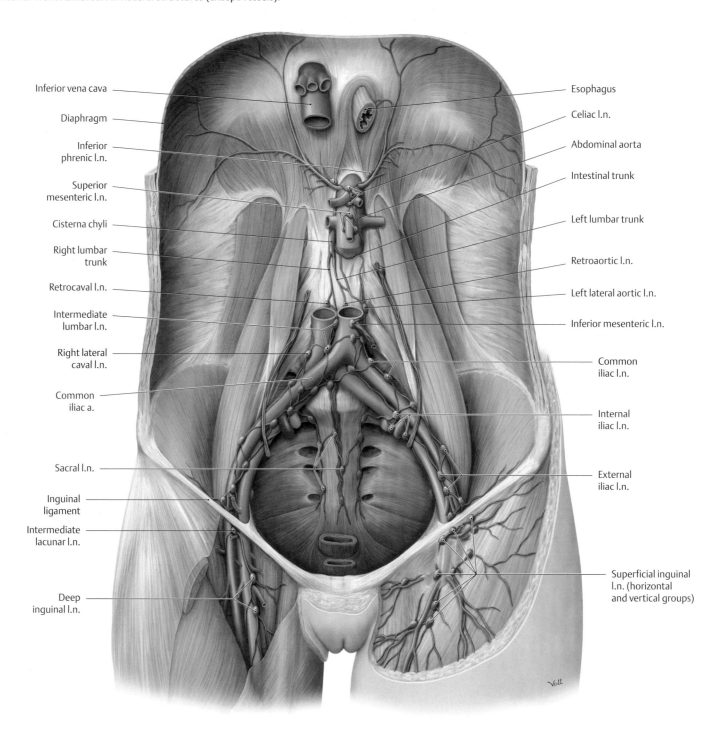

Inferior vena cava

Diaphragm

Inferior phrenic l.n.

Superior mesenteric l.n.

Cisterna chyli

Right lumbar trunk

Retrocaval l.n.

Intermediate lumbar l.n.

Right lateral caval l.n.

Common iliac a.

Sacral l.n.

Inguinal ligament

Intermediate lacunar l.n.

Deep inguinal l.n.

Esophagus

Celiac l.n.

Abdominal aorta

Intestinal trunk

Left lumbar trunk

Retroaortic l.n.

Left lateral aortic l.n.

Inferior mesenteric l.n.

Common iliac l.n.

Internal iliac l.n.

External iliac l.n.

Superficial inguinal l.n. (horizontal and vertical groups)

Fig. 16.7 Lymphatic nodes of the urinary organs
Anterior view.

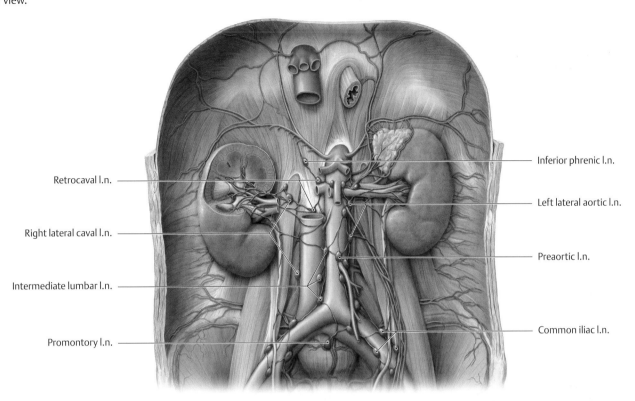

Retrocaval l.n.

Right lateral caval l.n.

Intermediate lumbar l.n.

Promontory l.n.

Inferior phrenic l.n.

Left lateral aortic l.n.

Preaortic l.n.

Common iliac l.n.

Fig. 16.8 Drainage of the kidneys (with pelvic organs)

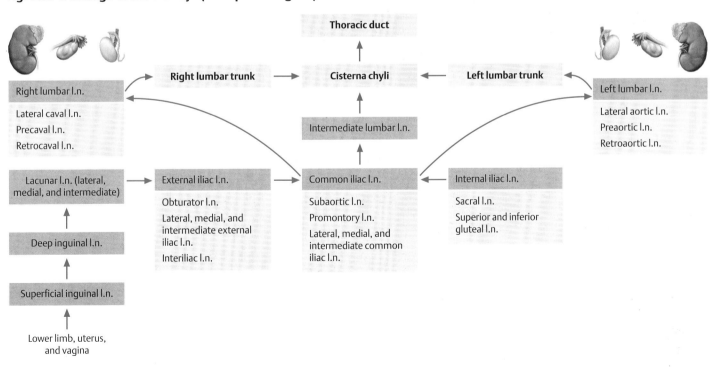

Thoracic duct

Right lumbar trunk → Cisterna chyli ← Left lumbar trunk

Right lumbar l.n.
Lateral caval l.n.
Precaval l.n.
Retrocaval l.n.

Left lumbar l.n.
Lateral aortic l.n.
Preaortic l.n.
Retroaortic l.n.

Intermediate lumbar l.n.

Lacunar l.n. (lateral, medial, and intermediate)

External iliac l.n.
Obturator l.n.
Lateral, medial, and intermediate external iliac l.n.
Interiliac l.n.

Common iliac l.n.
Subaortic l.n.
Promontory l.n.
Lateral, medial, and intermediate common iliac l.n.

Internal iliac l.n.
Sacral l.n.
Superior and inferior gluteal l.n.

Deep inguinal l.n.

Superficial inguinal l.n.

Lower limb, uterus, and vagina

Lymph Nodes of the Anterior Abdominal Organs

Fig. 16.9 **Lymph nodes of the stomach and liver**

Anterior view. *Removed:* Lesser omentum. *Opened:* Greater omentum.
Arrows show direction of lymphatic drainage.

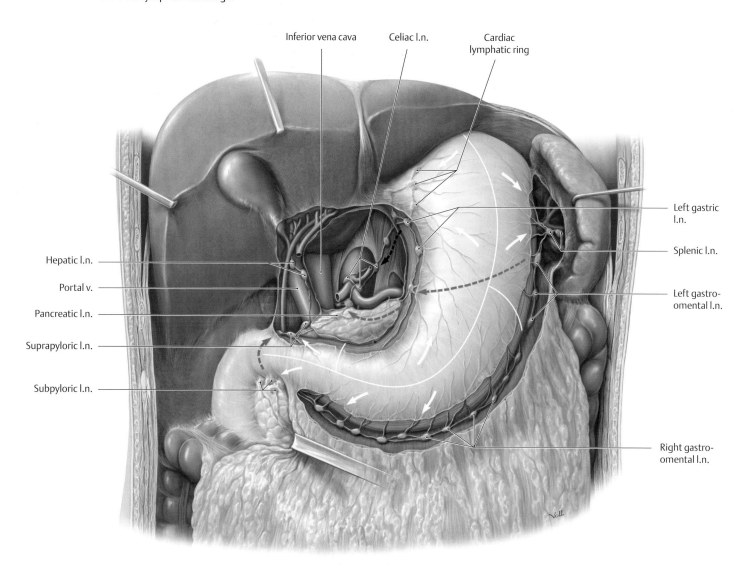

Inferior vena cava

Celiac l.n.

Cardiac lymphatic ring

Hepatic l.n.

Portal v.

Pancreatic l.n.

Suprapyloric l.n.

Subpyloric l.n.

Left gastric l.n.

Splenic l.n.

Left gastro-omental l.n.

Right gastro-omental l.n.

Fig. 16.10 Lymph nodes of the spleen, pancreas, and duodenum

Anterior view. *Removed:* Stomach and colon.

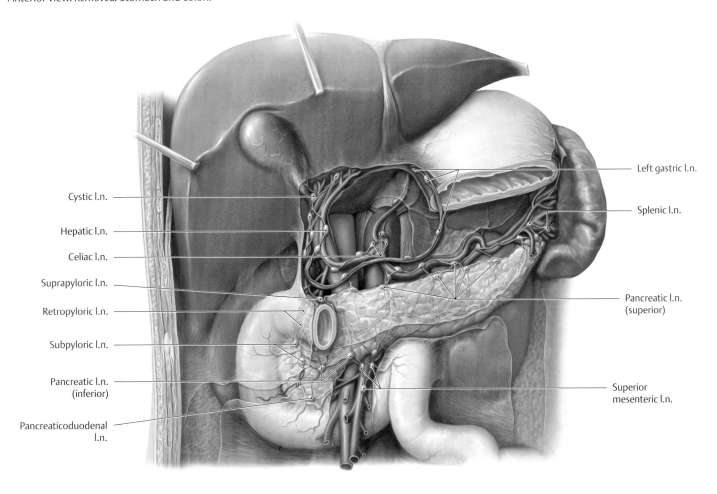

Cystic l.n.

Hepatic l.n.

Celiac l.n.

Suprapyloric l.n.

Retropyloric l.n.

Subpyloric l.n.

Pancreatic l.n. (inferior)

Pancreaticoduodenal l.n.

Left gastric l.n.

Splenic l.n.

Pancreatic l.n. (superior)

Superior mesenteric l.n.

Fig. 16.11 Lymphatic drainage of the stomach, liver, spleen, pancreas, and duodenum

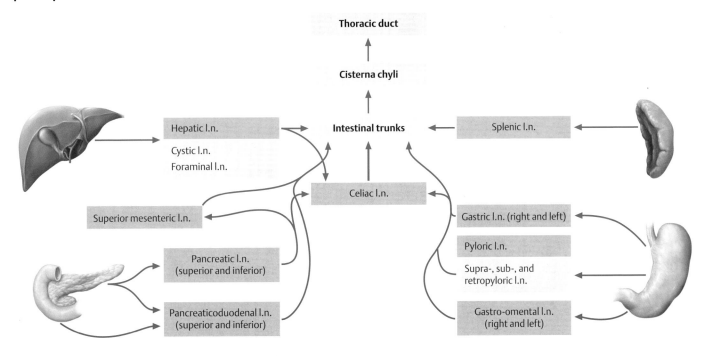

Thoracic duct

Cisterna chyli

Hepatic l.n.
Cystic l.n.
Foraminal l.n.

Intestinal trunks

Splenic l.n.

Superior mesenteric l.n.

Celiac l.n.

Gastric l.n. (right and left)

Pyloric l.n.

Supra-, sub-, and retropyloric l.n.

Pancreatic l.n. (superior and inferior)

Pancreaticoduodenal l.n. (superior and inferior)

Gastro-omental l.n. (right and left)

Lymph Nodes of the Intestines

Fig. 16.12 Lymph nodes of the jejunum and ileum
Anterior view. *Removed:* Stomach, liver, pancreas, and colon.

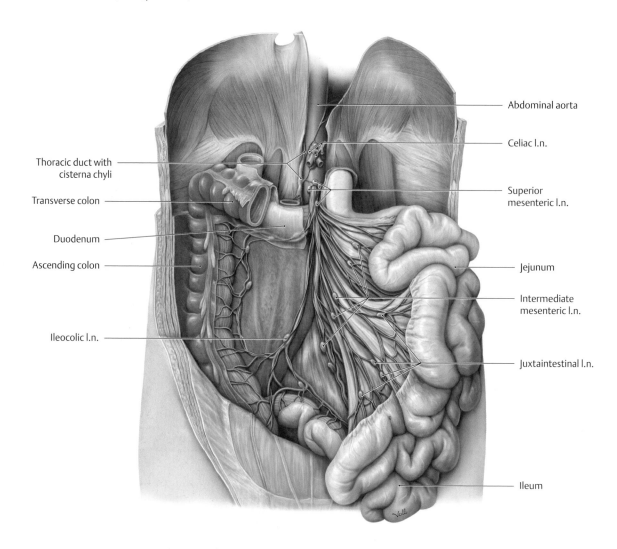

Thoracic duct with cisterna chyli

Transverse colon

Duodenum

Ascending colon

Ileocolic l.n.

Abdominal aorta

Celiac l.n.

Superior mesenteric l.n.

Jejunum

Intermediate mesenteric l.n.

Juxtaintestinal l.n.

Ileum

Fig. 16.13 Lymphatic drainage of the intestines

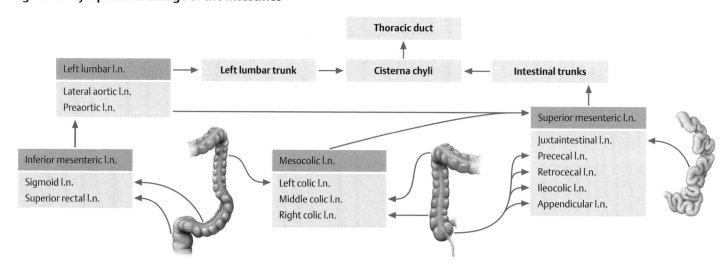

Fig. 16.14 Lymph nodes of the large intestine

Anterior view. *Reflected:* Transverse colon and greater omentum.

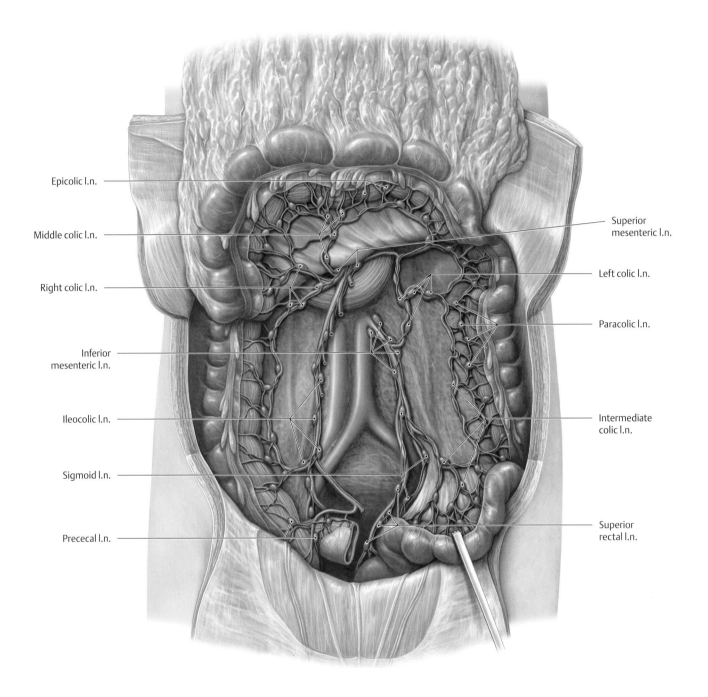

Epicolic l.n.

Middle colic l.n.

Right colic l.n.

Inferior
mesenteric l.n.

Ileocolic l.n.

Sigmoid l.n.

Prececal l.n.

Superior
mesenteric l.n.

Left colic l.n.

Paracolic l.n.

Intermediate
colic l.n.

Superior
rectal l.n.

Lymph Nodes of the Genitalia

Fig. 16.15 Lymph nodes of the male genitalia
Anterior view. *Removed:* Gastrointestinal tract (except rectal stump) and peritoneum.

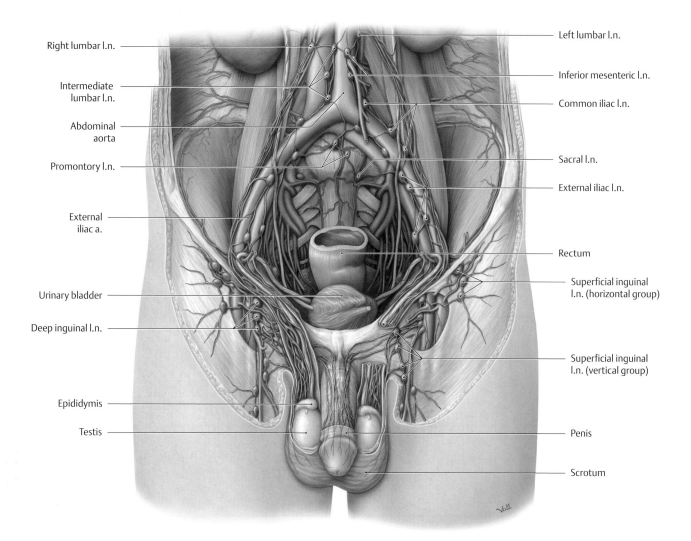

Right lumbar l.n.

Intermediate lumbar l.n.

Abdominal aorta

Promontory l.n.

External iliac a.

Urinary bladder

Deep inguinal l.n.

Epididymis

Testis

Left lumbar l.n.

Inferior mesenteric l.n.

Common iliac l.n.

Sacral l.n.

External iliac l.n.

Rectum

Superficial inguinal l.n. (horizontal group)

Superficial inguinal l.n. (vertical group)

Penis

Scrotum

Fig. 16.16 Lymph nodes of the female genitalia

Anterior view. *Removed:* Gastrointestinal tract (except rectal stump) and peritoneum. *Retracted:* Uterus.

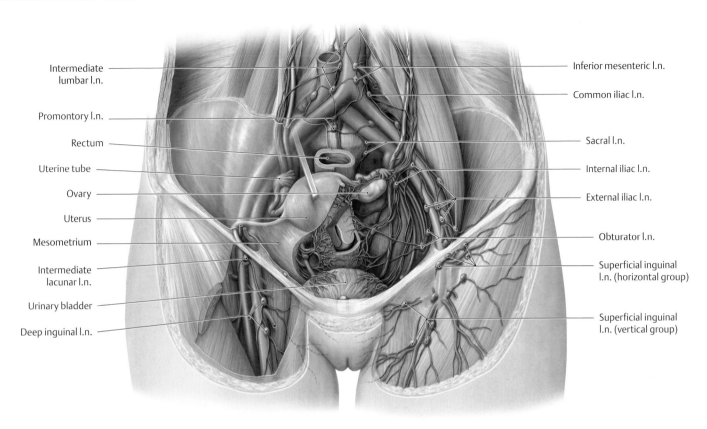

Intermediate lumbar l.n.
Promontory l.n.
Rectum
Uterine tube
Ovary
Uterus
Mesometrium
Intermediate lacunar l.n.
Urinary bladder
Deep inguinal l.n.

Inferior mesenteric l.n.
Common iliac l.n.
Sacral l.n.
Internal iliac l.n.
External iliac l.n.
Obturator l.n.
Superficial inguinal l.n. (horizontal group)
Superficial inguinal l.n. (vertical group)

Fig. 16.17 Lymphatic drainage of the pelvic organs

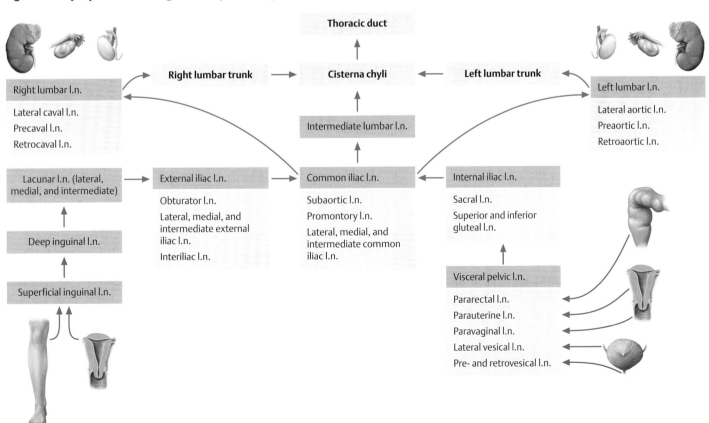

Thoracic duct

Right lumbar trunk → Cisterna chyli ← Left lumbar trunk

Right lumbar l.n.
Lateral caval l.n.
Precaval l.n.
Retrocaval l.n.

Intermediate lumbar l.n.

Left lumbar l.n.
Lateral aortic l.n.
Preaortic l.n.
Retroaortic l.n.

Lacunar l.n. (lateral, medial, and intermediate) → External iliac l.n.
Obturator l.n.
Lateral, medial, and intermediate external iliac l.n.
Interiliac l.n.

Common iliac l.n.
Subaortic l.n.
Promontory l.n.
Lateral, medial, and intermediate common iliac l.n.

Internal iliac l.n.
Sacral l.n.
Superior and inferior gluteal l.n.

Deep inguinal l.n.

Superficial inguinal l.n.

Visceral pelvic l.n.
Pararectal l.n.
Parauterine l.n.
Paravaginal l.n.
Lateral vesical l.n.
Pre- and retrovesical l.n.

235

Autonomic Plexuses

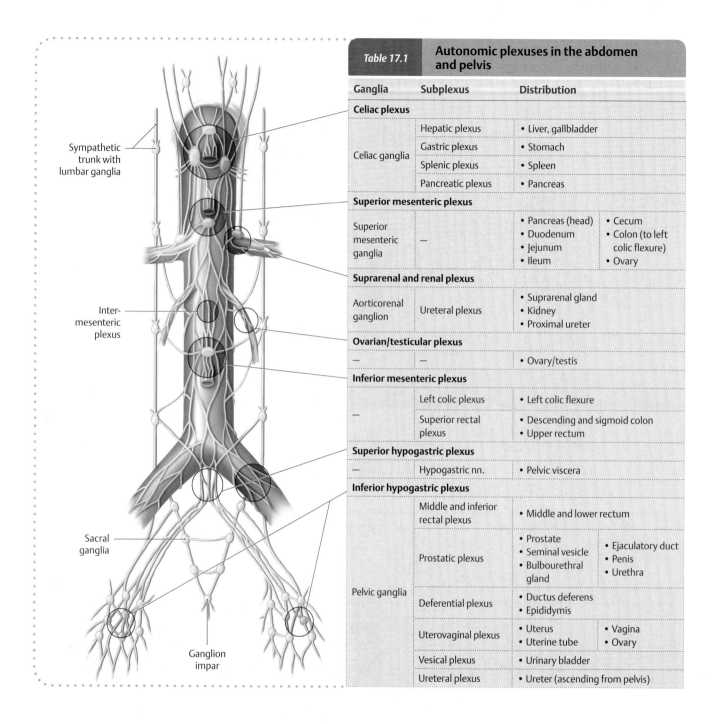

Sympathetic trunk with lumbar ganglia

Inter-mesenteric plexus

Sacral ganglia

Ganglion impar

Table 17.1	Autonomic plexuses in the abdomen and pelvis	

Ganglia	Subplexus	Distribution	
Celiac plexus			
Celiac ganglia	Hepatic plexus	• Liver, gallbladder	
	Gastric plexus	• Stomach	
	Splenic plexus	• Spleen	
	Pancreatic plexus	• Pancreas	
Superior mesenteric plexus			
Superior mesenteric ganglia	—	• Pancreas (head) • Duodenum • Jejunum • Ileum	• Cecum • Colon (to left colic flexure) • Ovary
Suprarenal and renal plexus			
Aorticorenal ganglion	Ureteral plexus	• Suprarenal gland • Kidney • Proximal ureter	
Ovarian/testicular plexus			
—	—	• Ovary/testis	
Inferior mesenteric plexus			
—	Left colic plexus	• Left colic flexure	
	Superior rectal plexus	• Descending and sigmoid colon • Upper rectum	
Superior hypogastric plexus			
—	Hypogastric nn.	• Pelvic viscera	
Inferior hypogastric plexus			
Pelvic ganglia	Middle and inferior rectal plexus	• Middle and lower rectum	
	Prostatic plexus	• Prostate • Seminal vesicle • Bulbourethral gland	• Ejaculatory duct • Penis • Urethra
	Deferential plexus	• Ductus deferens • Epididymis	
	Uterovaginal plexus	• Uterus • Uterine tube	• Vagina • Ovary
	Vesical plexus	• Urinary bladder	
	Ureteral plexus	• Ureter (ascending from pelvis)	

Fig. 17.1 Autonomic plexuses in the abdomen and pelvis

Anterior view of the male abdomen. *Removed:* Peritoneum and majority of the stomach.

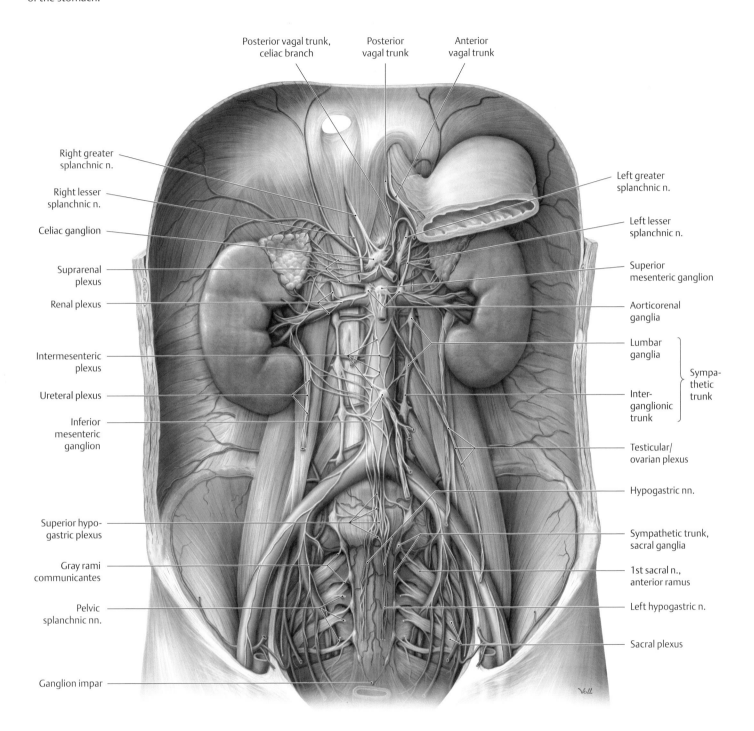

Posterior vagal trunk, celiac branch

Posterior vagal trunk

Anterior vagal trunk

Right greater splanchnic n.

Right lesser splanchnic n.

Celiac ganglion

Suprarenal plexus

Renal plexus

Intermesenteric plexus

Ureteral plexus

Inferior mesenteric ganglion

Superior hypo-gastric plexus

Gray rami communicantes

Pelvic splanchnic nn.

Ganglion impar

Left greater splanchnic n.

Left lesser splanchnic n.

Superior mesenteric ganglion

Aorticorenal ganglia

Lumbar ganglia

Inter-ganglionic trunk

Sympa-thetic trunk

Testicular/ ovarian plexus

Hypogastric nn.

Sympathetic trunk, sacral ganglia

1st sacral n., anterior ramus

Left hypogastric n.

Sacral plexus

Innervation of the Abdominal Organs

Fig. 17.2 **Innervation of the anterior abdominal organs**

Anterior view. *Removed:* Lesser omentum, ascending colon, and parts of the transverse colon. *Opened:* Lesser sac. The anterior and posterior vagal trunks each produce a celiac, hepatic, and pyloric branch, and a gastric plexus. See p. 245 for schematic.

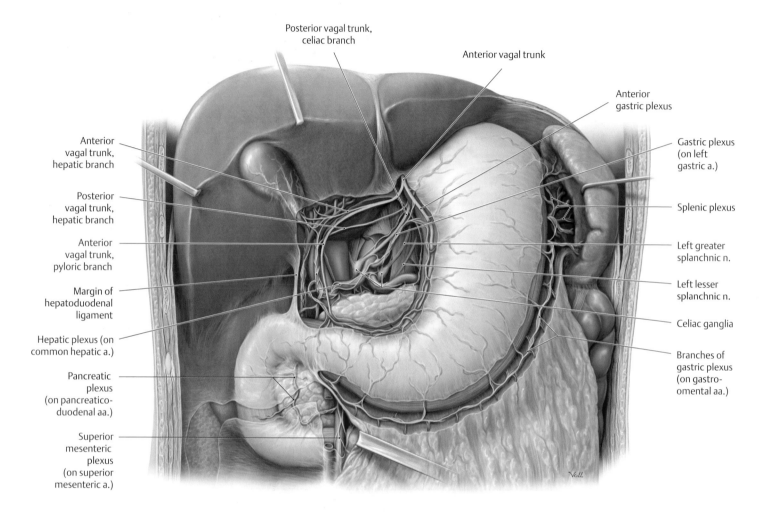

Fig. 17.3 **Innervation of the urinary organs**

Anterior view of the male abdomen and pelvis. *Removed:* Abdominal organs and peritoneum. See p. 246 for schematic.

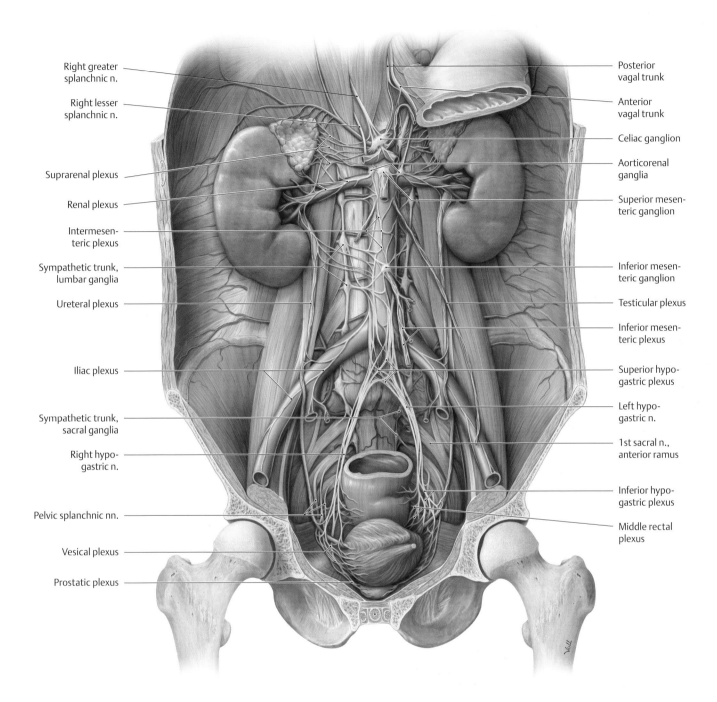

Right greater splanchnic n.

Right lesser splanchnic n.

Suprarenal plexus

Renal plexus

Intermesenteric plexus

Sympathetic trunk, lumbar ganglia

Ureteral plexus

Iliac plexus

Sympathetic trunk, sacral ganglia

Right hypogastric n.

Pelvic splanchnic nn.

Vesical plexus

Prostatic plexus

Posterior vagal trunk

Anterior vagal trunk

Celiac ganglion

Aorticorenal ganglia

Superior mesenteric ganglion

Inferior mesenteric ganglion

Testicular plexus

Inferior mesenteric plexus

Superior hypogastric plexus

Left hypogastric n.

1st sacral n., anterior ramus

Inferior hypogastric plexus

Middle rectal plexus

Innervation of the Intestines

Fig. 17.4 **Innervation of the small intestine**
Anterior view. *Partially removed:* Stomach, pancreas,
and transverse colon (distal part). See p. 245 for schematic.

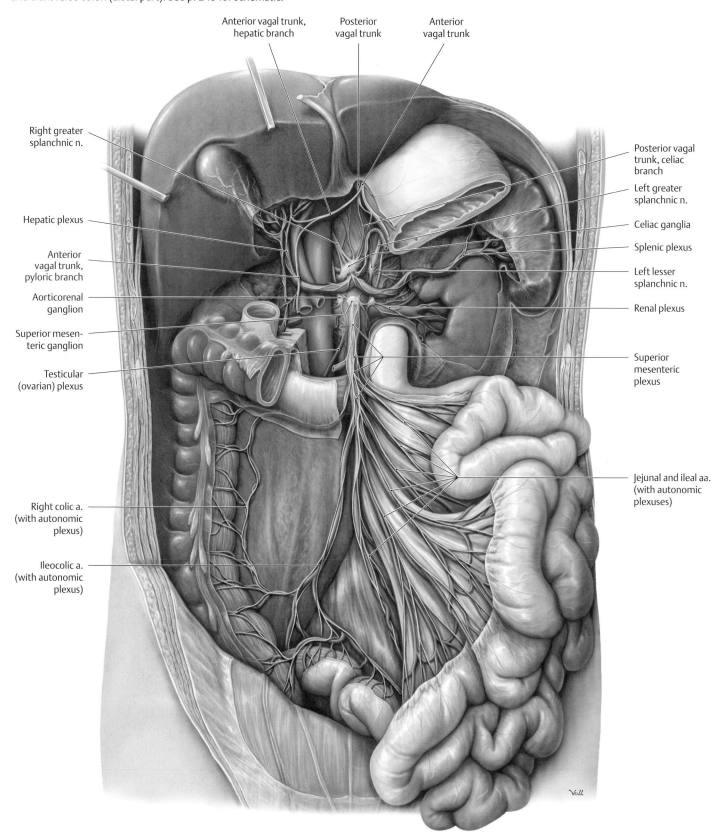

Anterior vagal trunk,
hepatic branch

Posterior
vagal trunk

Anterior
vagal trunk

Right greater
splanchnic n.

Posterior vagal
trunk, celiac
branch

Left greater
splanchnic n.

Hepatic plexus

Celiac ganglia

Splenic plexus

Anterior
vagal trunk,
pyloric branch

Left lesser
splanchnic n.

Aorticorenal
ganglion

Renal plexus

Superior mesen-
teric ganglion

Superior
mesenteric
plexus

Testicular
(ovarian) plexus

Jejunal and ileal aa.
(with autonomic
plexuses)

Right colic a.
(with autonomic
plexus)

Ileocolic a.
(with autonomic
plexus)

Fig. 17.5 **Innervation of the large intestine**

Anterior view. *Removed:* Jejunum and ileum. *Reflected:* Transverse and sigmoid colons. See p. 245 for schematic.

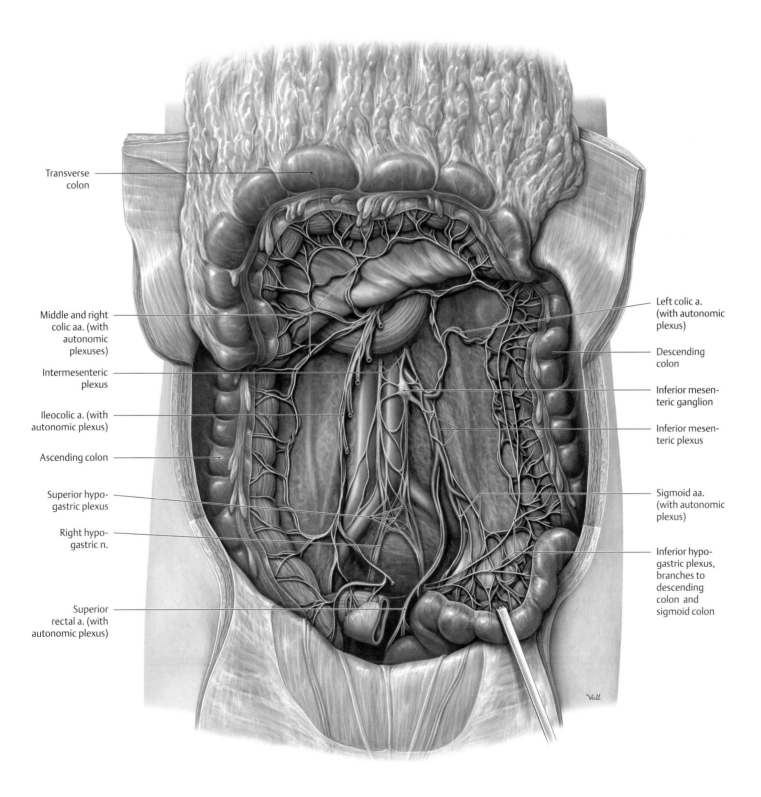

Transverse colon

Middle and right colic aa. (with autonomic plexuses)

Intermesenteric plexus

Ileocolic a. (with autonomic plexus)

Ascending colon

Superior hypogastric plexus

Right hypogastric n.

Superior rectal a. (with autonomic plexus)

Left colic a. (with autonomic plexus)

Descending colon

Inferior mesenteric ganglion

Inferior mesenteric plexus

Sigmoid aa. (with autonomic plexus)

Inferior hypogastric plexus, branches to descending colon and sigmoid colon

Innervation of the Pelvis

Fig. 17.6 **Innervation of the female pelvis**
Right pelvis, left lateral view. *Reflected:* Uterus and rectum.
See p. 247 for schematic.

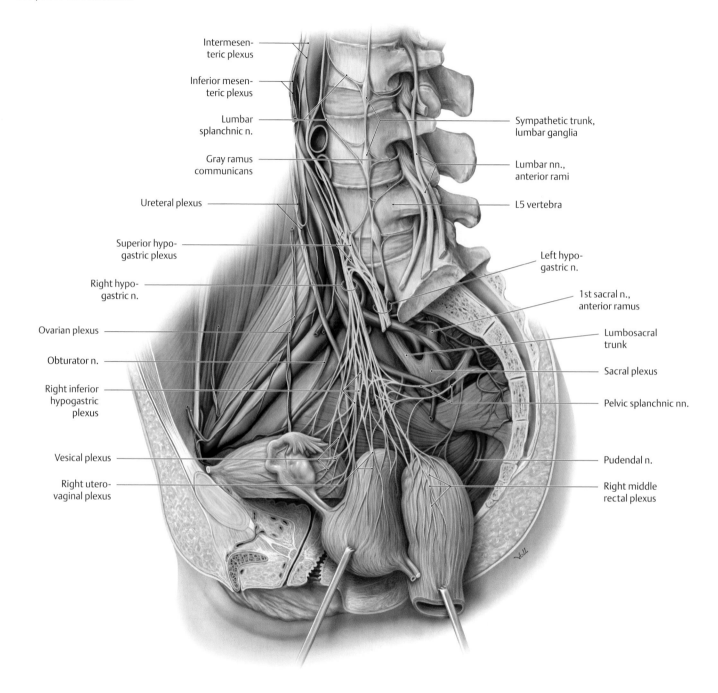

Intermesen-
teric plexus

Inferior mesen-
teric plexus

Lumbar
splanchnic n.

Gray ramus
communicans

Ureteral plexus

Superior hypo-
gastric plexus

Right hypo-
gastric n.

Ovarian plexus

Obturator n.

Right inferior
hypogastric
plexus

Vesical plexus

Right utero-
vaginal plexus

Sympathetic trunk,
lumbar ganglia

Lumbar nn.,
anterior rami

L5 vertebra

Left hypo-
gastric n.

1st sacral n.,
anterior ramus

Lumbosacral
trunk

Sacral plexus

Pelvic splanchnic nn.

Pudendal n.

Right middle
rectal plexus

Fig. 17.7 **Innervation of the male pelvis**

Right pelvis, left lateral view. See p. 247 for schematic.

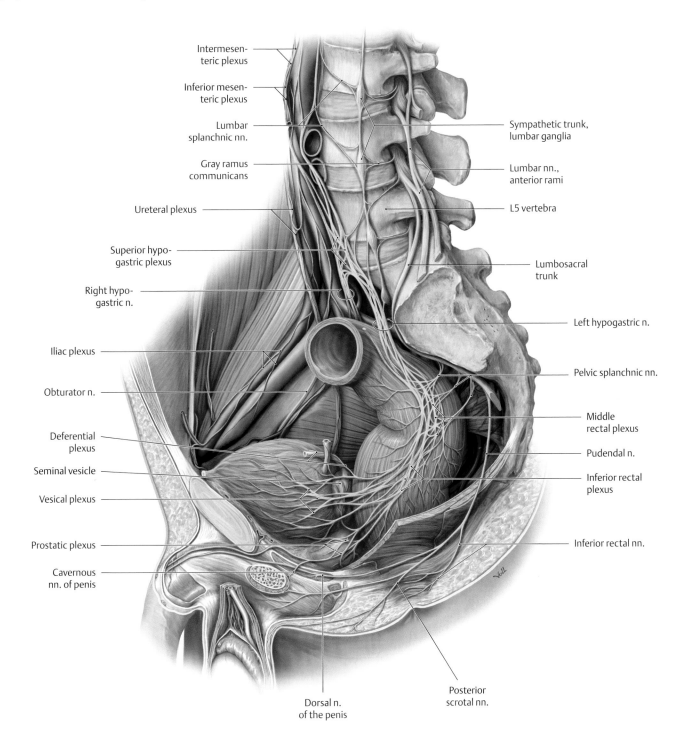

Intermesen-teric plexus

Inferior mesen-teric plexus

Lumbar splanchnic nn.

Gray ramus communicans

Ureteral plexus

Superior hypo-gastric plexus

Right hypo-gastric n.

Iliac plexus

Obturator n.

Deferential plexus

Seminal vesicle

Vesical plexus

Prostatic plexus

Cavernous nn. of penis

Dorsal n. of the penis

Posterior scrotal nn.

Sympathetic trunk, lumbar ganglia

Lumbar nn., anterior rami

L5 vertebra

Lumbosacral trunk

Left hypogastric n.

Pelvic splanchnic nn.

Middle rectal plexus

Pudendal n.

Inferior rectal plexus

Inferior rectal nn.

Autonomic Innervation: Overview

Fig. 17.8 Sympathetic and parasympathetic nervous systems in the abdomen and pelvis

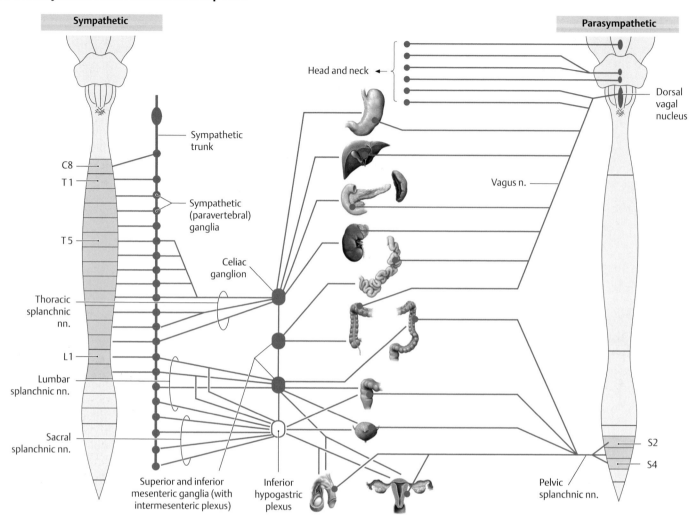

A Sympathetic nervous system.

B Parasympathetic nervous system.

Table 17.2	Effects of the autonomic nervous system in the abdomen and pelvis		
Organ (organ system)		**Sympathetic effect**	**Parasympathetic effect**
Gastrointestinal tract	Longitudinal and circular muscle fibers	↓ motility	↑ motility
	Sphincter muscles	Contraction	Relaxation
	Glands	↓ secretions	↑ secretions
Splenic capsule		Contraction	
Liver		↑ glycogenolysis/gluconeogenesis	No effect
Pancreas	Endocrine pancreas	↓ insulin secretion	
	Exocrine pancreas	↓ secretion	↑ secretion
Urinary bladder	Detrusor vesicae	Relaxation	Contraction
	Functional bladder sphincter	Contraction	Inhibits contraction
Seminal vesicle and ductus deferens		Contraction (ejaculation)	No effect
Uterus		Contraction or relaxation, depending on hormonal status	
Arteries		Vasoconstriction	Vasodilation of the arteries of the penis and clitoris (erection)
Suprarenal glands (medulla)		Release of adrenalin	No effect
Urinary tract	Kidney	Vasoconstriction (↓ urine formation)	Vasodilation

Fig. 17.9 **Autonomic innervation of the intraperitoneal organs**

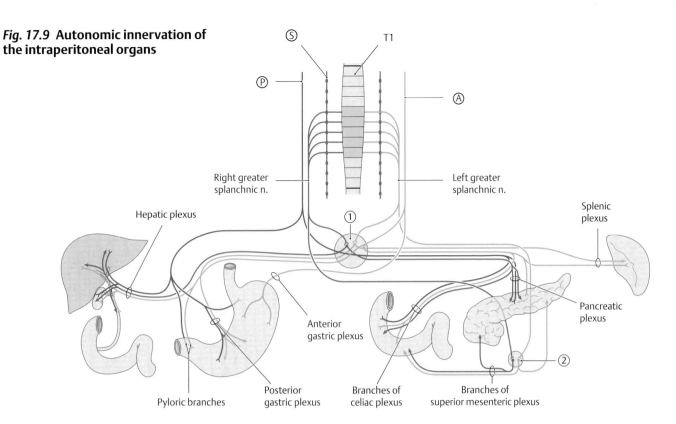

A Innervation of the foregut. As the left and right vagus nerves descend along the esophagus, they become the anterior and posterior vagal trunks, respectively. Each trunk produces a celiac, pyloric, and hepatic branch, and a gastric plexus.

Ⓢ	Sympathetic trunk
Ⓟ	Posterior vagal trunk (from right vagus n.)
Ⓐ	Anterior vagal trunk (from left vagus n.)
①	Celiac ganglia
②	Superior mesenteric ganglion
③	Inferior mesenteric ganglion
④	Greater splanchnic n. (T5–T9)
⑤	Lesser splanchnic n. (T10–T11)
⑥	Least splanchnic n. (T12)
⑦	Lumbar splanchnic nn. (L1–L2)
⑧	Lumbar splanchnic nn. (from 3rd to 5th lumbar ganglia)
⑨	Sacral splanchnic nn. (from 1st to 3rd sacral ganglia)
⑩	Pelvic splanchnic nn. (S2–S4)

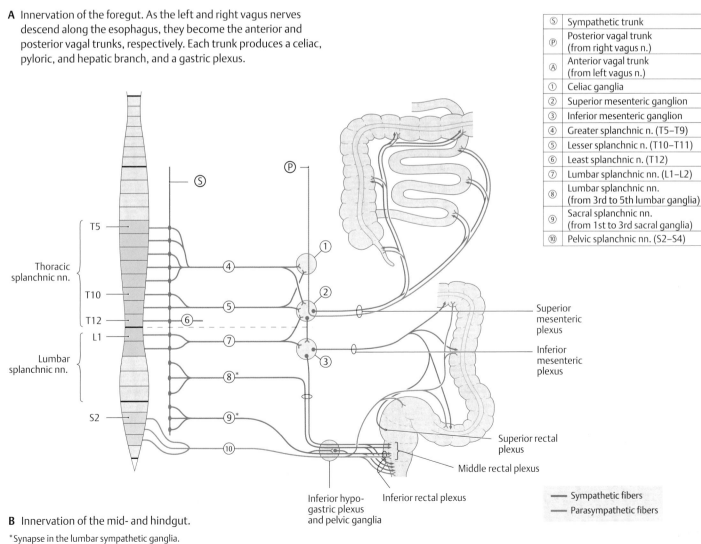

B Innervation of the mid- and hindgut.

*Synapse in the lumbar sympathetic ganglia.

Autonomic Innervation: Urinary & Genital Organs

Fig. 17.10 Autonomic innervation
of the urinary organs

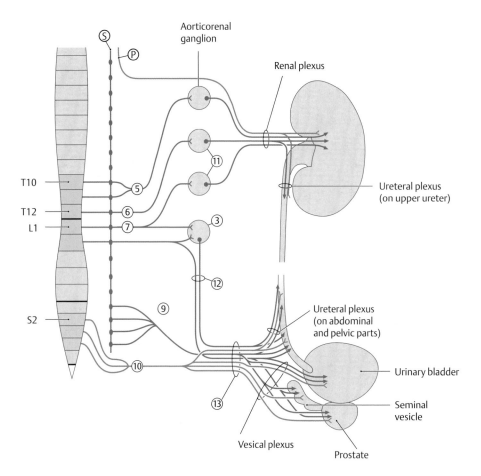

| — | Sympathetic fibers |
| — | Parasympathetic fibers |

Numbering continued from p. 245.	
Ⓢ	Sympathetic trunk
Ⓟ	Posterior vagal trunk (from right vagus n.)
③	Inferior mesenteric ganglion
⑤	Lesser splanchnic n. (T10–T11)
⑥	Least splanchnic n. (T12)
⑦	Lumbar splanchnic nn. (L1–L2)
⑨	Sacral splanchnic nn. (from 1st to 3rd sacral ganglia)
⑩	Pelvic splanchnic nn. (S2–S4)
⑪	Renal ganglia
⑫	Superior hypogastric plexus
⑬	Inferior hypogastric plexus

Clinical

Referred pain from the internal organs

The convergence of somatic and visceral afferent fibers to a common level of the spinal cord confuses the relationship between the perceived and actual sites of pain, a phenomenon known as referred pain. Pain impulses from a particular organ are consistently projected to the same well-defined skin area.

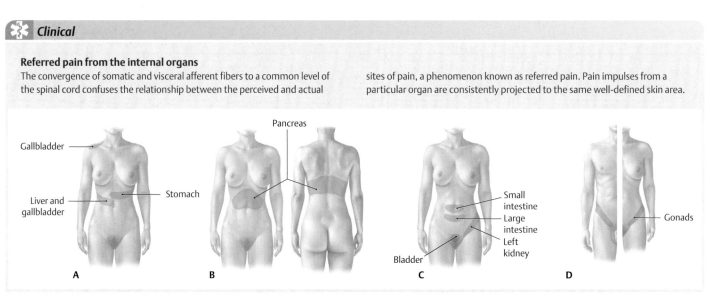

Fig. 17.11 Autonomic innervation of the genitalia

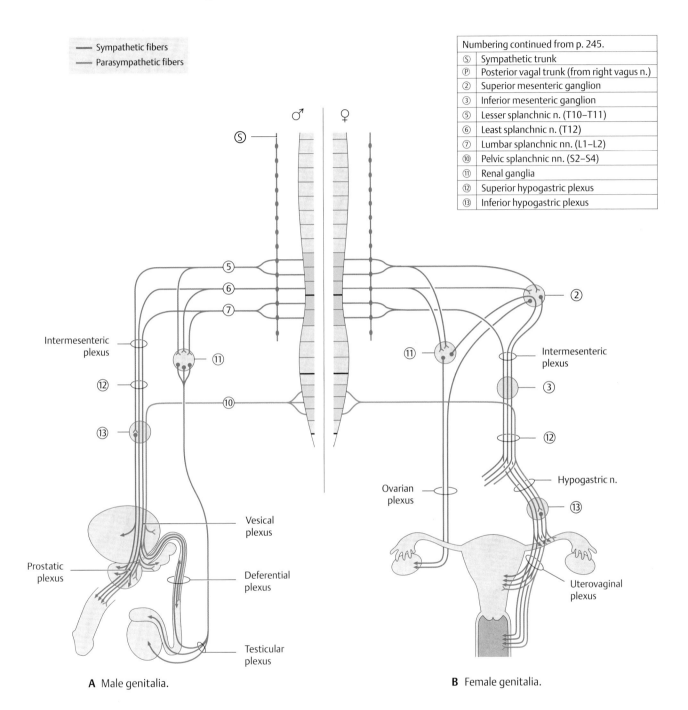

Numbering continued from p. 245.

Ⓢ	Sympathetic trunk
Ⓟ	Posterior vagal trunk (from right vagus n.)
②	Superior mesenteric ganglion
③	Inferior mesenteric ganglion
⑤	Lesser splanchnic n. (T10–T11)
⑥	Least splanchnic n. (T12)
⑦	Lumbar splanchnic nn. (L1–L2)
⑩	Pelvic splanchnic nn. (S2–S4)
⑪	Renal ganglia
⑫	Superior hypogastric plexus
⑬	Inferior hypogastric plexus

— Sympathetic fibers
— Parasympathetic fibers

Intermesenteric plexus

Prostatic plexus

Vesical plexus

Deferential plexus

Testicular plexus

A Male genitalia.

Intermesenteric plexus

Ovarian plexus

Hypogastric n.

Uterovaginal plexus

B Female genitalia.

Surface Anatomy

Fig. 18.1 **Palpable structures in the abdomen and pelvis**
Anterior view. See pp. 40–41 for structures of the back.

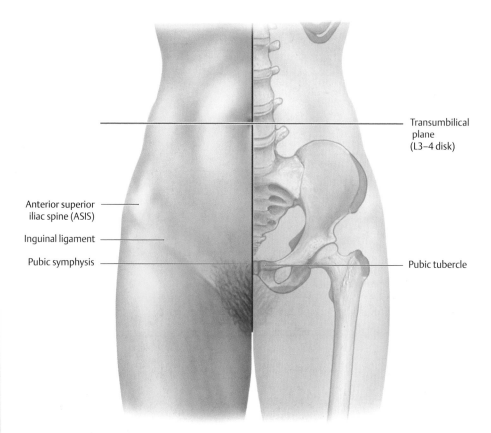

Transumbilical plane (L3–4 disk)

Anterior superior iliac spine (ASIS)

Inguinal ligament

Pubic symphysis

Pubic tubercle

A Bony prominences.

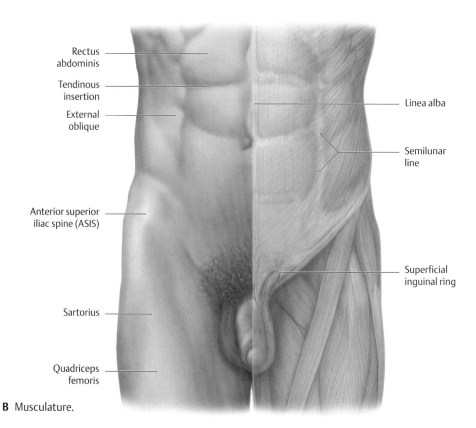

Rectus abdominis

Tendinous insertion

External oblique

Linea alba

Semilunar line

Anterior superior iliac spine (ASIS)

Superficial inguinal ring

Sartorius

Quadriceps femoris

B Musculature.

Fig. 18.2 **Surface anatomy of the abdomen and pelvis**
Anterior view. See pp. 40–41 for structures of the back.

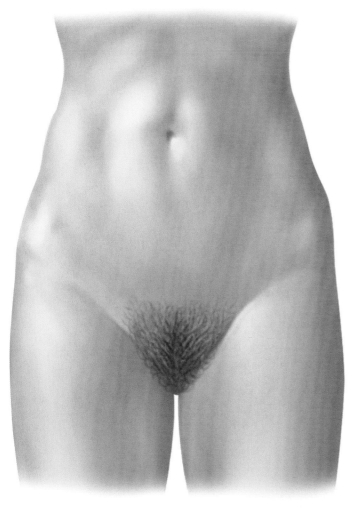

A Female abdomen and pelvis.

Q1: How would this patient's abdomen be subdivided for descriptive purposes into four quadrants? Name five organs in each quadrant.

Q2: A patient's inguinal region shows a slight swelling just superior to the middle of the inguinal region. What factors (age, anatomical) might assist you in determining if this is a direct or indirect inguinal hernia?

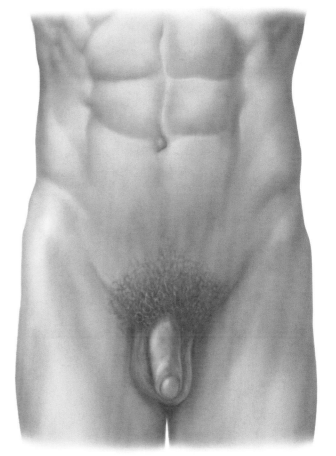

B Male abdomen and pelvis.

See answers beginning on p. 626.

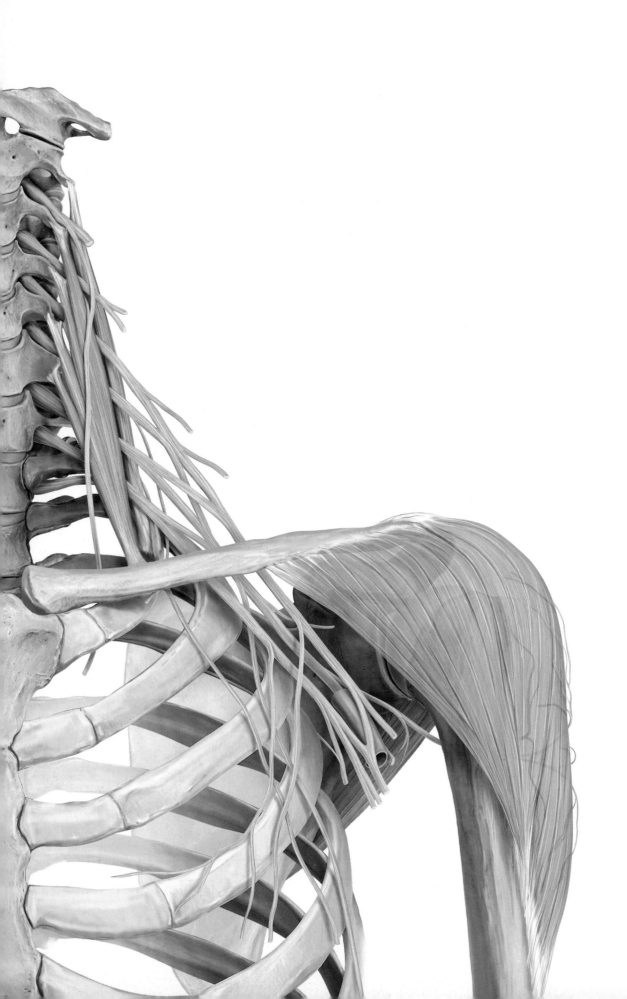

Upper Limb

Bones of the Upper Limb

Fig. 19.1 Skeleton of the upper limb

Right limb. The upper limb is subdivided into three regions: arm, fore-arm, and hand. The shoulder girdle (clavicle and scapula) joins the upper limb to the thorax at the sternoclavicular joint.

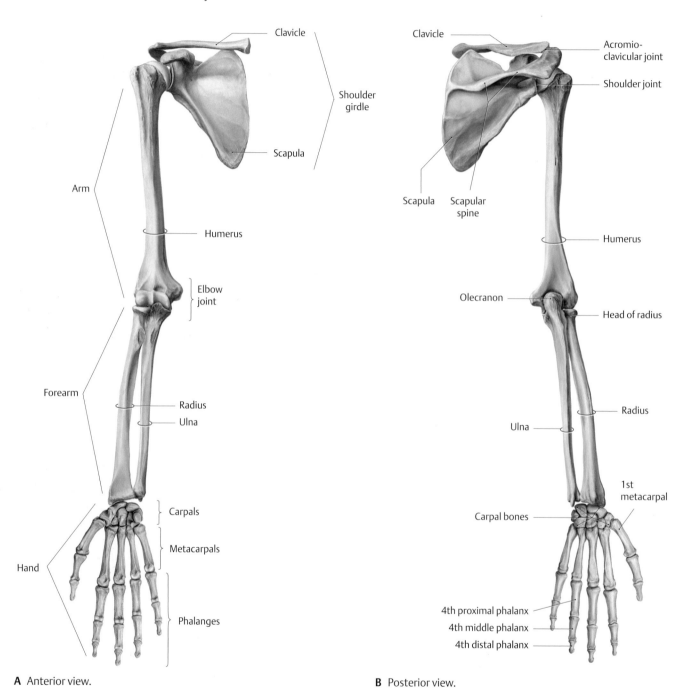

A Anterior view.

B Posterior view.

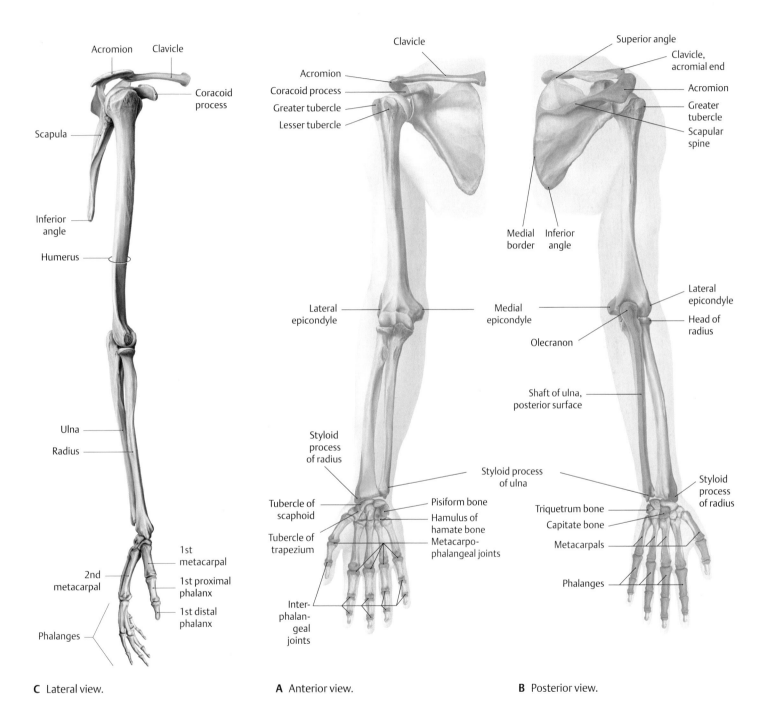

Fig. 19.2 **Palpable bony prominences**

Except for the lunate and trapezoid bones, all of the bones in the upper limb are palpable to some degree through the skin and soft tissues.

C Lateral view.

A Anterior view.

B Posterior view.

Clavicle & Scapula

 The shoulder girdle (clavicle and scapula) connects the bones of the upper limb to the thoracic cage. Whereas the pelvic girdle (paired hip bones) is firmly integrated into the axial skeleton (see p. 358), the shoulder girdle is extremely mobile.

Fig. 19.3 **Clavicle**

Right clavicle. The S-shaped clavicle is visible and palpable along its entire length (generally 12 to 15 cm). Its medial end articulates with the sternum at the sternoclavicular joint (see p. 258). Its lateral end articulates with the scapula at the acromioclavicular joint (see p. 259).

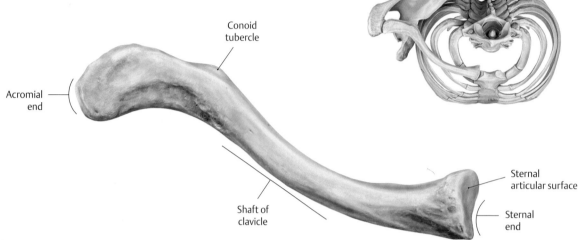

A Superior view.

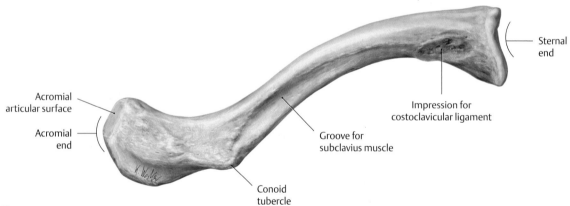

B Inferior view.

✚ *Clinical*

Scapular foramen

The superior transverse ligament of the scapula (see p. 259) may become ossified, transforming the scapular notch into an anomalous bony canal, the scapular foramen. This can lead to compression of the suprascapular nerve as it passes through the canal (see p. 333).

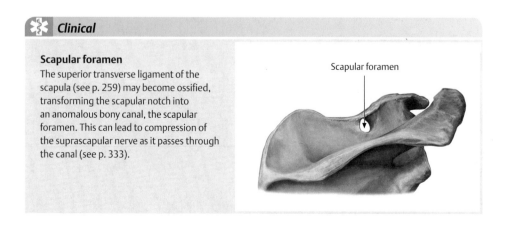

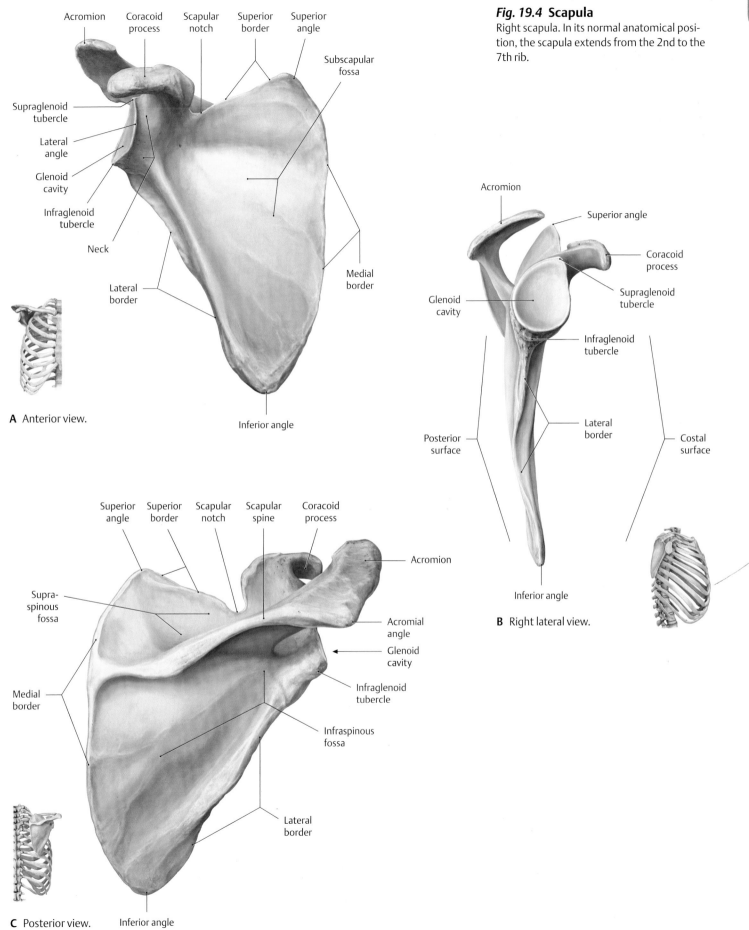

Fig. 19.4 Scapula

Right scapula. In its normal anatomical position, the scapula extends from the 2nd to the 7th rib.

Acromion
Coracoid process
Scapular notch
Superior border
Superior angle
Subscapular fossa
Supraglenoid tubercle
Lateral angle
Glenoid cavity
Infraglenoid tubercle
Neck
Lateral border
Medial border

A Anterior view.

Inferior angle

Acromion
Superior angle
Coracoid process
Supraglenoid tubercle
Glenoid cavity
Infraglenoid tubercle
Posterior surface
Lateral border
Costal surface
Inferior angle

B Right lateral view.

Superior angle
Superior border
Scapular notch
Scapular spine
Coracoid process
Acromion
Supra-spinous fossa
Acromial angle
Glenoid cavity
Medial border
Infraglenoid tubercle
Infraspinous fossa
Lateral border

C Posterior view.

Inferior angle

Humerus

Fig. 19.5 Humerus

Right humerus. The head of the humerus articulates with the scapula at the glenohumeral joint (see p. 258). The capitellum and trochlea of the humerus articulate with the radius and ulna, respectively, at the elbow (cubital) joint (see p. 282).

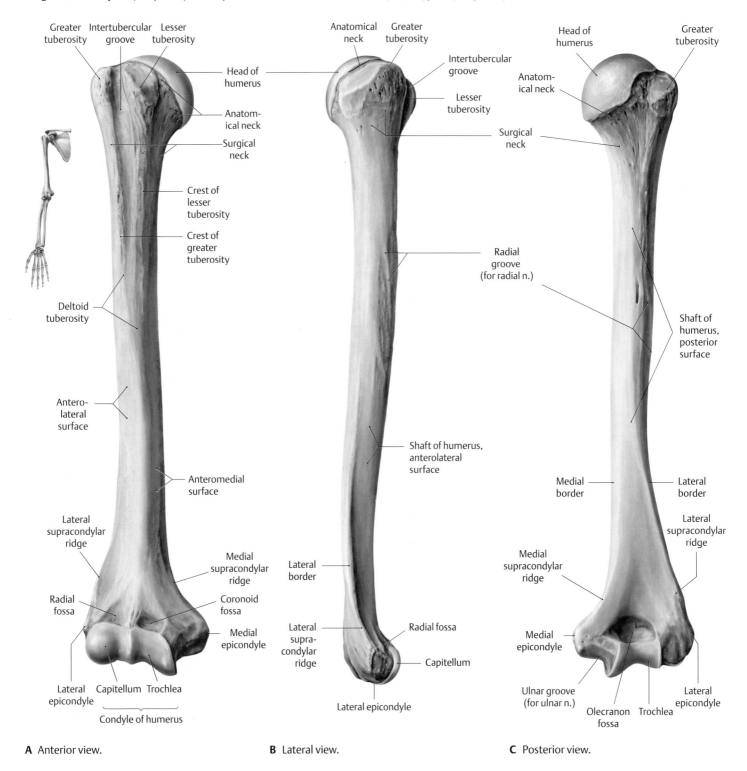

A Anterior view.

B Lateral view.

C Posterior view.

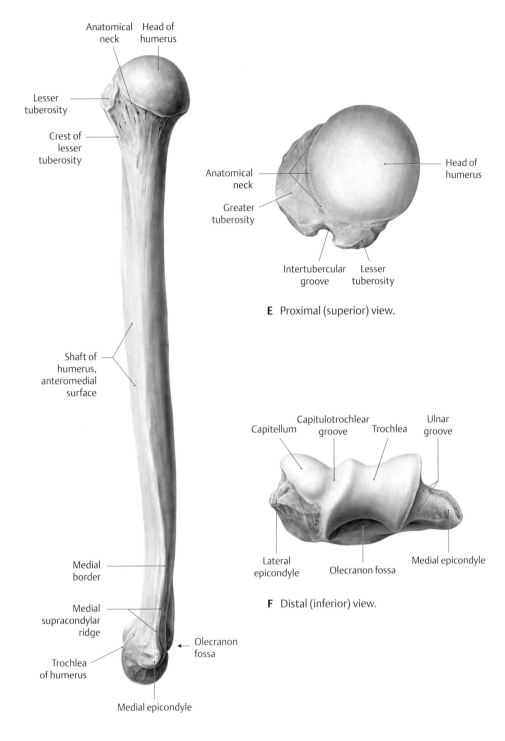

Anatomical neck Head of humerus

Lesser tuberosity

Crest of lesser tuberosity

Shaft of humerus, anteromedial surface

Medial border

Medial supracondylar ridge

Trochlea of humerus

Olecranon fossa

Medial epicondyle

D Medial view.

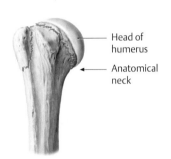

Anatomical neck

Greater tuberosity

Head of humerus

Intertubercular groove   Lesser tuberosity

E Proximal (superior) view.

Capitellum   Capitulotrochlear groove   Trochlea   Ulnar groove

Lateral epicondyle   Olecranon fossa   Medial epicondyle

F Distal (inferior) view.

✴ *Clinical*

Fractures of the humerus

Anterior view. Fractures of the proximal humerus are very common and occur predominantly in older patients who sustain a fall onto the outstretched arm or directly onto the shoulder. Three main types are distinguished.

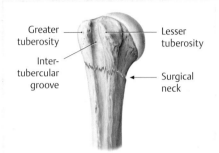

Greater tuberosity

Inter-tubercular groove

Lesser tuberosity

Surgical neck

A Extra-articular fracture.

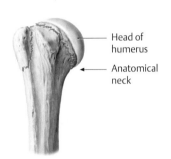

Head of humerus

Anatomical neck

B Intra-articular fracture.

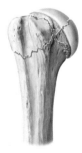

C Comminuted fracture.

Extra-articular fractures and intra-articular fractures are often accompanied by injuries of the blood vessels that supply the humeral head (anterior and posterior circumflex humeral arteries), with an associated risk of post-traumatic avascular necrosis.

Fractures of the humeral shaft and distal humerus are frequently associated with damage to the radial nerve.

Joints of the Shoulder

Fig. 19.6 Joints of the shoulder: Overview
Right shoulder, anterior view.

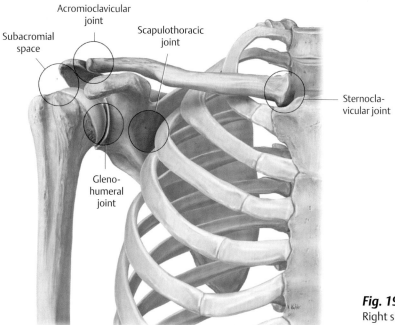

Fig. 19.7 Joints of the shoulder girdle
Right side, superior view.

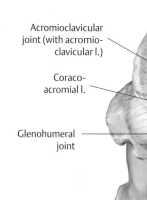

Fig. 19.8 Scapulothoracic joint
Right side, superior view. In all movements of the shoulder girdle, the scapula glides on a curved surface of loose connective tissue between the serratus anterior and the subscapularis muscles. This surface can be considered a scapulothoracic joint.

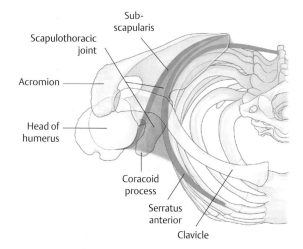

Fig. 19.9 **Sternoclavicular joint**

Anterior view with sternum coronally sectioned (left). *Note:* A fibrocartilaginous articular disk compensates for the mismatch of surfaces between the two saddle-shaped articular facets of the clavicle and manubrium sterni.

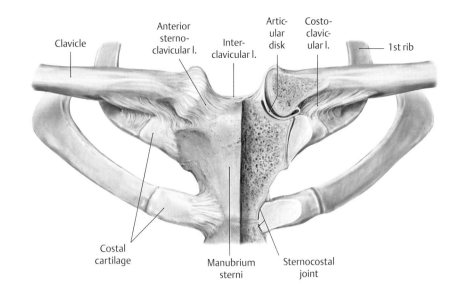

Fig. 19.10 **Acromioclavicular joint**

Anterior view. The acromioclavicular joint is a plane joint. Because the articulating surfaces are flat, they must be held in place by strong ligaments, greatly limiting the mobility of the joint.

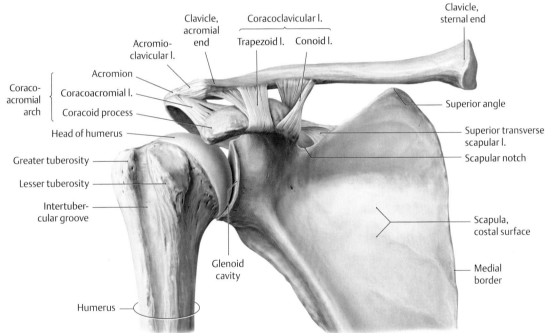

 Clinical

Injuries of the acromioclavicular joint

A fall onto the outstretched arm or shoulder frequently causes dislocation of the acromioclavicular joint and damage to the coracoclavicular ligaments.

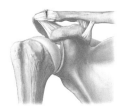

A Stretching of ligaments.

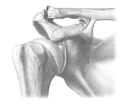

B Rupture of acromioclavicular ligament.

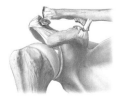

C Complete dislocation of acromioclavicular joint.

Joints of the Shoulder: Glenohumeral Joint

Fig. 19.11 **Glenohumeral joint: Bony elements**
Right shoulder.

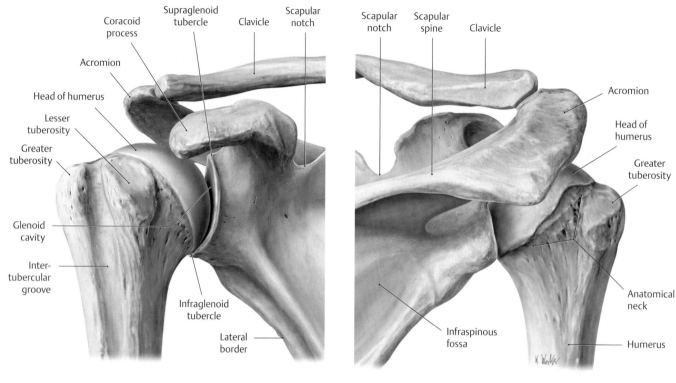

A Anterior view.

B Posterior view.

Fig. 19.12 **Radiograph of the shoulder**
Anteroposterior view.

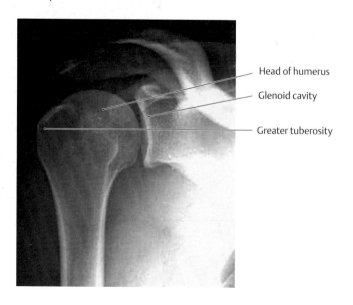

Fig. 19.13 Glenohumeral joint: Capsule and ligaments

Right shoulder.

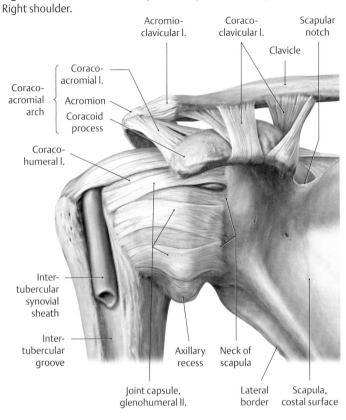

A Anterior view.

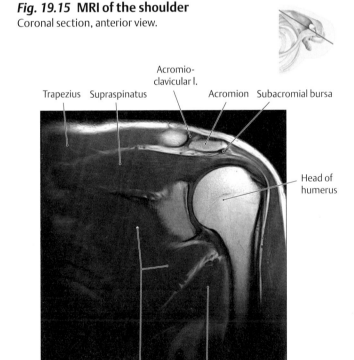

B Posterior view.

Fig. 19.14 Glenohumeral joint cavity

Anterior view.

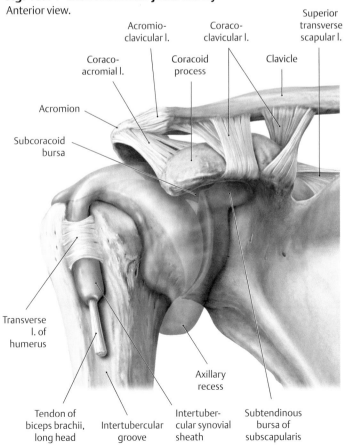

Fig. 19.15 MRI of the shoulder

Coronal section, anterior view.

Subacromial Space & Bursae

Fig. 19.16 Subacromial space
Right shoulder.

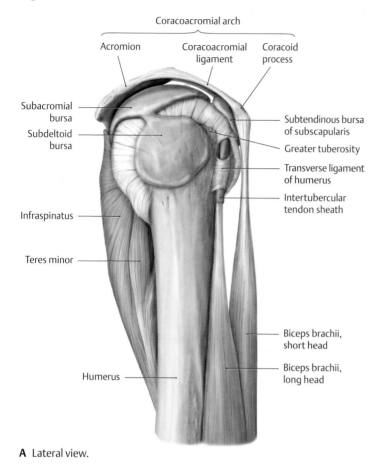

Coracoacromial arch

Acromion — Coracoacromial ligament — Coracoid process

Subacromial bursa

Subdeltoid bursa

Subtendinous bursa of subscapularis

Greater tuberosity

Transverse ligament of humerus

Intertubercular tendon sheath

Infraspinatus

Teres minor

Biceps brachii, short head

Biceps brachii, long head

Humerus

A Lateral view.

Fig. 19.17 Subacromial bursa and glenoid cavity
Right shoulder, lateral view of sagittal section with humerus removed.

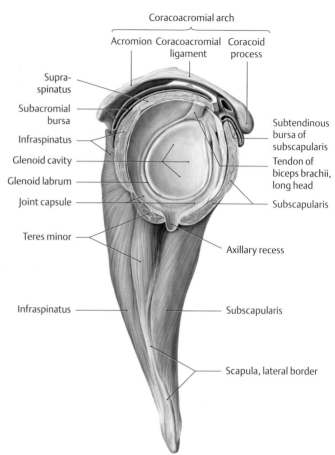

Coracoacromial arch

Acromion Coracoacromial ligament Coracoid process

Supra-spinatus

Subacromial bursa

Infraspinatus

Glenoid cavity

Glenoid labrum

Joint capsule

Teres minor

Infraspinatus

Subtendinous bursa of subscapularis

Tendon of biceps brachii, long head

Subscapularis

Axillary recess

Subscapularis

Scapula, lateral border

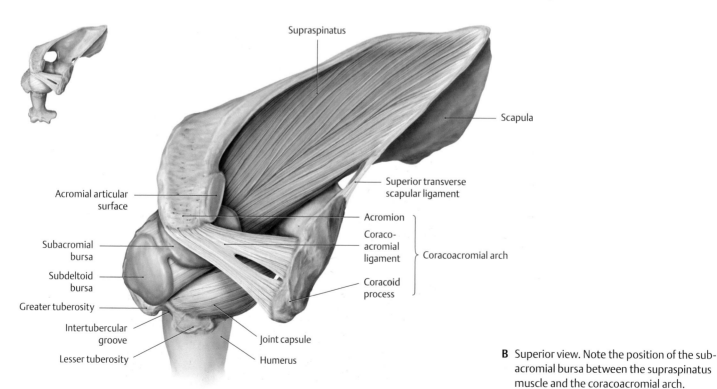

Supraspinatus

Scapula

Acromial articular surface

Superior transverse scapular ligament

Subacromial bursa

Acromion

Coraco-acromial ligament

Subdeltoid bursa

Coracoacromial arch

Greater tuberosity

Coracoid process

Intertubercular groove

Lesser tuberosity

Joint capsule

Humerus

B Superior view. Note the position of the subacromial bursa between the supraspinatus muscle and the coracoacromial arch.

Fig. 19.18 Subacromial and subdeltoid bursae

Right shoulder, anterior view.

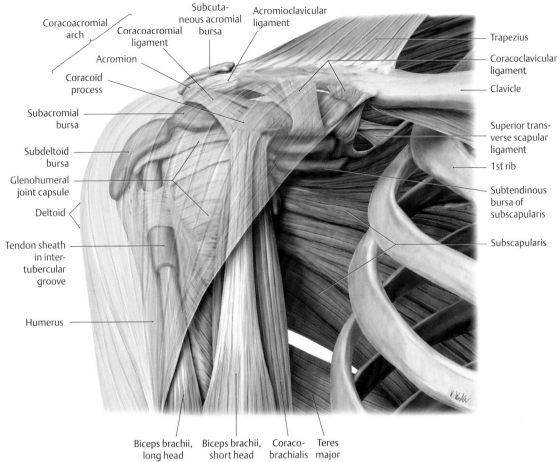

Coracoacromial arch
Coracoacromial ligament
Acromion
Coracoid process
Subacromial bursa
Subdeltoid bursa
Glenohumeral joint capsule
Deltoid
Tendon sheath in intertubercular groove
Humerus

Subcutaneous acromial bursa
Acromioclavicular ligament

Trapezius
Coracoclavicular ligament
Clavicle
Superior transverse scapular ligament
1st rib
Subtendinous bursa of subscapularis
Subscapularis

Biceps brachii, long head
Biceps brachii, short head
Coracobrachialis
Teres major

A Location of bursae.

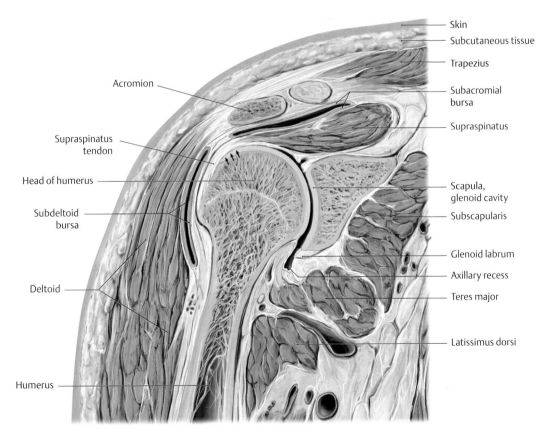

Acromion
Supraspinatus tendon
Head of humerus
Subdeltoid bursa
Deltoid
Humerus

Skin
Subcutaneous tissue
Trapezius
Subacromial bursa
Supraspinatus
Scapula, glenoid cavity
Subscapularis
Glenoid labrum
Axillary recess
Teres major
Latissimus dorsi

B Coronal section. The arrows are pointing at the supraspinatus tendon, which is frequently injured in a "rotator cuff tear" (for rotator cuff, see p. 273).

Anterior Muscles of the Shoulder & Arm (I)

Fig. 19.19 Anterior muscles

Right side, anterior view. Muscle origins (O) are shown in red, insertions (I) in blue.

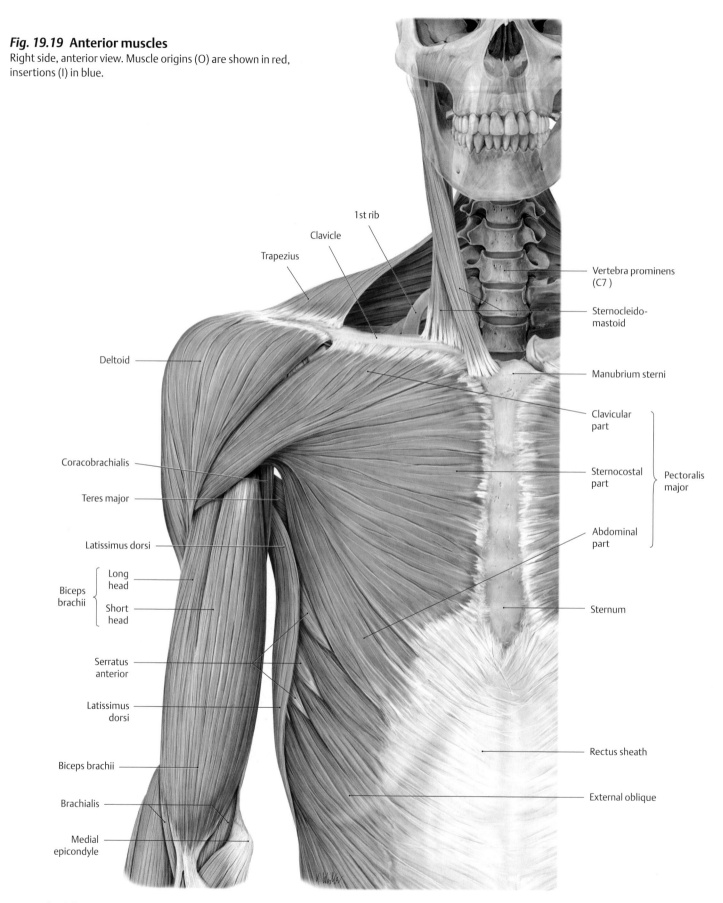

A Superficial dissection.

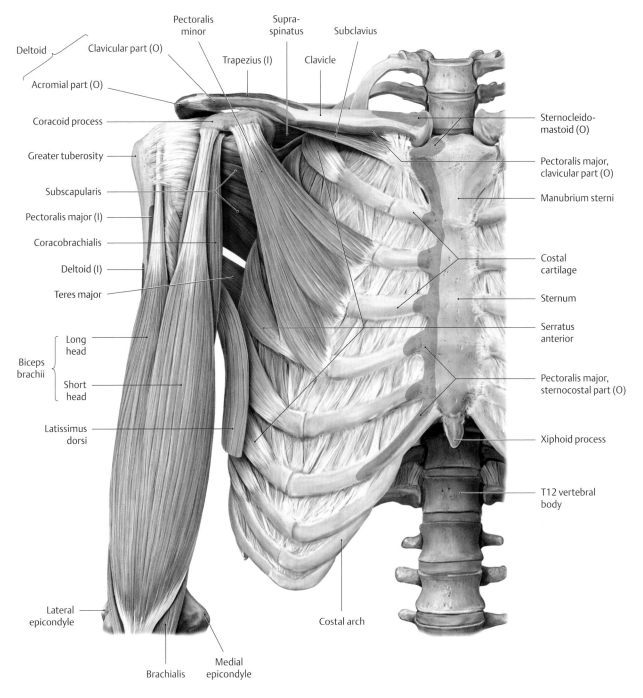

Deltoid

Clavicular part (O)

Pectoralis minor

Supra-spinatus

Subclavius

Acromial part (O)

Trapezius (I)

Clavicle

Coracoid process

Sternocleido-mastoid (O)

Greater tuberosity

Pectoralis major, clavicular part (O)

Subscapularis

Manubrium sterni

Pectoralis major (I)

Coracobrachialis

Costal cartilage

Deltoid (I)

Sternum

Teres major

Serratus anterior

Biceps brachii — Long head

Short head

Pectoralis major, sternocostal part (O)

Latissimus dorsi

Xiphoid process

T12 vertebral body

Lateral epicondyle

Costal arch

Brachialis

Medial epicondyle

B Deep dissection. *Removed:* Sternocleidomastoid, trapezius, pectoralis major, deltoid, and external oblique muscles.

Anterior Muscles of the Shoulder & Arm (II)

Fig. 19.20 **Anterior dissection**

Right arm, anterior view. Muscle origins (O) are shown in red, insertions (I) in blue.

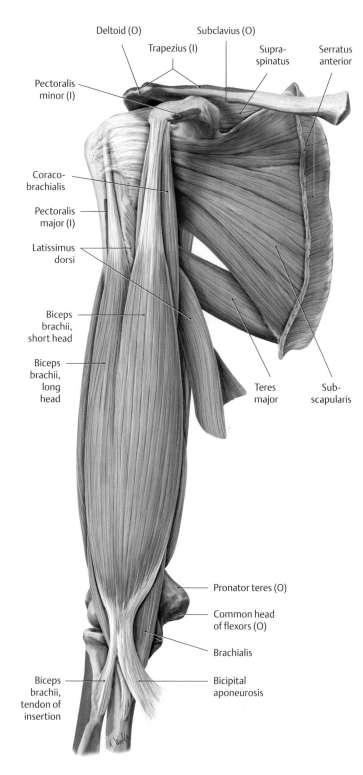

Deltoid (O) Subclavius (O) Trapezius (I) Supra-spinatus Serratus anterior Pectoralis minor (I) Coraco-brachialis Pectoralis major (I) Latissimus dorsi Biceps brachii, short head Biceps brachii, long head Teres major Sub-scapularis Pronator teres (O) Common head of flexors (O) Brachialis Biceps brachii, tendon of insertion Bicipital aponeurosis

A *Removed:* Thoracic skeleton. *Partially removed:* Latissimus dorsi and serratus anterior.

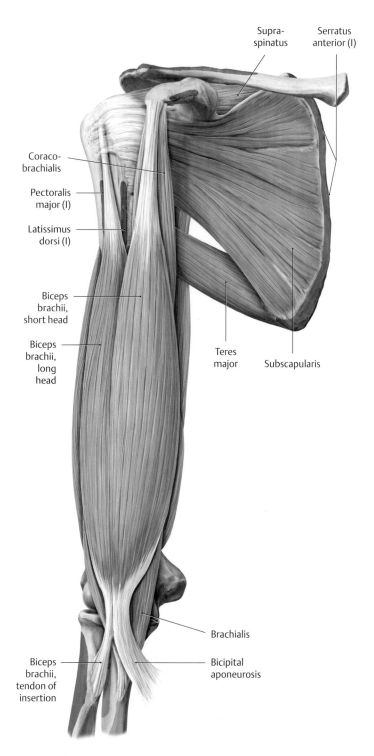

Supra-spinatus Serratus anterior (I) Coraco-brachialis Pectoralis major (I) Latissimus dorsi (I) Biceps brachii, short head Biceps brachii, long head Teres major Subscapularis Brachialis Biceps brachii, tendon of insertion Bicipital aponeurosis

B *Removed:* Latissimus dorsi and serratus anterior.

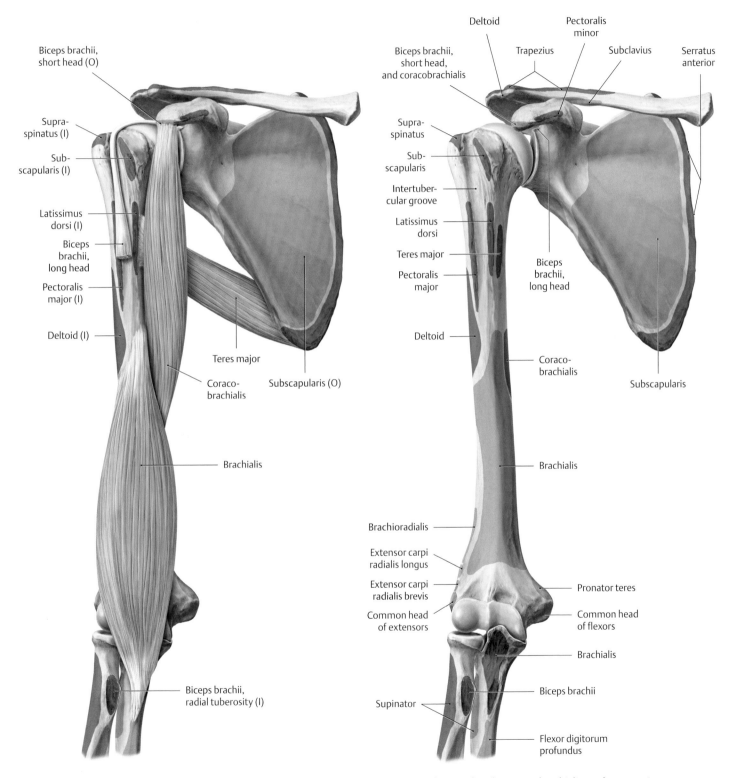

Biceps brachii,
short head (O)

Supra-
spinatus (I)

Sub-
scapularis (I)

Latissimus
dorsi (I)

Biceps
brachii,
long head

Pectoralis
major (I)

Deltoid (I)

Teres major

Coraco-
brachialis

Subscapularis (O)

Brachialis

Biceps brachii,
radial tuberosity (I)

Deltoid

Pectoralis
minor

Biceps brachii,
short head,
and coracobrachialis

Trapezius

Subclavius

Serratus
anterior

Supra-
spinatus

Sub-
scapularis

Intertuber-
cular groove

Latissimus
dorsi

Teres major

Pectoralis
major

Biceps
brachii,
long head

Deltoid

Coraco-
brachialis

Subscapularis

Brachialis

Brachioradialis

Extensor carpi
radialis longus

Extensor carpi
radialis brevis

Common head
of extensors

Pronator teres

Common head
of flexors

Brachialis

Biceps brachii

Supinator

Flexor digitorum
profundus

C *Removed:* Subscapularis and supraspinatus muscles. *Partially removed:* Biceps brachii.

D *Removed:* Biceps brachii, coracobrachialis, and teres major.

Posterior Muscles of the Shoulder & Arm (I)

***Fig. 19.21* Posterior muscles**
Right side, posterior view.

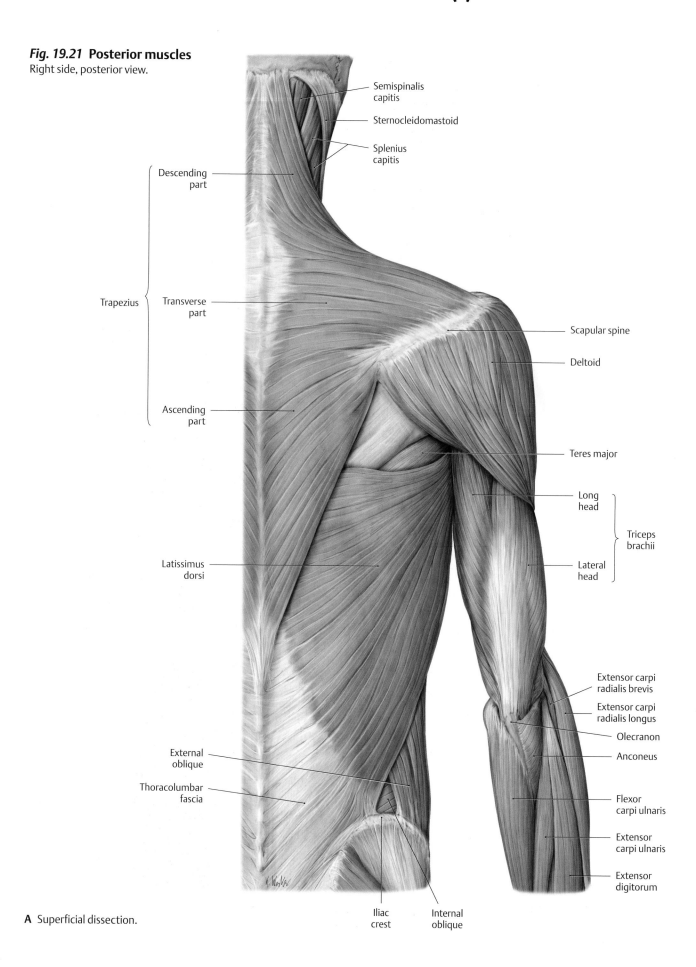

Semispinalis capitis

Sternocleidomastoid

Splenius capitis

Descending part

Trapezius

Transverse part

Scapular spine

Deltoid

Ascending part

Teres major

Long head

Triceps brachii

Lateral head

Latissimus dorsi

Extensor carpi radialis brevis

Extensor carpi radialis longus

Olecranon

Anconeus

External oblique

Flexor carpi ulnaris

Thoracolumbar fascia

Extensor carpi ulnaris

Extensor digitorum

Iliac crest

Internal oblique

A Superficial dissection.

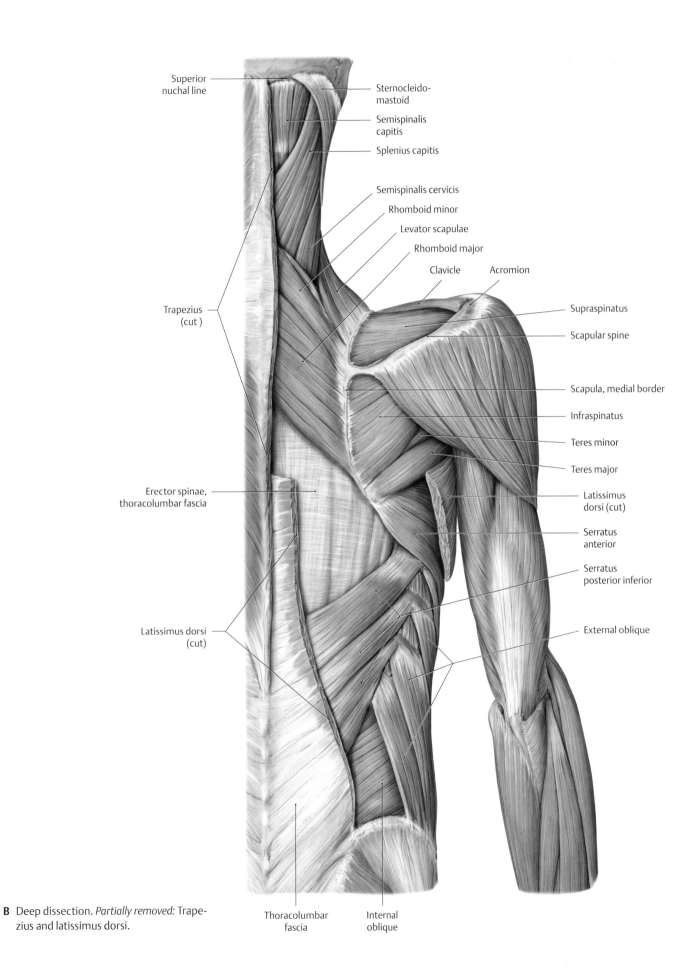

Superior
nuchal line

Sternocleido-
mastoid

Semispinalis
capitis

Splenius capitis

Semispinalis cervicis

Rhomboid minor

Levator scapulae

Rhomboid major

Clavicle   Acromion

Supraspinatus

Scapular spine

Trapezius
(cut)

Scapula, medial border

Infraspinatus

Teres minor

Teres major

Erector spinae,
thoracolumbar fascia

Latissimus
dorsi (cut)

Serratus
anterior

Serratus
posterior inferior

Latissimus dorsi
(cut)

External oblique

Thoracolumbar
fascia

Internal
oblique

B Deep dissection. *Partially removed:* Trapezius and latissimus dorsi.

Posterior Muscles of the Shoulder & Arm (II)

Fig. 19.22 **Posterior dissection**

Right arm, posterior view. Muscle origins (O) are shown in red, insertions (I) in blue.

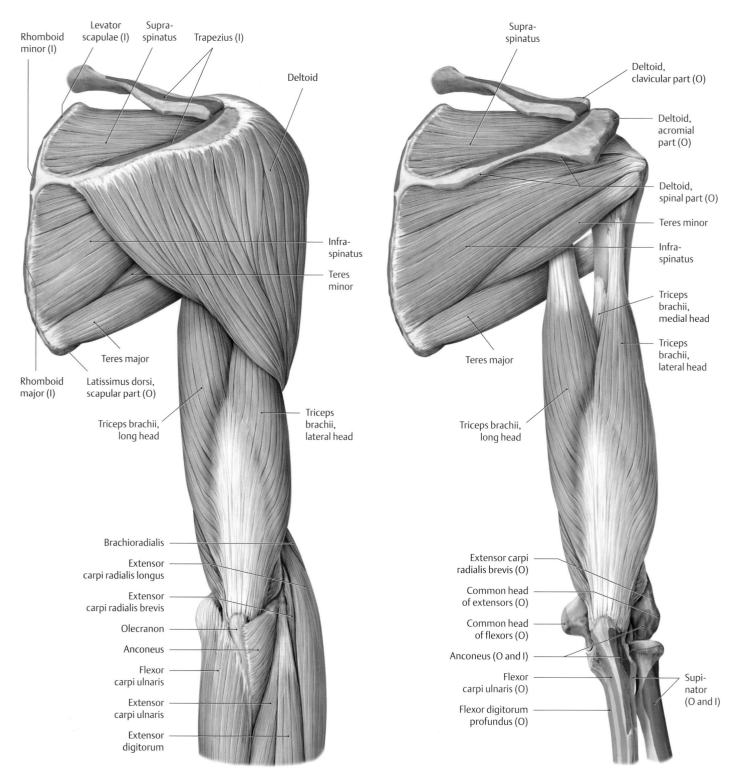

A *Removed:* Rhomboids major and minor, serratus anterior, and levator scapulae.

B *Removed:* Deltoid and forearm muscles.

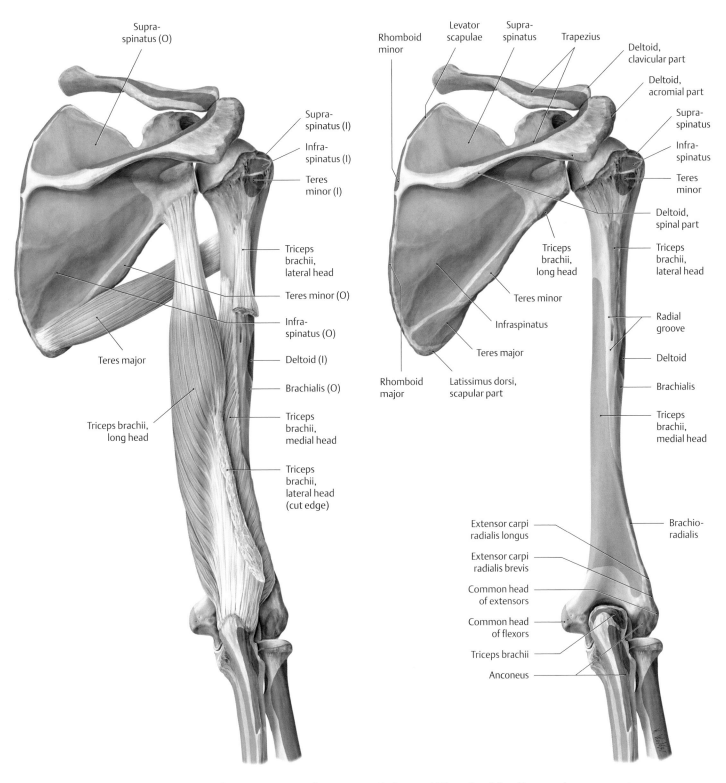

Supra-spinatus (O)

Supra-spinatus (I)

Infra-spinatus (I)

Teres minor (I)

Triceps brachii, lateral head

Teres minor (O)

Infra-spinatus (O)

Deltoid (I)

Brachialis (O)

Triceps brachii, medial head

Teres major

Triceps brachii, long head

Triceps brachii, lateral head (cut edge)

Rhomboid minor

Levator scapulae

Supra-spinatus

Trapezius

Deltoid, clavicular part

Deltoid, acromial part

Supra-spinatus

Infra-spinatus

Teres minor

Deltoid, spinal part

Triceps brachii, lateral head

Triceps brachii, long head

Teres minor

Infraspinatus

Teres major

Radial groove

Deltoid

Brachialis

Triceps brachii, medial head

Rhomboid major

Latissimus dorsi, scapular part

Extensor carpi radialis longus

Extensor carpi radialis brevis

Common head of extensors

Common head of flexors

Triceps brachii

Anconeus

Brachio-radialis

C *Removed:* Supraspinatus, infraspinatus, and teres minor. *Partially removed:* Triceps brachii.

D *Removed:* Triceps brachii and teres major.

Muscle Facts (I)

 The actions of the three parts of the deltoid muscle depend on their relationship to the position of the humerus and its axis of motion. At less than 60 degrees, the muscles act as adductors, but at greater than 60 degrees, they act as abductors. As a result, the parts of the deltoid can act antagonistically as well as synergistically.

Fig. 19.23 **Deltoid**
Right shoulder.

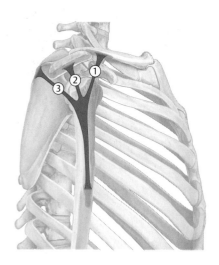

A Parts of the deltoid, right lateral view.

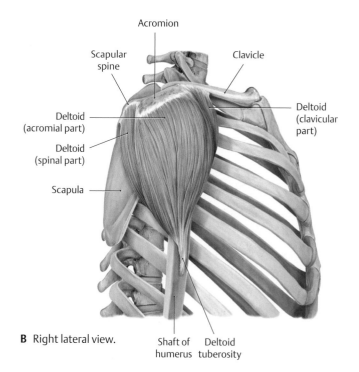

B Right lateral view.

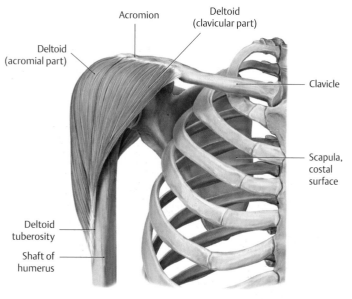

C Anterior view.

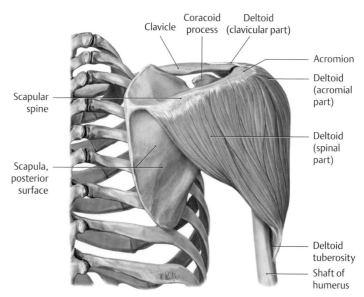

D Posterior view.

Table 19.2		Parts of the deltoid			
Muscle		**Origin**	**Insertion**	**Innervation**	**Action***
Deltoid	① Clavicular part	Lateral one third of clavicle	Humerus (deltoid tuberosity)	Axillary n. (C5, C6)	Flexion, internal rotation, adduction
	② Acromial part	Acromion			Abduction
	③ Spinal part	Scapular spine			Extension, external rotation, adduction
* Between 60 and 90 degrees of abduction, the clavicular and spinal parts assist the acromial part with abduction.					

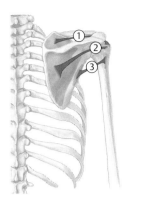

A Posterior view.

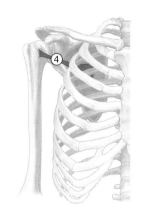

B Anterior view.

Fig. 19.24 Rotator cuff

Right shoulder. The rotator cuff consists of four muscles: supraspinatus, infraspinatus, teres minor, and subscapularis.

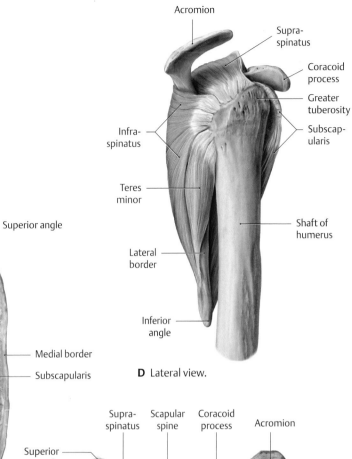

Acromion

Supra-
spinatus

Coracoid
process

Greater
tuberosity

Subscap-
ularis

Infra-
spinatus

Teres
minor

Shaft of
humerus

Lateral
border

Inferior
angle

D Lateral view.

Acromion

Coracoid
process

Scapular
notch

Supra-
spinatus

Superior
border

Superior angle

Greater
tuberosity

Lesser
tuberosity

Intertuber-
cular groove

Crest of greater
tuberosity

Crest of lesser
tuberosity

Shaft of humerus

Medial border

Subscapularis

Inferior angle

C Anterior view.

Supra-
spinatus

Scapular
spine

Coracoid
process

Acromion

Superior
angle

Greater
tuberosity

Medial
border

Teres
minor

Shaft of
humerus

Infra-
spinatus

Lateral border

Inferior angle

E Posterior view.

Table 19.3	Muscles of the rotator cuff				
Muscle	**Origin**	**Insertion**		**Innervation**	**Action**
① Supraspinatus	Scapula	Supraspinous fossa	Greater tuberosity	Suprascapular n. (C4–C6)	Abduction
② Infraspinatus		Infraspinous fossa			External rotation
③ Teres minor		Lateral border		Axillary n. (C5, C6)	External rotation, weak adduction
④ Subscapularis		Subscapular fossa	Lesser tuberosity	Subscapular n. (C5, C6)	Internal rotation

Muscle Facts (II)

Fig. 19.25 **Pectoralis major and coracobrachialis**
Anterior view.

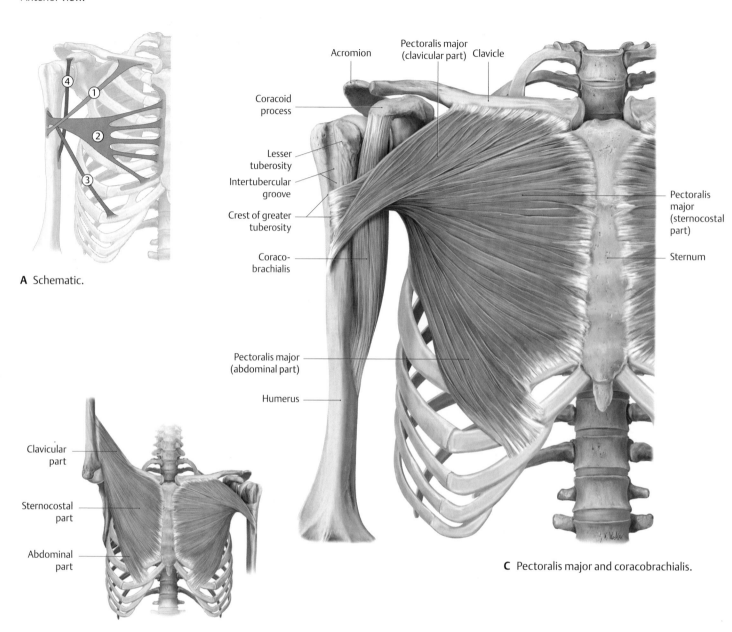

A Schematic.

B Pectoralis major in neutral position (left) and elevation (right).

C Pectoralis major and coracobrachialis.

Table 19.4		Pectoralis major and coracobrachialis			
Muscle		**Origin**	**Insertion**	**Innervation**	**Action**
Pectoralis major	① Clavicular part	Clavicle (medial half)	Humerus (crest of greater tuberosity)	Medial and lateral pectoral nn. (C5–T1)	Entire muscle: adduction, internal rotation Clavicular and sternocostal parts: flexion; assist in respiration when shoulder is fixed
	② Sternocostal part	Sternum and costal cartilages 1–6			
	③ Abdominal part	Rectus sheath (anterior layer)			
④ Coracobrachialis		Scapula (coracoid process)	Humerus (in line with crest of lesser tuberosity)	Musculocutaneous n. (C6, C7)	Flexion, adduction, internal rotation

Fig. 19.26 Subclavius and pectoralis minor

Right side, anterior view.

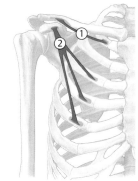

A Schematic.

Clavicle — 1st rib

Acromion

Coracoid process

Subclavius

Pectoralis minor

3rd through 5th ribs

B Subclavius and pectoralis minor.

Fig. 19.27 Serratus anterior

Right lateral view.

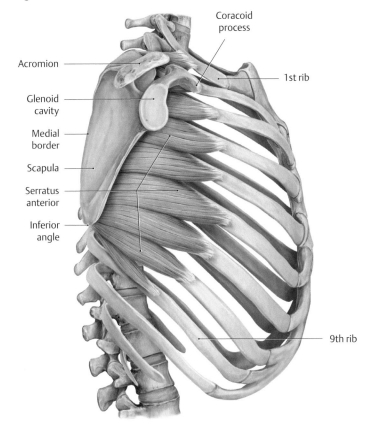

Coracoid process

Acromion

Glenoid cavity

Medial border

Scapula

Serratus anterior

Inferior angle

1st rib

9th rib

A Serratus anterior.

B Schematic.

Table 19.5		Subclavius, pectoralis minor, and serratus anterior				
Muscle		**Origin**	**Insertion**	**Innervation**	**Action**	
① Subclavius		1st rib	Clavicle (inferior surface)	N. to subclavius (C5, C6)	Steadies the clavicle in the sternoclavicular joint	
② Pectoralis minor		3rd to 5th ribs	Coracoid process	Medial and lateral pectoral nn. (C6–T1)	Draws scapula downward, causing inferior angle to move posteromedially; rotates glenoid inferiorly; assists in respiration	
Serratus anterior	③ Superior part	1st to 9th ribs	Scapula (medial border)	Long thoracic n. (C5–C7)	Superior part: lowers the raised arm	
	④ Intermediate part				Entire muscle: draws scapula laterally forward; elevates ribs when shoulder is fixed	
	⑤ Inferior part				Inferior part: rotates scapula laterally	

Muscle Facts (III)

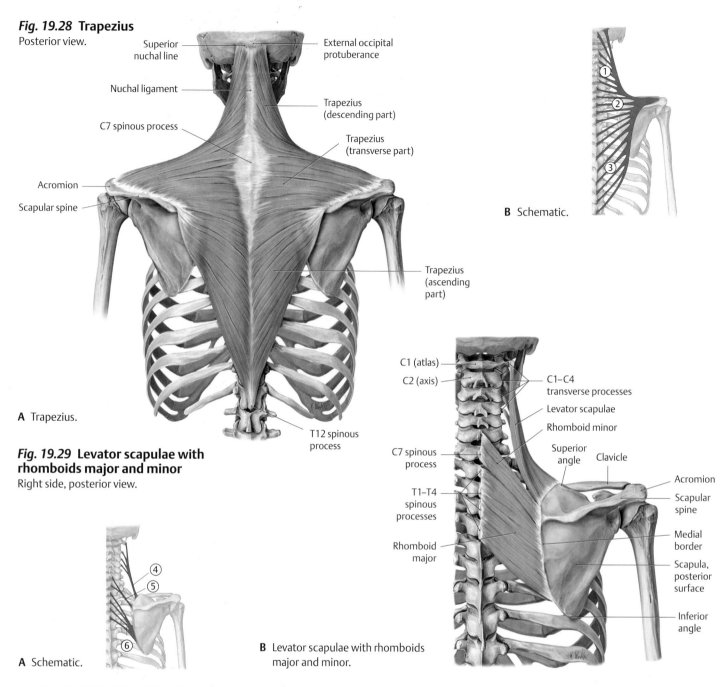

Fig. 19.28 Trapezius
Posterior view.

Superior nuchal line
External occipital protuberance
Nuchal ligament
Trapezius (descending part)
C7 spinous process
Trapezius (transverse part)
Acromion
Scapular spine
Trapezius (ascending part)

A Trapezius.

B Schematic.

T12 spinous process

Fig. 19.29 Levator scapulae with rhomboids major and minor
Right side, posterior view.

A Schematic.

B Levator scapulae with rhomboids major and minor.

C1 (atlas)
C2 (axis)
C1–C4 transverse processes
Levator scapulae
Rhomboid minor
Superior angle
Clavicle
C7 spinous process
Acromion
Scapular spine
T1–T4 spinous processes
Medial border
Rhomboid major
Scapula, posterior surface
Inferior angle

Table 19.6		Trapezius, levator scapulae, and rhomboids major and minor			
Muscle		**Origin**	**Insertion**	**Innervation**	**Action**
Trapezius	① Descending part	Occipital bone; spinous process of C1–C7	Clavicle (lateral one third)	Accessory n. (CN X); cervical plexus (C3–C4)	Draws scapula obliquely upward; rotates glenoid cavity superiorly; tilts head to same side and rotates it to opposite
	② Transverse part	Aponeurosis at T1–T4 spinous processes	Acromion		Draws scapula medially
	③ Ascending part	Spinous process of T5–T12	Scapular spine		Draws scapula medially downward
					Entire muscle: steadies scapula on thorax
④ Levator scapulae		Transverse process of C1–C4	Scapula (superior angle)	Dorsal scapular n. (C4–C5)	Draws scapula medially upward while moving inferior angle medially; inclines neck to same side
⑤ Rhomboid minor		Spinous process of C6, C7	Medial border of scapula above (minor) and below (major) scapular spine		Steadies scapula; draws scapula medially upward
⑥ Rhomboid major		Spinous process of T1–T4 vertebrae			

CN = cranial nerve.

Fig. 19.30 Latissimus dorsi and teres major

Posterior view.

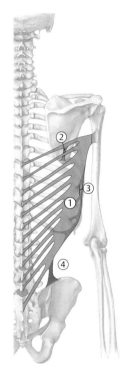

A Latissimus dorsi.

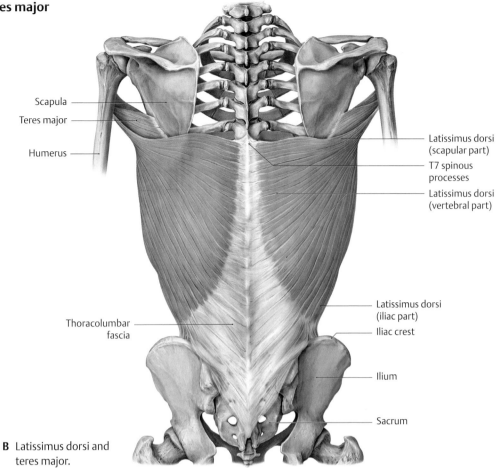

Scapula
Teres major
Humerus

Latissimus dorsi
(scapular part)

T7 spinous
processes

Latissimus dorsi
(vertebral part)

Thoracolumbar
fascia

Latissimus dorsi
(iliac part)

Iliac crest

Ilium

Sacrum

B Latissimus dorsi and
teres major.

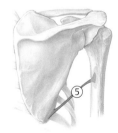

C Teres major.

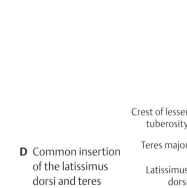

D Common insertion
of the latissimus
dorsi and teres
major, anterior view.

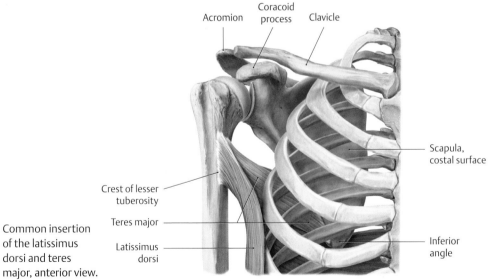

Acromion
Coracoid
process
Clavicle

Scapula,
costal surface

Crest of lesser
tuberosity

Teres major

Latissimus
dorsi

Inferior
angle

Table 19.7		Latissimus dorsi and teres major			
Muscle		**Origin**	**Insertion**	**Innervation**	**Action**
Latissimus dorsi	① Vertebral part	Spinous process of T7–T12 vertebrae; thoracolumbar fascia	Crest of lesser tuberosity of the humerus (anterior angle)	Thoracodorsal n. (C6–C8)	Internal rotation, adduction, extension, respiration ("cough muscle")
	② Scapular part	Scapula (inferior angle)			
	③ Costal part	9th to 12th ribs			
	④ Iliac part	Iliac crest (posterior one third)			
⑤ Teres major		Scapula (inferior angle)		Lower subscapular n. (C5–C7)	Internal rotation, adduction, extension

Muscle Facts (IV)

The anterior and posterior muscles of the arm may be classified respectively as flexors and extensors relative to the movement of the elbow joint. Although the coracobrachialis is topographically part of the anterior compartment, it is functionally grouped with the muscles of the shoulder (see p. 274).

(see p. 274).

Fig. 19.31 **Biceps brachii and brachialis**
Right arm, anterior view.

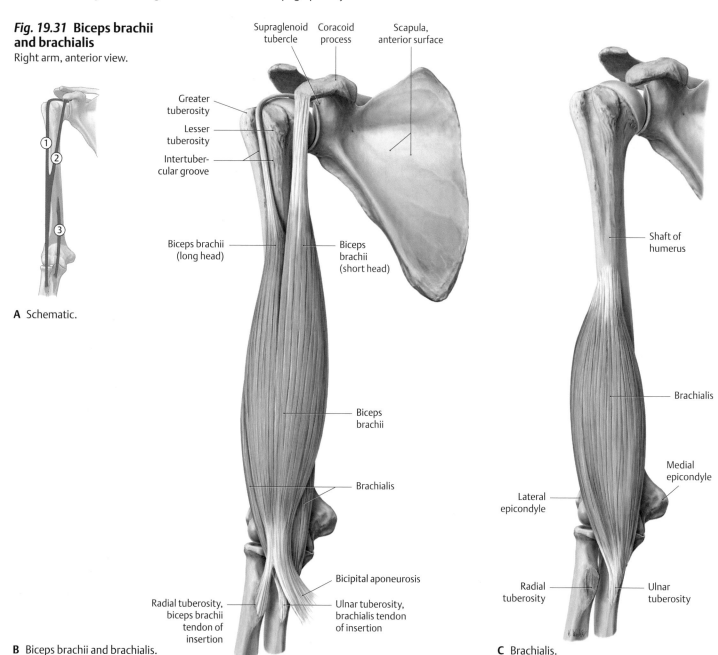

A Schematic.

B Biceps brachii and brachialis.

C Brachialis.

Table 19.8		Anterior group: Biceps brachii and brachialis			
Muscle		**Origin**	**Insertion**	**Innervation**	**Action**
Biceps brachii	① Long head	Supraglenoid tubercle of scapula	Radial tuberosity	Musculocutaneous n. (C5–C6)	Elbow joint: flexion; supination* Shoulder joint: flexion; stabilization of humeral head during deltoid contraction; abduction and internal rotation of the humerus
	② Short head	Coracoid process of scapula			
③ Brachialis		Humerus (distal half of anterior surface)	Ulnar tuberosity	Musculocutaneous n. (C5–C6) and radial n. (C7, minor)	Flexion at the elbow joint

Note: When the elbow is flexed, the biceps brachii acts as a powerful supinator because the lever arm is almost perpendicular to the axis of pronation/supination.

Fig. 19.32 Triceps brachii and anconeus

Right arm, posterior view.

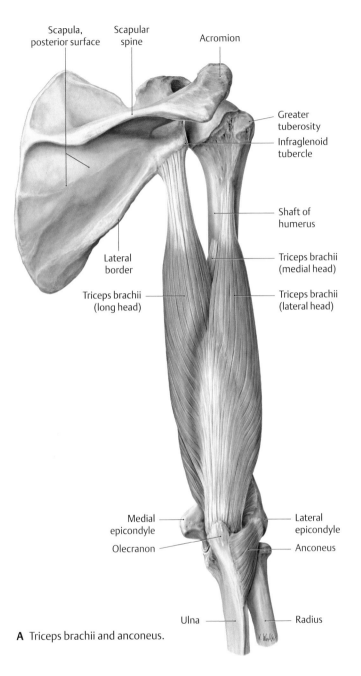

Scapula, posterior surface
Scapular spine
Acromion
Greater tuberosity
Infraglenoid tubercle
Shaft of humerus
Triceps brachii (medial head)
Triceps brachii (lateral head)
Lateral border
Triceps brachii (long head)
Medial epicondyle
Olecranon
Lateral epicondyle
Anconeus
Ulna
Radius

A Triceps brachii and anconeus.

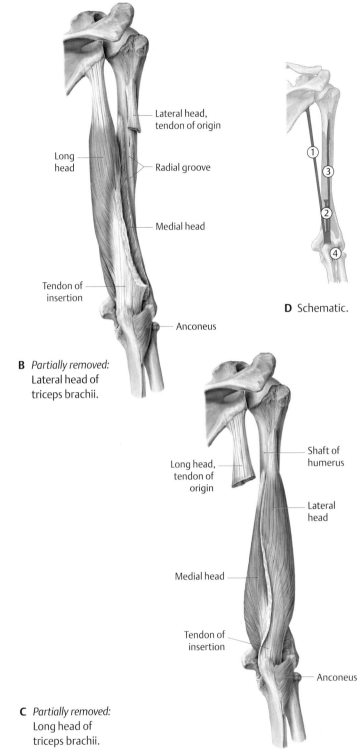

Lateral head, tendon of origin
Long head
Radial groove
Medial head
Tendon of insertion
Anconeus

B *Partially removed:* Lateral head of triceps brachii.

D Schematic.

Long head, tendon of origin
Shaft of humerus
Lateral head
Medial head
Tendon of insertion
Anconeus

C *Partially removed:* Long head of triceps brachii.

Table 19.9		Posterior group: Triceps brachii and anconeus			
Muscle		**Origin**	**Insertion**	**Innervation**	**Action**
Triceps brachii	① Long head	Scapula (infraglenoid tubercle)	Olecranon of ulna	Radial n. (C6–C8)	Elbow joint: extension Shoulder joint, long head: extension and adduction
	② Medial head	Posterior humerus, distal to radial groove; medial intermuscular septum			
	③ Lateral head	Posterior humerus, proximal to radial groove; lateral intermuscular septum			
④ Anconeus		Lateral epicondyle of humerus (variance: posterior joint capsule)	Olecranon of ulna (radial surface)		Extends the elbow and tightens its joint

Radius & Ulna

Fig. 20.1 Radius and ulna
Right forearm.

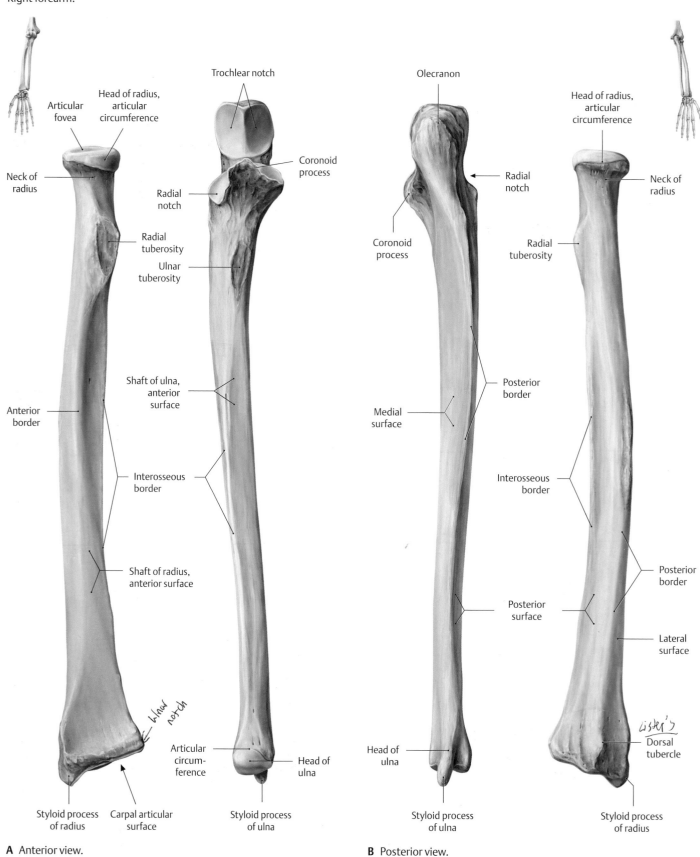

Trochlear notch

Head of radius,
articular
circumference

Articular
fovea

Neck of
radius

Radial
notch

Coronoid
process

Radial
tuberosity

Ulnar
tuberosity

Shaft of ulna,
anterior
surface

Anterior
border

Interosseous
border

Shaft of radius,
anterior surface

Ulnar notch

Styloid process
of radius

Carpal articular
surface

Articular
circum-
ference

Head of
ulna

Styloid process
of ulna

A Anterior view.

Olecranon

Head of radius,
articular
circumference

Coronoid
process

Radial
notch

Neck of
radius

Medial
surface

Radial
tuberosity

Posterior
border

Interosseous
border

Posterior
surface

Posterior
border

Lateral
surface

Head of
ulna

Lister's
Dorsal
tubercle

Styloid process
of ulna

Styloid process
of radius

B Posterior view.

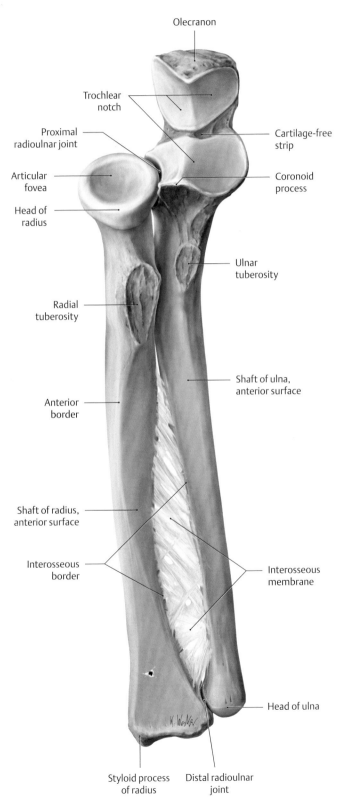

Olecranon

Trochlear notch

Proximal radioulnar joint

Articular fovea

Head of radius

Radial tuberosity

Anterior border

Shaft of radius, anterior surface

Interosseous border

Cartilage-free strip

Coronoid process

Ulnar tuberosity

Shaft of ulna, anterior surface

Interosseous membrane

Head of ulna

Styloid process of radius

Distal radioulnar joint

C Anterosuperior view.

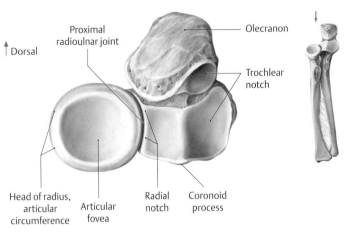

↑ Dorsal

Proximal radioulnar joint

Olecranon

Trochlear notch

Head of radius, articular circumference

Articular fovea

Radial notch

Coronoid process

D Proximal view.

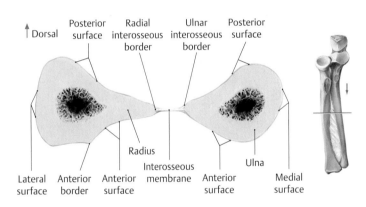

↑ Dorsal

Posterior surface

Radial interosseous border

Ulnar interosseous border

Posterior surface

Lateral surface

Anterior border

Anterior surface

Radius

Interosseous membrane

Anterior surface

Ulna

Medial surface

E Transverse section, proximal view.

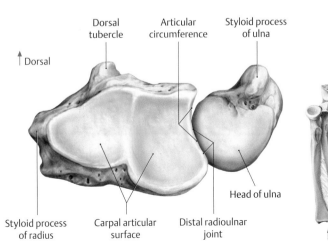

Dorsal tubercle

Articular circumference

Styloid process of ulna

↑ Dorsal

Styloid process of radius

Carpal articular surface

Distal radioulnar joint

Head of ulna

F Distal view.

Elbow Joint

Fig. 20.2 **Elbow (cubital) joint**
Right limb. The elbow consists of three articulations between the humerus, ulna, and radius: the humeroulnar, humeroradial, and proximal radioulnar joints.

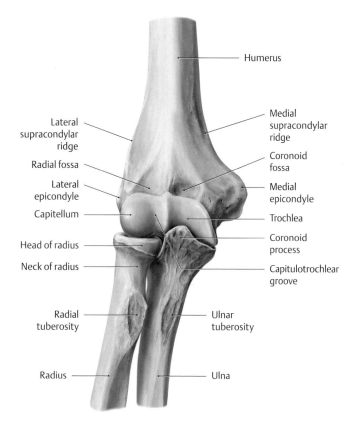

A Anterior view.

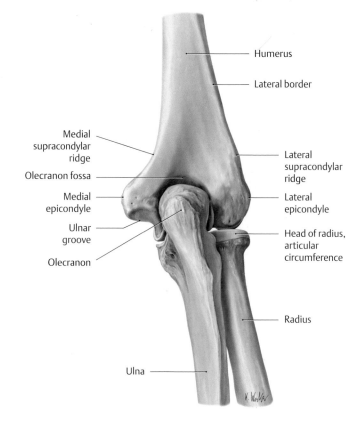

B Posterior view.

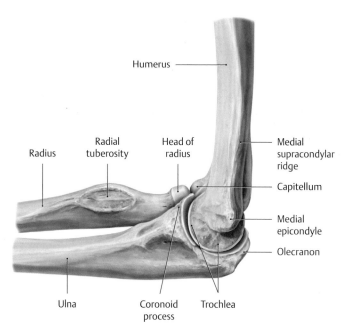

C Medial view.

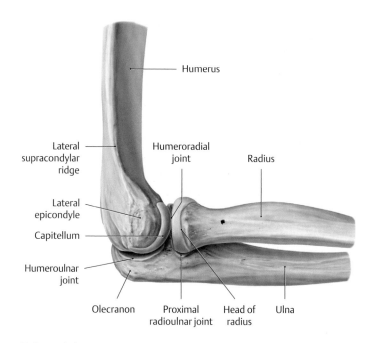

D Lateral view.

Fig. 20.3 MRI of the elbow joint

Sagittal section.

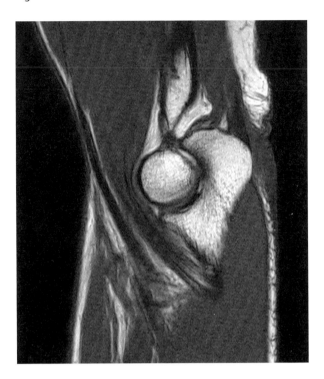

Fig. 20.4 Humeroulnar joint

Sagittal section through the humeroulnar joint, medial view.

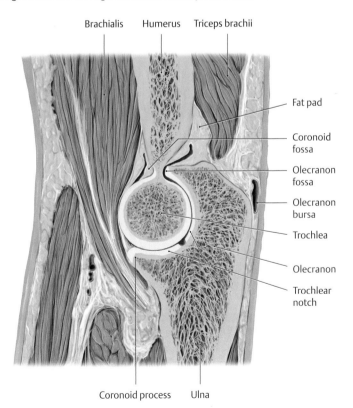

Clinical

Assessing elbow injuries

The fat pads between the fibrous capsule and synovial membrane are part of the normal anatomy of the elbow joint. The anterior pad is most readily seen on a sagittal MRI while the posterior pad is often hidden within the bony fossa (Fig. 20.3). With an effusion of the joint space, the inferior edge of the anterior pad appears concave as it gets pushed superiorly by the intra-articular fluid. This causes the pad to resemble the shape of a ship's sail, thus creating a characteristic "sail sign." The alignment of the prominences in the elbow also aids in the identification of fractures and dislocations.

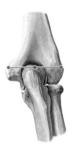

A Posterior view of extended elbow: The epicondyles and olecranon lie in a straight line.

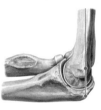

B Lateral view of flexed elbow: The epicondyles and olecranon lie in a straight line.

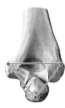

C Posterior view of flexed elbow: The two epicondyles and the tip of the olecranon form an equilateral triangle. Fractures and dislocations alter the shape of the triangle.

Ligaments of the Elbow Joint

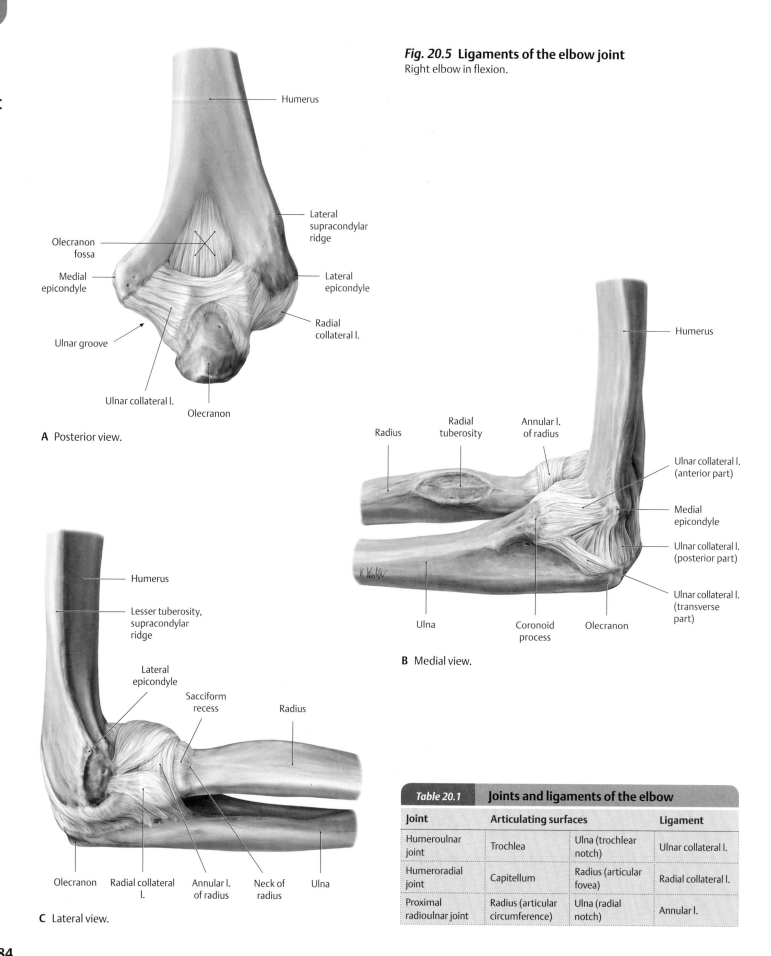

***Fig. 20.5* Ligaments of the elbow joint**
Right elbow in flexion.

A Posterior view.

B Medial view.

C Lateral view.

Table 20.1	Joints and ligaments of the elbow		
Joint	**Articulating surfaces**		**Ligament**
Humeroulnar joint	Trochlea	Ulna (trochlear notch)	Ulnar collateral l.
Humeroradial joint	Capitellum	Radius (articular fovea)	Radial collateral l.
Proximal radioulnar joint	Radius (articular circumference)	Ulna (radial notch)	Annular l.

Fig. 20.6 **Joint capsule of the elbow**
Right elbow in extension, anterior view.

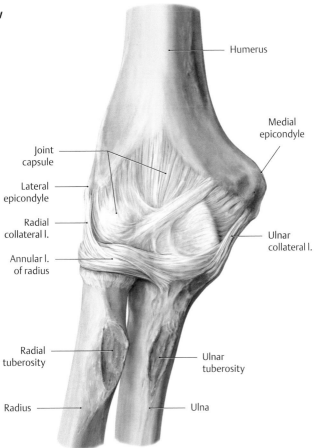

Humerus

Medial epicondyle

Joint capsule

Lateral epicondyle

Radial collateral l.

Ulnar collateral l.

Annular l. of radius

Radial tuberosity

Ulnar tuberosity

Radius

Ulna

A Intact joint capsule.

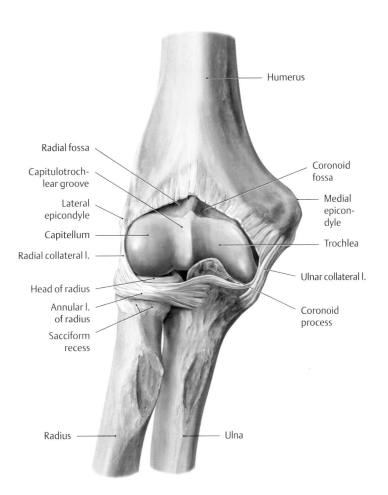

Humerus

Radial fossa

Coronoid fossa

Capitulotrochlear groove

Medial epicondyle

Lateral epicondyle

Capitellum

Trochlea

Radial collateral l.

Head of radius

Ulnar collateral l.

Annular l. of radius

Coronoid process

Sacciform recess

Radius

Ulna

B Windowed joint capsule.

Radioulnar Joints

 The proximal and distal radioulnar joints function together to enable pronation and supination movements of the hand. The joints are functionally linked by the interosseous membrane. The axis for pronation and supination runs obliquely from the center of the humeral capitellum through the center of the radial articular fovea down to the styloid process of the ulna.

Fig. 20.7 Supination
Right forearm, anterior view.

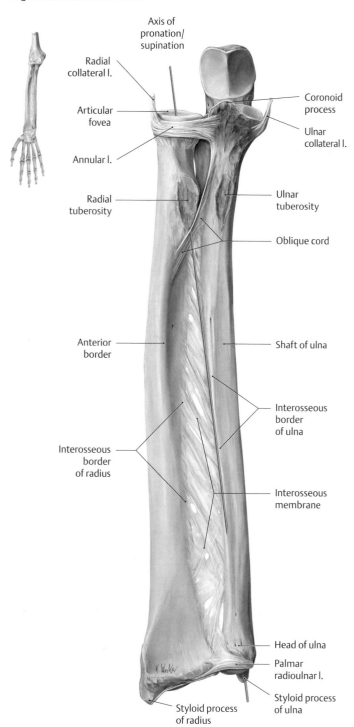

Fig. 20.8 Pronation
Right forearm, anterior view.

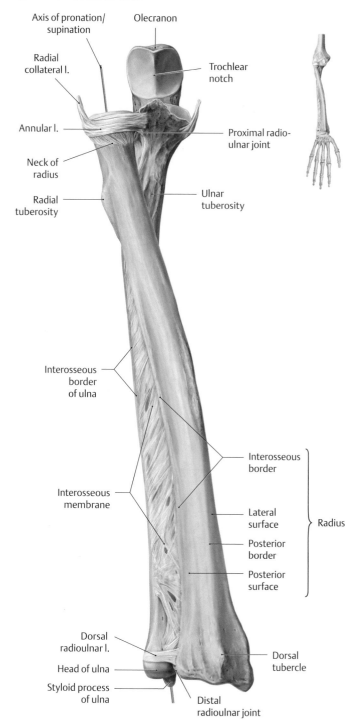

Subluxation of the radial head ("nursemaid's elbow")
When small children are abruptly pulled up by their arm, the immature head of the radius can dislocate from the annular ligament, resulting in painful pronation.

Fig. 20.9 Proximal radioulnar joint
Right elbow, proximal (superior) view.

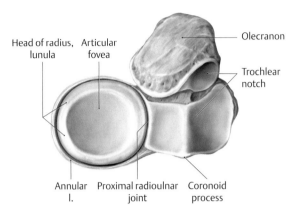

A Proximal articular surfaces of radius and ulna.

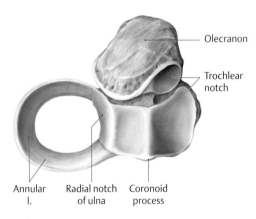

B Radius removed.

Radius fracture
Falls onto the outstretched arm often result in fractures of the distal radius. In a "Colles' fracture," the distal fragment is tilted dorsally.

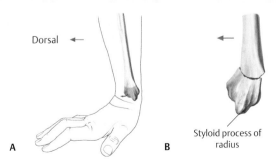

Fig. 20.10 Distal radioulnar joint rotation
Right forearm, distal view of articular surfaces of radius and ulna. The dorsal and palmar radioulnar ligaments stabilize the distal radioulnar joint.

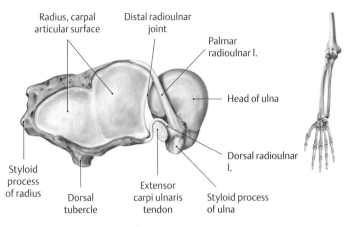

A Supination.

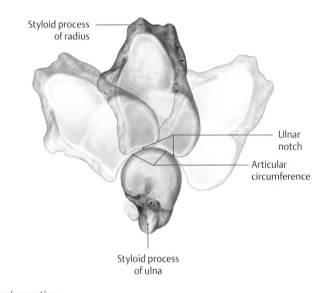

B Semipronation.

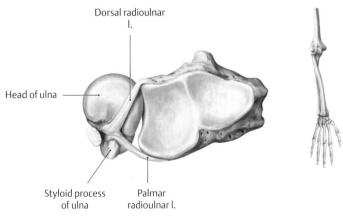

C Pronation.

Muscles of the Forearm (I)

Fig. 20.11 Anterior muscles
Right forearm, anterior view. Muscle origins (O) are shown in red, insertions (I) in blue.

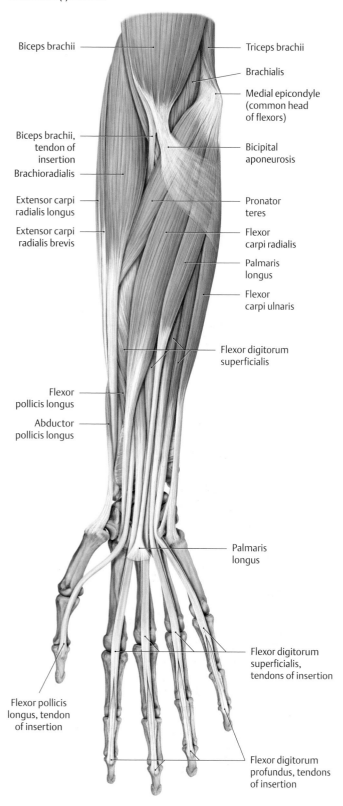

Biceps brachii

Triceps brachii

Brachialis

Medial epicondyle (common head of flexors)

Biceps brachii, tendon of insertion

Bicipital aponeurosis

Brachioradialis

Pronator teres

Extensor carpi radialis longus

Flexor carpi radialis

Extensor carpi radialis brevis

Palmaris longus

Flexor carpi ulnaris

Flexor digitorum superficialis

Flexor pollicis longus

Abductor pollicis longus

Palmaris longus

Flexor digitorum superficialis, tendons of insertion

Flexor pollicis longus, tendon of insertion

Flexor digitorum profundus, tendons of insertion

A Superficial flexors and radialis group.

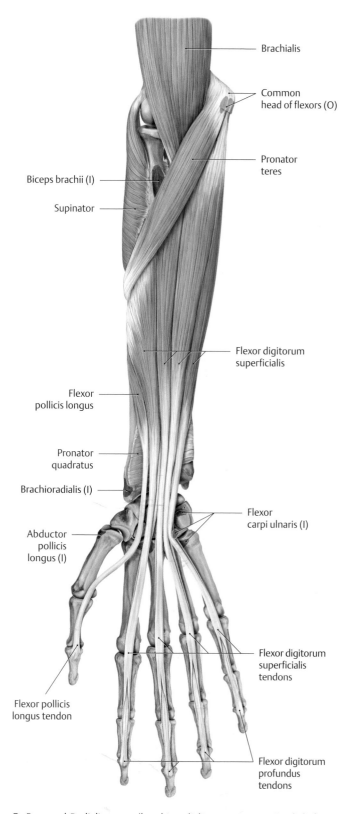

Brachialis

Common head of flexors (O)

Biceps brachii (I)

Pronator teres

Supinator

Flexor digitorum superficialis

Flexor pollicis longus

Pronator quadratus

Brachioradialis (I)

Flexor carpi ulnaris (I)

Abductor pollicis longus (I)

Flexor digitorum superficialis tendons

Flexor pollicis longus tendon

Flexor digitorum profundus tendons

B *Removed:* Radialis group (brachioradialis, extensor carpi radialis longus, and extensor carpi radialis brevis), flexor carpi radialis, flexor carpi ulnaris, abductor pollicis longus, palmaris longus, and biceps brachii.

288

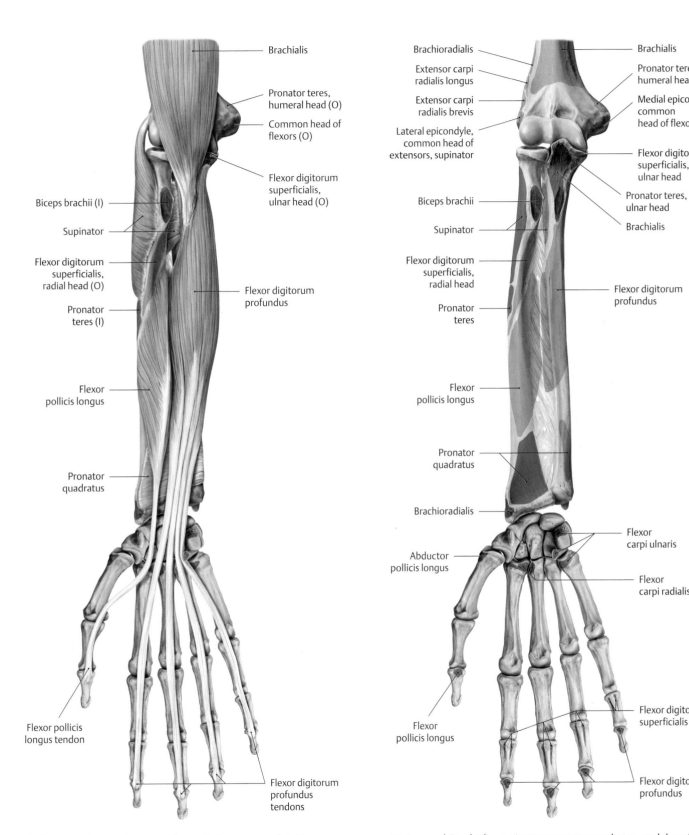

Brachialis

Pronator teres, humeral head (O)

Common head of flexors (O)

Flexor digitorum superficialis, ulnar head (O)

Biceps brachii (I)

Supinator

Flexor digitorum superficialis, radial head (O)

Pronator teres (I)

Flexor pollicis longus

Pronator quadratus

Flexor digitorum profundus

Flexor pollicis longus tendon

Flexor digitorum profundus tendons

Brachioradialis

Extensor carpi radialis longus

Extensor carpi radialis brevis

Lateral epicondyle, common head of extensors, supinator

Biceps brachii

Supinator

Flexor digitorum superficialis, radial head

Pronator teres

Flexor pollicis longus

Pronator quadratus

Brachioradialis

Abductor pollicis longus

Flexor pollicis longus

Brachialis

Pronator teres, humeral head

Medial epicondyle, common head of flexors

Flexor digitorum superficialis, ulnar head

Pronator teres, ulnar head

Brachialis

Flexor digitorum profundus

Flexor carpi ulnaris

Flexor carpi radialis

Flexor digitorum superficialis

Flexor digitorum profundus

C *Removed:* Pronator teres and flexor digitorum superficialis.

D *Removed:* Brachialis, supinator, pronator quadratus, and deep flexors.

289

Muscles of the Forearm (II)

***Fig. 20.12* Posterior muscles**

Right forearm, posterior view. Muscle origins (O) are shown in red, insertions (I) in blue.

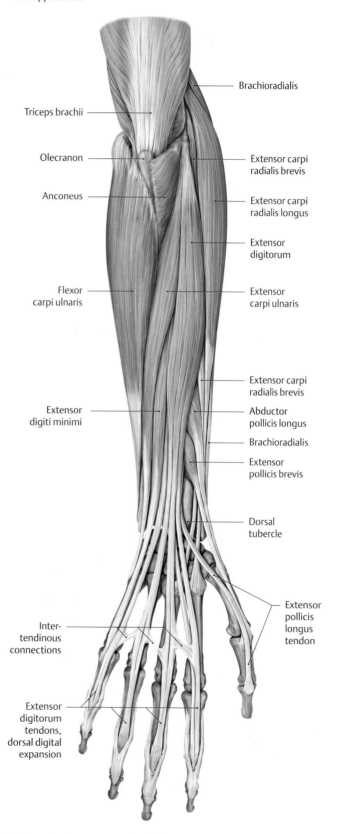

Brachioradialis

Triceps brachii

Olecranon

Anconeus

Flexor carpi ulnaris

Extensor digiti minimi

Extensor carpi radialis brevis

Extensor carpi radialis longus

Extensor digitorum

Extensor carpi ulnaris

Extensor carpi radialis brevis

Abductor pollicis longus

Brachioradialis

Extensor pollicis brevis

Dorsal tubercle

Inter-tendinous connections

Extensor digitorum tendons, dorsal digital expansion

Extensor pollicis longus tendon

A Superficial extensors and radialis group.

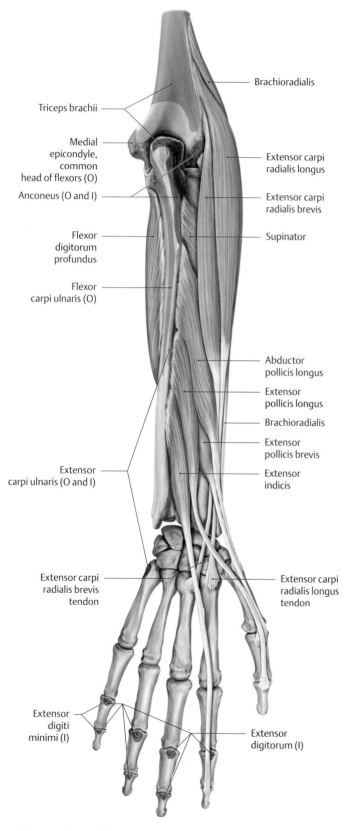

Brachioradialis

Triceps brachii

Medial epicondyle, common head of flexors (O)

Anconeus (O and I)

Flexor digitorum profundus

Flexor carpi ulnaris (O)

Extensor carpi ulnaris (O and I)

Extensor carpi radialis longus

Extensor carpi radialis brevis

Supinator

Abductor pollicis longus

Extensor pollicis longus

Brachioradialis

Extensor pollicis brevis

Extensor indicis

Extensor carpi radialis brevis tendon

Extensor carpi radialis longus tendon

Extensor digiti minimi (I)

Extensor digitorum (I)

B *Removed:* Triceps brachii, anconeus, flexor carpi ulnaris, extensor carpi ulnaris, and extensor digitorum.

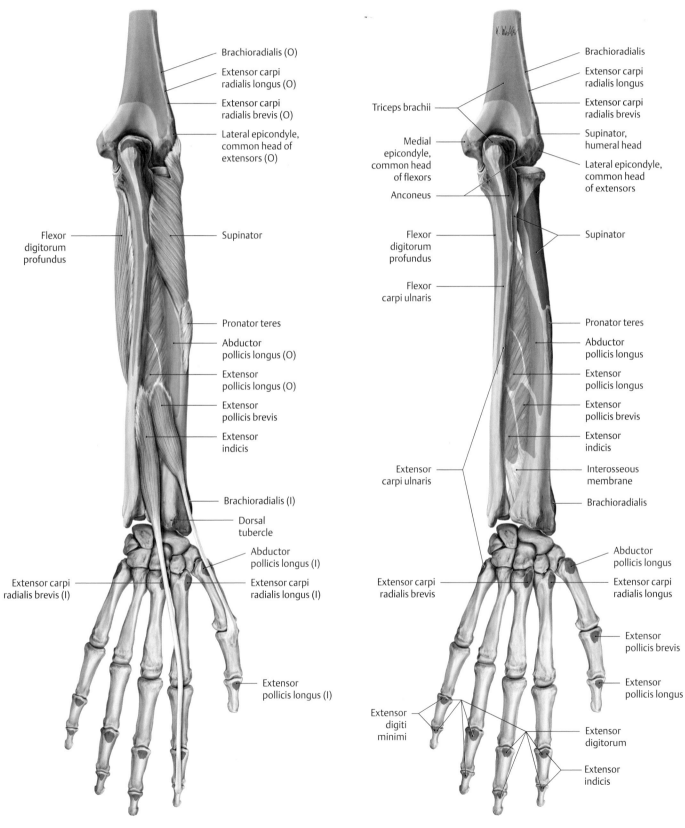

C *Removed:* Abductor pollicis longus, extensor pollicis longus, and radialis group.

D *Removed:* Flexor digitorum profundus, supinator, extensor pollicis brevis, and extensor indicis.

291

Muscle Facts (I)

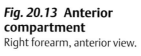

Fig. 20.13 Anterior compartment
Right forearm, anterior view.

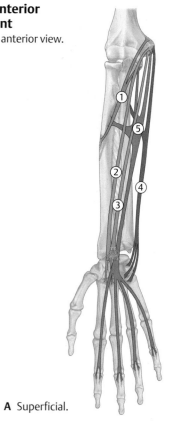

A Superficial.

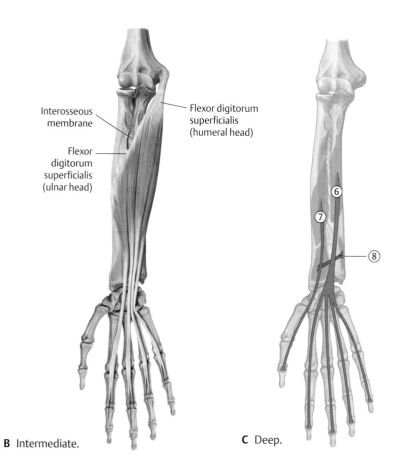

B Intermediate.

C Deep.

Interosseous membrane

Flexor digitorum superficialis (humeral head)

Flexor digitorum superficialis (ulnar head)

Table 20.2	Anterior compartment of the forearm			
Muscle	**Origin**	**Insertion**	**Innervation**	**Action**
Superficial group				
① Pronator teres	Humeral head: medial epicondyle of humerus Ulnar head: coronoid process	Lateral radius (distal to supinator insertion)	Median n. (C6, C7)	Elbow: weak flexor Forearm: pronation
② Flexor carpi radialis	Medial epicondyle of humerus	Base of 2nd metacarpal (variance: base of 3rd metacarpal)		Wrist: flexion and abduction (radial deviation) of hand
③ Palmaris longus		Palmar aponeurosis	Median n. (C7, C8)	Elbow: weak flexion Wrist: flexion tightens palmar aponeurosis
④ Flexor carpi ulnaris	Humeral head: medial epicondyle Ulnar head: olecranon	Pisiform; hook of hamate; base of 5th metacarpal	Ulnar n. (C7–T1)	Wrist: flexion and adduction (ulnar deviation) of hand
Intermediate group				
⑤ Flexor digitorum superficialis	Humeral head: medial epicondyle Ulnar head: coronoid process	Sides of middle phalanges of 2nd to 5th digits	Median n. (C8, T1)	Elbow: weak flexor Wrist, MCP, and PIP joints of 2nd to 5th digits: flexion
Deep group				
⑥ Flexor digitorum profundis	Ulna (two thirds of flexor surface) and interosseous membrane	Distal phalanges of 2nd to 5th digits (palmar surface)	Median n. (C8, T1) Ulnar n. (C8, T1)	Wrist, MCP, PIP, and DIP of 2nd to 5th digits: flexion
⑦ Flexor pollicis longus	Radius (midanterior surface) and adjacent interosseous membrane	Distal phalanx of thumb (palmar surface)	Median n. (C7, C8)	Wrist: flexion and abduction (radial deviation) of hand Carpometacarpal of thumb: flexion MCP and IP of thumb: flexion
⑧ Pronator quadratus	Distal quarter of ulna (anterior surface)	Distal quarter of radius (anterior surface)		Hand: pronation Distal radioulnar joint: stabilization

DIP = distal interphalangeal; IP = interphalangeal; MCP = metacarpophalangeal; PIP = proximal interphalangeal.

Fig. 20.14 Superficial and intermediate groups
Right forearm, anterior view.

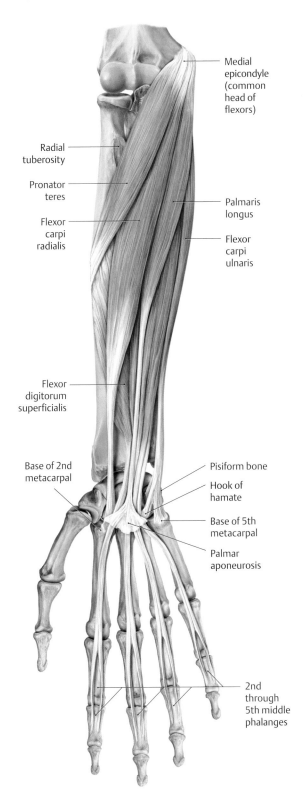

Medial epicondyle (common head of flexors)

Radial tuberosity

Pronator teres

Flexor carpi radialis

Flexor digitorum superficialis

Palmaris longus

Flexor carpi ulnaris

Base of 2nd metacarpal

Pisiform bone

Hook of hamate

Base of 5th metacarpal

Palmar aponeurosis

2nd through 5th middle phalanges

Fig. 20.15 Deep group
Right forearm, anterior view.

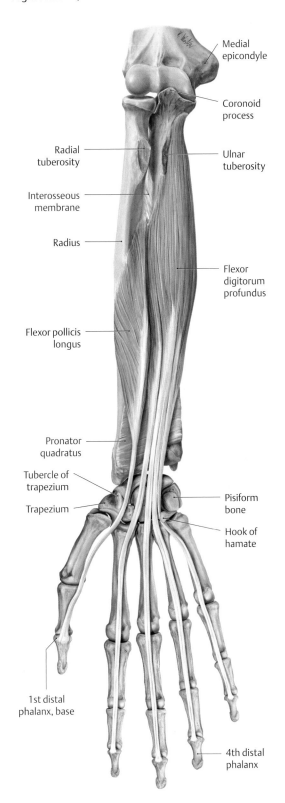

Medial epicondyle

Coronoid process

Radial tuberosity

Ulnar tuberosity

Interosseous membrane

Radius

Flexor digitorum profundus

Flexor pollicis longus

Pronator quadratus

Tubercle of trapezium

Trapezium

Pisiform bone

Hook of hamate

1st distal phalanx, base

4th distal phalanx

Muscle Facts (II)

Fig. 20.16 **Radialis group**
Right forearm, posterior view.

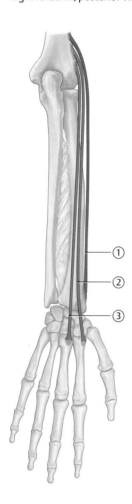

Table 20.3	Posterior compartment of the forearm: Radialis muscles			
Muscle	**Origin**	**Insertion**	**Innervation**	**Action**
① Brachioradialis	Distal humerus (distal surface), lateral intermuscular septum	Styloid process of the radius	Radial n. (C5, C6)	Elbow: flexion Forearm: semipronation
② Extensor carpi radialis longus	Lateral supracondylar ridge of distal humerus, lateral intermuscular septum	2nd metacarpal (base)	Radial n. (C6, C7)	Elbow: weak flexion Wrist: extension and abduction
③ Extensor carpi radialis brevis	Lateral epicondyle of humerus	3rd metacarpal (base)	Radial n. (C7, C8)	

Fig. 20.17 **Radialis muscles of the forearm**
Right forearm.

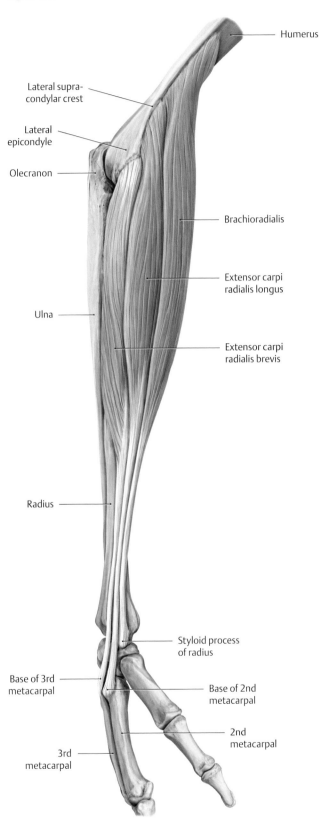

Humerus

Lateral supra-
condylar crest

Lateral
epicondyle

Olecranon

Brachioradialis

Extensor carpi
radialis longus

Ulna

Extensor carpi
radialis brevis

Radius

Styloid process
of radius

Base of 3rd
metacarpal

Base of 2nd
metacarpal

2nd
metacarpal

3rd
metacarpal

A Lateral (radial) view.

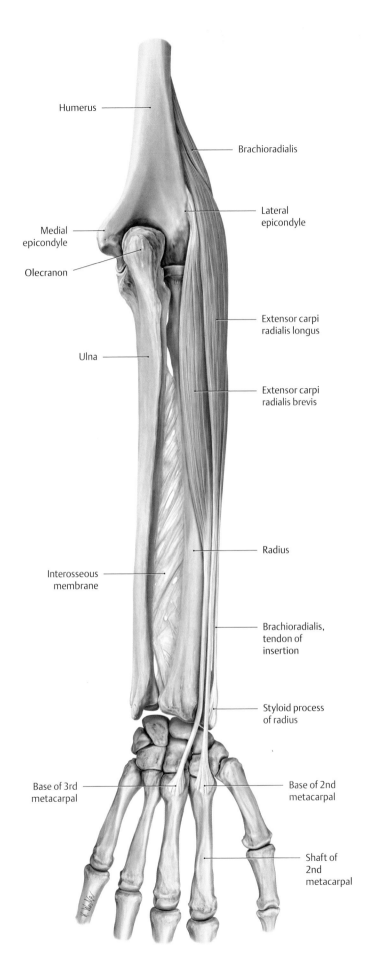

Humerus

Brachioradialis

Medial
epicondyle

Lateral
epicondyle

Olecranon

Ulna

Extensor carpi
radialis longus

Extensor carpi
radialis brevis

Radius

Interosseous
membrane

Brachioradialis,
tendon of
insertion

Styloid process
of radius

Base of 3rd
metacarpal

Base of 2nd
metacarpal

Shaft of
2nd
metacarpal

B Posterior view.

Muscle Facts (III)

Fig. 20.18 Superficial group
Right forearm, posterior view.

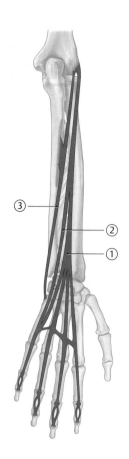

Fig. 20.19 Deep group
Right forearm, posterior view.

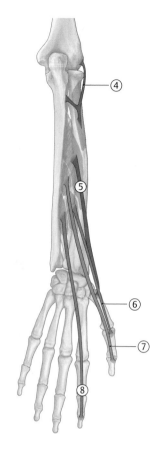

Table 20.4	Posterior compartment of the forearm			
Muscle	**Origin**	**Insertion**	**Innervation**	**Action**
Superficial group				
① Extensor digitorum	Common head (lateral epicondyle of humerus)	Dorsal digital expansion of 2nd to 5th digits	Radial n. (C7, C8)	Wrist: extension MCP, PIP, and DIP of 2nd to 5th digits: extension/abduction of fingers
② Extensor digiti minimi		Dorsal digital expansion of 5th digit		Wrist: extension, ulnar abduction of hand MCP, PIP, and DIP of 5th digit: extension and abduction of 5th digit
③ Extensor carpi ulnaris	Common head (lateral epicondyle of humerus) Ulnar head (dorsal surface)	Base of 5th metacarpal		Wrist: extension, adduction (ulnar deviation) of hand
Deep group				
④ Supinator	Olecranon, lateral epicondyle of humerus, radial collateral ligament, annular ligament of radius	Radius (between radial tuberosity and insertion of pronator teres)	Radial n. (C6, C7)	Radioulnar joints: supination
⑤ Abductor pollicis longus	Radius and ulna (dorsal surfaces, interosseous membrane)	Base of 1st metacarpal	Radial n. (C7, C8)	Radiocarpal joint: abduction of the hand Carpometacarpal joint of thumb: abduction
⑥ Extensor pollicis brevis	Radius (posterior surface) and interosseous membrane	Base of proximal phalanx of thumb		Radiocarpal joint: abduction (radial deviation) of hand Carpometacarpal and MCP of thumb: extension
⑦ Extensor pollicis longus	Ulna (posterior surface) and interosseous membrane	Base of distal phalanx of thumb		Wrist: extension and abduction (radial deviation) of hand Carpometacarpal of thumb: adduction MCP and IP of thumb: extension
⑧ Extensor indicis	Ulna (posterior surface) and interosseous membrane	Posterior digital extension of 2nd digit		Wrist: extension MCP, PIP, and DIP of 2nd digit: extension

DIP = distal interphalangeal; IP = interphalangeal; MCP = metacarpophalangeal; PIP = proximal interphalangeal.

Fig. 20.20 **Muscles of the posterior forearm**
Right forearm, posterior view.

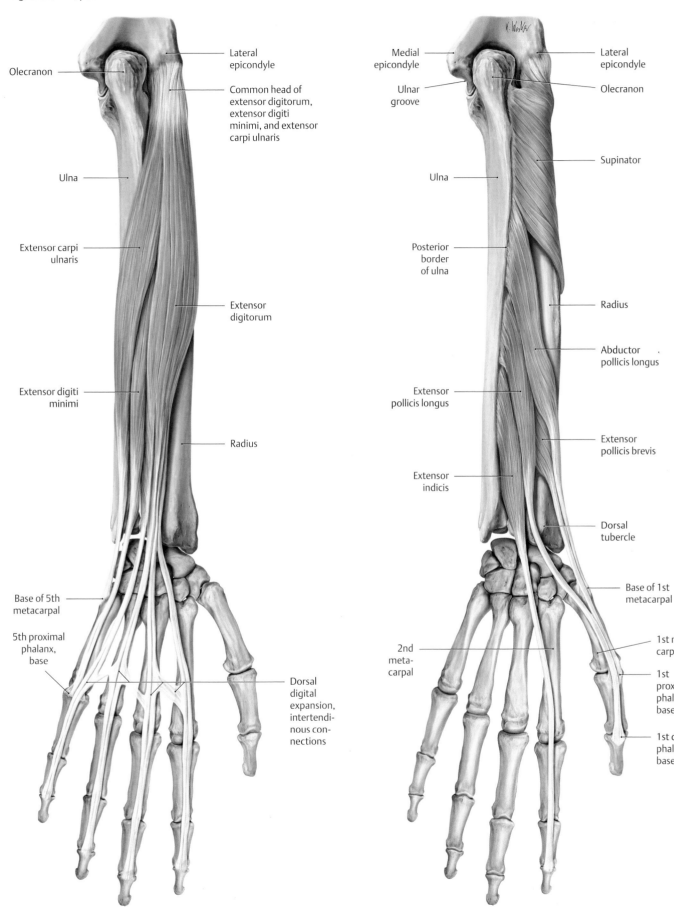

Olecranon

Lateral epicondyle

Common head of extensor digitorum, extensor digiti minimi, and extensor carpi ulnaris

Ulna

Extensor carpi ulnaris

Extensor digitorum

Extensor digiti minimi

Radius

Base of 5th metacarpal

5th proximal phalanx, base

Dorsal digital expansion, intertendinous connections

Medial epicondyle

Ulnar groove

Lateral epicondyle

Olecranon

Supinator

Ulna

Posterior border of ulna

Radius

Abductor pollicis longus

Extensor pollicis longus

Extensor pollicis brevis

Extensor indicis

Dorsal tubercle

Base of 1st metacarpal

2nd metacarpal

1st metacarpal

1st proximal phalanx, base

1st distal phalanx, base

A Superficial extensors.

B Deep extensors with supinator.

Bones of the Wrist & Hand

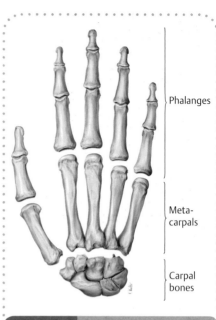

Phalanges

Meta-carpals

Carpal bones

Table 21.1	Bones of the wrist and hand	
Phalanges	1st to 5th proximal phalanges	
	2nd to 5th middle phalanges*	
	1st to 5th distal phalanges	
Metacarpal bones	1st to 5th metacarpals	
Carpal bones	Trapezium	Scaphoid
	Trapezoid	Lunate
	Capitate	Triquetrum
	Hamate	

*There are only four middle phalanges (the thumb has only a proximal and a distal phalanx).

Fig. 21.1 **Dorsal view**
Right hand.

2nd distal phalanx

2nd middle phalanx

2nd proximal phalanx

1st metacarpal

Trapezoid

Trapezium

Scaphoid

Styloid process of radius

Radius

Capitate

Hamate

Triquetrum

Lunate

Styloid process of ulna

Ulna

Fig. 21.2 Palmar view
Right hand.

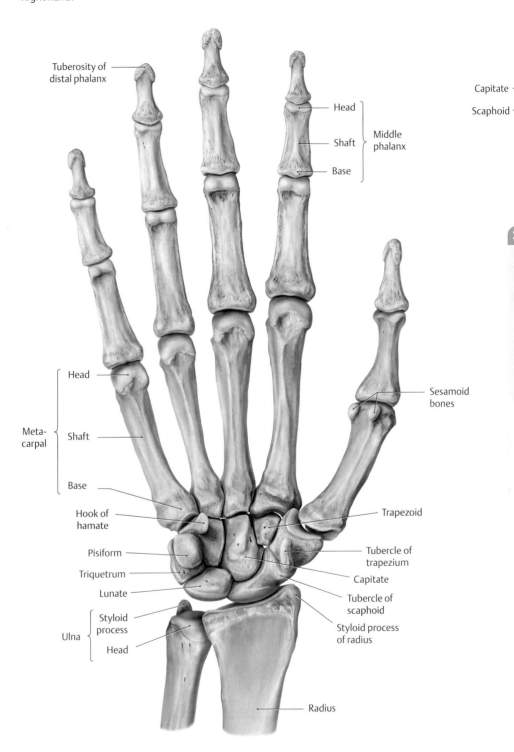

Tuberosity of distal phalanx

Head

Shaft — Middle phalanx

Base

Head

Meta-carpal { Shaft

Base

Hook of hamate

Pisiform

Triquetrum

Lunate

Ulna { Styloid process

Head

Sesamoid bones

Trapezoid

Tubercle of trapezium

Capitate

Tubercle of scaphoid

Styloid process of radius

Radius

Fig. 21.3 Radiograph of the wrist
Anteroposterior view of left limb.

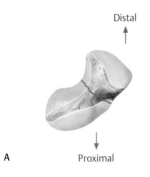

Capitate

Scaphoid

Hook of hamate

Pisiform

Triquetrum

Lunate

✦ Clinical

Scaphoid Fractures
Scaphoid fractures are the most common carpal bone fractures, generally occurring at the narrowed waist between the proximal and distal poles (**A**, right scaphoid). Because blood supply to the scaphoid is transmitted via the distal segment, fractures at the waist can compromise the supply to the proximal segment, often resulting in nonunion and avascular necrosis.

Distal

Proximal

A

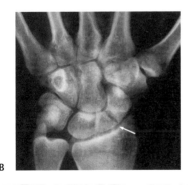

B

299

Joints of the Wrist & Hand

Fig. 21.4 **Joints of the wrist and hand**

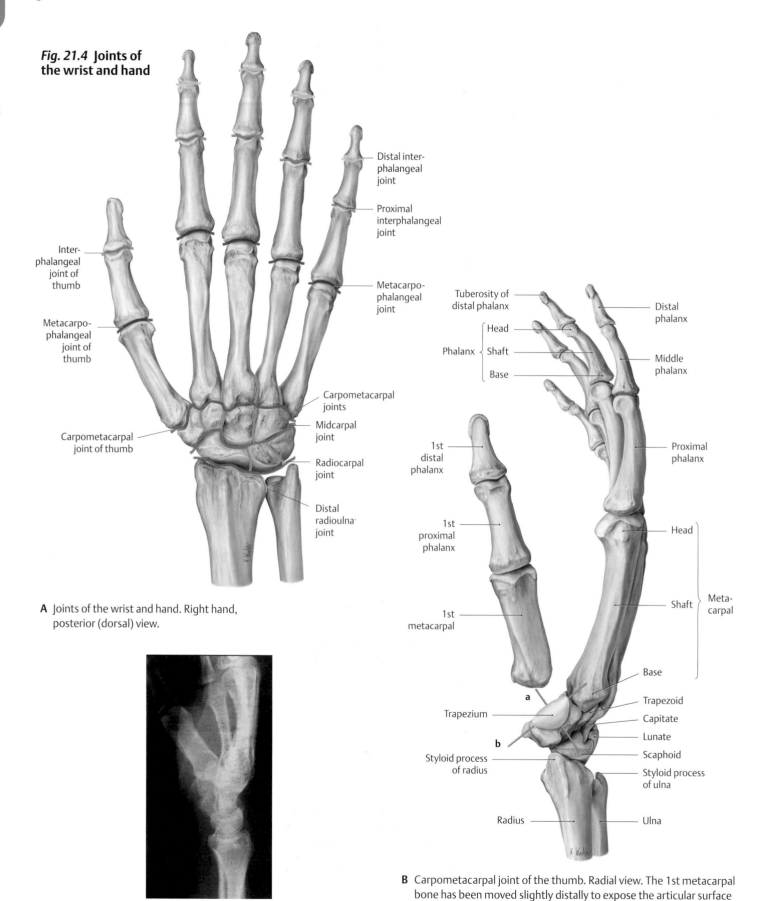

Distal inter-phalangeal joint

Proximal interphalangeal joint

Metacarpo-phalangeal joint

Inter-phalangeal joint of thumb

Metacarpo-phalangeal joint of thumb

Carpometacarpal joints

Midcarpal joint

Carpometacarpal joint of thumb

Radiocarpal joint

Distal radioulnar joint

A Joints of the wrist and hand. Right hand, posterior (dorsal) view.

Tuberosity of distal phalanx

Head

Phalanx { Shaft

Base

Distal phalanx

Middle phalanx

1st distal phalanx

1st proximal phalanx

1st metacarpal

Proximal phalanx

Head

Shaft } Meta-carpal

Base

Trapezoid

Capitate

Lunate

Scaphoid

Styloid process of ulna

Trapezium

a

b

Styloid process of radius

Radius

Ulna

B Carpometacarpal joint of the thumb. Radial view. The 1st metacarpal bone has been moved slightly distally to expose the articular surface of the trapezium. Two cardinal axes of motion are shown here: (**a**) flexion/extension and (**b**) abduction/adduction.

C Radiograph of wrist. Radial view.

Fig. 21.5 **Wrist and hand: Coronal section**
Right hand.

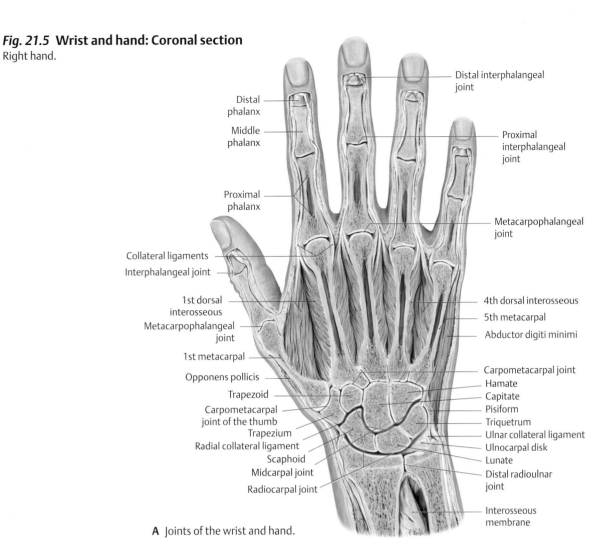

A Joints of the wrist and hand.

- Distal interphalangeal joint
- Distal phalanx
- Middle phalanx
- Proximal interphalangeal joint
- Proximal phalanx
- Metacarpophalangeal joint
- Collateral ligaments
- Interphalangeal joint
- 1st dorsal interosseous
- Metacarpophalangeal joint
- 1st metacarpal
- Opponens pollicis
- Trapezoid
- Carpometacarpal joint of the thumb
- Trapezium
- Radial collateral ligament
- Scaphoid
- Midcarpal joint
- Radiocarpal joint
- 4th dorsal interosseous
- 5th metacarpal
- Abductor digiti minimi
- Carpometacarpal joint
- Hamate
- Capitate
- Pisiform
- Triquetrum
- Ulnar collateral ligament
- Ulnocarpal disk
- Lunate
- Distal radioulnar joint
- Interosseous membrane

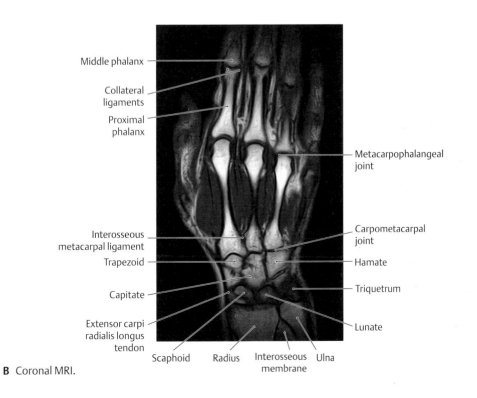

B Coronal MRI.

- Middle phalanx
- Collateral ligaments
- Proximal phalanx
- Metacarpophalangeal joint
- Interosseous metacarpal ligament
- Carpometacarpal joint
- Trapezoid
- Hamate
- Capitate
- Triquetrum
- Extensor carpi radialis longus tendon
- Lunate
- Scaphoid
- Radius
- Interosseous membrane
- Ulna

Ligaments of the Wrist & Hand

Fig. 21.6 **Ligaments of the hand**
Right hand.

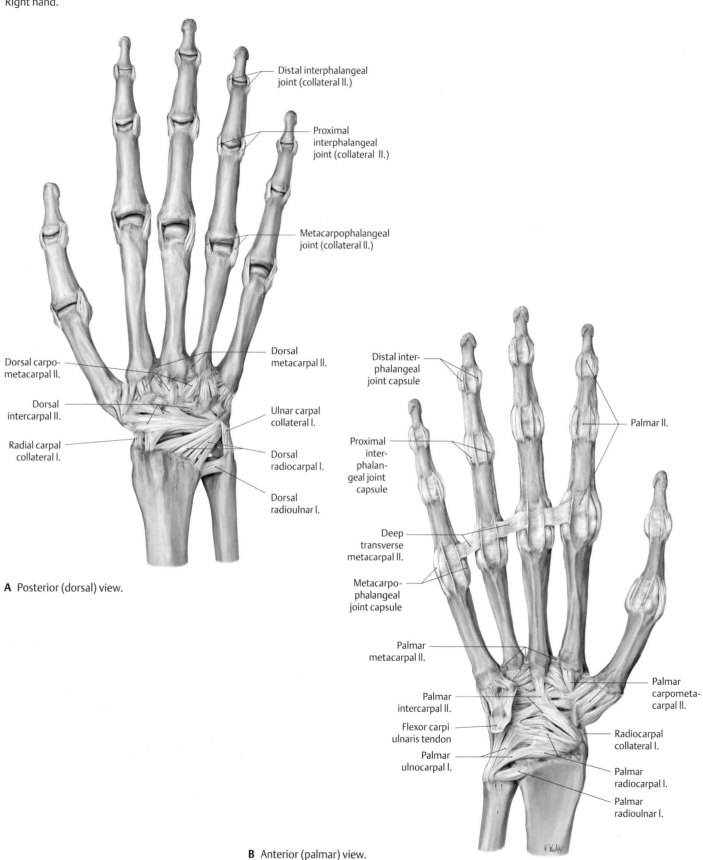

Distal interphalangeal
joint (collateral ll.)

Proximal
interphalangeal
joint (collateral ll.)

Metacarpophalangeal
joint (collateral ll.)

Dorsal carpo-
metacarpal ll.

Dorsal
metacarpal ll.

Dorsal
intercarpal ll.

Ulnar carpal
collateral l.

Radial carpal
collateral l.

Dorsal
radiocarpal l.

Dorsal
radioulnar l.

A Posterior (dorsal) view.

Distal inter-
phalangeal
joint capsule

Palmar ll.

Proximal
inter-
phalan-
geal joint
capsule

Deep
transverse
metacarpal ll.

Metacarpo-
phalangeal
joint capsule

Palmar
metacarpal ll.

Palmar
carpometa-
carpal ll.

Palmar
intercarpal ll.

Flexor carpi
ulnaris tendon

Radiocarpal
collateral l.

Palmar
ulnocarpal l.

Palmar
radiocarpal l.

Palmar
radioulnar l.

B Anterior (palmar) view.

Fig. 21.7 Ligaments of the carpal tunnel

Right hand, anterior view.

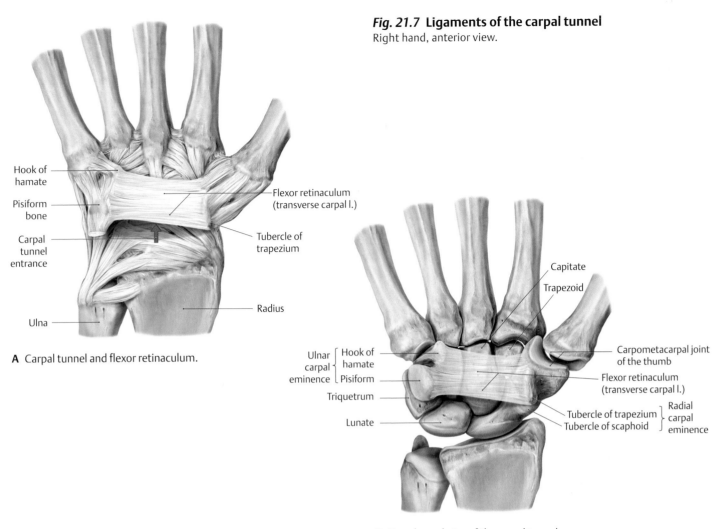

Hook of hamate

Pisiform bone

Carpal tunnel entrance

Ulna

Flexor retinaculum (transverse carpal l.)

Tubercle of trapezium

Radius

A Carpal tunnel and flexor retinaculum.

Capitate

Trapezoid

Ulnar carpal eminence { Hook of hamate / Pisiform }

Triquetrum

Lunate

Carpometacarpal joint of the thumb

Flexor retinaculum (transverse carpal l.)

Tubercle of trapezium } Radial carpal eminence
Tubercle of scaphoid

B Bony boundaries of the carpal tunnel.

Fig. 21.8 Carpal tunnel

Transverse section. The contents of the carpal tunnel are discussed on p. 342. See p. 343 for the ulnar tunnel and palmar carpal ligament.

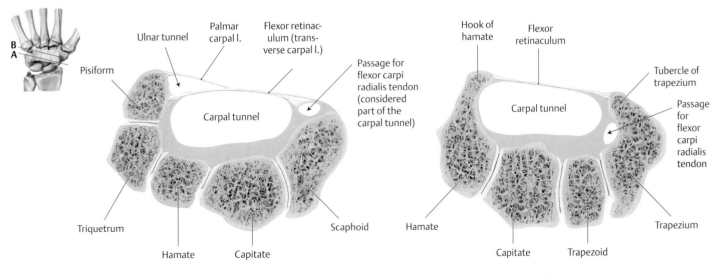

Ulnar tunnel

Palmar carpal l.

Flexor retinaculum (transverse carpal l.)

Pisiform

Passage for flexor carpi radialis tendon (considered part of the carpal tunnel)

Carpal tunnel

Triquetrum

Hamate

Capitate

Scaphoid

A Proximal part of the carpal tunnel.

Hook of hamate

Flexor retinaculum

Tubercle of trapezium

Passage for flexor carpi radialis tendon

Carpal tunnel

Hamate

Capitate

Trapezoid

Trapezium

B Distal part of the carpal tunnel.

Ligaments of the Fingers

Fig. 21.9 Ligaments of the fingers: Lateral view

Right middle finger. The outer fibrous layer of the tendon sheaths (stratum fibrosum) is strengthened by the annular and cruciform ligaments, which also bind the sheaths to the palmar surface of the phalanx and prevent palmar deviation of the sheaths during flexion.

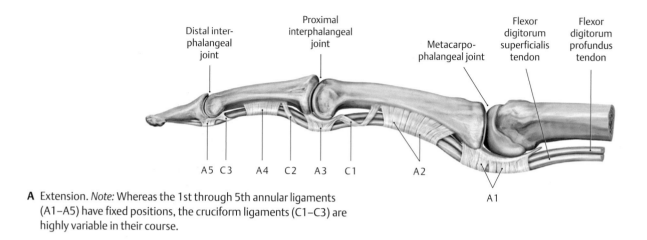

A Extension. *Note:* Whereas the 1st through 5th annular ligaments (A1–A5) have fixed positions, the cruciform ligaments (C1–C3) are highly variable in their course.

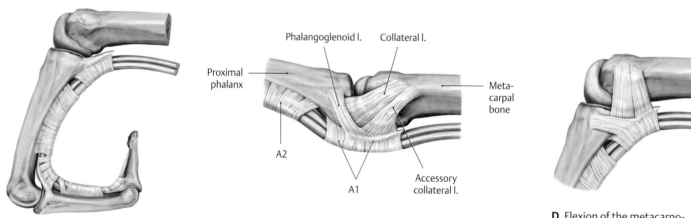

B Flexion.

C Extension of the metacarpophalangeal joint. *Note:* The collateral ligament is lax.

D Flexion of the metacarpophalangeal joint. *Note:* The collateral ligament is taut.

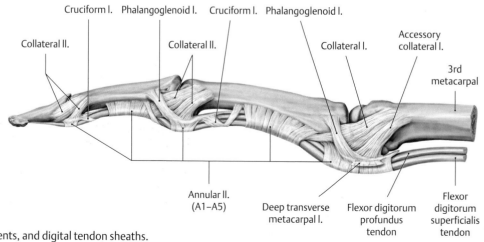

E Joint capsules, ligaments, and digital tendon sheaths.

Fig. 21.10 Anterior view

Right middle finger, palmar view.

Fig. 21.11 Third metacarpal: Transverse section

Proximal view.

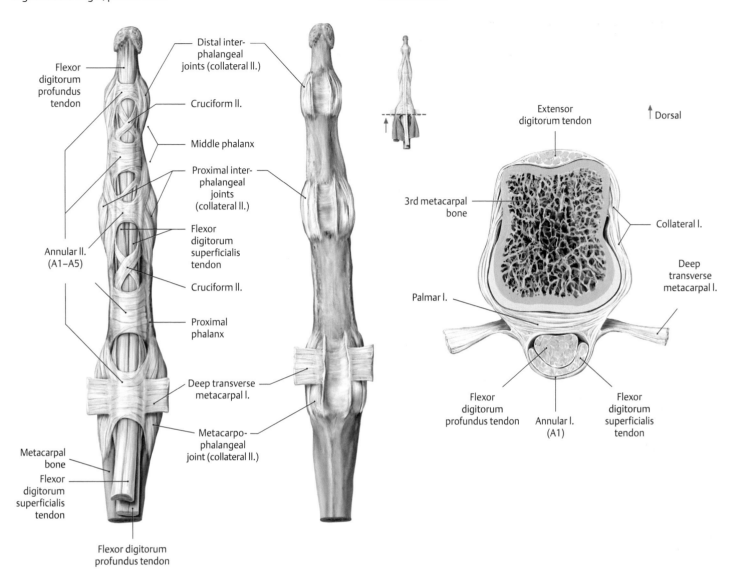

A Superficial ligaments.

B Deep ligaments with digital tendon sheath removed.

Fig. 21.12 Fingertip: Longitudinal section

The palmar articular surfaces of the phalanges are enlarged proximally at the joints by the palmar ligament. This fibrocartilaginous plate, also known as the volar plate, forms the floor of the digital tendon sheaths.

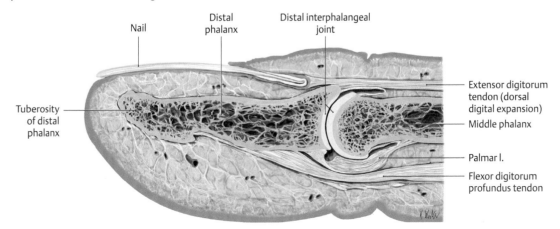

Muscles of the Hand: Superficial & Middle Layers

Fig. 21.13 Intrinsic muscles of the hand: Superficial and middle layers

Right hand, palmar surface.

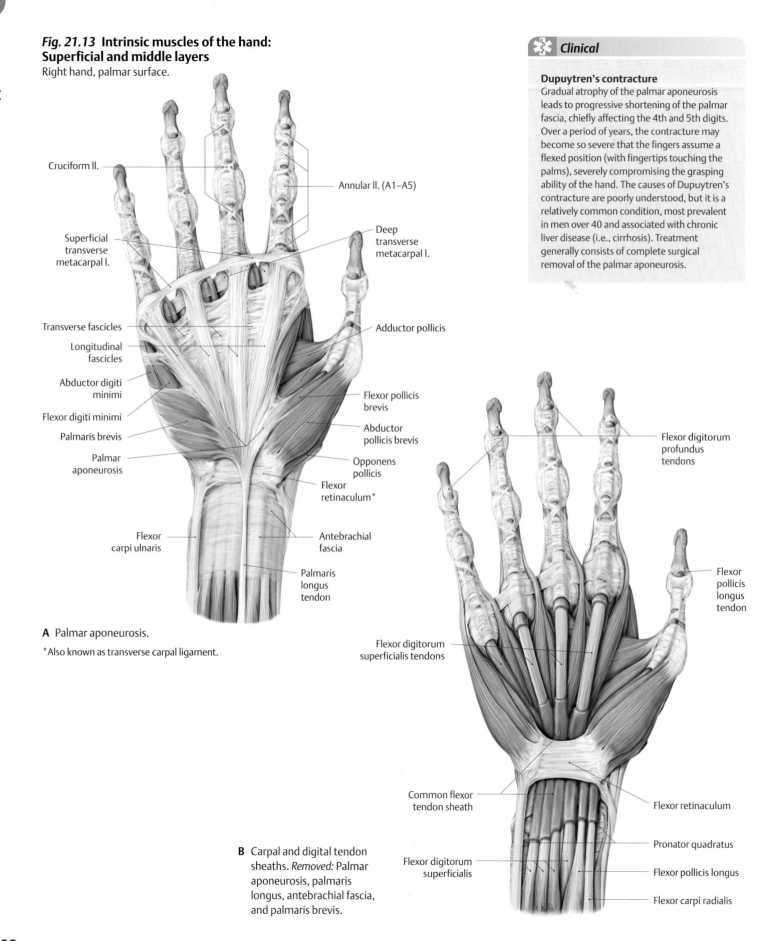

Cruciform ll.

Annular ll. (A1–A5)

Superficial transverse metacarpal l.

Deep transverse metacarpal l.

Transverse fascicles

Adductor pollicis

Longitudinal fascicles

Abductor digiti minimi

Flexor pollicis brevis

Flexor digiti minimi

Abductor pollicis brevis

Palmaris brevis

Palmar aponeurosis

Opponens pollicis

Flexor retinaculum*

Flexor carpi ulnaris

Antebrachial fascia

Palmaris longus tendon

A Palmar aponeurosis.

*Also known as transverse carpal ligament.

Flexor digitorum profundus tendons

Flexor pollicis longus tendon

Flexor digitorum superficialis tendons

Common flexor tendon sheath

Flexor retinaculum

Pronator quadratus

Flexor digitorum superficialis

Flexor pollicis longus

Flexor carpi radialis

B Carpal and digital tendon sheaths. *Removed:* Palmar aponeurosis, palmaris longus, antebrachial fascia, and palmaris brevis.

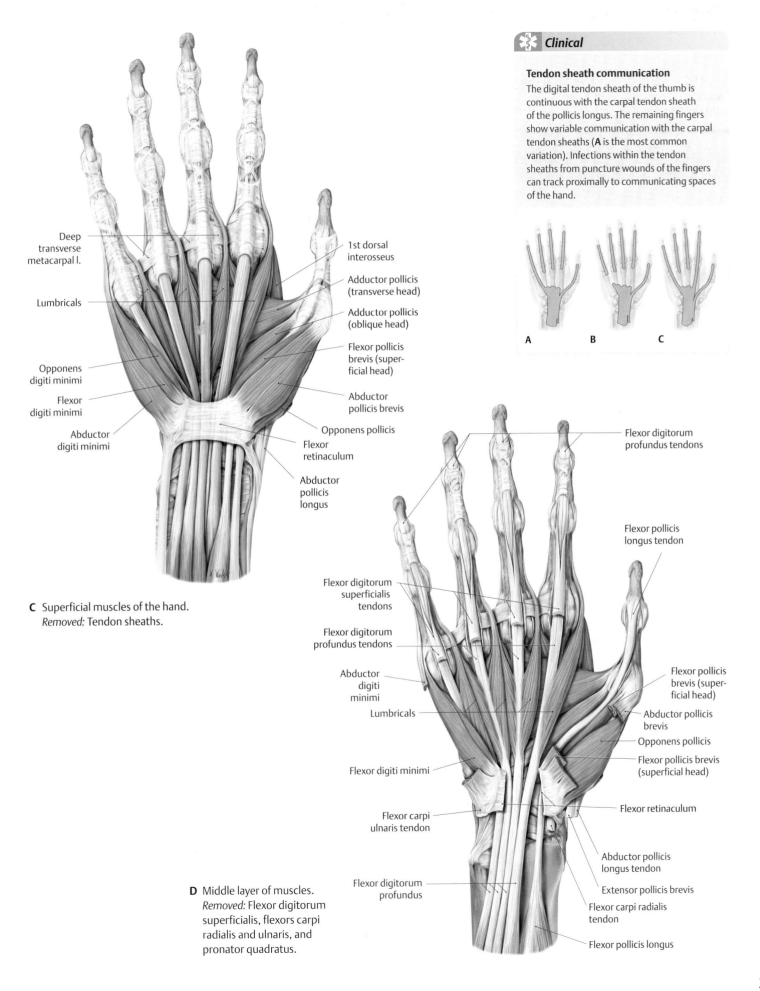

Deep transverse metacarpal l.

Lumbricals

Opponens digiti minimi

Flexor digiti minimi

Abductor digiti minimi

1st dorsal interosseus

Adductor pollicis (transverse head)

Adductor pollicis (oblique head)

Flexor pollicis brevis (superficial head)

Abductor pollicis brevis

Opponens pollicis

Flexor retinaculum

Abductor pollicis longus

C Superficial muscles of the hand.
Removed: Tendon sheaths.

✳ Clinical

Tendon sheath communication

The digital tendon sheath of the thumb is continuous with the carpal tendon sheath of the pollicis longus. The remaining fingers show variable communication with the carpal tendon sheaths (**A** is the most common variation). Infections within the tendon sheaths from puncture wounds of the fingers can track proximally to communicating spaces of the hand.

A   **B**   **C**

Flexor digitorum profundus tendons

Flexor pollicis longus tendon

Flexor digitorum superficialis tendons

Flexor digitorum profundus tendons

Abductor digiti minimi

Lumbricals

Flexor digiti minimi

Flexor carpi ulnaris tendon

Flexor digitorum profundus

Flexor pollicis brevis (superficial head)

Abductor pollicis brevis

Opponens pollicis

Flexor pollicis brevis (superficial head)

Flexor retinaculum

Abductor pollicis longus tendon

Extensor pollicis brevis

Flexor carpi radialis tendon

Flexor pollicis longus

D Middle layer of muscles.
Removed: Flexor digitorum superficialis, flexors carpi radialis and ulnaris, and pronator quadratus.

307

Muscles of the Hand: Middle & Deep Layers

Fig. 21.14 Intrinsic muscles: Middle and deep layers
Right hand, palmar surface.

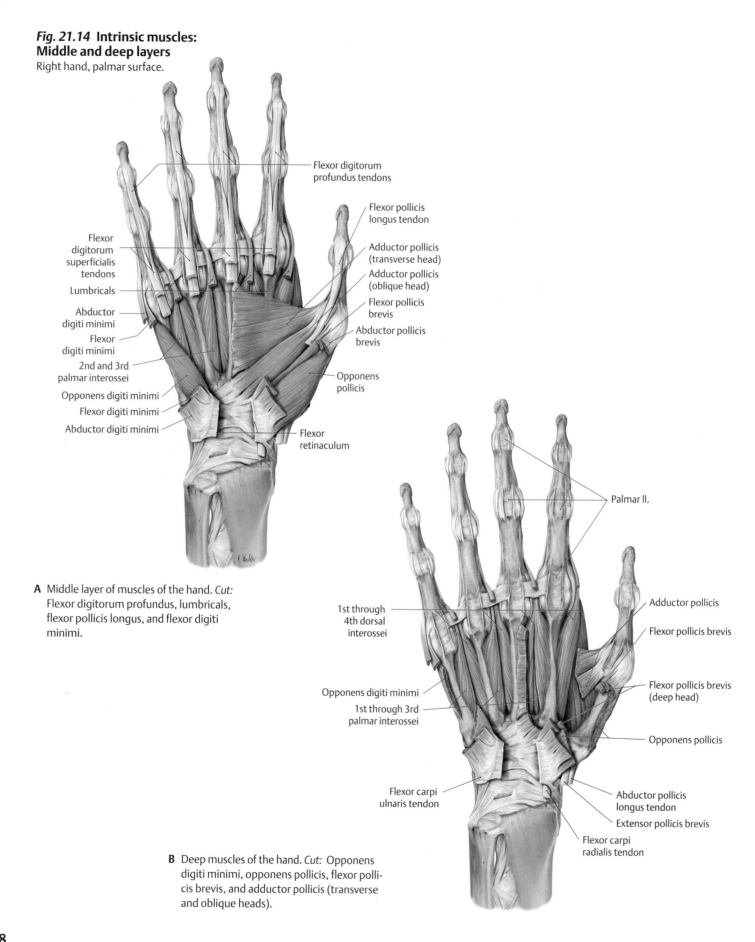

Flexor digitorum profundus tendons

Flexor pollicis longus tendon

Adductor pollicis (transverse head)

Adductor pollicis (oblique head)

Flexor pollicis brevis

Abductor pollicis brevis

Opponens pollicis

Flexor digitorum superficialis tendons

Lumbricals

Abductor digiti minimi

Flexor digiti minimi

2nd and 3rd palmar interossei

Opponens digiti minimi

Flexor digiti minimi

Abductor digiti minimi

Flexor retinaculum

A Middle layer of muscles of the hand. *Cut:* Flexor digitorum profundus, lumbricals, flexor pollicis longus, and flexor digiti minimi.

Palmar II.

1st through 4th dorsal interossei

Adductor pollicis

Flexor pollicis brevis

Flexor pollicis brevis (deep head)

Opponens digiti minimi

1st through 3rd palmar interossei

Opponens pollicis

Flexor carpi ulnaris tendon

Abductor pollicis longus tendon

Extensor pollicis brevis

Flexor carpi radialis tendon

B Deep muscles of the hand. *Cut:* Opponens digiti minimi, opponens pollicis, flexor pollicis brevis, and adductor pollicis (transverse and oblique heads).

Fig. 21.15 Origins and insertions

Right hand. Muscle origins shown in red, insertions in blue.

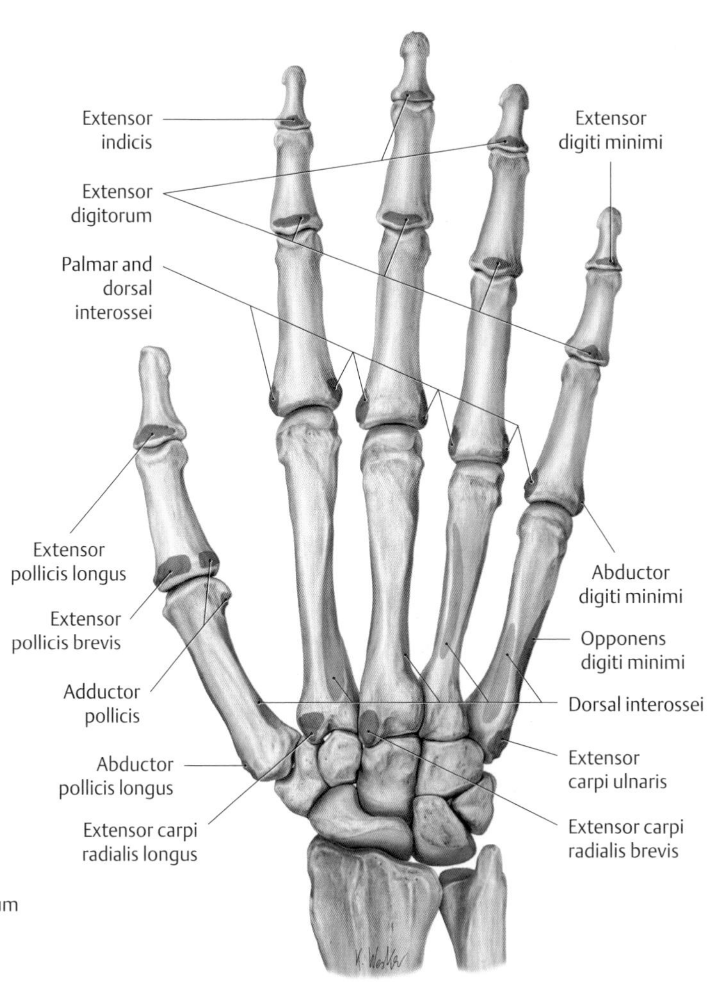

Extensor indicis

Extensor digitorum

Palmar and dorsal interossei

Extensor pollicis longus

Extensor pollicis brevis

Adductor pollicis

Abductor pollicis longus

Extensor carpi radialis longus

Extensor digiti minimi

Abductor digiti minimi

Opponens digiti minimi

Dorsal interossei

Extensor carpi ulnaris

Extensor carpi radialis brevis

A Dorsal (posterior) view.

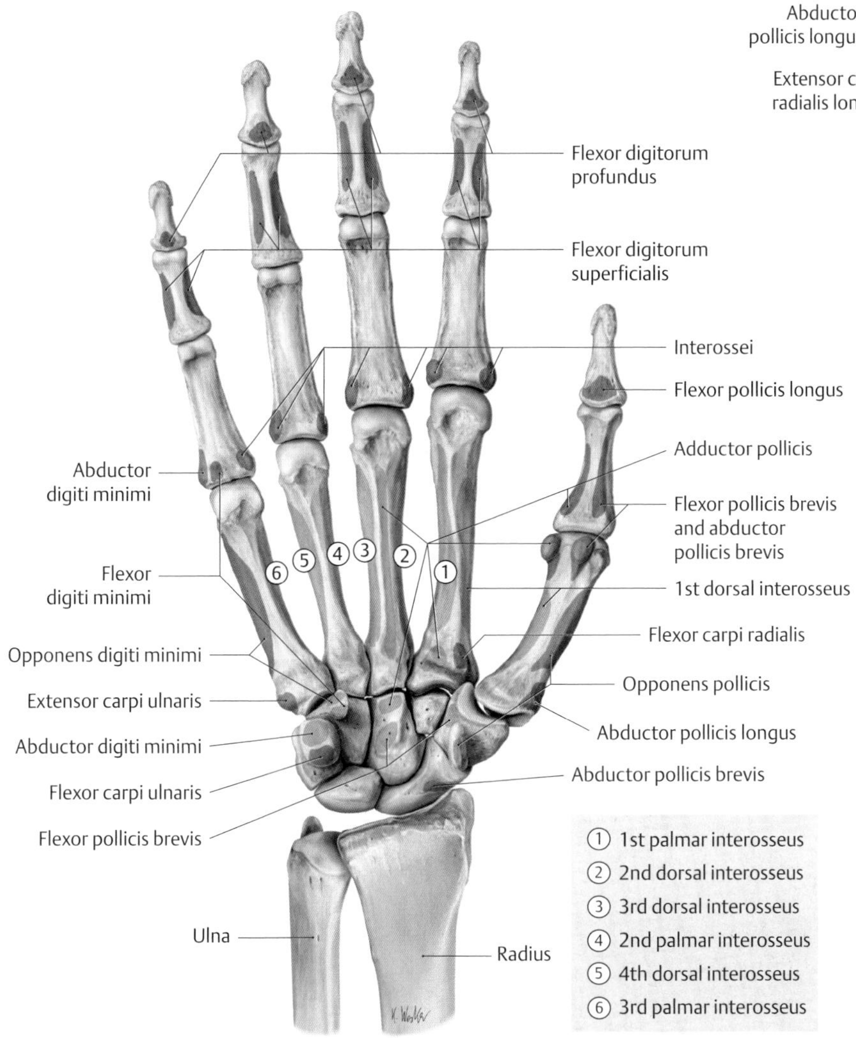

Flexor digitorum profundus

Flexor digitorum superficialis

Interossei

Flexor pollicis longus

Adductor pollicis

Flexor pollicis brevis and abductor pollicis brevis

1st dorsal interosseus

Flexor carpi radialis

Opponens pollicis

Abductor pollicis longus

Abductor pollicis brevis

Abductor digiti minimi

Flexor digiti minimi

Opponens digiti minimi

Extensor carpi ulnaris

Abductor digiti minimi

Flexor carpi ulnaris

Flexor pollicis brevis

Ulna

Radius

① 1st palmar interosseus
② 2nd dorsal interosseus
③ 3rd dorsal interosseus
④ 2nd palmar interosseus
⑤ 4th dorsal interosseus
⑥ 3rd palmar interosseus

B Palmar (anterior) view.

309

Dorsum of the Hand

Fig. 21.16 **Extensor retinaculum and dorsal carpal tendon sheaths**

Right hand, posterior (dorsal) view.

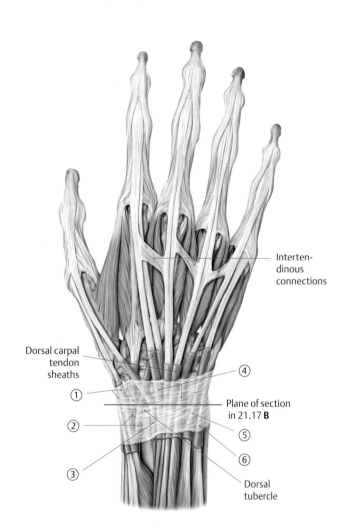

Fig. 21.17 **Muscles and tendons of the dorsum**

Right hand.

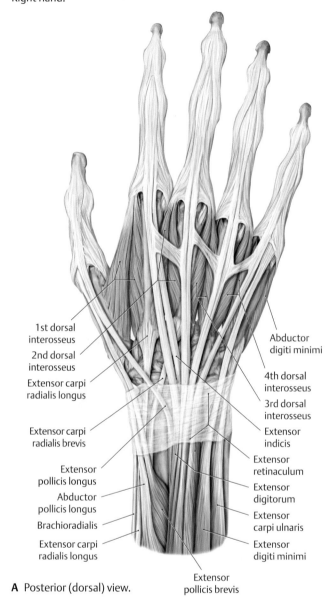

A Posterior (dorsal) view.

Table 21.2	Dorsal compartments for extensor tendons
①	Abductor pollicis longus
	Extensor pollicis brevis
②	Extensor carpi radialis longus
	Extensor carpi radialis brevis
③	Extensor pollicis longus
④	Extensor digitorum
	Extensor indicis
⑤	Extensor digiti minimi
⑥	Extensor carpi ulnaris

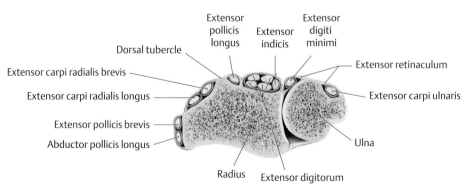

B Dorsal compartments, proximal view of section in Fig. 21.16.

Fig. 21.18 Dorsal digital expansion

Right hand, middle finger. The dorsal digital expansion permits the long digital flexors and the short muscles of the hand to act on all three finger joints.

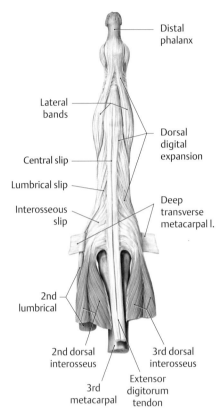

A Posterior view.

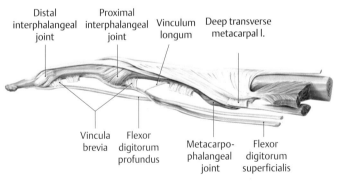

B Cross section through 3rd metacarpal head, proximal view.

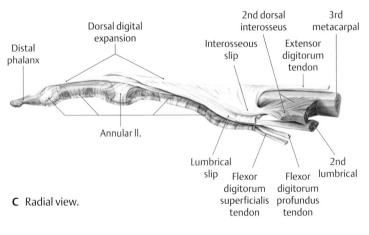

C Radial view.

D Radial view with common tendon sheath of flexor digitorum superficialis and profundus opened.

Muscle Facts (I)

The intrinsic muscles of the hand are divided into three groups: the thenar, hypothenar, and metacarpal muscles (see p. 314).

The thenar muscles are responsible for movement of the thumb, while the hypothenar muscles move the 5th digit.

Table 21.3   **Thenar muscles**

Muscle	Origin	Insertion		Innervation		Action
① Adductor pollicis	Transverse head: 3rd metacarpal (palmar surface)	Thumb (base of proximal phalanx)	Via the ulnar sesamoid	Ulnar n.	C8, T1	CMC joint of thumb: adduction MCP joint of thumb: flexion
	Oblique head: capitate bone, 2nd and 3rd metacarpals (bases)					
② Abductor pollicis brevis	Scaphoid bone and trapezium, flexor retinaculum		Via the radial sesamoid	Median n.		CMC joint of thumb: abduction
③ Flexor pollicis brevis	Superficial head: flexor retinaculum			Superficial head: median n.		CMC joint of thumb: flexion
	Deep head: capitate bone, trapezium			Deep head: ulnar n.		
④ Opponens pollicis	Trapezium	First metacarpal (radial border)		Median n.		CMC joint of thumb: opposition

CMC = carpometacarpal; MCP = metacarpophalangeal.

Fig. 21.19 Thenar and hypothenar muscles

Right hand, palmar (anterior) view.

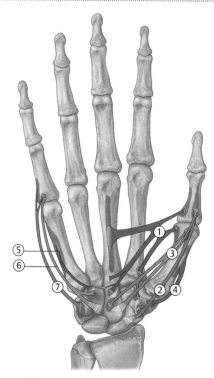

Table 21.4   **Hypothenar muscles**

Muscle	Origin	Insertion	Innervation	Action
⑤ Opponens digiti minimi	Hook of hamate, flexor retinaculum	5th metacarpal (ulnar border)	Ulnar n. (C8, T1)	Draws metacarpal in palmar direction (opposition)
⑥ Flexor digiti minimi		5th proximal phalanx (base)		MCP joint of little finger: flexion
⑦ Abductor digiti minimi	Pisiform bone	5th proximal phalanx (ulnar base) and dorsal digital expansion of 5th digit		MCP joint of little finger: flexion and abduction of little finger PIP and DIP joints of little finger: extension
Palmaris brevis	Palmar aponeurosis (ulnar border)	Skin of hypothenar eminence		Tightens the palmar aponeurosis (protective function)

DIP = distal interphalangeal; MCP = metacarpophalangeal; PIP = proximal interphalangeal.

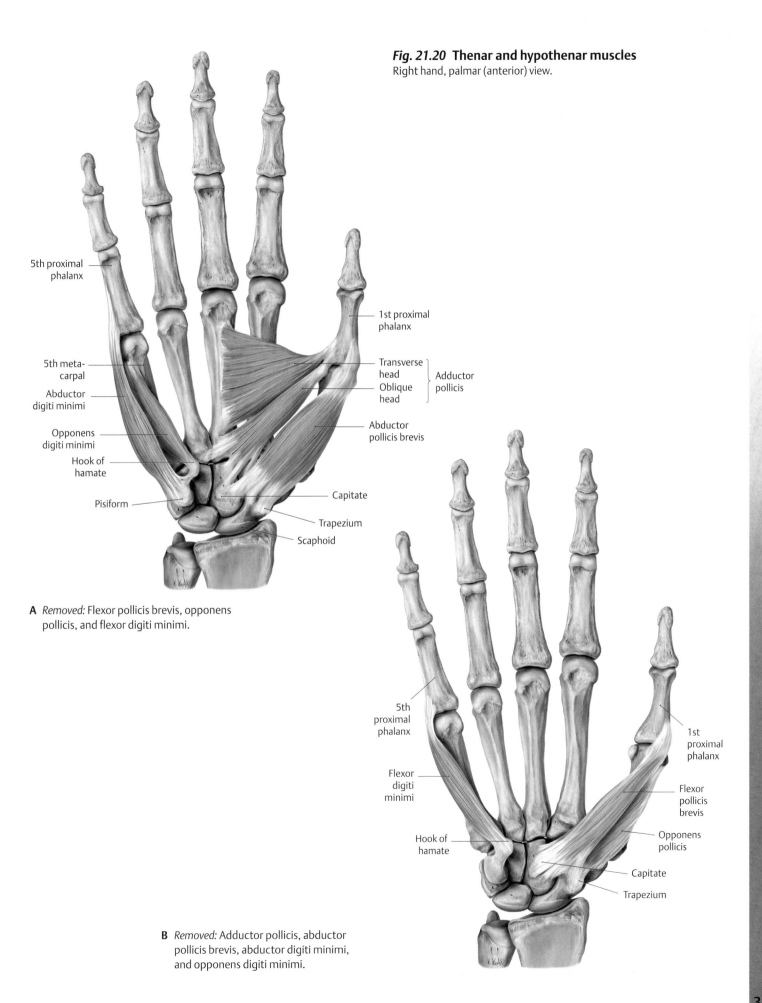

Fig. 21.20 **Thenar and hypothenar muscles**
Right hand, palmar (anterior) view.

5th proximal phalanx

5th meta-carpal

Abductor digiti minimi

Opponens digiti minimi

Hook of hamate

Pisiform

1st proximal phalanx

Transverse head
Oblique head
} Adductor pollicis

Abductor pollicis brevis

Capitate

Trapezium

Scaphoid

A *Removed:* Flexor pollicis brevis, opponens pollicis, and flexor digiti minimi.

5th proximal phalanx

Flexor digiti minimi

Hook of hamate

1st proximal phalanx

Flexor pollicis brevis

Opponens pollicis

Capitate

Trapezium

B *Removed:* Adductor pollicis, abductor pollicis brevis, abductor digiti minimi, and opponens digiti minimi.

313

Muscle Facts (II)

 The metacarpal muscles of the hand consist of the lumbricals and interossei. They are responsible for the movement of the digits (with the hypothenars, which act on the 5th digit).

Fig. 21.21 **Lumbricals**
Right hand, palmar view.

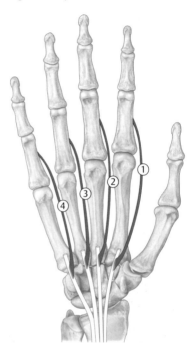

Fig. 21.22 **Dorsal interossei**
Right hand, palmar view.

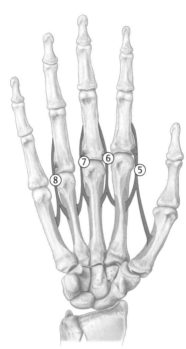

Fig. 21.23 **Palmar interossei**
Right hand, palmar view.

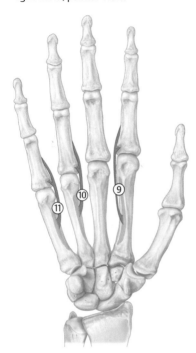

Table 21.5		Metacarpal muscles			
Muscle group	**Muscle**	**Origin**	**Insertion**	**Innervation**	**Action**
Lumbricals	① 1st	Tendons of flexor digitorum profundus (radial sides)	2nd digit (dde)	Median n. (C8, T1)	2nd to 5th digits: • MCP joints: flexion • Proximal and distal IP joints: extension
	② 2nd		3rd digit (dde)		
	③ 3rd	Tendons of flexor digitorum profundus (bipennate from medial and lateral sides)	4th digit (dde)		
	④ 4th		5th digit (dde)		
Dorsal interossei	⑤ 1st	1st and 2nd metacarpals (adjacent sides, two heads)	2nd digit (dde) 2nd proximal phalanx (radial side)	Ulnar n. (C8, T1)	2nd to 4th digits: • MCP joints: flexion • Proximal and distal IP joints: extension and abduction from 3rd digit
	⑥ 2nd	2nd and 3rd metacarpals (adjacent sides, two heads)	3rd digit (dde) 3rd proximal phalanx (radial side)		
	⑦ 3rd	3rd and 4th metacarpals (adjacent sides, two heads)	3rd digit (dde) 3rd proximal phalanx (ulnar side)		
	⑧ 4th	4th and 5th metacarpals (adjacent sides, two heads)	4th digit (dde) 4th proximal phalanx (ulnar side)		
Palmar interossei	⑨ 1st	2nd metacarpal (ulnar side)	2nd digit (dde) 2nd proximal phalanx (base)		2nd, 4th, and 5th digits: • MCP joints: flexion • Proximal and distal IP joints: extension and adduction toward 3rd digit
	⑩ 2nd	4th metacarpal (radial side)	4th digit (dde) 4th proximal phalanx (base)		
	⑪ 3rd	5th metacarpal (radial side)	5th digit (dde) 5th proximal phalanx (base)		

dde = dorsal digital expansion; IP = interphalangeal; MCP = metacarpophalangeal.

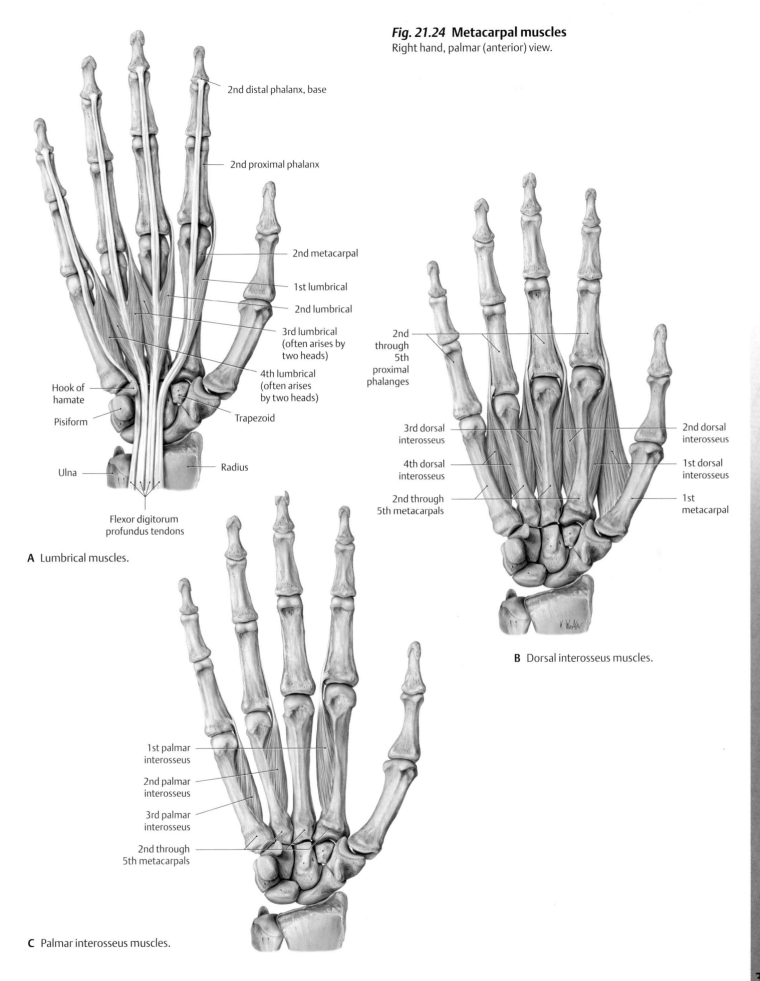

Fig. 21.24 Metacarpal muscles
Right hand, palmar (anterior) view.

2nd distal phalanx, base

2nd proximal phalanx

2nd metacarpal

1st lumbrical

2nd lumbrical

3rd lumbrical (often arises by two heads)

4th lumbrical (often arises by two heads)

Trapezoid

Hook of hamate

Pisiform

Ulna

Radius

Flexor digitorum profundus tendons

A Lumbrical muscles.

2nd through 5th proximal phalanges

3rd dorsal interosseus

4th dorsal interosseus

2nd through 5th metacarpals

2nd dorsal interosseus

1st dorsal interosseus

1st metacarpal

B Dorsal interosseus muscles.

1st palmar interosseus

2nd palmar interosseus

3rd palmar interosseus

2nd through 5th metacarpals

C Palmar interosseus muscles.

315

Arteries of the Upper Limb

Fig. 22.1 Arteries of the upper limb
Right limb, anterior view.

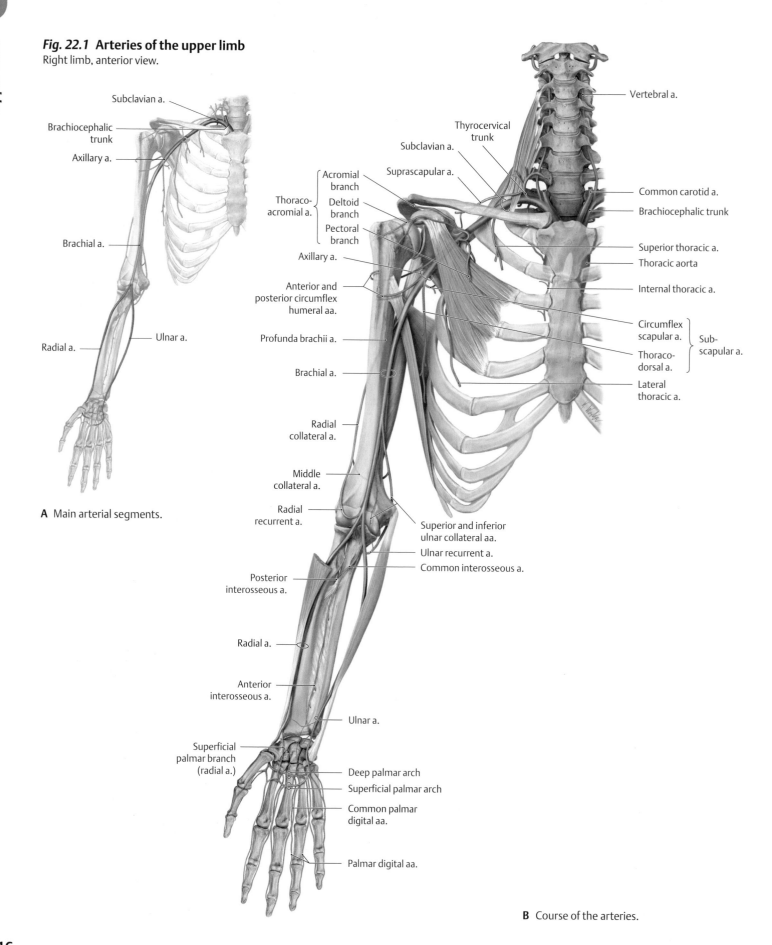

A Main arterial segments.

Subclavian a.

Brachiocephalic trunk

Axillary a.

Brachial a.

Radial a.

Ulnar a.

Thyrocervical trunk

Subclavian a.

Suprascapular a.

Acromial branch

Deltoid branch

Pectoral branch

Thoraco-acromial a.

Axillary a.

Anterior and posterior circumflex humeral aa.

Profunda brachii a.

Brachial a.

Radial collateral a.

Middle collateral a.

Radial recurrent a.

Posterior interosseous a.

Radial a.

Anterior interosseous a.

Ulnar a.

Superficial palmar branch (radial a.)

Vertebral a.

Common carotid a.

Brachiocephalic trunk

Superior thoracic a.

Thoracic aorta

Internal thoracic a.

Circumflex scapular a.

Thoraco-dorsal a.

Lateral thoracic a.

Sub-scapular a.

Superior and inferior ulnar collateral aa.

Ulnar recurrent a.

Common interosseous a.

Deep palmar arch

Superficial palmar arch

Common palmar digital aa.

Palmar digital aa.

B Course of the arteries.

316

22 Neurovasculature

Fig. 22.2 Branches of the subclavian artery

Right side, anterior view.

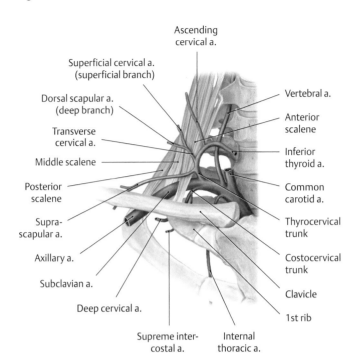

- Ascending cervical a.
- Superficial cervical a. (superficial branch)
- Dorsal scapular a. (deep branch)
- Transverse cervical a.
- Middle scalene
- Posterior scalene
- Supra-scapular a.
- Axillary a.
- Subclavian a.
- Deep cervical a.
- Supreme inter-costal a.
- Internal thoracic a.
- Vertebral a.
- Anterior scalene
- Inferior thyroid a.
- Common carotid a.
- Thyrocervical trunk
- Costocervical trunk
- Clavicle
- 1st rib

Fig. 22.3 Scapular arcade

Right side, posterior view.

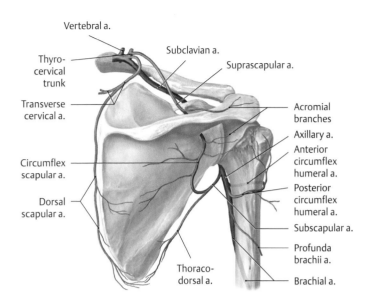

- Vertebral a.
- Thyro-cervical trunk
- Transverse cervical a.
- Circumflex scapular a.
- Dorsal scapular a.
- Thoraco-dorsal a.
- Subclavian a.
- Suprascapular a.
- Acromial branches
- Axillary a.
- Anterior circumflex humeral a.
- Posterior circumflex humeral a.
- Subscapular a.
- Profunda brachii a.
- Brachial a.

Fig. 22.4 Arteries of the forearm and hand

Right limb. The ulnar and radial arteries are interconnected by the superficial and deep palmar arches, the perforating branches, and the dorsal carpal network.

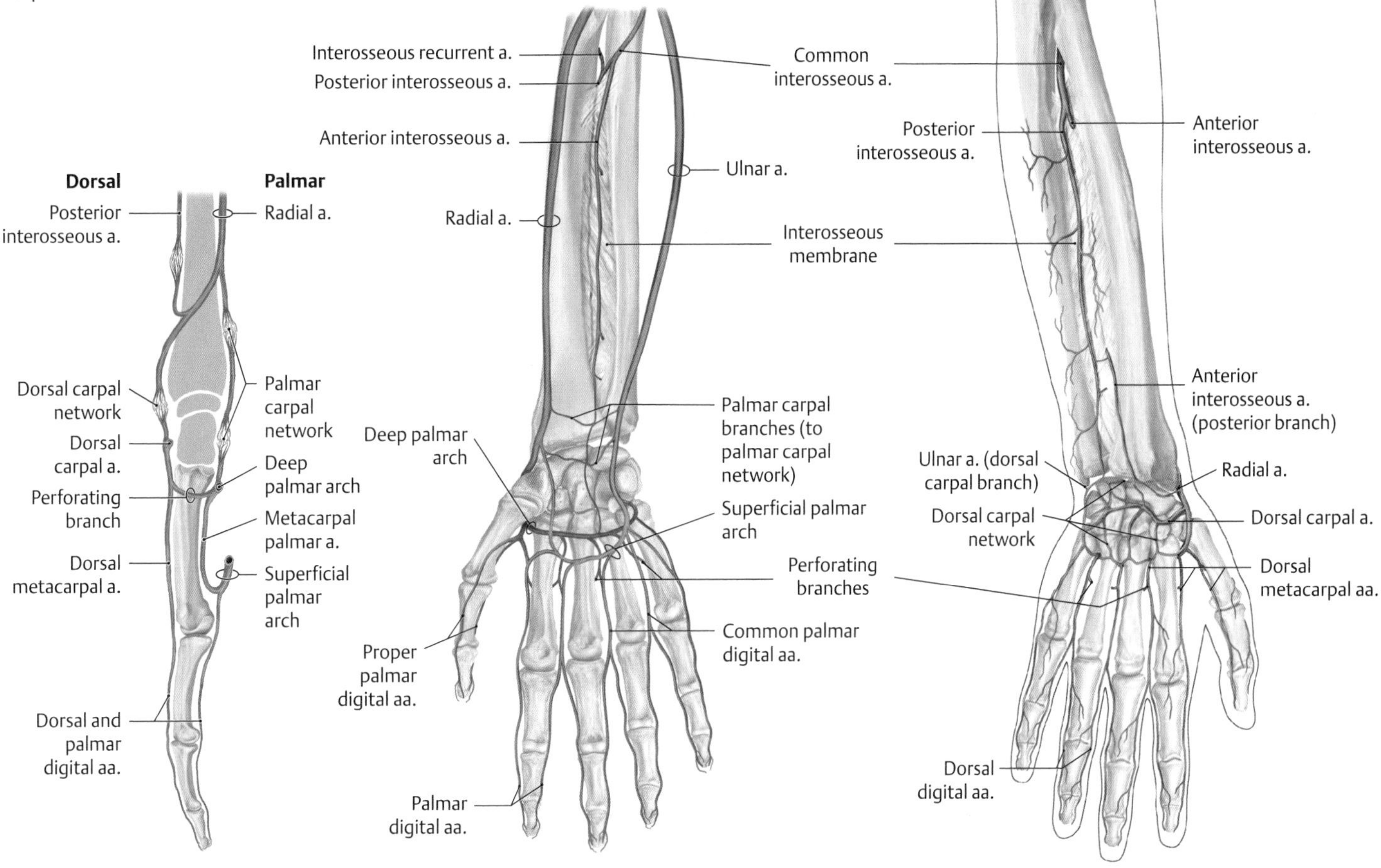

- Interosseous recurrent a.
- Posterior interosseous a.
- Anterior interosseous a.
- Common interosseous a.
- Posterior interosseous a.
- Anterior interosseous a.
- Ulnar a.
- Radial a.
- Interosseous membrane
- Anterior interosseous a. (posterior branch)

Dorsal / **Palmar**

- Posterior interosseous a.
- Radial a.
- Dorsal carpal network
- Dorsal carpal a.
- Perforating branch
- Dorsal metacarpal a.
- Dorsal and palmar digital aa.
- Palmar carpal network
- Deep palmar arch
- Metacarpal palmar a.
- Superficial palmar arch
- Deep palmar arch
- Proper palmar digital aa.
- Palmar digital aa.
- Palmar carpal branches (to palmar carpal network)
- Superficial palmar arch
- Perforating branches
- Common palmar digital aa.
- Ulnar a. (dorsal carpal branch)
- Dorsal carpal network
- Radial a.
- Dorsal carpal a.
- Dorsal metacarpal aa.
- Dorsal digital aa.

A Right middle finger, lateral view.   **B** Anterior (palmar) view.   **C** Posterior (dorsal) view.

317

Veins & Lymphatics of the Upper Limb

Fig. 22.5 Veins of the upper limb
Right limb, anterior view.

Deltopectoral groove
Cephalic v.
Basilic hiatus
Basilic v.
Median cubital v.
Median antebrachial v.
Cephalic v.
Median basilic v.
Perforator vv.
Superficial palmar venous arch
Intercapitular vv.

A Superficial veins.

Subclavian v.
Axillary v.
Thoraco-epigastric v.
Thoraco-dorsal v.
Brachial vv.
Anterior interosseous vv.
Radial vv.
Ulnar vv.
Deep palmar venous arch
Palmar metacarpal vv.
Palmar digital vv.

B Deep veins.

Fig. 22.6 Veins of the dorsum
Right hand, posterior view.

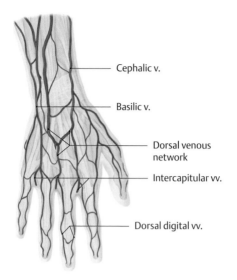

Cephalic v.
Basilic v.
Dorsal venous network
Intercapitular vv.
Dorsal digital vv.

✴ Clinical

Venipuncture
The veins of the cubital fossa are frequently used when drawing blood. In preparation, a tourniquet is applied. This allows arterial blood to flow, but blocks the return of venous blood. The resulting swelling makes the veins more visible and palpable.

Fig. 22.7 Cubital fossa
Right limb, anterior view. The subcutaneous veins of the cubital fossa have a highly variable course.

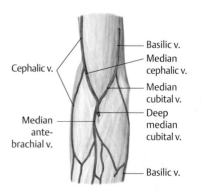

Cephalic v.
Basilic v.
Median cephalic v.
Median cubital v.
Deep median cubital v.
Median antebrachial v.
Basilic v.

A M-shaped.

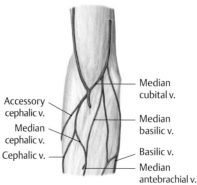

Accessory cephalic v.
Median cephalic v.
Cephalic v.
Median cubital v.
Median basilic v.
Basilic v.
Median antebrachial v.

B Accessory cephalic vein.

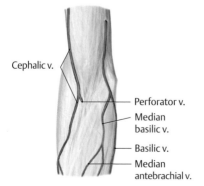

Cephalic v.
Perforator v.
Median basilic v.
Basilic v.
Median antebrachial v.

C Absent median cubital vein.

Lymph from the upper limb and breast drains to the axillary lymph nodes. The superficial lymphatics of the upper limb lie in the subcutaneous tissue, while the deep lymphatics accompany the arteries and deep veins. Numerous anastomoses exist between the two systems.

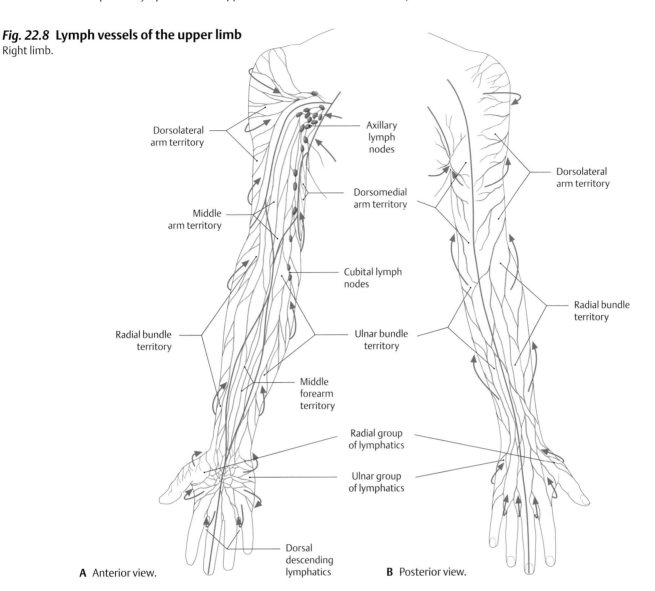

Fig. 22.8 Lymph vessels of the upper limb
Right limb.

Dorsolateral arm territory

Axillary lymph nodes

Dorsomedial arm territory

Middle arm territory

Cubital lymph nodes

Radial bundle territory

Ulnar bundle territory

Middle forearm territory

Radial group of lymphatics

Ulnar group of lymphatics

Dorsal descending lymphatics

Dorsolateral arm territory

Radial bundle territory

A Anterior view.

B Posterior view.

Fig. 22.9 Lymphatic drainage of the hand
Right hand, radial view. Most of the hand drains to the axillary nodes via cubital nodes. However, the thumb, index finger, and dorsum of the hand drain directly.

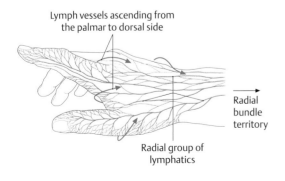

Lymph vessels ascending from the palmar to dorsal side

Radial bundle territory

Radial group of lymphatics

Fig. 22.10 Axillary lymph nodes
Right side, anterior view. The axillary lymph nodes are divided into three levels with respect to the pectoralis minor. They have major clinical importance in breast cancer (see p. 65).

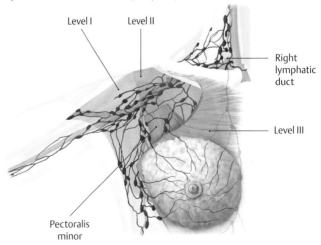

Level I

Level II

Right lymphatic duct

Level III

Pectoralis minor

Nerves of the Brachial Plexus

 Almost all muscles in the upper limb are innervated by the brachial plexus, which arises from spinal cord segments C5 to T1. The anterior rami of the spinal nerves give off direct branches (supraclavicular part of the brachial plexus) and merge to form three trunks, six divisions (three anterior and three posterior), and three cords. The infraclavicular part of the brachial plexus consists of short branches that arise directly from the cords and long (terminal) branches that traverse the limb.

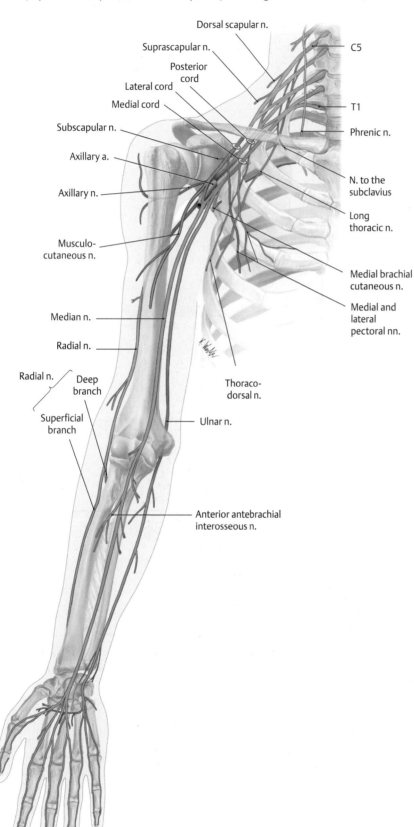

Table 22.1	Nerves of the brachial plexus		
Supraclavicular part			
Direct branches from the anterior rami or plexus trunks			
●	Dorsal scapular n.		C4–C5
	Suprascapular n.		C4–C6
	N. to the subclavius		C5–C6
	Long thoracic n.		C5–C7
Infraclavicular part			
Short and long branches from the plexus cords			
● **Lateral cord**	Lateral pectoral n.		C5–C7
	Musculocutaneous n.		
●	Median n.	Lateral root	C6–C7
		Medial root	
	Medial pectoral n.		C8–T1
● **Medial cord**	Median antebrachial cutaneous n.		
	Medial brachial cutaneous n.		T1
	Ulnar n.		C7–T1
● **Posterior cord**	Upper subscapular n.		C5–C6
	Thoracodorsal n.		C6–C8
	Lower subscapular n.		C5–C6
	Axillary n.		
	Radial n.		C5–T1

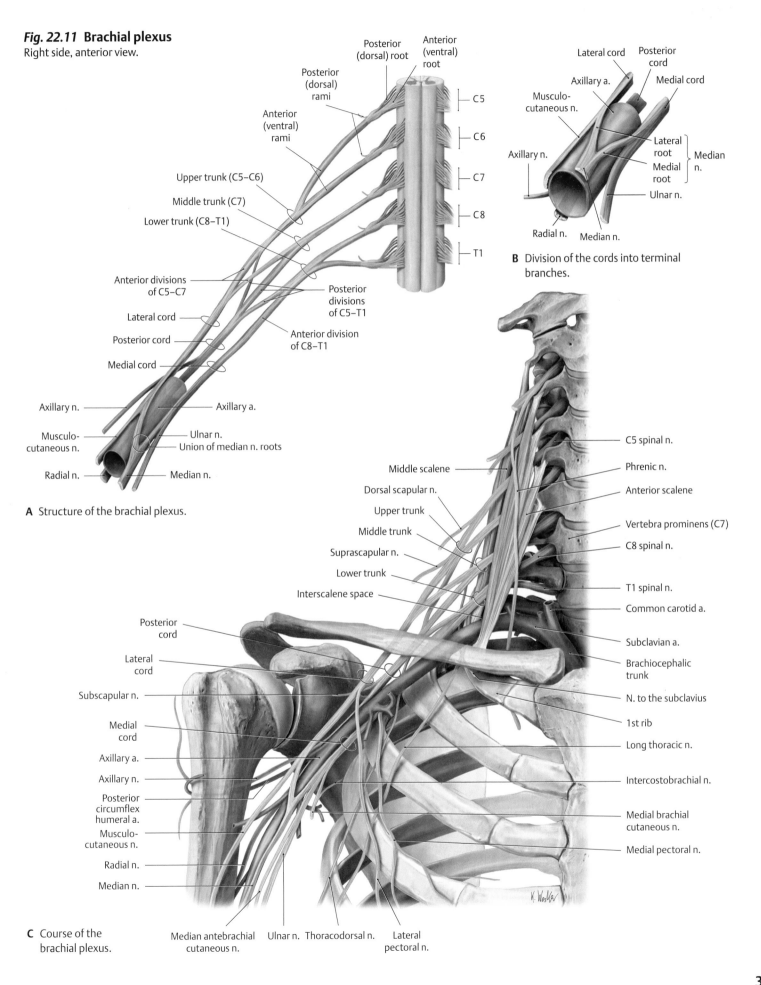

Fig. 22.11 Brachial plexus
Right side, anterior view.

A Structure of the brachial plexus.

Posterior (dorsal) root
Anterior (ventral) root
Posterior (dorsal) rami
Anterior (ventral) rami
C5
C6
C7
C8
T1
Upper trunk (C5–C6)
Middle trunk (C7)
Lower trunk (C8–T1)
Anterior divisions of C5–C7
Posterior divisions of C5–T1
Lateral cord
Posterior cord
Medial cord
Anterior division of C8–T1
Axillary n.
Axillary a.
Musculo-cutaneous n.
Ulnar n.
Union of median n. roots
Radial n.
Median n.

B Division of the cords into terminal branches.

Lateral cord
Posterior cord
Axillary a.
Medial cord
Musculo-cutaneous n.
Axillary n.
Lateral root
Medial root
Median n.
Ulnar n.
Radial n.
Median n.

C Course of the brachial plexus.

Middle scalene
Dorsal scapular n.
Upper trunk
Middle trunk
Suprascapular n.
Lower trunk
Interscalene space
Posterior cord
Lateral cord
Subscapular n.
Medial cord
Axillary a.
Axillary n.
Posterior circumflex humeral a.
Musculo-cutaneous n.
Radial n.
Median n.
Median antebrachial cutaneous n.
Ulnar n.
Thoracodorsal n.
Lateral pectoral n.
C5 spinal n.
Phrenic n.
Anterior scalene
Vertebra prominens (C7)
C8 spinal n.
T1 spinal n.
Common carotid a.
Subclavian a.
Brachiocephalic trunk
N. to the subclavius
1st rib
Long thoracic n.
Intercostobrachial n.
Medial brachial cutaneous n.
Medial pectoral n.

Supraclavicular Branches & Posterior Cord

Fig. 22.12 **Supraclavicular branches**
Right shoulder.

 The supraclavicular branches of the brachial plexus arise directly from the plexus roots (anterior rami of the spinal nerves) or from the plexus trunks in the lateral cervical triangle.

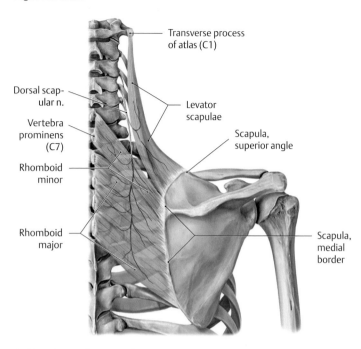

Transverse process of atlas (C1)

Dorsal scapular n.

Levator scapulae

Vertebra prominens (C7)

Scapula, superior angle

Rhomboid minor

Rhomboid major

Scapula, medial border

A Dorsal scapular nerve. Posterior view.

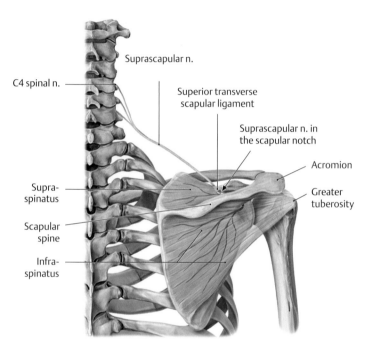

Suprascapular n.

C4 spinal n.

Superior transverse scapular ligament

Suprascapular n. in the scapular notch

Acromion

Supra-spinatus

Greater tuberosity

Scapular spine

Infra-spinatus

B Suprascapular nerve. Posterior view.

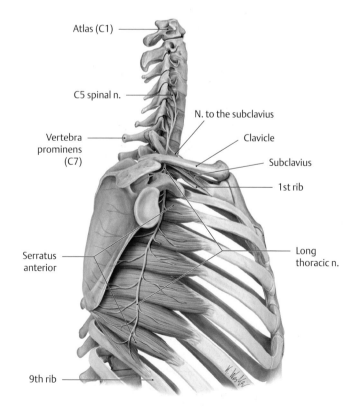

Atlas (C1)

C5 spinal n.

N. to the subclavius

Clavicle

Vertebra prominens (C7)

Subclavius

1st rib

Serratus anterior

Long thoracic n.

9th rib

C Long thoracic nerve and nerve to the sub-clavius. Right lateral view.

Table 22.2	**Supraclavicular branches**	
Nerve	**Level**	**Innervated muscle**
Dorsal scapular n.	C4–C5	Levator scapulae Rhomboids major and minor
Suprascapular n.	C4–C6	Supraspinatus Infraspinatus
Nerve to the subclavius	C5–C6	Subclavius Intercostobrachial nn.
Long thoracic n.	C5–C7	Serratus anterior

Fig. 22.13 Posterior cord: Short branches

Right shoulder.

 The posterior cord gives off three short branches (arising at the level of the plexus cords) and two long branches (terminal nerves, see pp. 324–325).

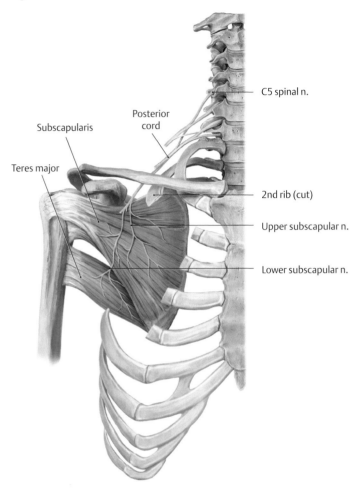

A Subscapular nerves. Anterior view.

Table 22.3	Branches of the posterior cord	
Nerve	**Level**	**Innervated muscle**
Short branches		
Upper subscapular n.	C5–C6	Subscapularis
Lower subscapular n.		Subscapularis Teres major
Thoracodorsal n.	C6–C8	Latissimus dorsi
Long (terminal) branches		
Axillary n.	C5–C6	See p. 324
Radial n.	C5–T1	See p. 325

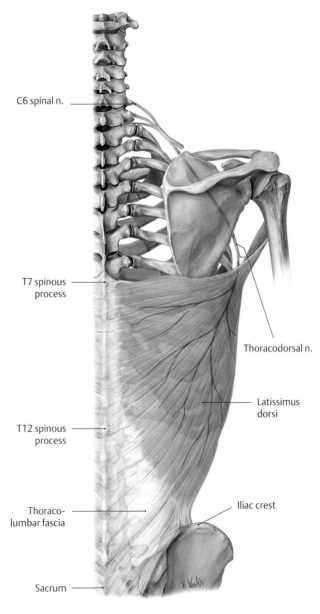

B Thoracodorsal nerve. Posterior view.

Posterior Cord: Axillary & Radial Nerves

Fig. 22.14 Axillary nerve: Sensory distribution
Right limb.

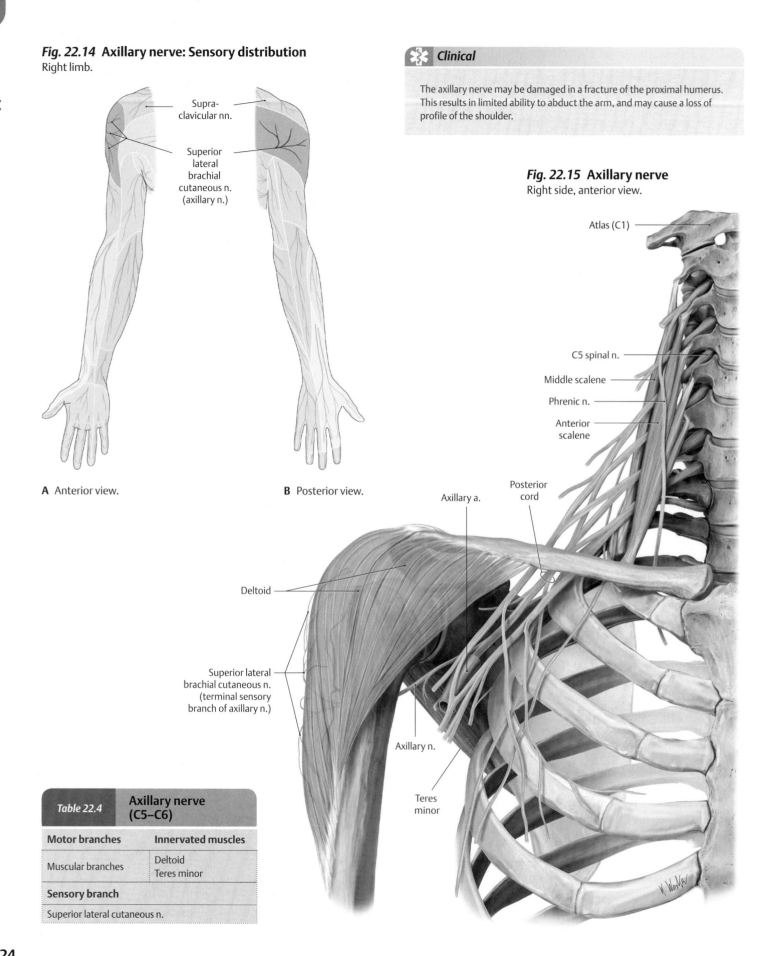

Supra-clavicular nn.

Superior lateral brachial cutaneous n. (axillary n.)

A Anterior view.

B Posterior view.

Fig. 22.15 Axillary nerve
Right side, anterior view.

Atlas (C1)

C5 spinal n.

Middle scalene

Phrenic n.

Anterior scalene

Posterior cord

Axillary a.

Deltoid

Superior lateral brachial cutaneous n. (terminal sensory branch of axillary n.)

Axillary n.

Teres minor

Table 22.4	**Axillary nerve (C5–C6)**
Motor branches	**Innervated muscles**
Muscular branches	Deltoid Teres minor
Sensory branch	
Superior lateral cutaneous n.	

Fig. 22.16 Radial nerve: Sensory distribution

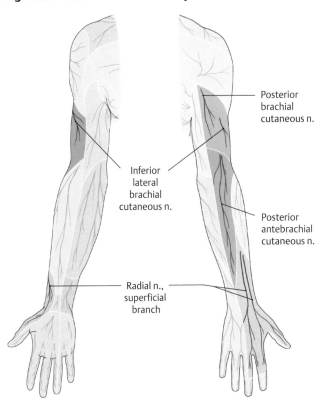

- Posterior brachial cutaneous n.
- Inferior lateral brachial cutaneous n.
- Posterior antebrachial cutaneous n.
- Radial n., superficial branch

A Anterior view. **B** Posterior view.

Fig. 22.17 Radial nerve

Right limb, anterior view with forearm pronated.

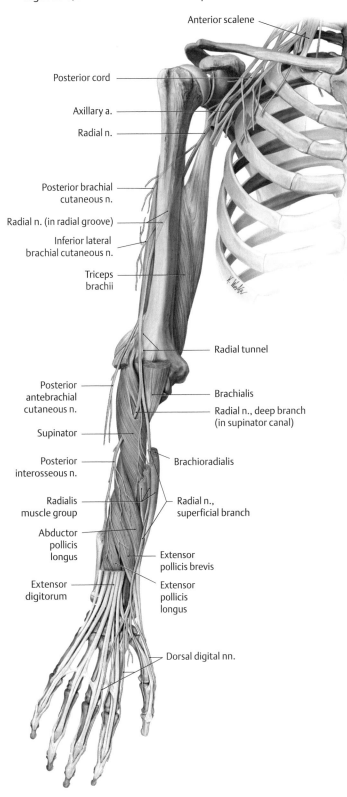

- Anterior scalene
- Posterior cord
- Axillary a.
- Radial n.
- Posterior brachial cutaneous n.
- Radial n. (in radial groove)
- Inferior lateral brachial cutaneous n.
- Triceps brachii
- Radial tunnel
- Posterior antebrachial cutaneous n.
- Brachialis
- Radial n., deep branch (in supinator canal)
- Supinator
- Posterior interosseous n.
- Brachioradialis
- Radialis muscle group
- Radial n., superficial branch
- Abductor pollicis longus
- Extensor pollicis brevis
- Extensor digitorum
- Extensor pollicis longus
- Dorsal digital nn.

Table 22.5	Radial nerve (C5–T1)
Motor branches	**Innervated muscles**
Muscular branches	Brachialis (partial)
	Triceps brachii
	Anconeus
	Brachioradialis
	Extensors carpi radialis longus and brevis
Deep branch (terminal branch: posterior interosseous n.)	Supinator
	Extensor digitorum
	Extensor digiti minimi
	Extensor carpi ulnaris
	Extensors pollicis brevis and longus
	Extensor indicis
	Abductor pollicis longus
Sensory branches	
Articular branches from radial n.: Capsule of the shoulder joint	
Articular branches from posterior interosseous n.: Joint capsule of the wrist and four radial metacarpophalangeal joints	
Posterior brachial cutaneous n.	
Inferior lateral brachial cutaneous n.	
Posterior antebrachial cutaneous n.	
Superficial branches	Dorsal digital nn.
	Ulnar communicating branch

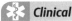 **Clinical**

Chronic radial nerve compression in the axilla (e.g., due to extended/improper crutch use) may cause loss of sensation or motor function in the hand, forearm, and posterior arm. More distal injuries (e.g., during anesthesia) affect fewer muscles, potentially resulting in wrist drop with intact triceps brachii function.

Medial & Lateral Cords

👉 The medial and lateral cords give off four short branches. The intercostobrachial nerves are included with the short branches

of the brachial plexus, although they are actually the cutaneous branches of the 2nd and 3rd intercostal nerves.

Table 22.6	Branches of the medial and lateral cords		
Nerve	**Level**	**Cord**	**Innervated muscle**
Short branches			
Lateral pectoral n.	C5–C7	Lateral cord	Pectoralis major
Medial pectoral n.	C8–T1	Medial cord	Pectoralis major and minor
Medial brachial cutaneous n.	T1	Medial cord	— (sensory branches)
Medial antebrachial cutaneous n.	C8–T1	Medial cord	— (sensory branches)
Intercostobrachial nn.	T2–T3		
Long (terminal) branches			
Musculocutaneous n.	C5–C7	Lateral cord	Coracobrachialis, Biceps brachii, Brachialis
Median n.	C6–T1		See p. 328
Ulnar n.	C7–T1	Medial cord	See p. 329

Fig. 22.18 Medial and lateral cords: Short branches
Right side, anterior view.

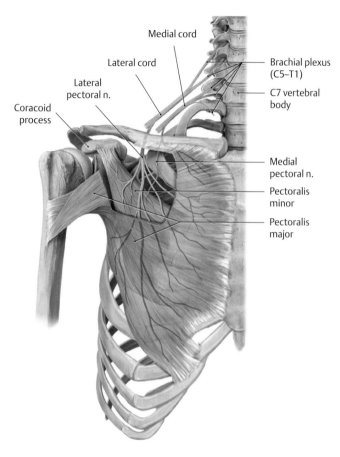

A Medial and lateral pectoral nerves.

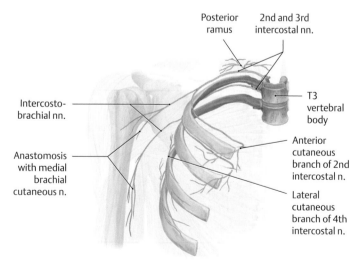

B Intercostobrachial nerves.

Fig. 22.19 Short branches: Sensory distribution

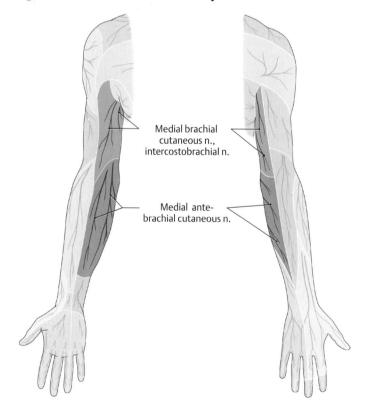

A Anterior view. **B** Posterior view.

Fig. 22.20 Musculocutaneous nerve

Right limb, anterior view.

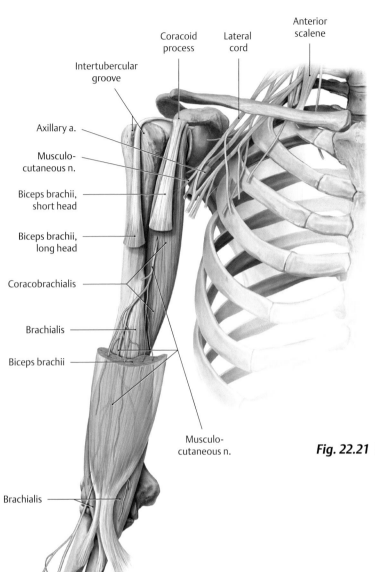

Anterior scalene

Coracoid process

Lateral cord

Intertubercular groove

Axillary a.

Musculocutaneous n.

Biceps brachii, short head

Biceps brachii, long head

Coracobrachialis

Brachialis

Biceps brachii

Musculocutaneous n.

Brachialis

Lateral antebrachial cutaneous n.

Ulna

Radius

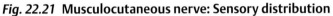

Table 22.7	Musculocutaneous nerve (C5–C7)	
Motor branches	**Innervated muscles**	
Muscular branches	Coracobrachialis	
	Biceps brachii	
	Brachialis	
Sensory branches		
Lateral antebrachial cutaneous n.		
Articular branches: Joint capsule of the elbow (anterior part)		
Note: Musculocutaneous nerve innervation of the arm is purely motor; innervation of the forearm is purely sensory.		

Fig. 22.21 Musculocutaneous nerve: Sensory distribution

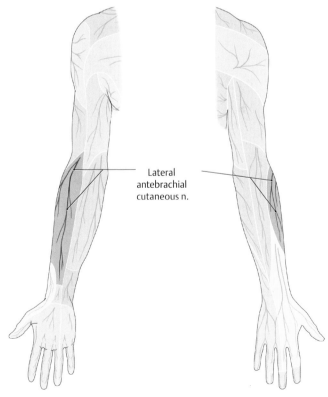

Lateral antebrachial cutaneous n.

A Anterior view.

B Posterior view.

Median & Ulnar Nerves

 The median nerve is a terminal branch arising from both the medial and lateral cords. The ulnar nerve arises exclusively from the medial cord.

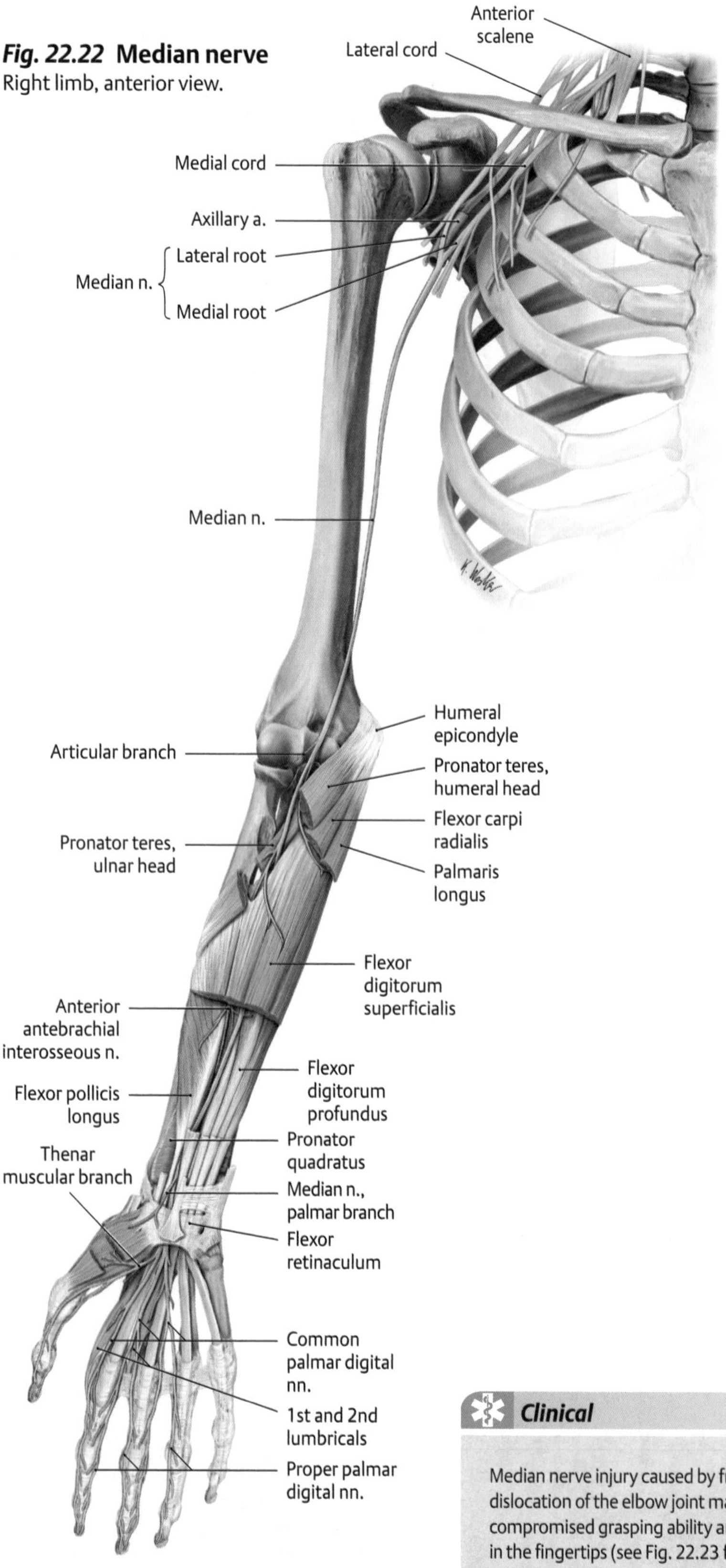

Fig. 22.22 **Median nerve**
Right limb, anterior view.

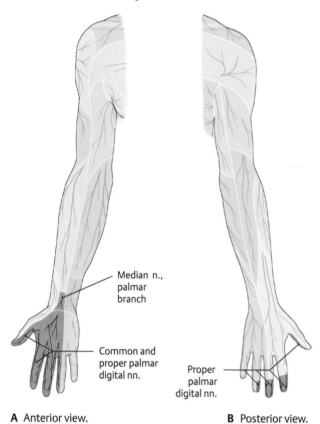

Fig. 22.23 **Median nerve: Sensory distribution**

A Anterior view.

B Posterior view.

Table 22.8	**Median nerve (C6–T1)**
Motor branches	**Innervated muscles**
Direct muscular branches	Pronator teres
	Flexor carpi radialis
	Palmaris longus
	Flexor digitorum superficialis
Muscular branches from anterior antebrachial interosseous n.	Pronator quadratus
	Flexor pollicis longus
	Flexor digitorum profundus (radial half)
Thenar muscular branch	Abductor pollicis brevis
	Flexor pollicis brevis (superficial head)
	Opponens pollicis
Muscular branches from common palmar digital nn.	1st and 2nd lumbricals
Sensory branches	
Articular branches: Capsules of the elbow and wrist joints	
Palmar branch of median n. (thenar eminence)	
Communicating branch to ulnar n.	
Common palmar digital nn.	

✚ **Clinical**

Median nerve injury caused by fracture/dislocation of the elbow joint may result in compromised grasping ability and sensory loss in the fingertips (see Fig. 22.23 for territories). See also carpal tunnel syndrome (p. 343).

Fig. 22.24 Ulnar nerve: Sensory distribution

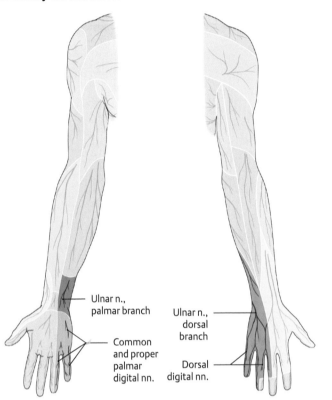

A Anterior view.

B Posterior view.

Ulnar n., palmar branch

Common and proper palmar digital nn.

Ulnar n., dorsal branch

Dorsal digital nn.

Fig. 22.25 Ulnar nerve
Right limb, anterior view.

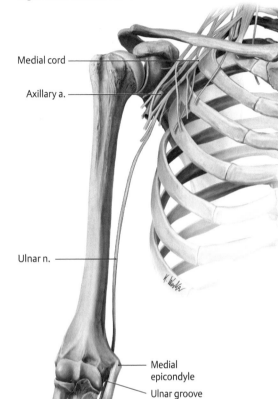
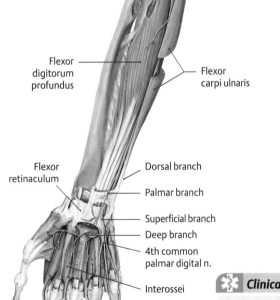

Medial cord

Axillary a.

Ulnar n.

Medial epicondyle

Ulnar groove

Flexor digitorum profundus

Flexor carpi ulnaris

Flexor retinaculum

Dorsal branch

Palmar branch

Superficial branch

Deep branch

4th common palmar digital n.

Interossei

Proper palmar digital nn.

Table 22.9	Ulnar nerve (C7–T1)
Motor branches	**Innervated muscles**
Direct muscular branches	Flexor carpi ulnaris
	Flexor digitorum profundus (ulnar half)
Muscular branch from superior ulnar n.	Palmaris brevis
Muscular branches from deep ulnar n.	Abductor digiti minimi
	Flexor digiti minimi
	Opponens digiti minimi
	3rd and 4th lumbricals
	Palmar and dorsal interosseous muscles
	Adductor pollicis
	Flexor pollicis brevis (deep head)

Sensory branches

Articular branches: Capsules of the elbow, carpal, and metacarpophalangeal joints

Dorsal branch (terminal branches: dorsal digital nn.)

Palmar branch

Proper palmar digital n. (from superficial branch)

Common palmar digital n. (from superficial branch; terminal branches: proper palmar digital nn.)

✚ Clinical

Ulnar nerve palsy is the most common peripheral nerve damage. The ulnar nerve is most vulnerable to trauma or chronic compression in the elbow joint and ulnar tunnel (see p. 343). Nerve damage causes "clawing" of the hand and atrophy of the interossei. Sensory losses are often limited to the 5th digit.

Superficial Veins & Nerves of the Upper Limb

Fig. 22.26 Cutaneous innervation of the upper limb: Anterior view

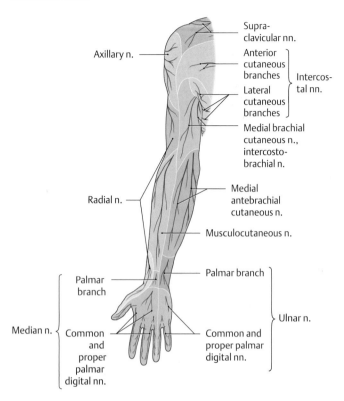

- Supra-clavicular nn.
- Axillary n.
- Anterior cutaneous branches
- Lateral cutaneous branches
- Intercostal nn.
- Medial brachial cutaneous n., intercosto-brachial n.
- Radial n.
- Medial antebrachial cutaneous n.
- Musculocutaneous n.
- Palmar branch
- Palmar branch
- Median n.
- Common and proper palmar digital nn.
- Common and proper palmar digital nn.
- Ulnar n.

A Peripheral sensory cutaneous innervation.

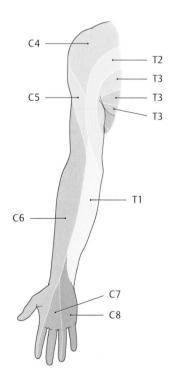

- C4
- T2
- T3
- C5
- T3
- T3
- T1
- C6
- C7
- C8

B Segmental, radicular cutaneous innervation (dermatomes).

Fig. 22.27 Superficial cutaneous veins and nerves of the upper limb

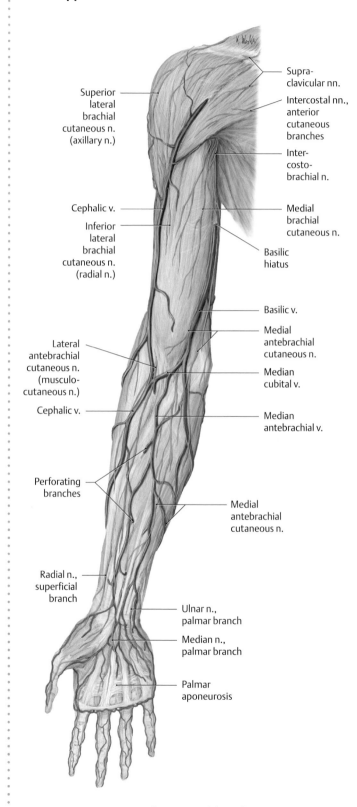

- Superior lateral brachial cutaneous n. (axillary n.)
- Supra-clavicular nn.
- Intercostal nn., anterior cutaneous branches
- Inter-costo-brachial n.
- Cephalic v.
- Inferior lateral brachial cutaneous n. (radial n.)
- Medial brachial cutaneous n.
- Basilic hiatus
- Lateral antebrachial cutaneous n. (musculo-cutaneous n.)
- Basilic v.
- Medial antebrachial cutaneous n.
- Median cubital v.
- Cephalic v.
- Median antebrachial v.
- Perforating branches
- Medial antebrachial cutaneous n.
- Radial n., superficial branch
- Ulnar n., palmar branch
- Median n., palmar branch
- Palmar aponeurosis

A Anterior view. See p. 344 for nerves of the palm.

Fig. 22.28 Cutaneous innervation of the upper limb: Posterior view

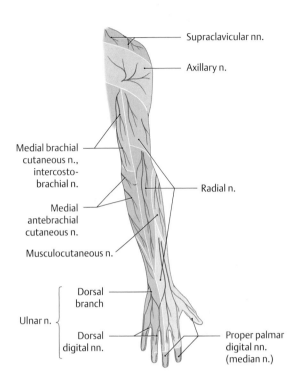

Supraclavicular nn.

Axillary n.

Medial brachial cutaneous n., intercosto-brachial n.

Radial n.

Medial antebrachial cutaneous n.

Musculocutaneous n.

Ulnar n. { Dorsal branch

Dorsal digital nn.

Proper palmar digital nn. (median n.)

A Peripheral sensory cutaneous innervation.

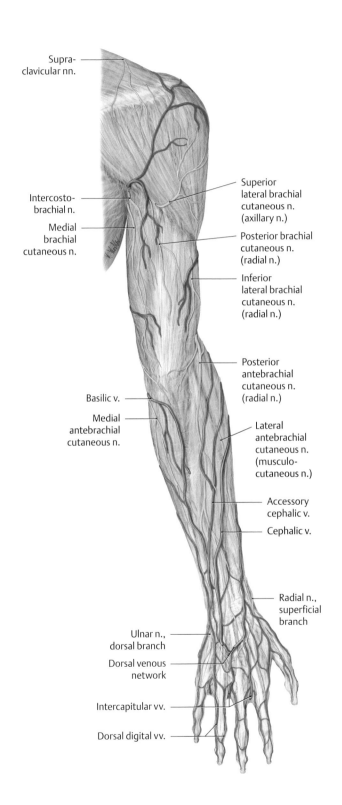

Supra-clavicular nn.

Intercosto-brachial n.

Medial brachial cutaneous n.

Superior lateral brachial cutaneous n. (axillary n.)

Posterior brachial cutaneous n. (radial n.)

Inferior lateral brachial cutaneous n. (radial n.)

Posterior antebrachial cutaneous n. (radial n.)

Basilic v.

Medial antebrachial cutaneous n.

Lateral antebrachial cutaneous n. (musculo-cutaneous n.)

Accessory cephalic v.

Cephalic v.

Radial n., superficial branch

Ulnar n., dorsal branch

Dorsal venous network

Intercapitular vv.

Dorsal digital vv.

B Posterior view. See p. 346 for nerves of the dorsum.

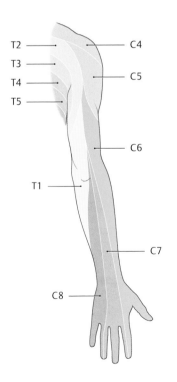

T2

T3

T4

T5

C4

C5

C6

T1

C7

C8

B Segmental, radicular cutaneous innervation (dermatomes).

Posterior Shoulder & Axilla

Fig. 22.29 Posterior shoulder
Right shoulder, posterior view. *Raised:* Trapezius (transverse part).
Windowed: Supraspinatus. *Revealed:* Suprascapular region.

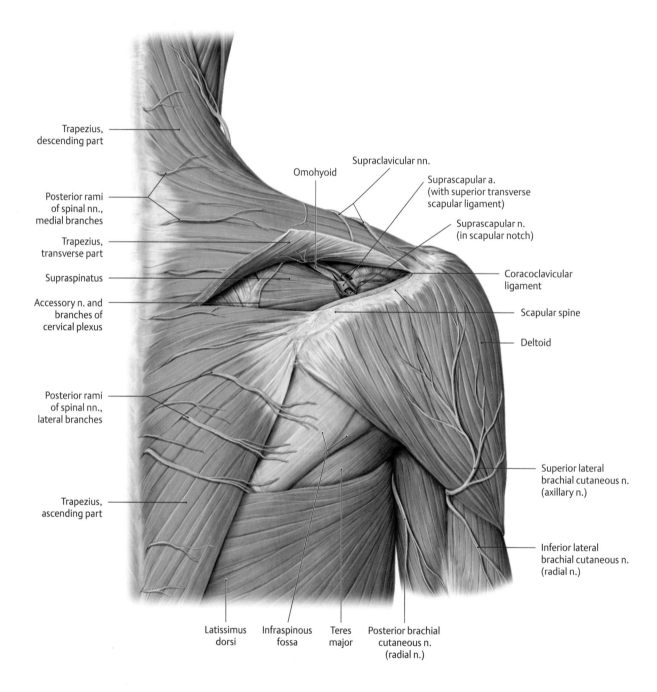

Trapezius, descending part

Posterior rami of spinal nn., medial branches

Trapezius, transverse part

Supraspinatus

Accessory n. and branches of cervical plexus

Posterior rami of spinal nn., lateral branches

Trapezius, ascending part

Omohyoid

Supraclavicular nn.

Suprascapular a. (with superior transverse scapular ligament)

Suprascapular n. (in scapular notch)

Coracoclavicular ligament

Scapular spine

Deltoid

Superior lateral brachial cutaneous n. (axillary n.)

Inferior lateral brachial cutaneous n. (radial n.)

Latissimus dorsi

Infraspinous fossa

Teres major

Posterior brachial cutaneous n. (radial n.)

Table 22.10 | **Neurovascular tracts of the scapula**

	Passageway	Boundaries	Transmitted structures
①	Scapular notch	Superior transverse scapular ligament, scapula	Suprascapular a. and n.
②	Medial border	Scapula	Dorsal scapular a. and n.
③	Triangular space	Teres major and minor	Circumflex scapular a.
④	Triceps hiatus	Triceps brachii, humerus, teres major	Profunda brachii a. and radial n.
⑤	Quadrangular space	Teres major and minor, triceps brachii, humerus	Posterior circumflex humeral a. and axillary n.

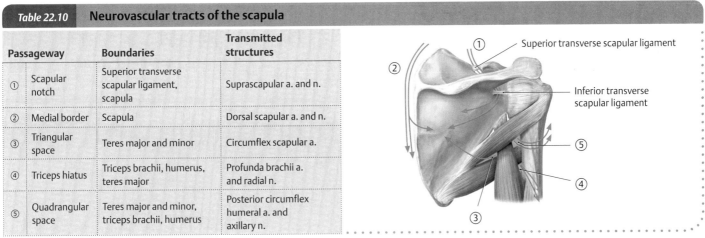

Fig. 22.30 **Axilla: Triangular and quadrangular spaces**
Right shoulder, posterior view.

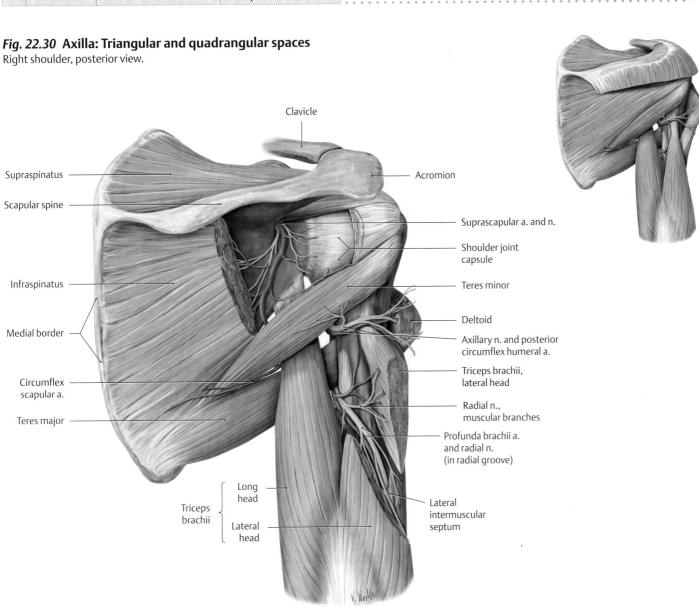

Anterior Shoulder

Fig. 22.31 **Anterior shoulder: Superficial dissection**
Right shoulder.

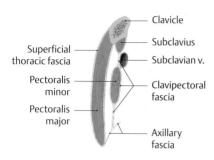

- Clavicle
- Subclavius
- Subclavian v.
- Superficial thoracic fascia
- Pectoralis minor
- Clavipectoral fascia
- Pectoralis major
- Axillary fascia

A Sagittal section through anterior wall.

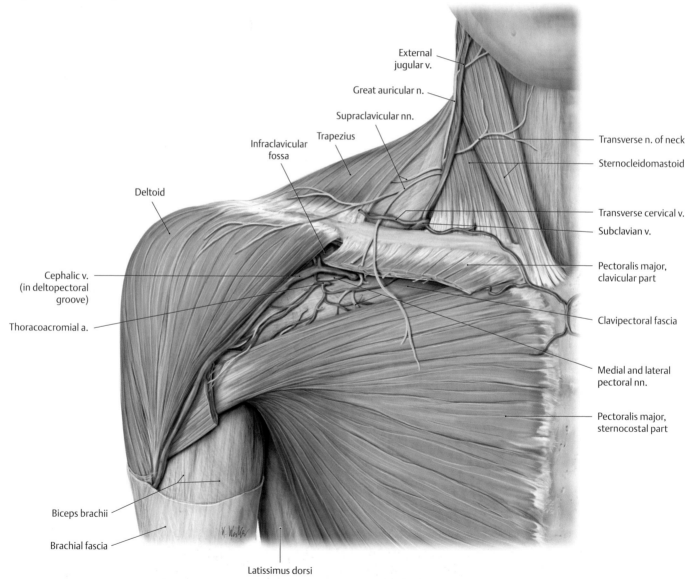

- External jugular v.
- Great auricular n.
- Supraclavicular nn.
- Infraclavicular fossa
- Trapezius
- Transverse n. of neck
- Sternocleidomastoid
- Deltoid
- Transverse cervical v.
- Subclavian v.
- Pectoralis major, clavicular part
- Cephalic v. (in deltopectoral groove)
- Thoracoacromial a.
- Clavipectoral fascia
- Medial and lateral pectoral nn.
- Pectoralis major, sternocostal part
- Biceps brachii
- Brachial fascia
- Latissimus dorsi

B Anterior view. *Removed:* Platysma, muscle fasciae, superficial layer of cervical fascia, and pectoralis major (clavicular part). *Revealed:* Clavipectoral triangle.

Fig. 22.32 Shoulder: Transverse section

Right shoulder, inferior view.

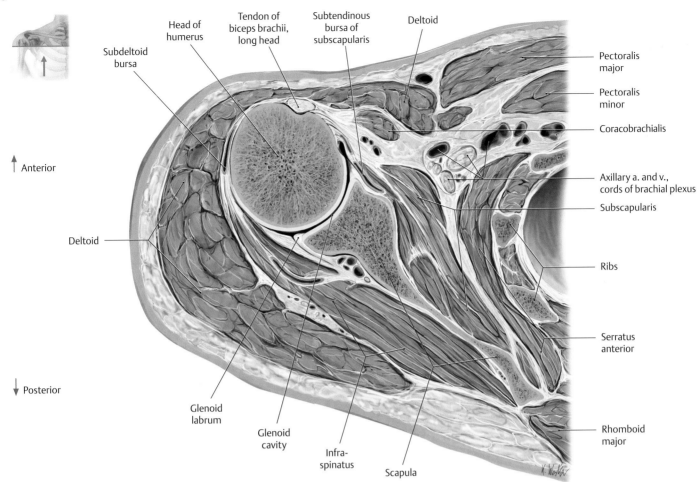

Labels on figure:
- Subdeltoid bursa
- Head of humerus
- Tendon of biceps brachii, long head
- Subtendinous bursa of subscapularis
- Deltoid
- Pectoralis major
- Pectoralis minor
- Coracobrachialis
- Axillary a. and v., cords of brachial plexus
- Subscapularis
- Ribs
- Anterior
- Deltoid
- Posterior
- Glenoid labrum
- Glenoid cavity
- Infra-spinatus
- Scapula
- Serratus anterior
- Rhomboid major

Fig. 22.33 Anterior shoulder: Deep dissection

Right limb, anterior view. *Removed:* Sternocleidomastoid, omohyoid, and pectoralis major. This dissection reveals the neurovascular contents of the lateral cervical triangle (see pp. 580–581) and axilla (see pp. 336–337).

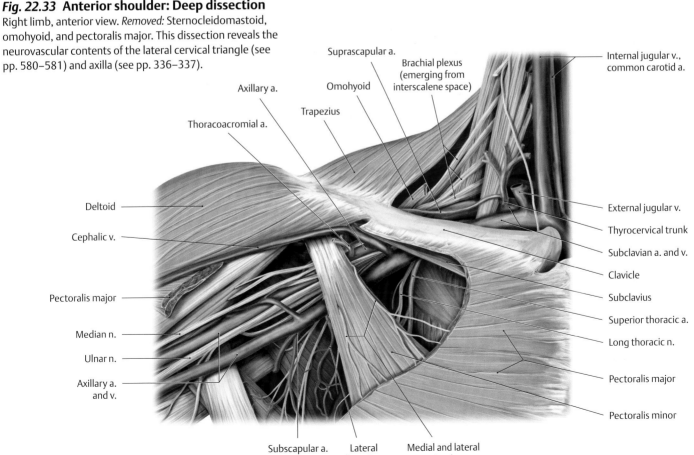

Labels on figure:
- Suprascapular a.
- Brachial plexus (emerging from interscalene space)
- Omohyoid
- Axillary a.
- Trapezius
- Thoracoacromial a.
- Internal jugular v., common carotid a.
- Deltoid
- Cephalic v.
- External jugular v.
- Thyrocervical trunk
- Subclavian a. and v.
- Clavicle
- Subclavius
- Pectoralis major
- Median n.
- Superior thoracic a.
- Long thoracic n.
- Ulnar n.
- Pectoralis major
- Axillary a. and v.
- Pectoralis minor
- Subscapular a.
- Lateral thoracic a.
- Medial and lateral pectoral nn.

335

Topography of the Axilla

Fig. 22.34 Dissection of the axilla
Right shoulder, anterior view.

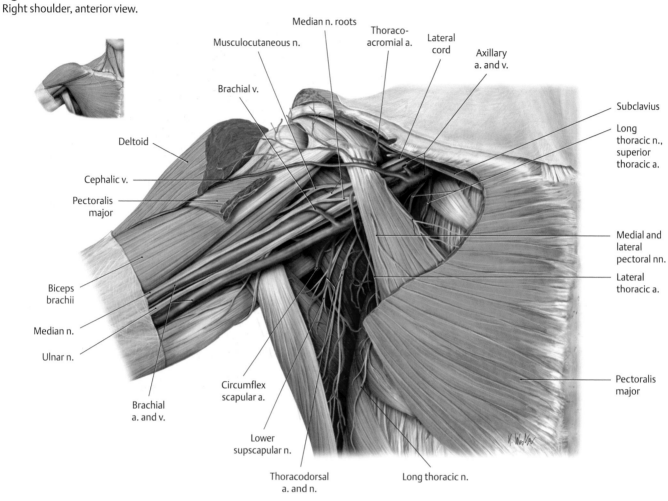

A *Removed:* Pectoralis major and clavipectoral fascia.

Table 22.11	Walls of the axilla
Anterior wall	Pectoralis major Pectoralis minor Clavipectoral fascia
Lateral wall	Intertubercular groove of humerus
Posterior wall	Subscapularis Teres major Latissimus dorsi
Medial wall	Lateral thoracic wall Serratus anterior

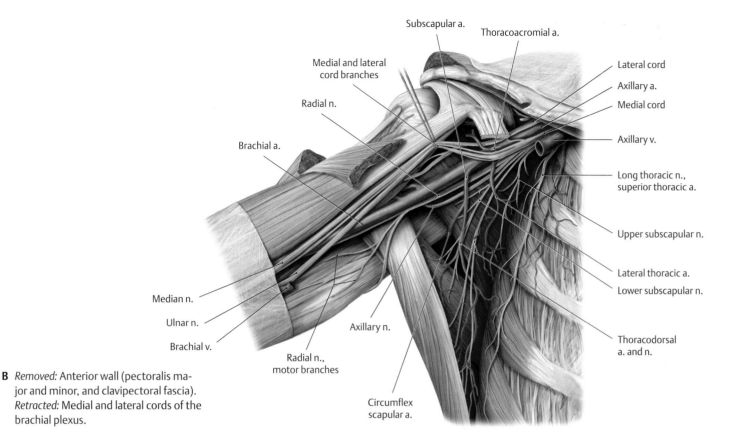

Subscapular a.
Thoracoacromial a.
Medial and lateral cord branches
Radial n.
Brachial a.
Lateral cord
Axillary a.
Medial cord
Axillary v.
Long thoracic n., superior thoracic a.
Upper subscapular n.
Lateral thoracic a.
Lower subscapular n.
Median n.
Ulnar n.
Brachial v.
Axillary n.
Thoracodorsal a. and n.
Radial n., motor branches
Circumflex scapular a.

B *Removed:* Anterior wall (pectoralis major and minor, and clavipectoral fascia). *Retracted:* Medial and lateral cords of the brachial plexus.

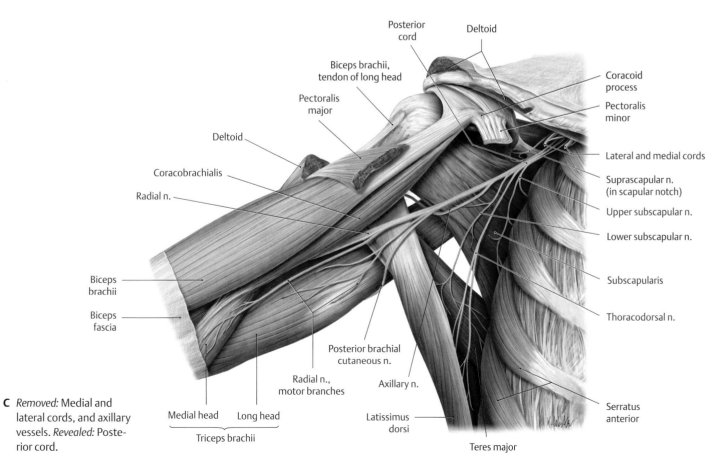

Posterior cord
Deltoid
Biceps brachii, tendon of long head
Pectoralis major
Coracoid process
Pectoralis minor
Deltoid
Coracobrachialis
Radial n.
Lateral and medial cords
Suprascapular n. (in scapular notch)
Upper subscapular n.
Lower subscapular n.
Biceps brachii
Biceps fascia
Subscapularis
Thoracodorsal n.
Posterior brachial cutaneous n.
Radial n., motor branches
Axillary n.
Medial head
Long head
Latissimus dorsi
Serratus anterior
Triceps brachii
Teres major

C *Removed:* Medial and lateral cords, and axillary vessels. *Revealed:* Posterior cord.

Topography of the Brachial & Cubital Regions

Fig. 22.35 Brachial region
Right arm, anterior view. *Removed:* Deltoid, pectoralis major and minor. *Revealed:* Medial bicipital groove.

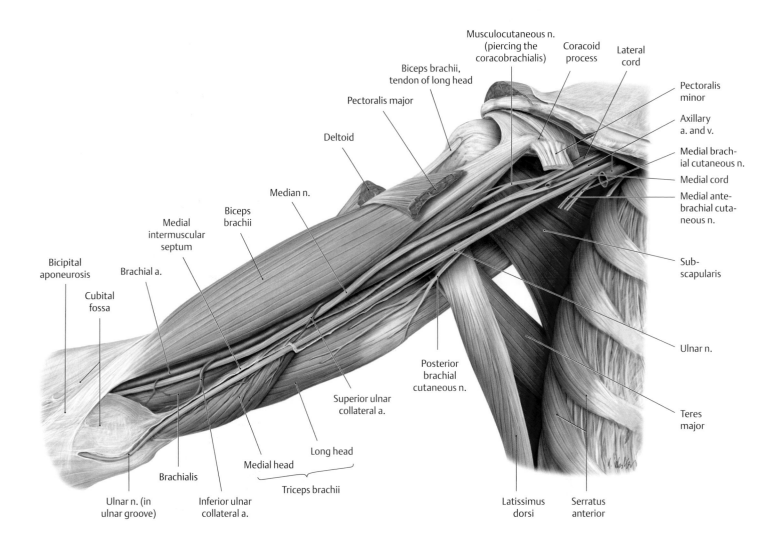

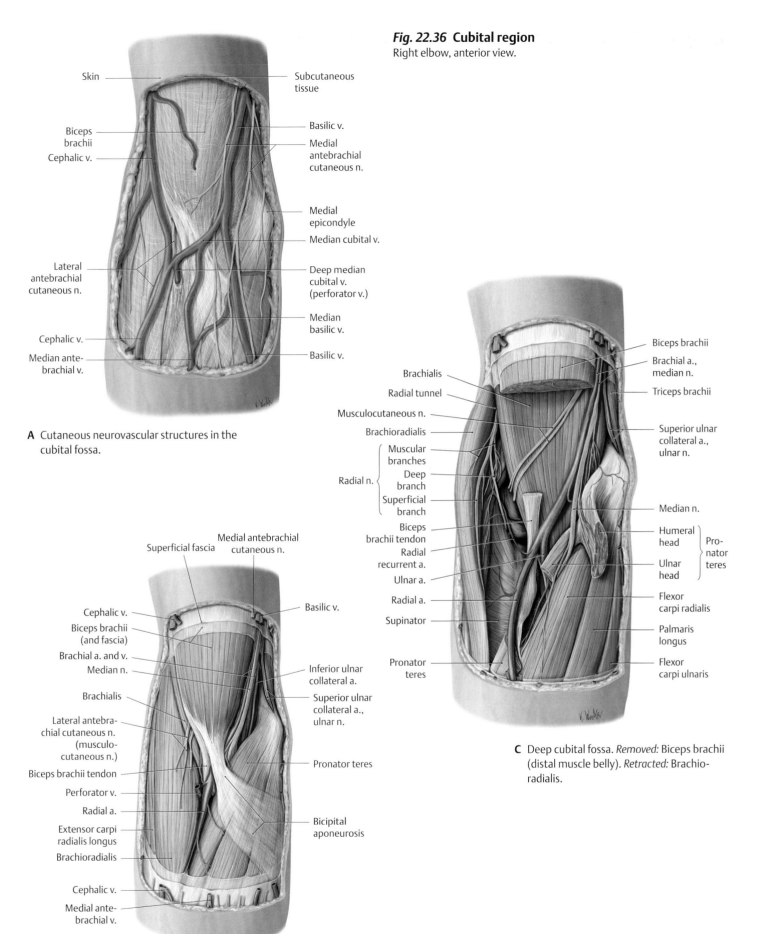

Fig. 22.36 Cubital region
Right elbow, anterior view.

A Cutaneous neurovascular structures in the cubital fossa.

B Superficial cubital fossa. *Removed:* Fasciae and epifascial neurovascular structures.

C Deep cubital fossa. *Removed:* Biceps brachii (distal muscle belly). *Retracted:* Brachioradialis.

339

Topography of the Forearm

Fig. 22.37 Anterior forearm

Right forearm, anterior view.

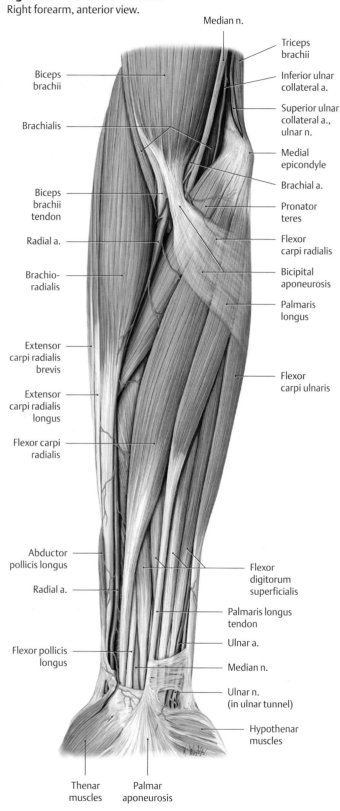

A Superficial layer. *Removed:* Fasciae and superficial neurovasculature.

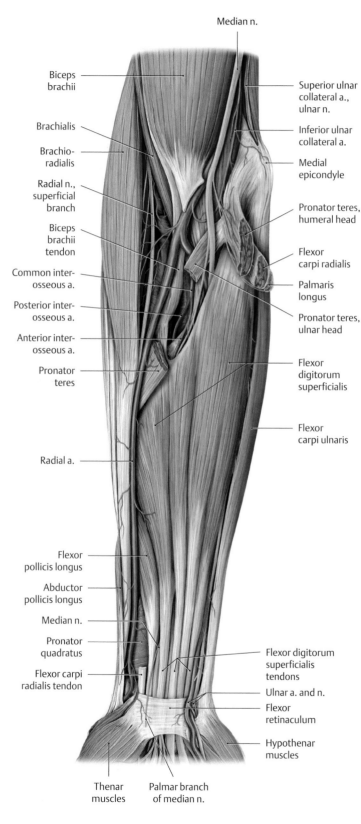

B Middle layer. *Partially removed:* Superficial flexors (pronator teres, flexor digitorum superficialis, palmaris longus, and flexor carpi radialis).

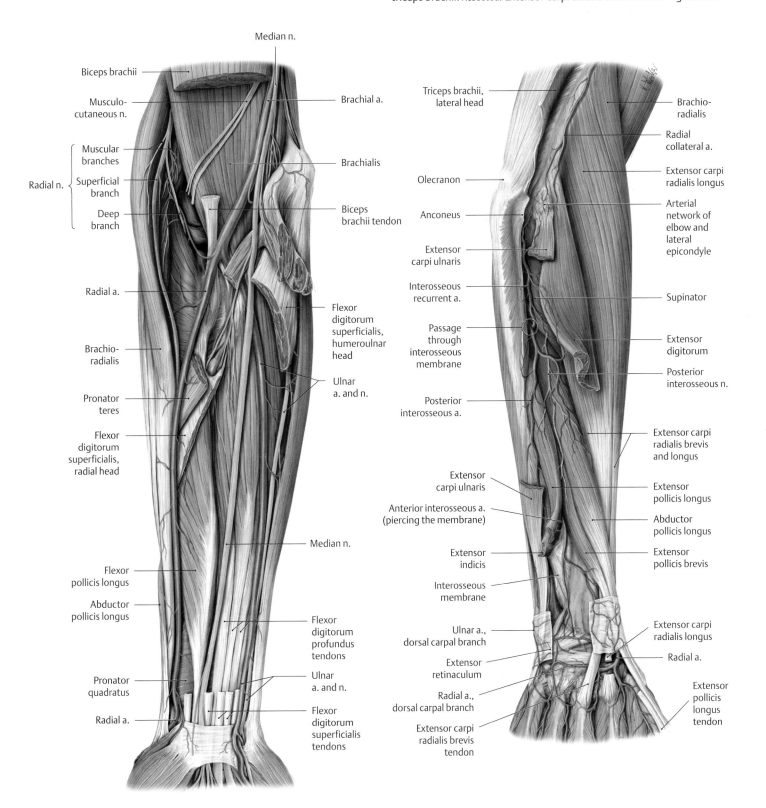

Fig. 22.38 Posterior forearm

Right forearm, anterior view during pronation. *Reflected:* Anconeus and triceps brachii. *Resected:* Extensor carpi ulnaris and extensor digitorum.

Median n.

Biceps brachii

Musculo-cutaneous n.

Brachial a.

Radial n. {
Muscular branches

Superficial branch

Deep branch
}

Brachialis

Radial a.

Biceps brachii tendon

Brachio-radialis

Flexor digitorum superficialis, humeroulnar head

Pronator teres

Ulnar a. and n.

Flexor digitorum superficialis, radial head

Flexor pollicis longus

Median n.

Abductor pollicis longus

Pronator quadratus

Flexor digitorum profundus tendons

Radial a.

Ulnar a. and n.

Flexor digitorum superficialis tendons

Triceps brachii, lateral head

Brachio-radialis

Radial collateral a.

Olecranon

Extensor carpi radialis longus

Anconeus

Arterial network of elbow and lateral epicondyle

Extensor carpi ulnaris

Interosseous recurrent a.

Supinator

Passage through interosseous membrane

Extensor digitorum

Posterior interosseous n.

Posterior interosseous a.

Extensor carpi radialis brevis and longus

Extensor carpi ulnaris

Extensor pollicis longus

Anterior interosseous a. (piercing the membrane)

Abductor pollicis longus

Extensor indicis

Extensor pollicis brevis

Interosseous membrane

Ulnar a., dorsal carpal branch

Extensor carpi radialis longus

Extensor retinaculum

Radial a.

Radial a., dorsal carpal branch

Extensor pollicis longus tendon

Extensor carpi radialis brevis tendon

C Deep layer. *Removed:* Deep flexors.

Topography of the Carpal Region

***Fig. 22.39* Anterior carpal region**
Right hand, anterior (palmar) view.

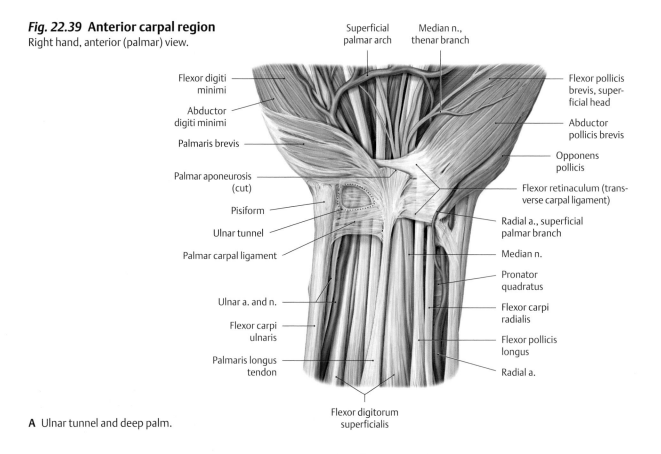

Flexor digiti minimi

Abductor digiti minimi

Palmaris brevis

Palmar aponeurosis (cut)

Pisiform

Ulnar tunnel

Palmar carpal ligament

Ulnar a. and n.

Flexor carpi ulnaris

Palmaris longus tendon

Superficial palmar arch

Median n., thenar branch

Flexor pollicis brevis, superficial head

Abductor pollicis brevis

Opponens pollicis

Flexor retinaculum (transverse carpal ligament)

Radial a., superficial palmar branch

Median n.

Pronator quadratus

Flexor carpi radialis

Flexor pollicis longus

Radial a.

Flexor digitorum superficialis

A Ulnar tunnel and deep palm.

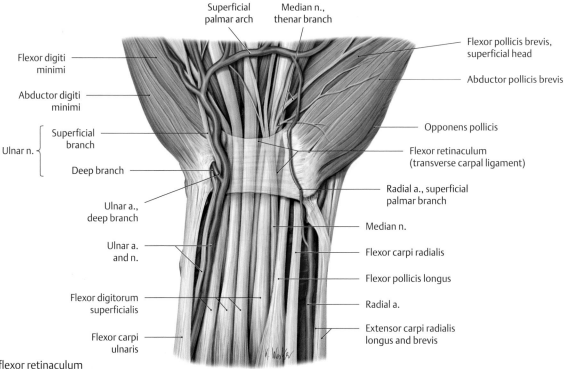

Superficial palmar arch

Median n., thenar branch

Flexor digiti minimi

Abductor digiti minimi

Ulnar n. {
Superficial branch

Deep branch
}

Ulnar a., deep branch

Ulnar a. and n.

Flexor digitorum superficialis

Flexor carpi ulnaris

Flexor pollicis brevis, superficial head

Abductor pollicis brevis

Opponens pollicis

Flexor retinaculum (transverse carpal ligament)

Radial a., superficial palmar branch

Median n.

Flexor carpi radialis

Flexor pollicis longus

Radial a.

Extensor carpi radialis longus and brevis

B Carpal tunnel with flexor retinaculum windowed.

Fig. 22.40 Ulnar tunnel

Right hand, anterior (palmar) view.

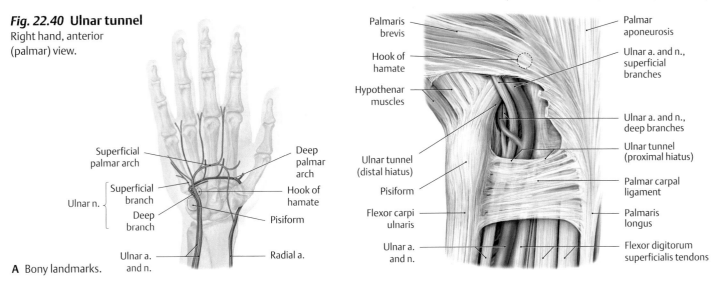

A Bony landmarks.

B Apertures and walls of the ulnar tunnel.

Fig. 22.41 Carpal tunnel: Cross section

Right hand, proximal view. The tight fit of sensitive neurovascular structures with closely apposed, frequently moving tendons in the carpal tunnel often causes problems (carpal tunnel syndrome) when any of the structures swell or degenerate.

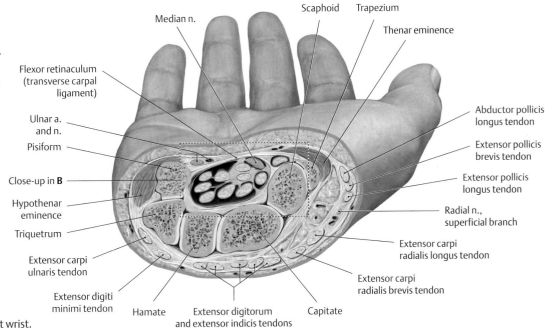

A Cross section through the right wrist.

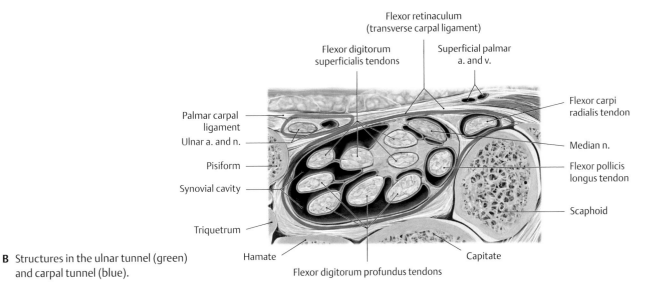

B Structures in the ulnar tunnel (green) and carpal tunnel (blue).

Topography of the Palm of the Hand

Fig. 22.42 Superficial neurovascular structures of the palm

Right hand, anterior view.

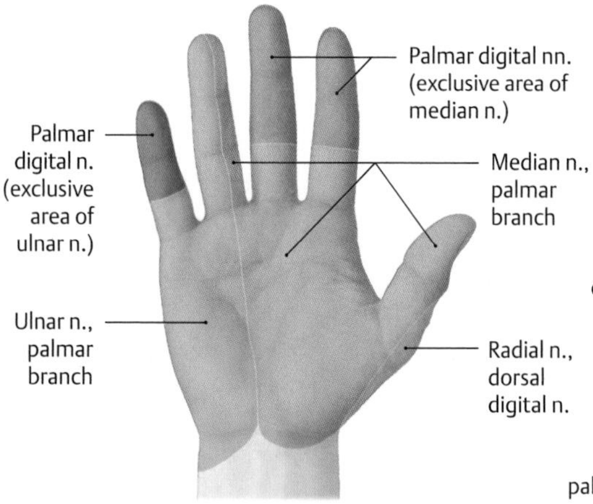

A Sensory territories. Extensive overlap exists between adjacent areas. *Exclusive* nerve territories indicated with darker shading.

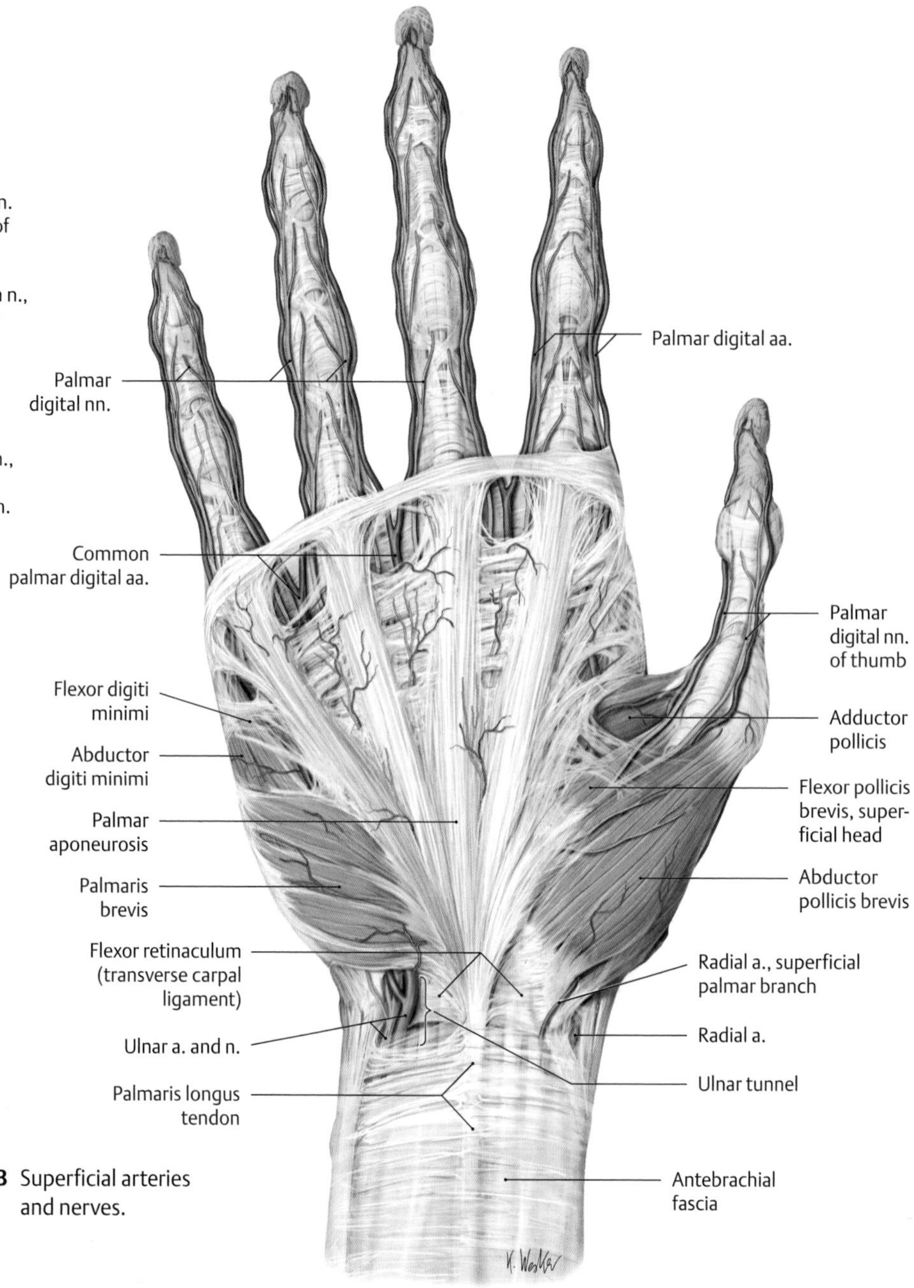

Palmar digital nn. (exclusive area of median n.)

Palmar digital n. (exclusive area of ulnar n.)

Median n., palmar branch

Ulnar n., palmar branch

Radial n., dorsal digital n.

Palmar digital nn.

Palmar digital aa.

Common palmar digital aa.

Palmar digital nn. of thumb

Flexor digiti minimi

Adductor pollicis

Abductor digiti minimi

Flexor pollicis brevis, superficial head

Palmar aponeurosis

Abductor pollicis brevis

Palmaris brevis

Flexor retinaculum (transverse carpal ligament)

Radial a., superficial palmar branch

Radial a.

Ulnar a. and n.

Ulnar tunnel

Palmaris longus tendon

Antebrachial fascia

B Superficial arteries and nerves.

Fig. 22.43 Neurovasculature of the finger

Right middle finger, lateral view.

Palmar digital n., dorsal branch

Metacarpophalangeal joint

Dorsal digital a. and n.

Palmar digital n.

Proper palmar digital a. and n.

Common palmar digital a.

A Nerves and arteries.

Palmar digital a.

Digitopalmar branches

Metacarpal

Vincula brevia

Vincula longa

Flexor digitorum profundus

Flexor digitorum superficialis

B Blood supply to the flexor tendons in the tendon sheath.

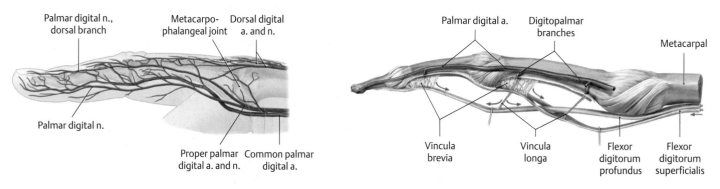

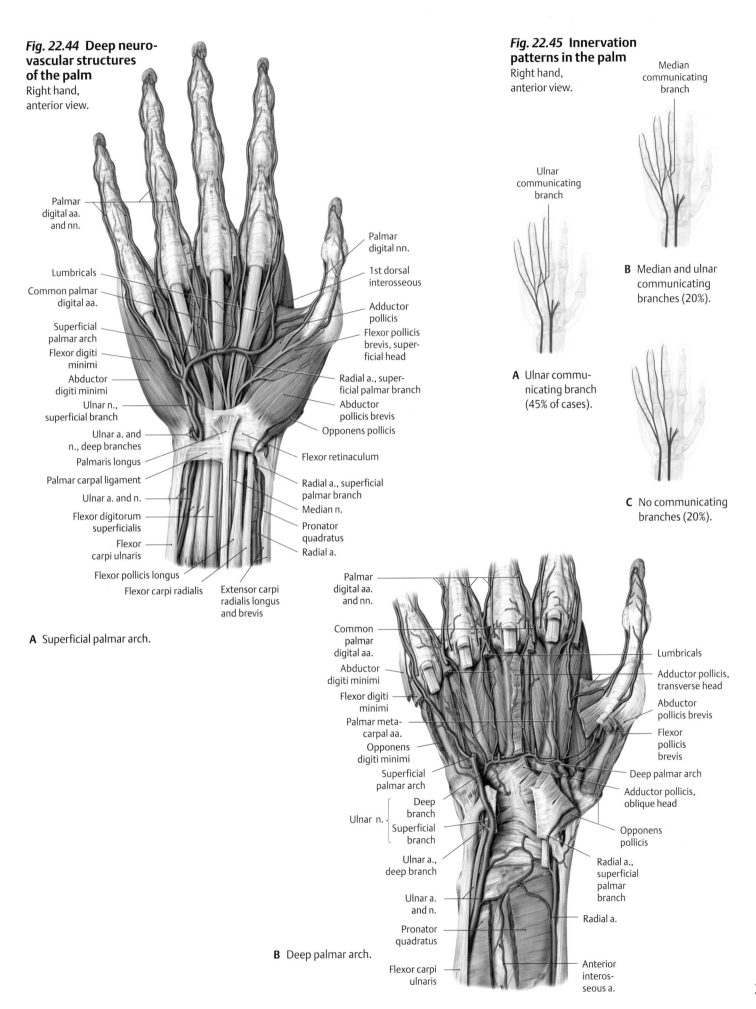

Fig. 22.44 Deep neuro-vascular structures of the palm
Right hand, anterior view.

Palmar digital aa. and nn.

Lumbricals

Common palmar digital aa.

Superficial palmar arch

Flexor digiti minimi

Abductor digiti minimi

Ulnar n., superficial branch

Ulnar a. and n., deep branches

Palmaris longus

Palmar carpal ligament

Ulnar a. and n.

Flexor digitorum superficialis

Flexor carpi ulnaris

Flexor pollicis longus

Flexor carpi radialis

Palmar digital nn.

1st dorsal interosseous

Adductor pollicis

Flexor pollicis brevis, superficial head

Radial a., superficial palmar branch

Abductor pollicis brevis

Opponens pollicis

Flexor retinaculum

Radial a., superficial palmar branch

Median n.

Pronator quadratus

Radial a.

Extensor carpi radialis longus and brevis

A Superficial palmar arch.

Fig. 22.45 Innervation patterns in the palm
Right hand, anterior view.

Median communicating branch

Ulnar communicating branch

B Median and ulnar communicating branches (20%).

A Ulnar communicating branch (45% of cases).

C No communicating branches (20%).

Palmar digital aa. and nn.

Common palmar digital aa.

Abductor digiti minimi

Flexor digiti minimi

Palmar metacarpal aa.

Opponens digiti minimi

Superficial palmar arch

Ulnar n. { Deep branch / Superficial branch }

Ulnar a., deep branch

Ulnar a. and n.

Pronator quadratus

Flexor carpi ulnaris

Lumbricals

Adductor pollicis, transverse head

Abductor pollicis brevis

Flexor pollicis brevis

Deep palmar arch

Adductor pollicis, oblique head

Opponens pollicis

Radial a., superficial palmar branch

Radial a.

Anterior interosseous a.

B Deep palmar arch.

345

Topography of the Dorsum of the Hand

Fig. 22.46 **Sensory innervation of the dorsum**
Right hand, posterior view.

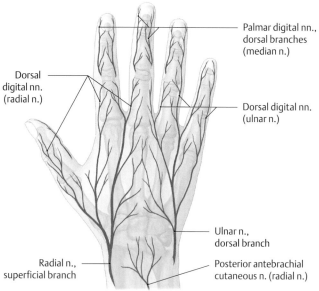

Palmar digital nn., dorsal branches (median n.)

Dorsal digital nn. (radial n.)

Dorsal digital nn. (ulnar n.)

Ulnar n., dorsal branch

Radial n., superficial branch

Posterior antebrachial cutaneous n. (radial n.)

A Nerves of the dorsum.

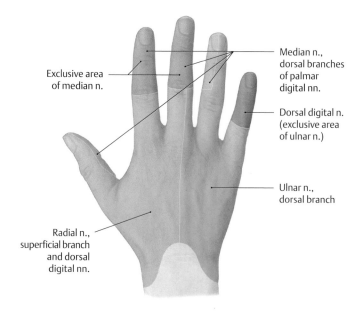

Median n., dorsal branches of palmar digital nn.

Exclusive area of median n.

Dorsal digital n. (exclusive area of ulnar n.)

Ulnar n., dorsal branch

Radial n., superficial branch and dorsal digital nn.

B Sensory territories. Extensive overlap exists between adjacent areas. *Exclusive* nerve territories indicated with darker shading.

Fig. 22.47 **Anatomic snuffbox**
Right hand, radial view. The three-sided "anatomic snuffbox" is bounded by the tendons of insertion of the abductor pollicis longus and extensors pollicis brevis and longus.

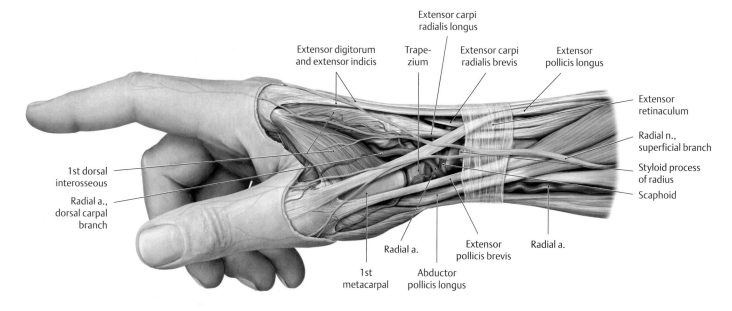

Extensor carpi radialis longus

Extensor digitorum and extensor indicis

Trapezium

Extensor carpi radialis brevis

Extensor pollicis longus

Extensor retinaculum

Radial n., superficial branch

Styloid process of radius

Scaphoid

1st dorsal interosseous

Radial a., dorsal carpal branch

Radial a.

Extensor pollicis brevis

Radial a.

1st metacarpal

Abductor pollicis longus

Fig. 22.48 Neurovascular structures of the dorsum

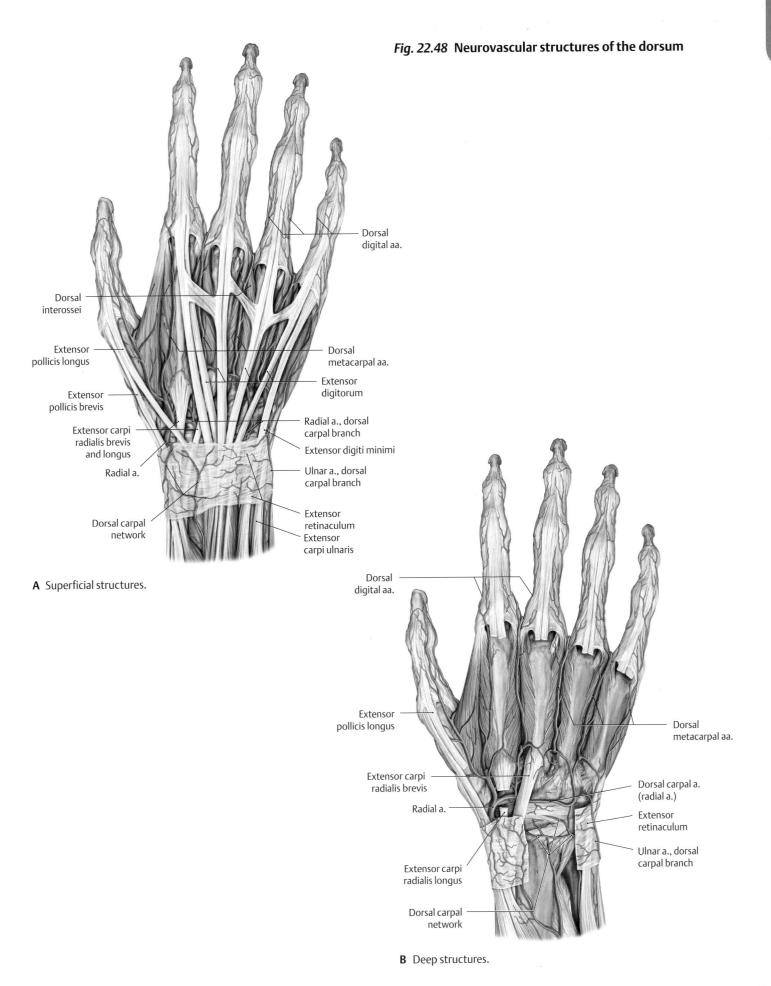

Dorsal digital aa.

Dorsal interossei

Extensor pollicis longus

Extensor pollicis brevis

Extensor carpi radialis brevis and longus

Radial a.

Dorsal carpal network

Dorsal metacarpal aa.

Extensor digitorum

Radial a., dorsal carpal branch

Extensor digiti minimi

Ulnar a., dorsal carpal branch

Extensor retinaculum

Extensor carpi ulnaris

A Superficial structures.

Dorsal digital aa.

Extensor pollicis longus

Extensor carpi radialis brevis

Radial a.

Extensor carpi radialis longus

Dorsal carpal network

Dorsal metacarpal aa.

Dorsal carpal a. (radial a.)

Extensor retinaculum

Ulnar a., dorsal carpal branch

B Deep structures.

Transverse Sections

Fig. 22.49 **Windowed dissection**
Right limb, anterior view.

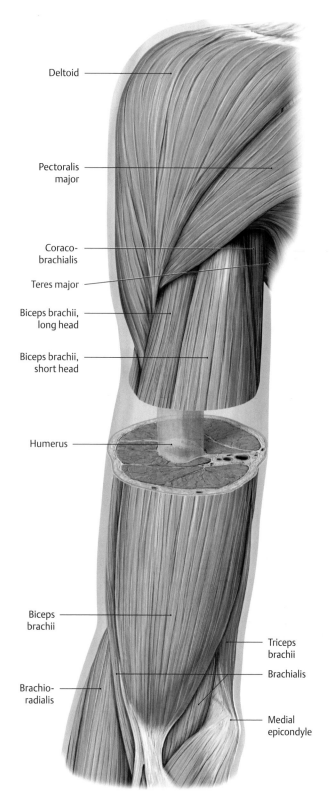

A Dissection of the arm.

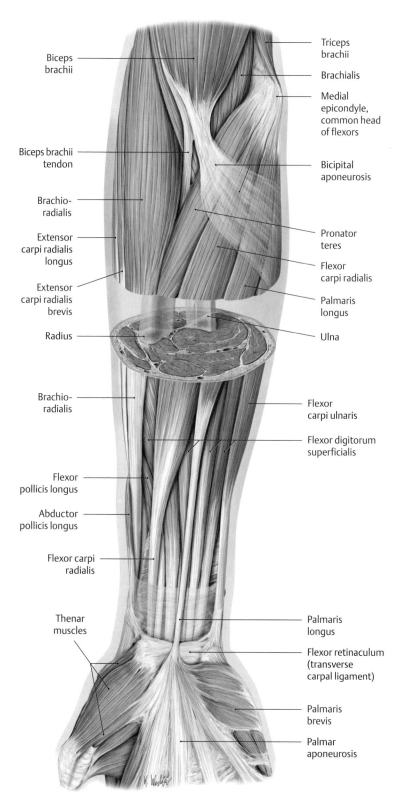

B Dissection of the forearm.

Fig. 22.50 Transverse sections

Right limb, proximal (superior) view.

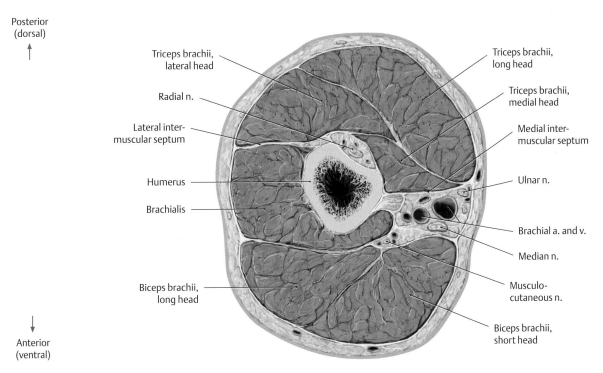

Posterior
(dorsal)

Triceps brachii,
lateral head

Radial n.

Lateral inter-
muscular septum

Humerus

Brachialis

Biceps brachii,
long head

Anterior
(ventral)

Triceps brachii,
long head

Triceps brachii,
medial head

Medial inter-
muscular septum

Ulnar n.

Brachial a. and v.

Median n.

Musculo-
cutaneous n.

Biceps brachii,
short head

A Arm (plane of section in Fig. 22.49A).

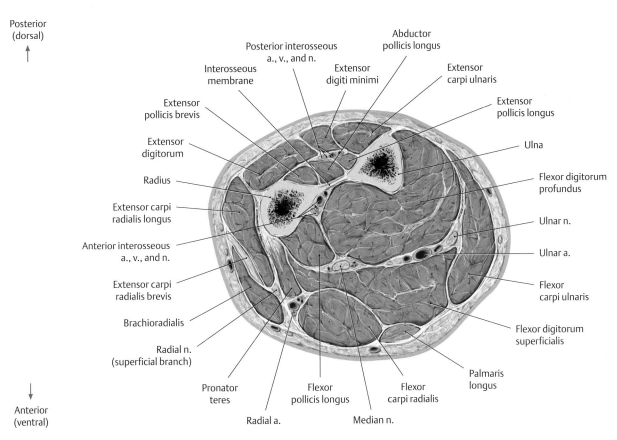

Posterior
(dorsal)

Posterior interosseous
a., v., and n.

Interosseous
membrane

Extensor
pollicis brevis

Extensor
digitorum

Radius

Extensor carpi
radialis longus

Anterior interosseous
a., v., and n.

Extensor carpi
radialis brevis

Brachioradialis

Radial n.
(superficial branch)

Abductor
pollicis longus

Extensor
digiti minimi

Extensor
carpi ulnaris

Extensor
pollicis longus

Ulna

Flexor digitorum
profundus

Ulnar n.

Ulnar a.

Flexor
carpi ulnaris

Flexor digitorum
superficialis

Palmaris
longus

Pronator
teres

Flexor
pollicis longus

Flexor
carpi radialis

Median n.

Radial a.

Anterior
(ventral)

B Forearm (plane of section in Fig. 22.49B).

Surface Anatomy (I)

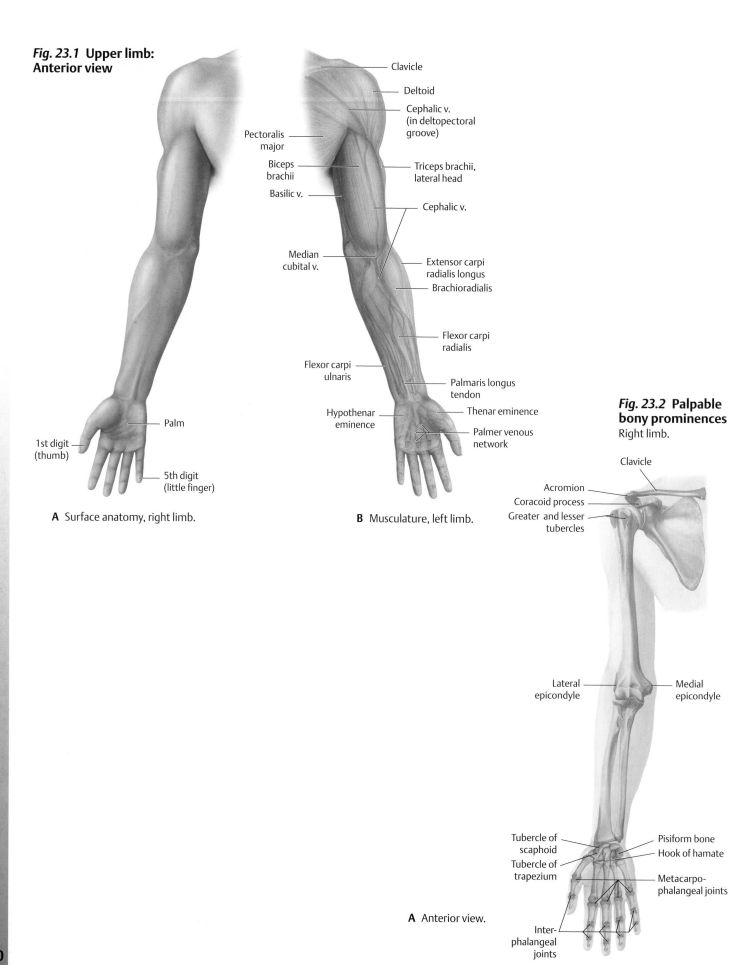

Fig. 23.1 Upper limb: Anterior view

Clavicle

Deltoid

Cephalic v. (in deltopectoral groove)

Pectoralis major

Biceps brachii

Triceps brachii, lateral head

Basilic v.

Cephalic v.

Median cubital v.

Extensor carpi radialis longus

Brachioradialis

Flexor carpi radialis

Flexor carpi ulnaris

Palmaris longus tendon

Hypothenar eminence

Thenar eminence

Palmer venous network

Palm

1st digit (thumb)

5th digit (little finger)

A Surface anatomy, right limb.

B Musculature, left limb.

Fig. 23.2 Palpable bony prominences
Right limb.

Clavicle

Acromion

Coracoid process

Greater and lesser tubercles

Lateral epicondyle

Medial epicondyle

Tubercle of scaphoid

Pisiform bone

Hook of hamate

Tubercle of trapezium

Metacarpo-phalangeal joints

Inter-phalangeal joints

A Anterior view.

Q1: Which cutaneous nerves are most vulnerable during intravenous punctures (e.g., drawing blood, injections)?

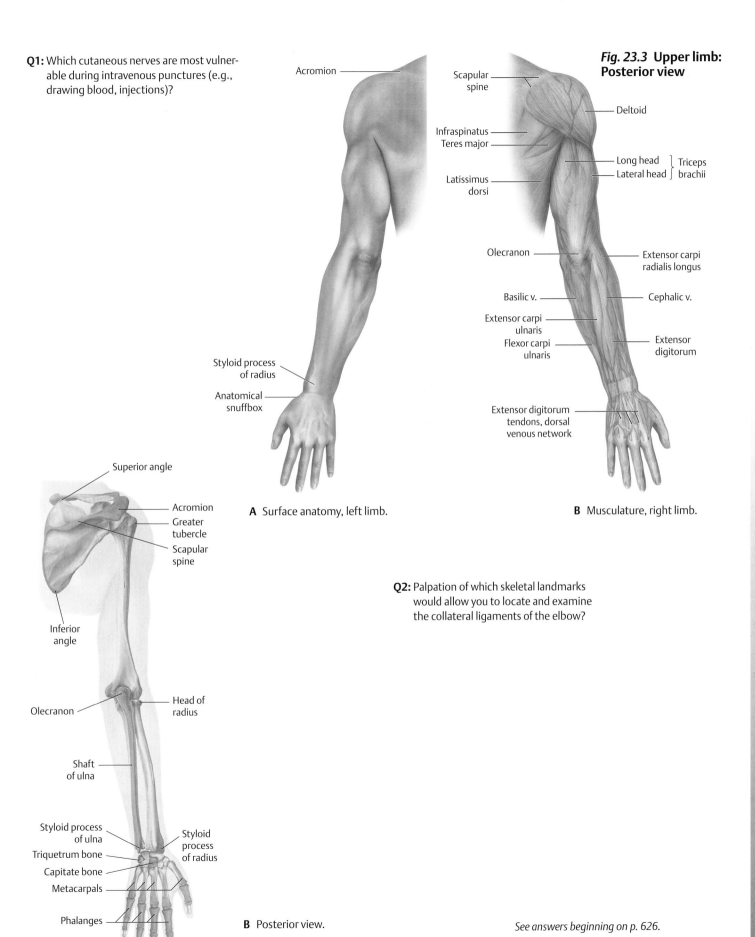

***Fig. 23.3* Upper limb: Posterior view**

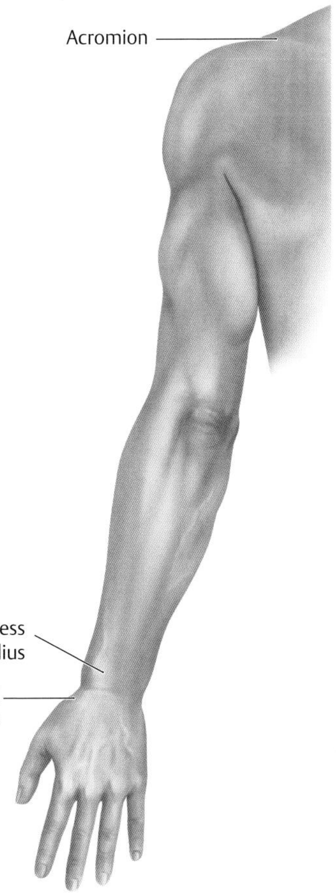
Acromion
Styloid process of radius
Anatomical snuffbox

A Surface anatomy, left limb.

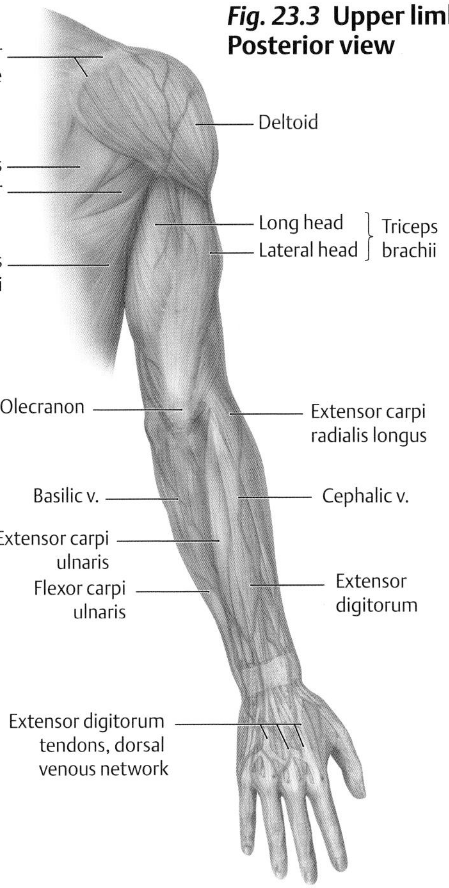
Scapular spine
Deltoid
Infraspinatus
Teres major
Long head
Lateral head
Triceps brachii
Latissimus dorsi
Olecranon
Extensor carpi radialis longus
Basilic v.
Cephalic v.
Extensor carpi ulnaris
Flexor carpi ulnaris
Extensor digitorum
Extensor digitorum tendons, dorsal venous network

B Musculature, right limb.

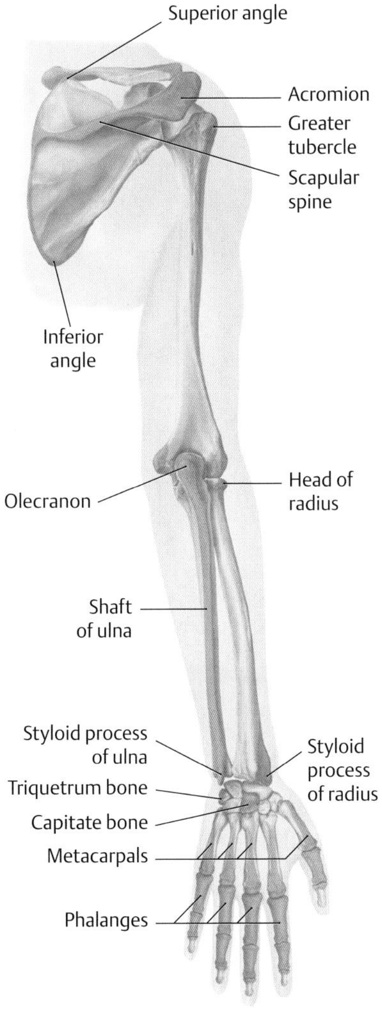
Superior angle
Acromion
Greater tubercle
Scapular spine
Inferior angle
Olecranon
Head of radius
Shaft of ulna
Styloid process of ulna
Styloid process of radius
Triquetrum bone
Capitate bone
Metacarpals
Phalanges

B Posterior view.

Q2: Palpation of which skeletal landmarks would allow you to locate and examine the collateral ligaments of the elbow?

See answers beginning on p. 626.

Surface Anatomy (II)

Fig. 23.4 Palpable bony structures
Left hand.

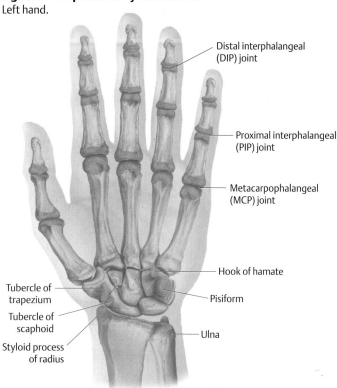

A Anterior (palmar) view.

Distal interphalangeal (DIP) joint

Proximal interphalangeal (PIP) joint

Metacarpophalangeal (MCP) joint

Hook of hamate

Tubercle of trapezium

Pisiform

Tubercle of scaphoid

Ulna

Styloid process of radius

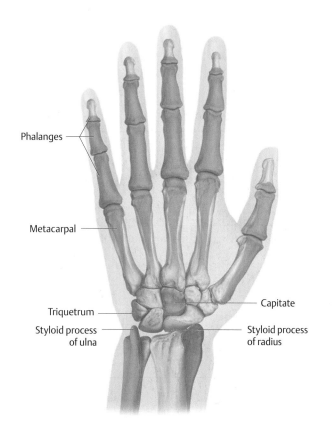

B Posterior (dorsal) view.

Phalanges

Metacarpal

Triquetrum

Styloid process of ulna

Capitate

Styloid process of radius

Fig. 23.5 Surface anatomy of the wrist
Left wrist, oblique anterolateral view.

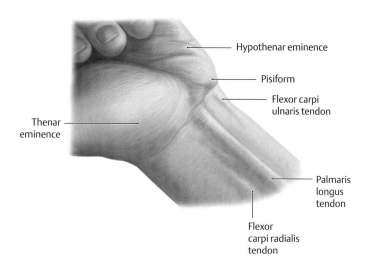

Hypothenar eminence

Pisiform

Flexor carpi ulnaris tendon

Thenar eminence

Palmaris longus tendon

Flexor carpi radialis tendon

Q3: How can the palpable tendons in the wrist be used to determine the location of key arteries and nerves?

Fig. 23.6 Anatomic snuffbox
Left hand, oblique posterolateral view.

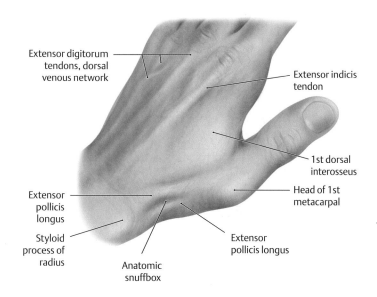

Extensor digitorum tendons, dorsal venous network

Extensor indicis tendon

1st dorsal interosseus

Head of 1st metacarpal

Extensor pollicis longus

Extensor pollicis longus

Styloid process of radius

Anatomic snuffbox

Q4: Tenderness in the base of the anatomic snuffbox can suggest a fracture of which of the carpal bones?

See answers beginning on p. 626.

Fig. 23.7 Palm

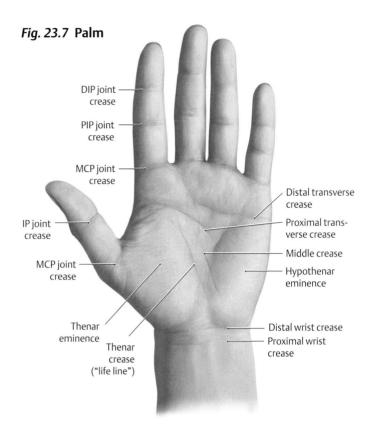

DIP joint crease
PIP joint crease
MCP joint crease
IP joint crease
MCP joint crease
Distal transverse crease
Proximal transverse crease
Middle crease
Hypothenar eminence
Thenar eminence
Thenar crease ("life line")
Distal wrist crease
Proximal wrist crease

A Surface anatomy, left palm.

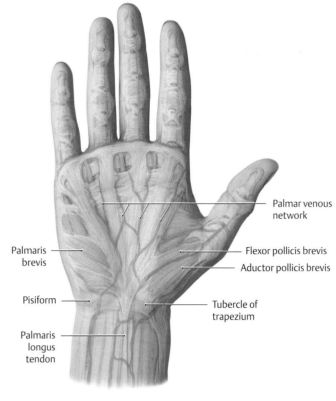

Palmaris brevis
Pisiform
Palmaris longus tendon
Palmar venous network
Flexor pollicis brevis
Aductor pollicis brevis
Tubercle of trapezium

B Musculature, right palm.

Fig. 23.8 Dorsum

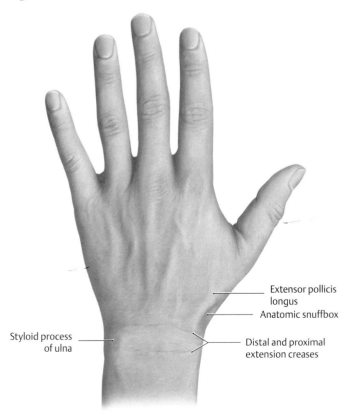
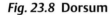

Extensor pollicis longus
Anatomic snuffbox
Styloid process of ulna
Distal and proximal extension creases

A Surface anatomy, left hand.

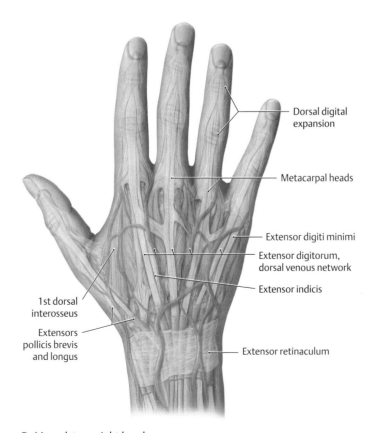

Dorsal digital expansion
Metacarpal heads
1st dorsal interosseus
Extensors pollicis brevis and longus
Extensor digiti minimi
Extensor digitorum, dorsal venous network
Extensor indicis
Extensor retinaculum

B Musculature, right hand.

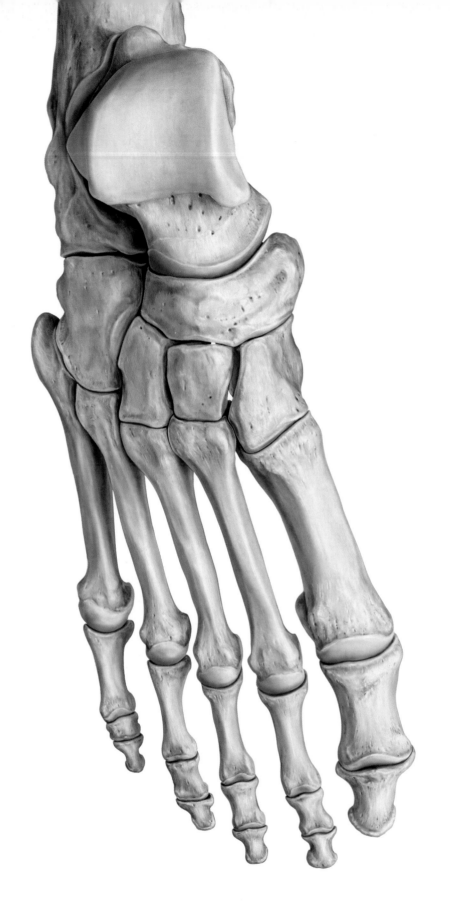

Lower Limb

Bones of the Lower Limb

Fig. 24.1 **Bones of the lower limb**

Right limb. The skeleton of the lower limb consists of a limb girdle and an attached free limb. The free limb is divided into the thigh (femur), leg (tibia and fibula), and foot. It is connected to the pelvic girdle by the hip joint.

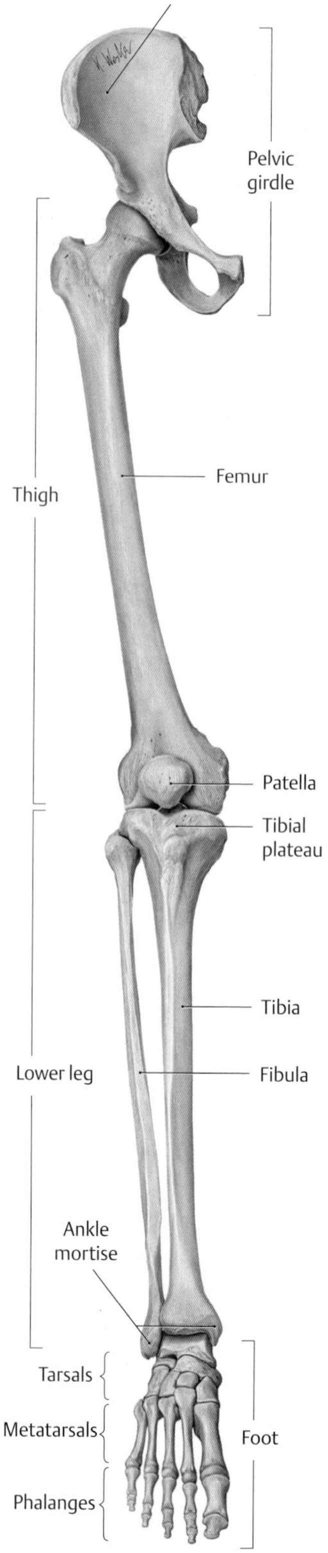

A Anterior view.

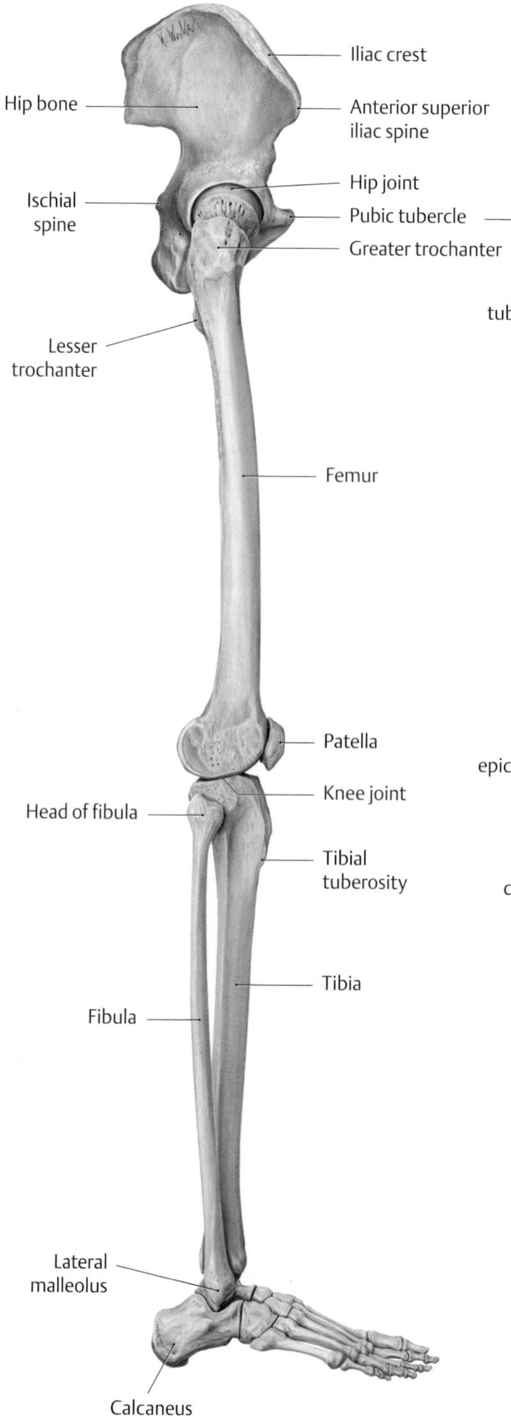

B Right lateral view.

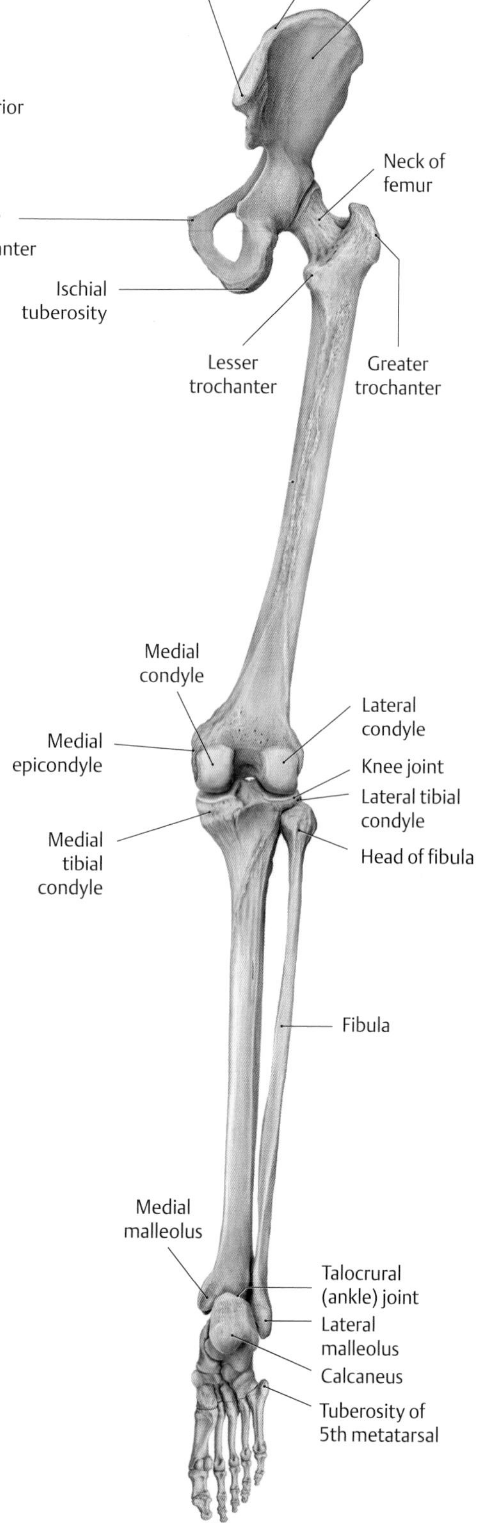

C Posterior view.

Fig. 24.2 Line of gravity

Right lateral view. The line of gravity runs vertically from the whole-body center of gravity to the ground with characteristic points of intersection.

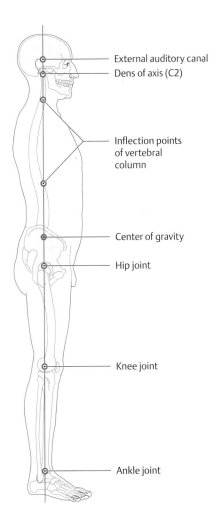

External auditory canal
Dens of axis (C2)

Inflection points of vertebral column

Center of gravity

Hip joint

Knee joint

Ankle joint

Fig. 24.3 Palpable bony prominences in the lower limb

Most skeletal elements of the lower limb have bony prominences, margins, or surfaces (e.g., medial or tibial surfaces) that can be palpated through the skin and soft tissues.

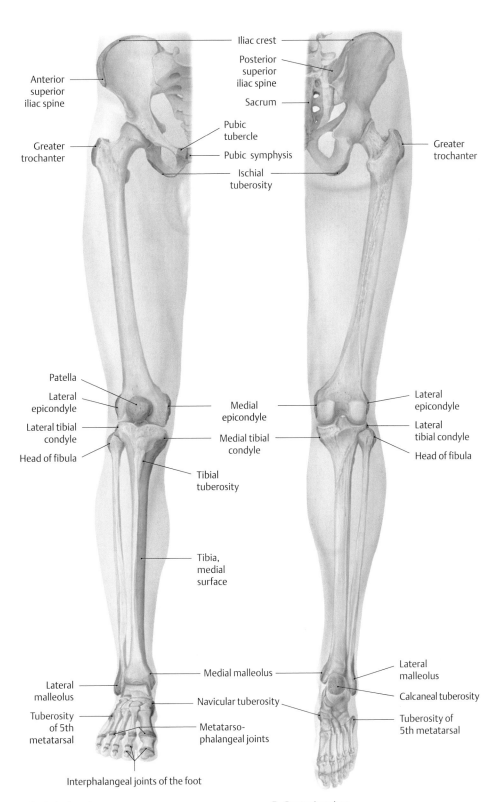

Iliac crest

Posterior superior iliac spine

Anterior superior iliac spine

Sacrum

Pubic tubercle

Greater trochanter

Pubic symphysis

Ischial tuberosity

Greater trochanter

Patella

Lateral epicondyle

Medial epicondyle

Lateral epicondyle

Lateral tibial condyle

Head of fibula

Medial tibial condyle

Lateral tibial condyle

Head of fibula

Tibial tuberosity

Tibia, medial surface

Medial malleolus

Lateral malleolus

Lateral malleolus

Navicular tuberosity

Calcaneal tuberosity

Tuberosity of 5th metatarsal

Metatarso-phalangeal joints

Tuberosity of 5th metatarsal

Interphalangeal joints of the foot

A Anterior view.

B Posterior view.

Pelvic Girdle & Hip Bone

Fig. 24.4 **Pelvic girdle**
Anterior view. Pelvic ring in red.

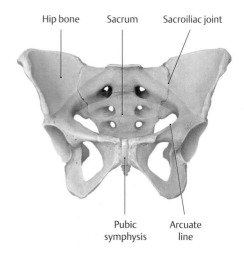

Hip bone   Sacrum   Sacroiliac joint

Pubic symphysis   Arcuate line

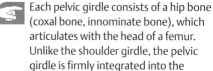

Each pelvic girdle consists of a hip bone (coxal bone, innominate bone), which articulates with the head of a femur. Unlike the shoulder girdle, the pelvic girdle is firmly integrated into the axial skeleton: the paired hip bones are connected to each other at the cartilaginous pubic symphysis and to the sacrum via the sacroiliac joints. These attachments create the bony pelvic ring (red), permitting very little motion. This stability is an important prerequisite for the transfer of trunk loads to the lower limb (necessary for normal gait).

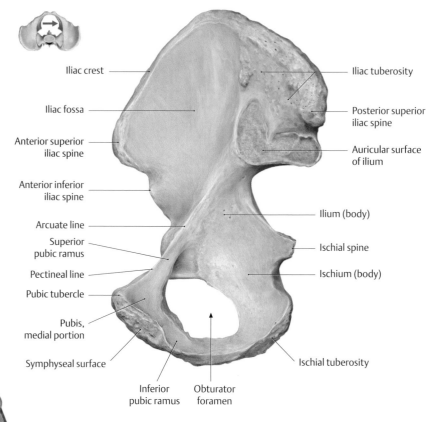

Iliac crest

Iliac fossa

Anterior superior iliac spine

Anterior inferior iliac spine

Arcuate line

Superior pubic ramus

Pectineal line

Pubic tubercle

Pubis, medial portion

Symphyseal surface

Inferior pubic ramus   Obturator foramen

Iliac tuberosity

Posterior superior iliac spine

Auricular surface of ilium

Ilium (body)

Ischial spine

Ischium (body)

Ischial tuberosity

B Medial view.

Fig. 24.5 **Right hip bone**

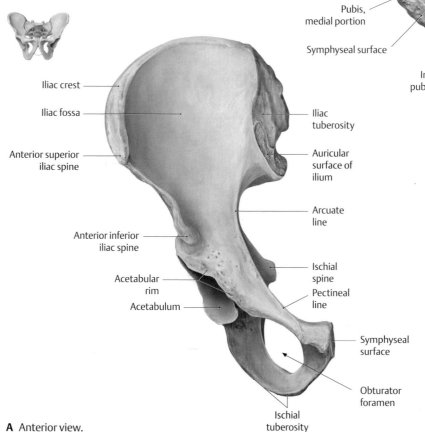

Iliac crest

Iliac fossa

Anterior superior iliac spine

Anterior inferior iliac spine

Acetabular rim

Acetabulum

Iliac tuberosity

Auricular surface of ilium

Arcuate line

Ischial spine

Pectineal line

Symphyseal surface

Obturator foramen

Ischial tuberosity

A Anterior view.

Fig. 24.6 Components of the hip bone

Right hip bone. The three bony elements of the hip bone (ilium, ischium, and pubis) come together at the acetabulum. Definitive fusion of the Y-shaped growth plate (triradiate cartilage) occurs between the 14th and 16th years of life.

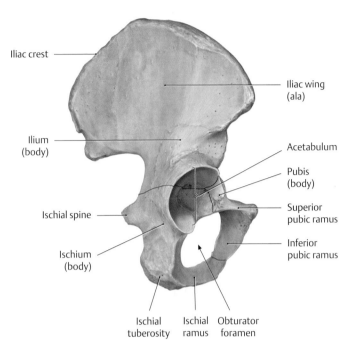

Iliac crest — Iliac wing (ala) — Ilium (body) — Acetabulum — Pubis (body) — Superior pubic ramus — Ischial spine — Inferior pubic ramus — Ischium (body) — Ischial tuberosity — Ischial ramus — Obturator foramen

A Triradiate cartilage of the hip bone. Lateral view.

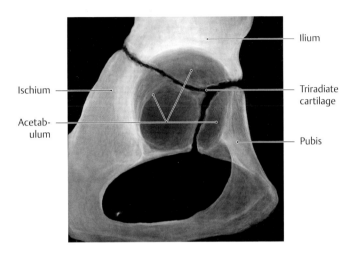

Ischium — Ilium — Triradiate cartilage — Acetabulum — Pubis

B Radiograph of right acetabulum of a child.

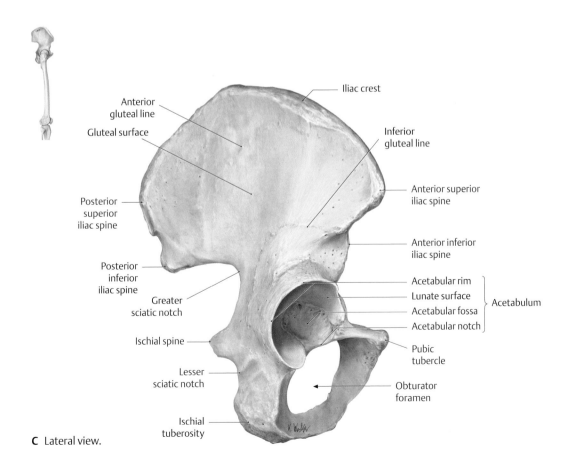

Anterior gluteal line — Iliac crest — Gluteal surface — Inferior gluteal line — Posterior superior iliac spine — Anterior superior iliac spine — Posterior inferior iliac spine — Anterior inferior iliac spine — Greater sciatic notch — Acetabular rim — Lunate surface — Acetabular fossa — Acetabular notch — Acetabulum — Ischial spine — Pubic tubercle — Lesser sciatic notch — Obturator foramen — Ischial tuberosity

C Lateral view.

Femur

Fig. 24.7 **Right femur**

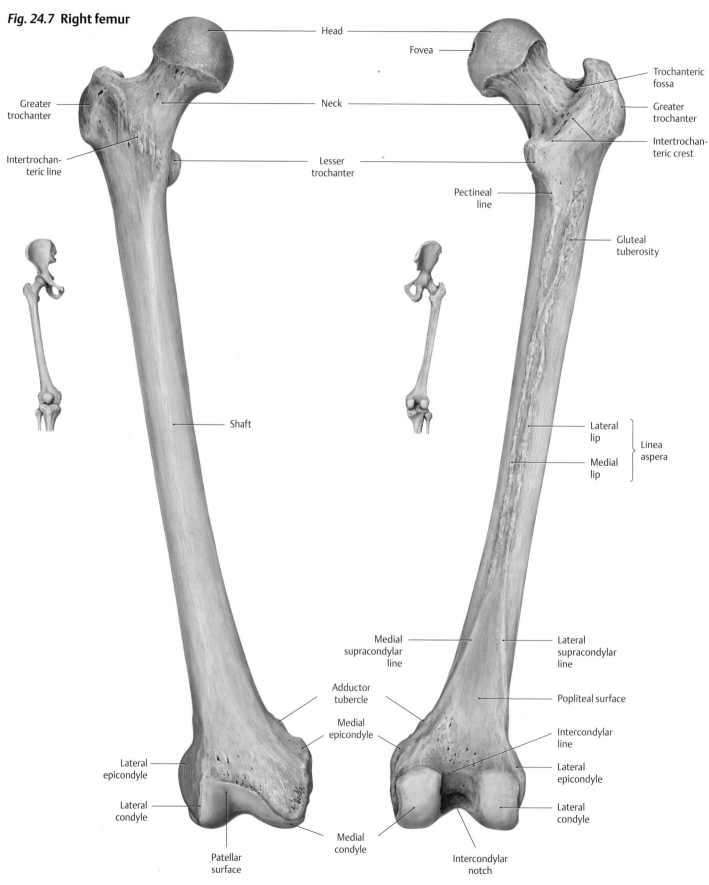

Head

Fovea

Trochanteric fossa

Greater trochanter

Neck

Greater trochanter

Intertrochanteric crest

Intertrochanteric line

Lesser trochanter

Pectineal line

Gluteal tuberosity

Shaft

Lateral lip

Linea aspera

Medial lip

Medial supracondylar line

Lateral supracondylar line

Adductor tubercle

Popliteal surface

Medial epicondyle

Intercondylar line

Lateral epicondyle

Lateral condyle

Lateral epicondyle

Medial condyle

Lateral condyle

Patellar surface

Intercondylar notch

A Anterior view.

B Posterior view.

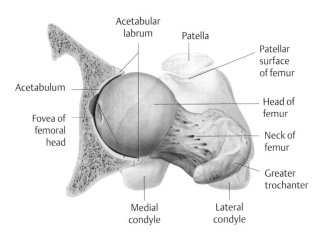

C Proximal view. The acetabulum has been sectioned in the horizontal plane.

Clinical

Fractures of the femur

Femoral fractures caused by falls in patients with osteoporosis are most frequently located in the neck of the femur. Femoral shaft fractures are less frequent and are usually caused by strong trauma (e.g., a car accident).

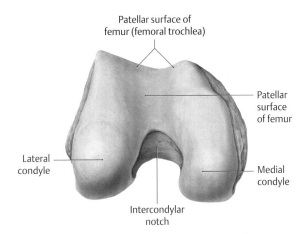

D Distal view. See pp. 382–383 for the knee joint.

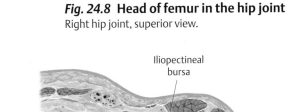

Fig. 24.8 **Head of femur in the hip joint**
Right hip joint, superior view.

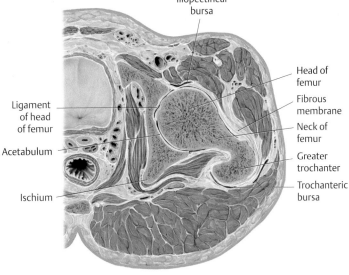

A Transverse section.

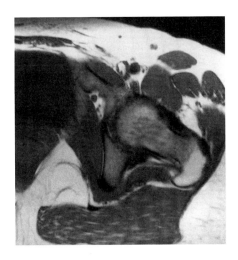

B T1-weighted MRI.

Hip Joint: Overview

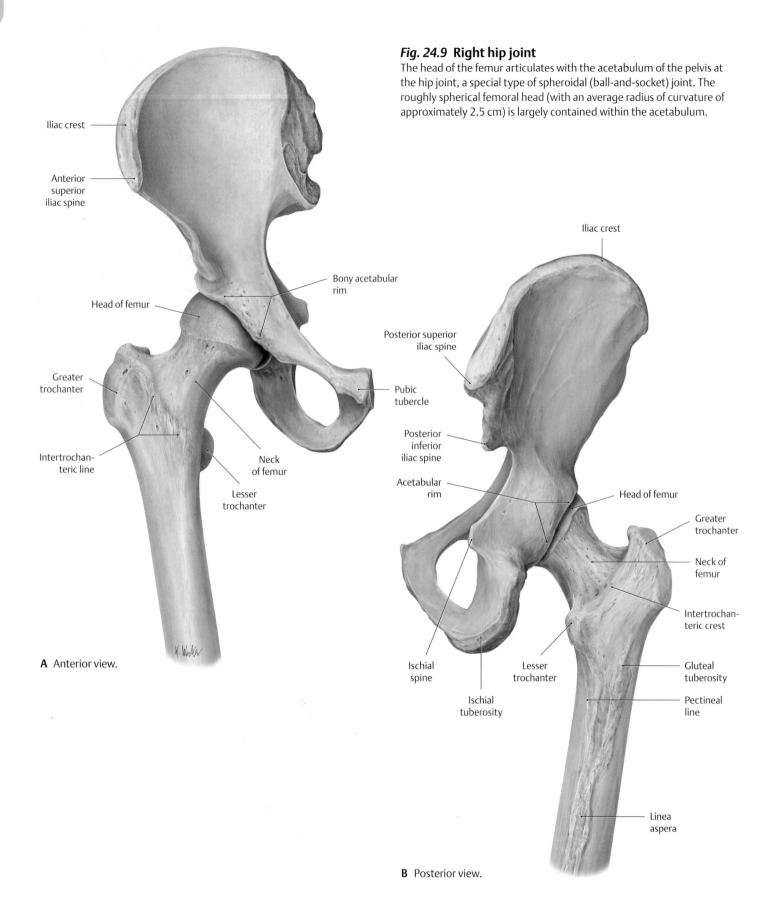

Fig. 24.9 Right hip joint

The head of the femur articulates with the acetabulum of the pelvis at the hip joint, a special type of spheroidal (ball-and-socket) joint. The roughly spherical femoral head (with an average radius of curvature of approximately 2.5 cm) is largely contained within the acetabulum.

Iliac crest

Anterior superior iliac spine

Bony acetabular rim

Head of femur

Greater trochanter

Intertrochanteric line

Lesser trochanter

Neck of femur

Pubic tubercle

Posterior superior iliac spine

Posterior inferior iliac spine

Acetabular rim

Head of femur

Greater trochanter

Neck of femur

Intertrochanteric crest

Ischial spine

Ischial tuberosity

Lesser trochanter

Gluteal tuberosity

Pectineal line

Linea aspera

Iliac crest

A Anterior view.

B Posterior view.

Fig. 24.10 Hip joint: Coronal section

Right hip joint, anterior view.

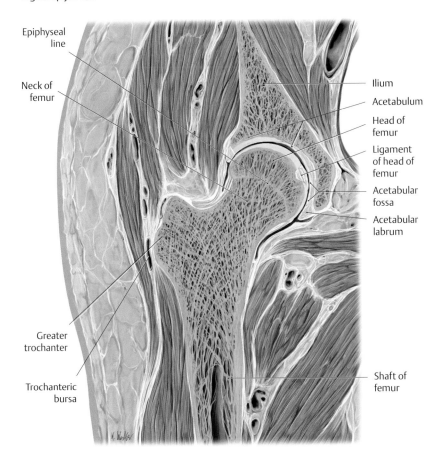

Epiphyseal line

Neck of femur

Ilium

Acetabulum

Head of femur

Ligament of head of femur

Acetabular fossa

Acetabular labrum

Greater trochanter

Trochanteric bursa

Shaft of femur

A Coronal section.

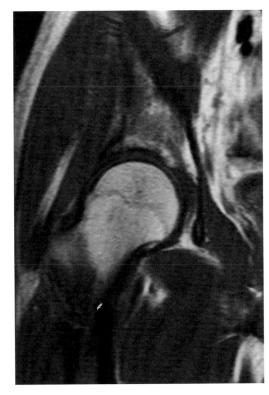

B T1-weighted MRI.

✳ Clinical

Diagnosing hip dysplasia and dislocation

Ultrasonography, the most important imaging method for screening the infant hip, is used to identify morphological changes such as hip dysplasia and dislocation. Clinically, hip dislocation presents itself with instability and limited abduction of the hip joint, and leg shortening with asymmetry of the gluteal folds.

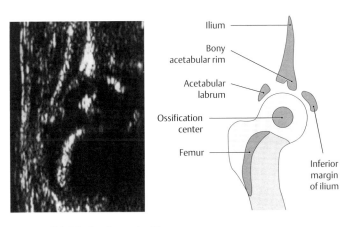

Ilium

Bony acetabular rim

Acetabular labrum

Ossification center

Femur

Inferior margin of ilium

A Normal hip joint in a 5-month-old.

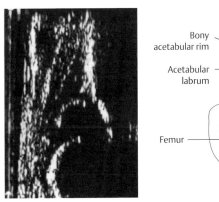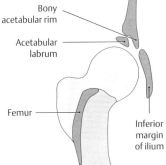

Bony acetabular rim

Acetabular labrum

Femur

Inferior margin of ilium

B Hip dislocation and dysplasia in a 3-month-old.

Hip Joint: Ligaments & Capsule

The hip joint has three major ligaments: iliofemoral, pubofemoral, and ischiofemoral. The zona orbicularis (annular ligament) is not visible externally and encircles the femoral neck like a buttonhole.

Fig. 24.11 **Hip joint: Lateral view**

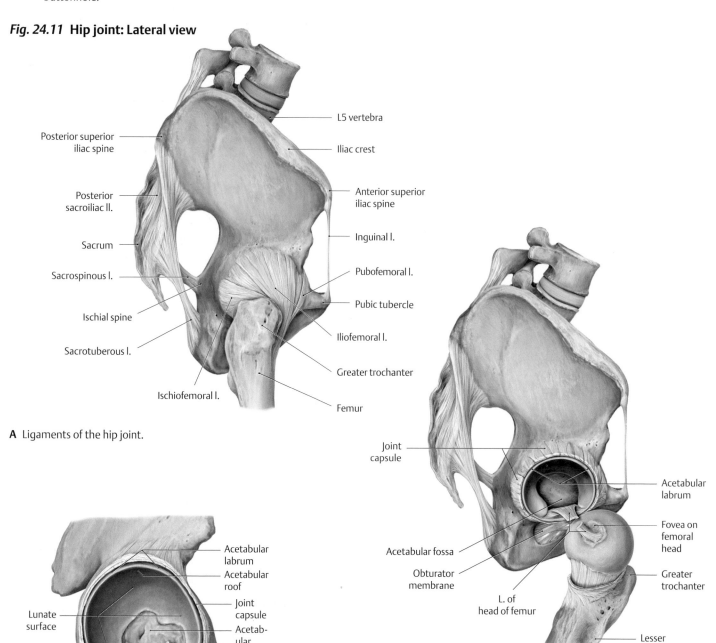

A Ligaments of the hip joint.

C Acetabulum of right hip joint. *Note:* The ligament of the femoral head (cut) transmits branches from the obturator artery that nourish the femoral head (see p. 421).

B Joint capsule. The capsule has been divided and the femoral head dislocated to expose the cut ligament of the head of the femur.

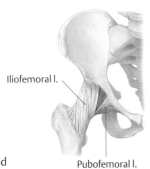

Iliofemoral l.

Pubofemoral l.

A Ligaments and weak spot (red).

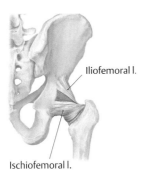

Synovial membrane

Reflection of synovial membrane

Neck of femur

Greater trochanter

Intertrochanteric line

Fibrous membrane

Lesser trochanter

C Joint capsule. *Removed:* Fibrous membrane (at level of femoral neck). *Exposed:* Synovial membrane.

Fig. 24.12 Hip joint: Anterior view

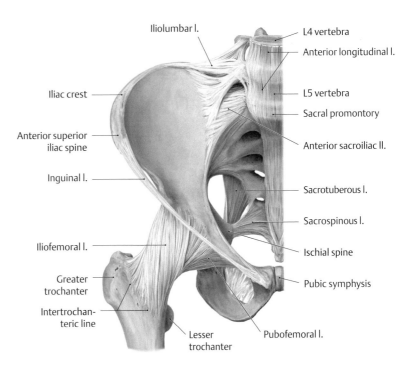

Iliolumbar l.

L4 vertebra

Anterior longitudinal l.

Iliac crest

L5 vertebra

Sacral promontory

Anterior superior iliac spine

Anterior sacroiliac ll.

Inguinal l.

Sacrotuberous l.

Sacrospinous l.

Iliofemoral l.

Ischial spine

Greater trochanter

Pubic symphysis

Intertrochanteric line

Lesser trochanter

Pubofemoral l.

B Ligaments of the hip joint.

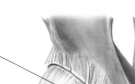

Iliofemoral l.

Ischiofemoral l.

A Ligaments and weak spot (red).

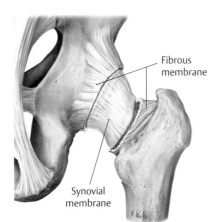

Fibrous membrane

Synovial membrane

C Joint capsule.

Fig. 24.13 Hip Joint: Posterior view

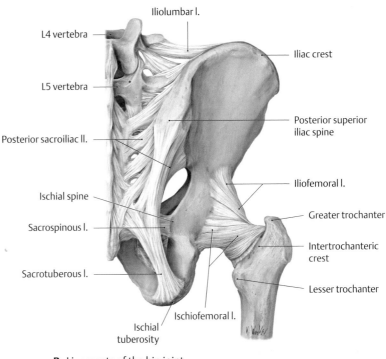

Iliolumbar l.

L4 vertebra

Iliac crest

L5 vertebra

Posterior superior iliac spine

Posterior sacroiliac ll.

Iliofemoral l.

Ischial spine

Greater trochanter

Sacrospinous l.

Intertrochanteric crest

Sacrotuberous l.

Lesser trochanter

Ischiofemoral l.

Ischial tuberosity

B Ligaments of the hip joint.

Anterior Muscles of the Thigh, Hip & Gluteal Region (I)

***Fig. 24.14* Muscles of the hip and thigh: Anterior view (I)**
Right limb. Muscle origins (O) are shown in red, insertions (I) in blue.

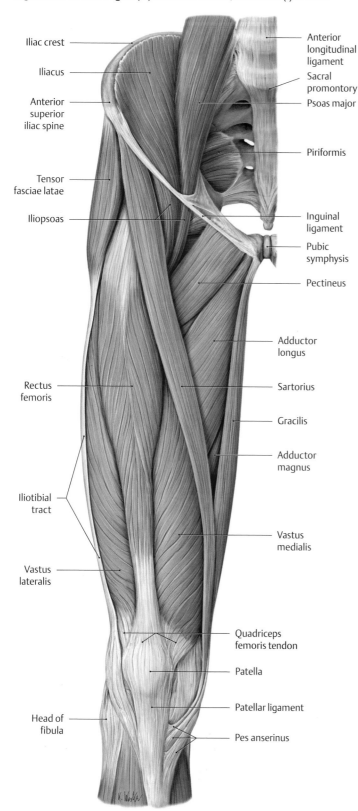

Iliac crest
Iliacus
Anterior superior iliac spine
Tensor fasciae latae
Iliopsoas
Rectus femoris
Iliotibial tract
Vastus lateralis
Head of fibula

Anterior longitudinal ligament
Sacral promontory
Psoas major
Piriformis
Inguinal ligament
Pubic symphysis
Pectineus
Adductor longus
Sartorius
Gracilis
Adductor magnus
Vastus medialis
Quadriceps femoris tendon
Patella
Patellar ligament
Pes anserinus

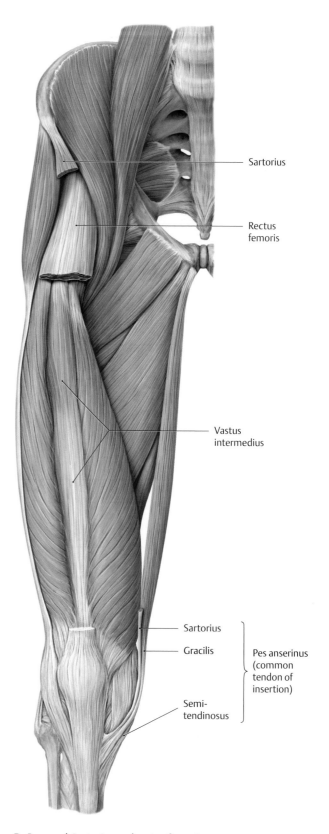

Sartorius
Rectus femoris
Vastus intermedius
Sartorius
Gracilis
Pes anserinus (common tendon of insertion)
Semi-tendinosus

A *Removed:* Fascia lata of thigh (to the lateral iliotibial tract).

B *Removed:* Sartorius and rectus femoris.

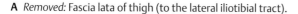

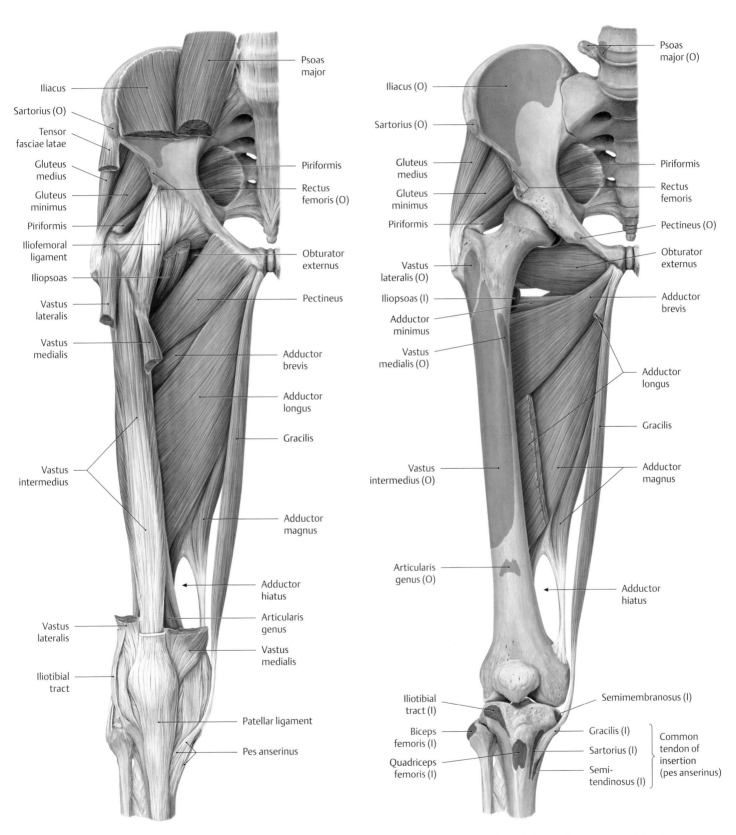

Psoas
major

Iliacus

Sartorius (O)

Tensor
fasciae latae

Gluteus
medius

Gluteus
minimus

Piriformis

Iliofemoral
ligament

Iliopsoas

Vastus
lateralis

Vastus
medialis

Vastus
intermedius

Vastus
lateralis

Iliotibial
tract

Piriformis

Rectus
femoris (O)

Obturator
externus

Pectineus

Adductor
brevis

Adductor
longus

Gracilis

Adductor
magnus

Adductor
hiatus

Articularis
genus

Vastus
medialis

Patellar ligament

Pes anserinus

Psoas
major (O)

Iliacus (O)

Sartorius (O)

Gluteus
medius

Gluteus
minimus

Piriformis

Vastus
lateralis (O)

Iliopsoas (I)

Adductor
minimus

Vastus
medialis (O)

Vastus
intermedius (O)

Articularis
genus (O)

Iliotibial
tract (I)

Biceps
femoris (I)

Quadriceps
femoris (I)

Piriformis

Rectus
femoris

Pectineus (O)

Obturator
externus

Adductor
brevis

Adductor
longus

Gracilis

Adductor
magnus

Adductor
hiatus

Semimembranosus (I)

Gracilis (I)

Sartorius (I)

Semi-
tendinosus (I)

Common
tendon of
insertion
(pes anserinus)

C *Removed:* Rectus femoris (completely), vastus lateralis, vastus medialis, iliopsoas, and tensor fasciae latae.

D *Removed:* Quadriceps femoris (rectus femoris, vastus lateralis, vastus
medialis, vastus intermedius), iliopsoas, tensor fasciae latae, pectineus,
and midportion of adductor longus.

Anterior Muscles of the Thigh, Hip & Gluteal Region (II)

Fig. 24.15 **Muscles of the hip and thigh: Anterior view (II)**
Right limb. Muscle origins (O) are shown in red, insertions (I) in blue.

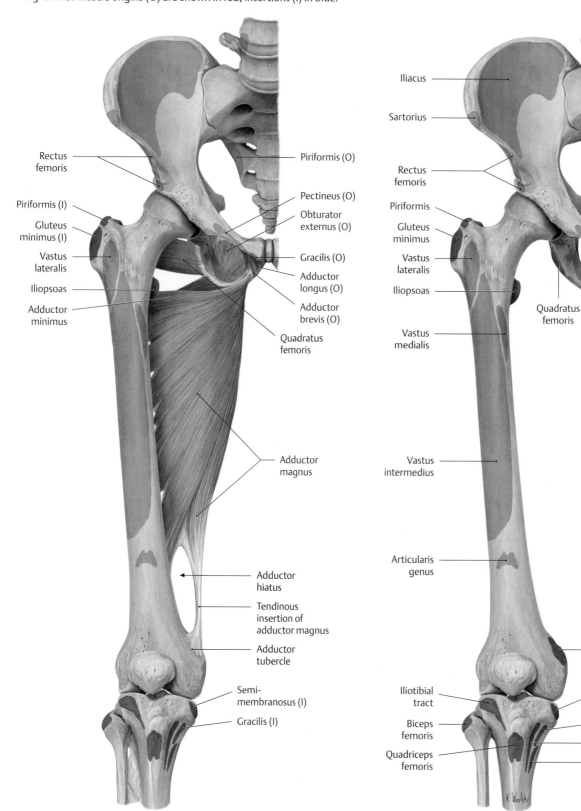

A *Removed:* Gluteus medius and minimus, piriformis, obturator externus, adductor brevis and longus, and gracilis.

B *Removed:* All muscles.

Fig. 24.16 Muscles of the hip, thigh, and gluteal region: Medial view
Midsagittal section.

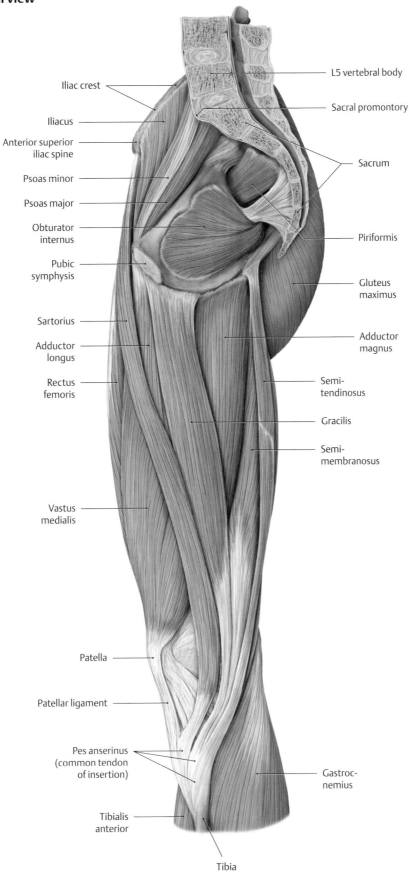

Iliac crest

Iliacus

Anterior superior iliac spine

Psoas minor

Psoas major

Obturator internus

Pubic symphysis

Sartorius

Adductor longus

Rectus femoris

Vastus medialis

Patella

Patellar ligament

Pes anserinus (common tendon of insertion)

Tibialis anterior

Tibia

L5 vertebral body

Sacral promontory

Sacrum

Piriformis

Gluteus maximus

Adductor magnus

Semi-tendinosus

Gracilis

Semi-membranosus

Gastroc-nemius

Posterior Muscles of the Thigh, Hip & Gluteal Region (I)

***Fig. 24.17* Muscles of the hip, thigh, and gluteal region: Posterior view (I)**
Right limb. Muscle origins (O) are shown in red, insertions (I) in blue.

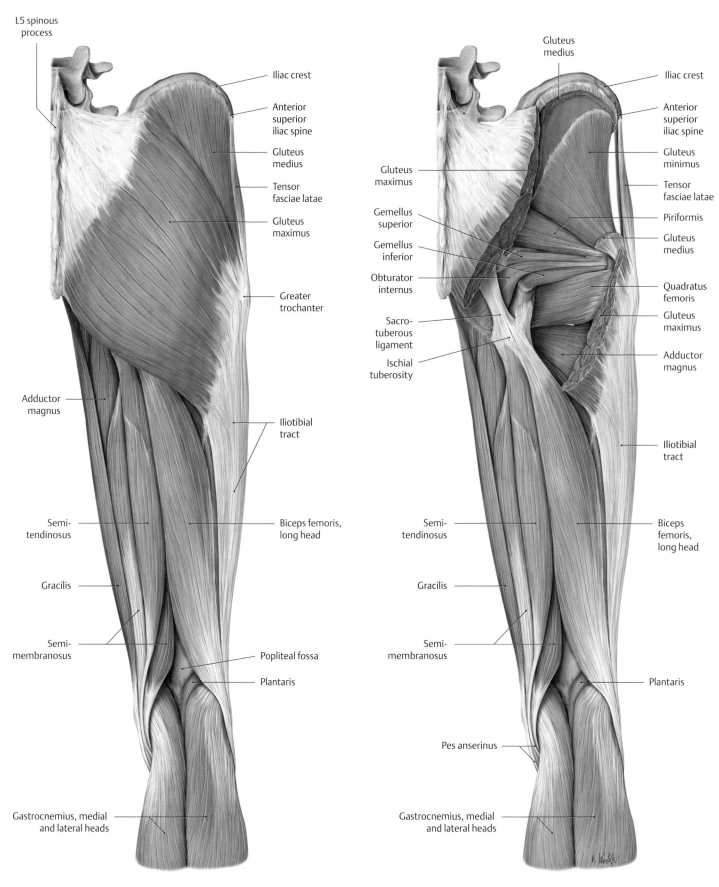

A *Removed:* Fascia lata (to iliotibial tract).

B *Partially removed:* Gluteus maximus and medius.

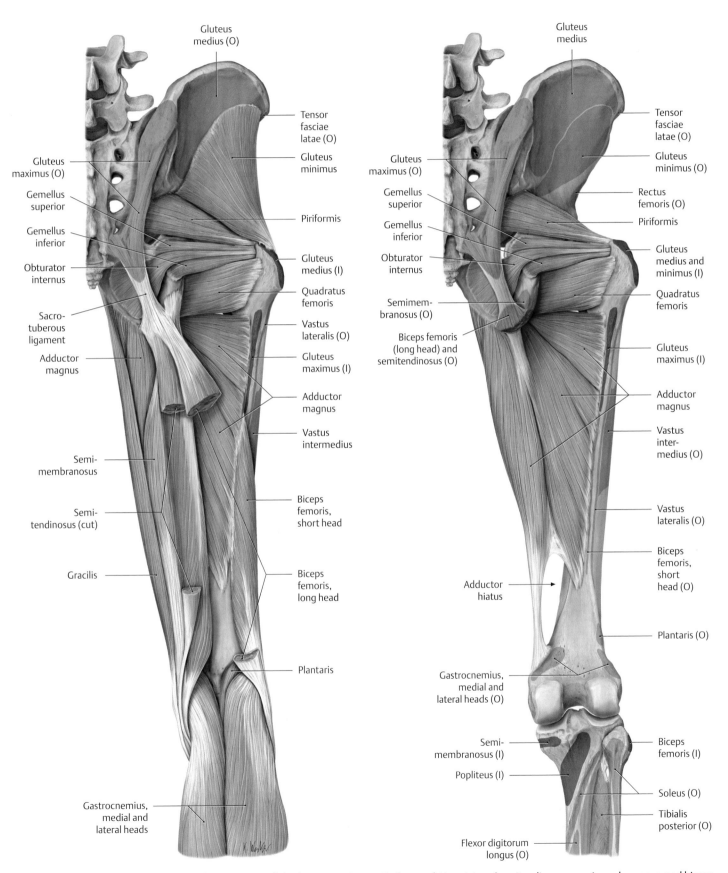

Gluteus medius (O)

Tensor fasciae latae (O)

Gluteus minimus

Gluteus maximus (O)

Gemellus superior

Gemellus inferior

Obturator internus

Piriformis

Gluteus medius (I)

Quadratus femoris

Vastus lateralis (O)

Gluteus maximus (I)

Sacro-tuberous ligament

Adductor magnus

Adductor magnus

Vastus intermedius

Semi-membranosus

Semi-tendinosus (cut)

Gracilis

Biceps femoris, short head

Biceps femoris, long head

Plantaris

Gastrocnemius, medial and lateral heads

Gluteus medius

Tensor fasciae latae (O)

Gluteus minimus (O)

Rectus femoris (O)

Piriformis

Gluteus medius and minimus (I)

Quadratus femoris

Gluteus maximus (I)

Adductor magnus

Vastus inter-medius (O)

Vastus lateralis (O)

Biceps femoris, short head (O)

Plantaris (O)

Gluteus maximus (O)

Gemellus superior

Gemellus inferior

Obturator internus

Semimem-branosus (O)

Biceps femoris (long head) and semitendinosus (O)

Adductor hiatus

Gastrocnemius, medial and lateral heads (O)

Semi-membranosus (I)

Popliteus (I)

Flexor digitorum longus (O)

Biceps femoris (I)

Soleus (O)

Tibialis posterior (O)

C *Removed:* Semitendinosus and biceps femoris (partially); gluteus maximus and medius (completely).

D *Removed:* Hamstrings (semitendinosus, semimembranosus, and biceps femoris), gluteus minimus, gastrocnemius, and muscles of the leg.

Posterior Muscles of the Thigh, Hip & Gluteal Region (II)

***Fig. 24.18* Muscles of the hip, thigh, and gluteal region: Posterior view (II)**
Right limb. Muscle origins (O) are shown in red, insertions (I) in blue.

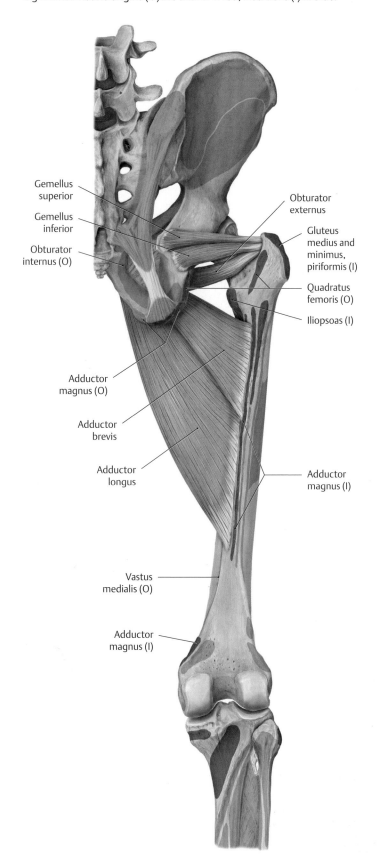

Gluteus medius

Gemellus superior

Gemellus inferior

Obturator internus (O)

Obturator externus

Gluteus medius and minimus, piriformis (I)

Quadratus femoris (O)

Iliopsoas (I)

Adductor magnus (O)

Adductor brevis

Adductor longus

Adductor magnus (I)

Vastus medialis (O)

Adductor magnus (I)

Gluteus maximus

Gemellus superior

Gemellus inferior

Obturator internus

Semi-membranosus

Biceps femoris (long head) and semitendinosus

Adductor magnus

Iliopsoas

Vastus medialis

Adductor longus

Adductor magnus

Gastrocnemius, medial and lateral heads

Semi-membranosus

Popliteus

Flexor digitorum longus

Tensor fasciae latae

Gluteus minimus

Rectus femoris

Obturator internus and externus, gemellus superior and inferior

Gluteus medius and minimus, piriformis

Quadratus femoris

Gluteus maximus

Pectineus

Vastus lateralis

Adductor brevis

Vastus intermedius

Adductor magnus

Biceps femoris, short head

Plantaris

Biceps femoris

Soleus

Tibialis posterior

A *Removed:* Piriformis, obturator internus, quadratus femoris, and adductor magnus.

B *Removed:* All muscles.

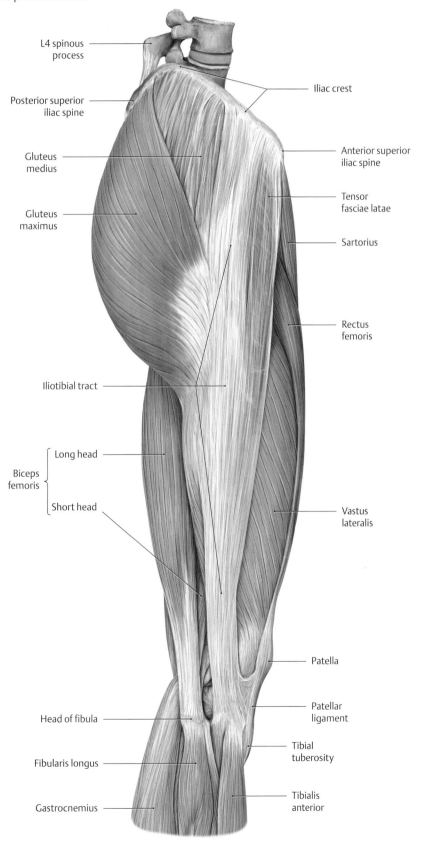

Fig. 24.19 Muscles of the hip, thigh, and gluteal region: Lateral view

Note: The iliotibial tract (the thickened band of fascia lata) functions as a tension band to reduce the bending loads on the proximal femur.

L4 spinous process

Iliac crest

Posterior superior iliac spine

Gluteus medius

Anterior superior iliac spine

Tensor fasciae latae

Gluteus maximus

Sartorius

Rectus femoris

Iliotibial tract

Long head

Biceps femoris

Short head

Vastus lateralis

Patella

Patellar ligament

Head of fibula

Tibial tuberosity

Fibularis longus

Tibialis anterior

Gastrocnemius

Muscle Facts (I)

Table 24.1 Psoas and iliacus muscles

Muscles		Origin	Insertion	Innervation	Action
③ Iliopsoas	Psoas minor	T12–L1 vertebrae and intervertebral disk (lateral surfaces)	Iliopectineal arch	Direct branches from the lumbar plexus (psoas) (L2–L4)	Assists in upward rotation of the pelvis
	① Psoas major	*Superficial:* T12–L4 and associated intervertebral disks (lateral surfaces) *Deep:* L1–L5 vertebrae (transverse processes)	Lesser trochanter		• Hip joint: flexion and external rotation • Lumbar spine: *unilateral* contraction (with the femur fixed) bends the trunk laterally to the same side; *bilateral* contraction raises the trunk from the supine position
	② Iliacus	Iliac fossa		Femoral n. (L2–L4)	

Fig. 24.20 Muscles of the hip
Right side.

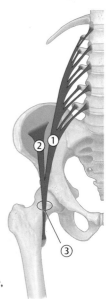

A Iliopsoas muscle, anterior view.

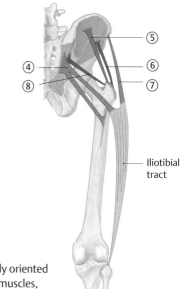

Iliotibial tract

B Vertically oriented gluteal muscles, posterior view.

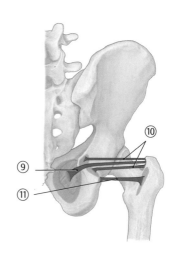

C Horizontally oriented gluteal muscles, posterior view.

Table 24.2 Gluteal muscles

Muscle	Origin	Insertion	Innervation	Action
④ Gluteus maximus	Sacrum (dorsal surface, lateral part), ilium (gluteal surface, posterior part), thoracolumbar fascia, sacrotuberous ligament	• Upper fibers: iliotibial tract • Lower fibers: gluteal tuberosity	Inferior gluteal n. (L5–S2)	• Entire muscle: extends and externally rotates the hip in sagittal and coronal planes • Upper fibers: abduction • Lower fibers: adduction
⑤ Gluteus medius	Ilium (gluteal surface below the iliac crest between the anterior and posterior gluteal line)	Greater trochanter of the femur (lateral surface)	Superior gluteal n. (L4–S1)	• Entire muscle: abducts the hip, stabilizes the pelvis in the coronal plane • Anterior part: flexion and internal rotation • Posterior part: extension and external rotation
⑥ Gluteus minimus	Ilium (gluteal surface below the origin of gluteus medius)	Greater trochanter of the femur (anterolateral surface)		
⑦ Tensor fasciae latae	Anterior superior iliac spine	Iliotibial tract		• Tenses the fascia lata • Hip joint: abduction, flexion, and internal rotation
⑧ Piriformis	Pelvic surface of the sacrum	Apex of the greater trochanter of the femur	Direct branches from the sacral plexus (S1–S2)	• External rotation, abduction, and extension of the hip joint • Stabilizes the hip joint
⑨ Obturator internus	Inner surface of the obturator membrane and its bony boundaries	Medial surface of the greater trochanter	Direct branches from the sacral plexus (L5, S1)	External rotation, adduction, and extension of the hip joint (also active in abduction, depending on the joint's position)
⑩ Gemelli	• Gemellus superior: ischial spine • Gemellus inferior: ischial tuberosity	Jointly with obturator internus tendon (medial surface, greater trochanter)		
⑪ Quadratus femoris	Lateral border of the ischial tuberosity	Intertrochanteric crest of the femur		External rotation and adduction of the hip joint

Fig. 24.21 Psoas and iliacus muscles

Right side, anterior view.

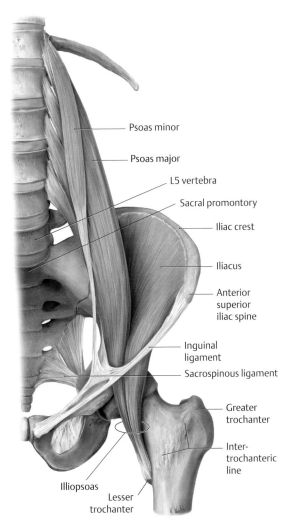

- Psoas minor
- Psoas major
- L5 vertebra
- Sacral promontory
- Iliac crest
- Iliacus
- Anterior superior iliac spine
- Inguinal ligament
- Sacrospinous ligament
- Greater trochanter
- Intertrochanteric line
- Illiopsoas
- Lesser trochanter

Fig. 24.22 Superficial muscles of the gluteal region

Right side, posterior view.

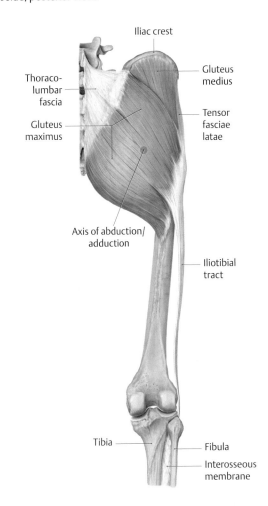

- Iliac crest
- Thoraco-lumbar fascia
- Gluteus medius
- Gluteus maximus
- Tensor fasciae latae
- Axis of abduction/adduction
- Iliotibial tract
- Tibia
- Fibula
- Interosseous membrane

Fig. 24.23 Deep muscles of the gluteal region

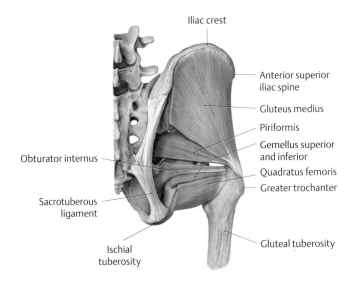

- Iliac crest
- Anterior superior iliac spine
- Gluteus medius
- Piriformis
- Gemellus superior and inferior
- Quadratus femoris
- Greater trochanter
- Obturator internus
- Sacrotuberous ligament
- Gluteal tuberosity
- Ischial tuberosity

A Deep layer with gluteus maximus removed.

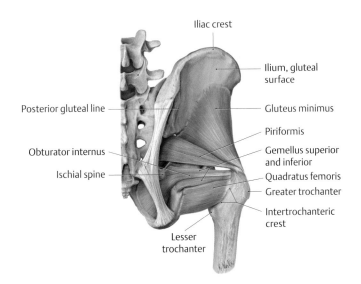

- Iliac crest
- Ilium, gluteal surface
- Posterior gluteal line
- Gluteus minimus
- Piriformis
- Obturator internus
- Gemellus superior and inferior
- Ischial spine
- Quadratus femoris
- Greater trochanter
- Intertrochanteric crest
- Lesser trochanter

B Deep layer with gluteus medius removed.

Muscle Facts (II)

Functionally, the medial thigh muscles are considered the adductors of the hip.

Fig. 24.24 **Medial group: Superficial layer**
Right side, anterior view.

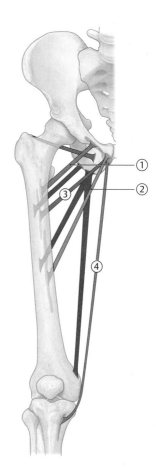

A Schematic.

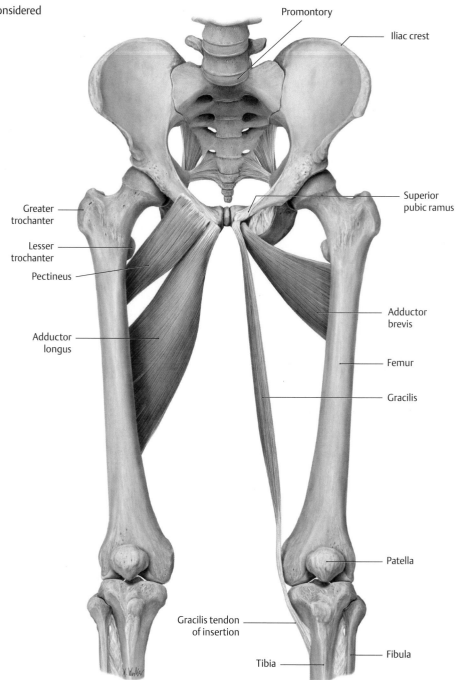

B Superficial adductor group.

Table 24.3	**Medial thigh muscles: Superficial layer**			
Muscle	**Origin**	**Insertion**	**Innervation**	**Action**
① Pectineus	Pecten pubis	Femur (pectineal line and the proximal linea aspera)	Femoral n., obturator n. (L2, L3)	• Hip joint: adduction, external rotation, and slight flexion • Stabilizes the pelvis in the coronal and sagittal planes
② Adductor longus	Superior pubic ramus and anterior side of the symphysis	Femur (linea aspera, medial lip in the middle third of the femur)	Obturator n. (L2–L4)	• Hip joint: adduction and flexion (up to 70 degrees); extension (past 80 degrees of flexion) • Stabilizes the pelvis in the coronal and sagittal planes
③ Adductor brevis	Inferior pubic ramus			
④ Gracilis	Inferior pubic ramus below the symphysis	Tibia (medial border of the tuberosity, along with the tendons of sartorius and semitendinosus)	Obturator n. (L2, L3)	• Hip joint: adduction and flexion • Knee joint: flexion and internal rotation

Fig. 24.25 Medial group: Deep layer

Right side, anterior view.

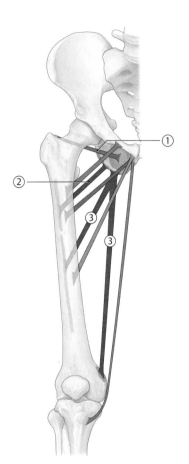

A Schematic.

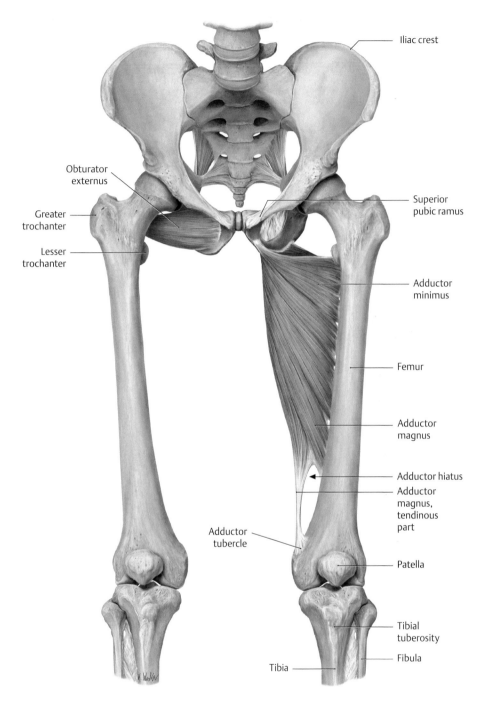

B Deep adductor group.

Table 24.4	Medial thigh muscles: Deep layer			
Muscle	**Origin**	**Insertion**	**Innervation**	**Action**
① Obturator externus	Outer surface of the obturator membrane and its bony boundaries	Trochanteric fossa of the femur	Obturator n. (L3, L4)	• Hip joint: adduction and external rotation • Stabilizes the pelvis in the sagittal plane
② Adductor minimus	Inferior pubic ramus	Medial lip of the linea aspera	Obturator n. (L2–L4)	Hip joint: adduction extension, and slight flexion of the hip joint
③ Adductor magnus	Inferior pubic ramus, ischial ramus, and ischial tuberosity	• Deep part ("fleshy insertion"): medial lip of the linea spine • Superficial part ("tendinous insertion"): adductor tubercle of the femur	• Deep part: obturator n. (L2–L4) • Superficial part: tibial n. (L4)	• Hip joint: adduction, extention, and slight flexion (the tendinous insertion is also active in internal rotation) • Stabilizes the pelvis in the coronal and sagittal plane

377

Muscle Facts (III)

The anterior and posterior muscles of the thigh can be classified as extensors and flexors, respectively, with regard to the knee joint.

Fig. 24.26 Anterior thigh muscles

Right side, anterior view.

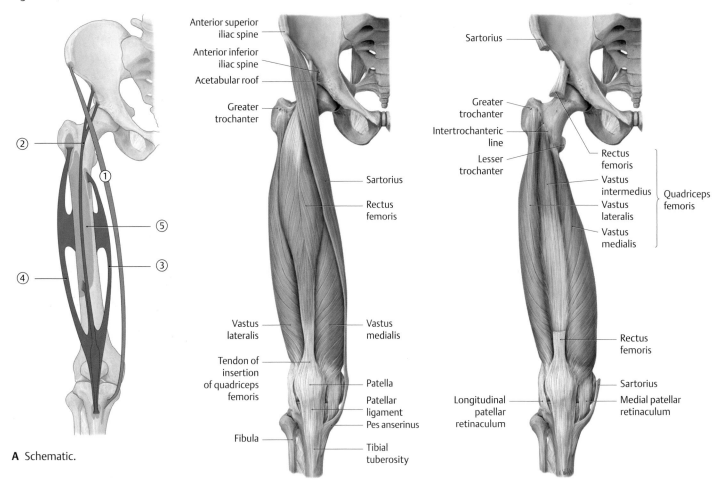

A Schematic.

B Superficial group.

C Deep group. *Removed:* Sartorius and rectus femoris.

Table 24.5		Anterior thigh muscles			
Muscle		**Origin**	**Insertion**	**Innervation**	**Action**
① Sartorius		Anterior superior iliac spine	Medial to the tibial tuberosity (together with gracilis and semitendinosus)	Femoral n. (L2, L3)	• Hip joint: flexion, abduction, and external rotation • Knee joint: flexion and internal rotation
Quadriceps femoris*	② Rectus femoris	Anterior inferior iliac spine, acetabular roof of hip joint	Tibial tuberosity (via patellar ligament)	Femoral n. (L2–L4)	• Hip joint: flexion • Knee joint: extension
	③ Vastus medialis	Linea aspera (medial lip), intertrochanteric line (distal part)	Both sides of tuberosity on the medial and lateral condyles (via the medial and longitudinal patellar retinacula)		Knee joint: extension
	④ Vastus lateralis	Linea aspera (lateral lip), greater trochanter (lateral surface)			
	⑤ Vastus intermedius	Femoral shaft (anterior side)	Tibial tuberosity (via patellar ligament)		
	Articularis genus (distal fibers of vastus intermedius)	Anterior side of femoral shaft at level of the suprapatellar recess	Suprapatellar recess of knee joint capsule		Knee joint: extension; prevents entrapment of capsule
*The entire muscle inserts on the tibial tuberosity via the patellar ligament.					

Fig. 24.27 Posterior thigh muscles

Right side, posterior view.

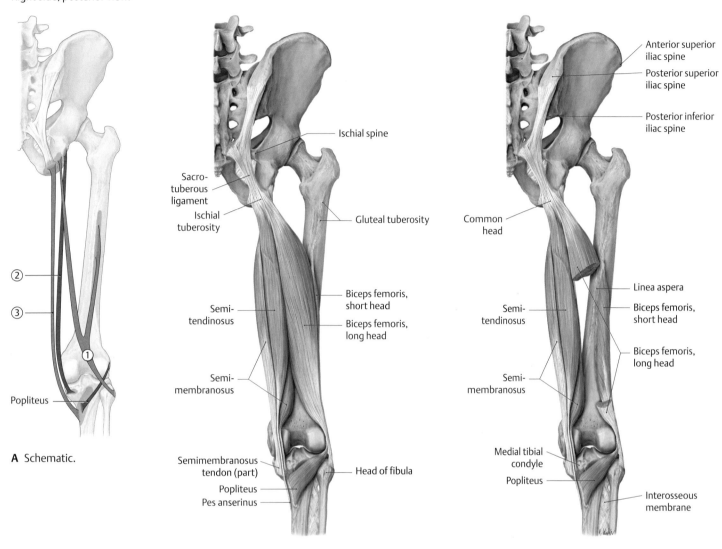

A Schematic.

B Superficial group.

C Deep group. *Removed:* Biceps femoris (long head) and semitendinosus.

Table 24.6	Posterior thigh muscles			
Muscle	**Origin**	**Insertion**	**Innervation**	**Action**
① Biceps femoris	Long head: ischial tuberosity, sacrotuberous ligament (common head with semitendinosus)	Head of fibula	Tibial n. (L5–S2)	• Hip joint (long head): extends the hip, stabilizes the pelvis in the sagittal plane • Knee joint: flexion and external rotation
	Short head: lateral lip of the linea aspera in the middle third of the femur		Common fibular n. (L5–S2)	Knee joint: flexion and external rotation
② Semimembranosus	Ischial tuberosity	Medial tibial condyle, oblique popliteal ligament, popliteus fascia	Tibial n. (L5–S2)	• Hip joint: extends the hip, stabilizes the pelvis in the sagittal plane • Knee joint: flexion and internal rotation
③ Semitendinosus	Ischial tuberosity and sacrotuberous ligament (common head with long head of biceps femoris)	Medial to the tibial tuberosity in the pes anserinus (along with the tendons of gracilis and sartorius)		
See p. 399 for popliteus.				

Tibia & Fibula

 The tibia and fibula articulate at two joints, allowing limited motion (rotation). The crural interosseous membrane is a sheet of tough connective tissue that serves as an origin for several muscles in the leg. It also acts with the tibiofibular syndesmosis to stabilize the ankle joint.

Fig. 25.1 **Tibia and fibula**
Right leg.

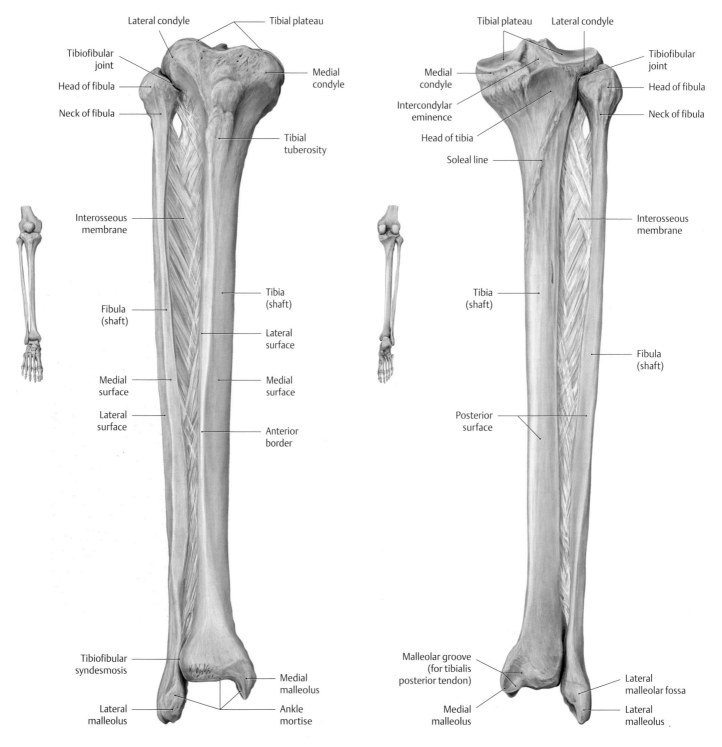

A Anterior view.

B Posterior view.

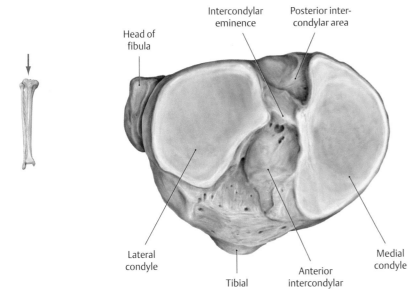

C Proximal view.

Labels: Head of fibula; Intercondylar eminence; Posterior inter-condylar area; Lateral condyle; Tibial tuberosity; Anterior intercondylar area; Medial condyle

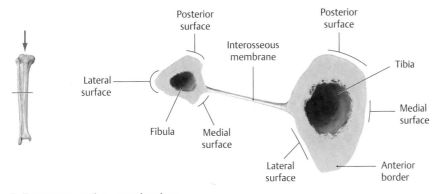

D Transverse section, superior view.

Labels: Posterior surface; Posterior surface; Interosseous membrane; Tibia; Lateral surface; Medial surface; Fibula; Medial surface; Lateral surface; Anterior border

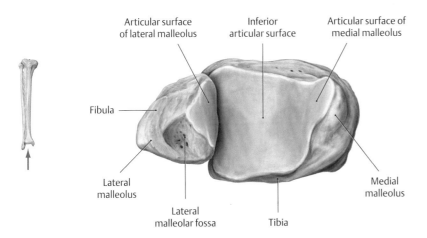

E Distal view.

Labels: Articular surface of lateral malleolus; Inferior articular surface; Articular surface of medial malleolus; Fibula; Lateral malleolus; Lateral malleolar fossa; Tibia; Medial malleolus

✳ *Clinical*

Fibular fracture

When diagnosing a fibular fracture, it is important to determine whether the syndesmosis (see p. 380) is disrupted. Fibular fractures may occur distal to, level with, or proximal to the syndesmosis; the latter two frequently involve tearing of the syndesmosis.

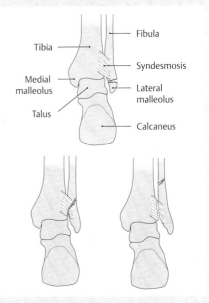

Labels: Tibia; Fibula; Syndesmosis; Medial malleolus; Lateral malleolus; Talus; Calcaneus

In this fracture, located proximal to the syndesmosis, the syndesmosis is torn, as indicated by the widened medial joint space of the upper ankle joint (see p. 405).

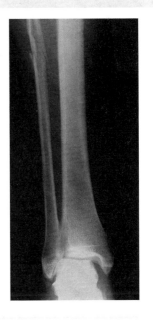

Knee Joint: Overview

In the knee joint, the femur articulates with the tibia and patella. Both joints are contained within a common capsule and have communicating articular cavities. *Note:* The fibula is not included in the knee joint (contrast to the humerus in the elbow; see p. 282). Instead, it forms a separate rigid articulation with the tibia.

Fig. 25.2 **Right knee joint**

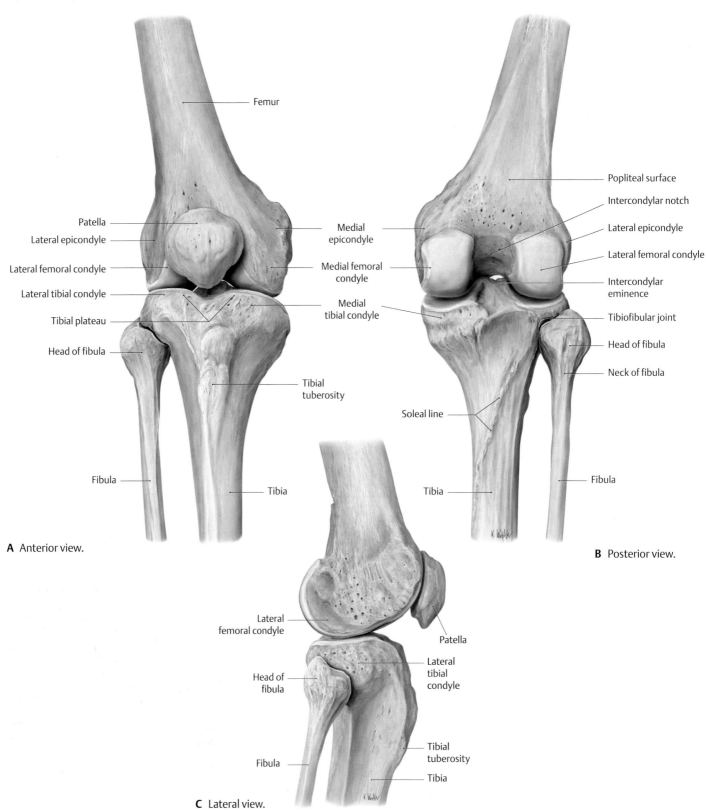

A Anterior view.

B Posterior view.

C Lateral view.

Fig. 25.4 Patella

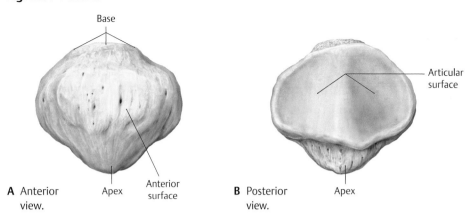

Base

A Anterior view. — Apex — Anterior surface

B Posterior view. — Apex — Articular surface

Fig. 25.3 Knee joint: Radiographs

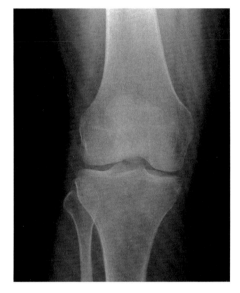

A Anteroposterior projection.

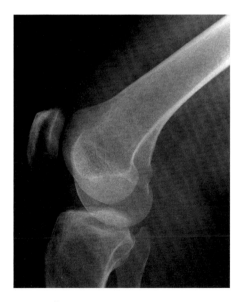

B Lateral projection.

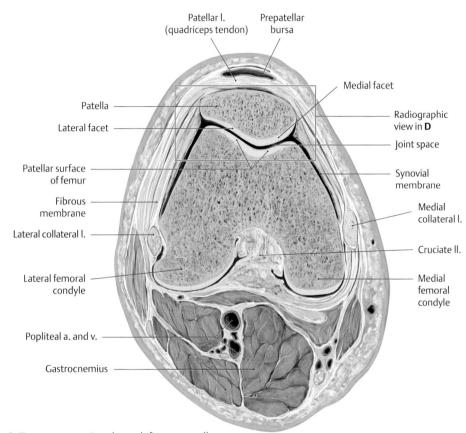

Patellar l. (quadriceps tendon) — Prepatellar bursa — Medial facet — Radiographic view in **D** — Joint space — Synovial membrane — Medial collateral l. — Cruciate ll. — Medial femoral condyle

Patella — Lateral facet — Patellar surface of femur — Fibrous membrane — Lateral collateral l. — Lateral femoral condyle — Popliteal a. and v. — Gastrocnemius

C Transverse section through femoropatellar joint. Distal view with right knee in slight flexion.

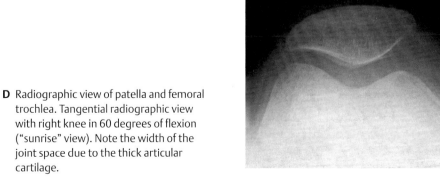

D Radiographic view of patella and femoral trochlea. Tangential radiographic view with right knee in 60 degrees of flexion ("sunrise" view). Note the width of the joint space due to the thick articular cartilage.

Knee Joint: Capsule, Ligaments & Bursae

Table 25.1	Ligaments of the knee joint
Extrinsic ligaments	
Anterior side	Patellar l.
	Medial longitudinal patellar retinaculum
	Lateral longitudinal patellar retinaculum
	Medial transverse patellar retinaculum
	Lateral transverse patellar retinaculum
Medial and lateral sides	Medial (tibial) collateral l.
	Lateral (fibular) collateral l.
Posterior side	Oblique popliteal l.
	Arcuate popliteal l.
Intrinsic ligaments	
Anterior cruciate l.	
Posterior cruciate l.	
Transverse l. of knee	
Posterior meniscofemoral l.	

***Fig. 25.5* Ligaments of the knee joint**
Anterior view of right knee.

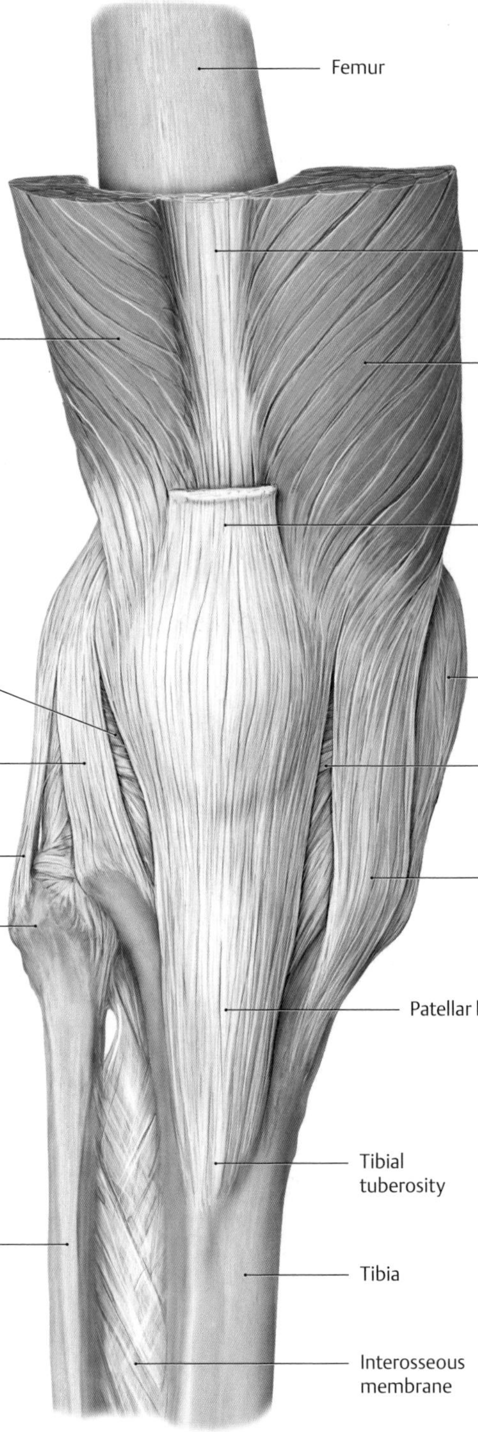

Fig. 25.6 Capsule, ligaments, and periarticular bursae

Posterior view of right knee. The joint cavity communicates with periarticular bursae at the subpopliteal recess, semimembranosus bursa, and medial subtendinous bursa of the gastrocnemius.

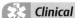

Gastrocnemio-semimembranosus bursa (Baker's cyst)
Painful swelling behind the knee may be caused by a cystic outpouching of the joint capsule (synovial popliteal cyst). This frequently results from a rise in intra-articular pressure (e.g., in rheumatoid arthritis).

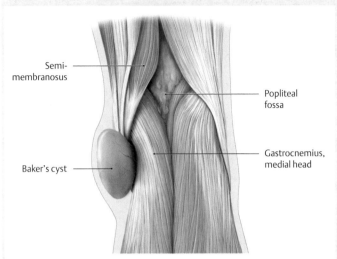

A Baker's cyst in the right popliteal fossa. Baker's cysts often occur in the medial part of the popliteal fossa between the semimembranosus tendon and the medial head of the gastrocnemius at the level of the posteromedial femoral condyle.

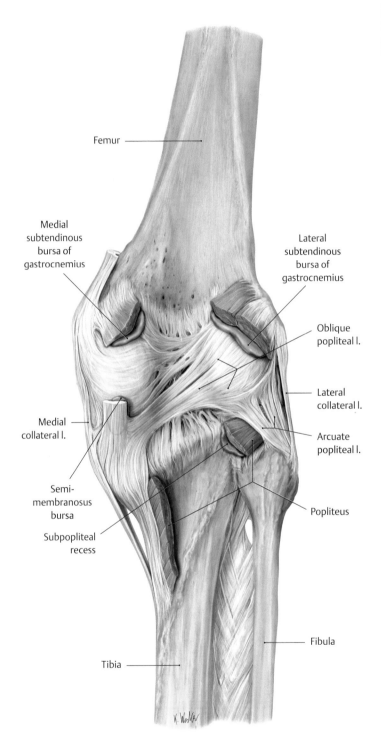

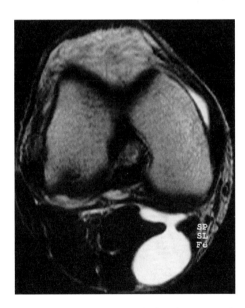

B Axial magnetic resonance imaging (MRI) of a Baker's cyst in the popliteal fossa, inferior view.

Knee Joint: Ligaments & Menisci

Fig. 25.7 Collateral and patellar ligaments of the knee joint

Right knee joint. Each knee joint has medial and lateral collateral ligaments. The medial collateral ligament is attached to both the capsule and the medial meniscus, whereas the lateral collateral ligament has no direct contact with either the capsule or the lateral meniscus. Both collateral ligaments are taut when the knee is in extension and stabilize the joint in the coronal plane.

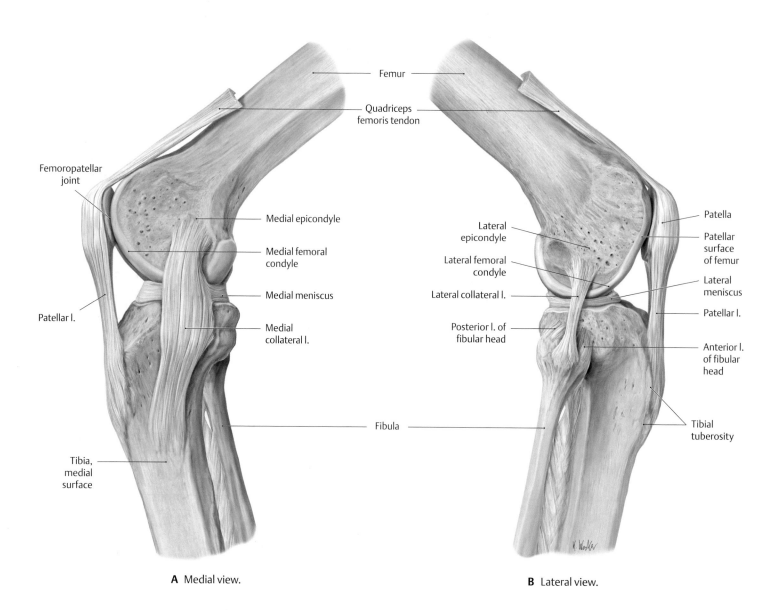

Femur

Quadriceps femoris tendon

Femoropatellar joint

Medial epicondyle

Medial femoral condyle

Medial meniscus

Patellar l.

Medial collateral l.

Tibia, medial surface

Fibula

Lateral epicondyle

Lateral femoral condyle

Lateral collateral l.

Posterior l. of fibular head

Patella

Patellar surface of femur

Lateral meniscus

Patellar l.

Anterior l. of fibular head

Tibial tuberosity

A Medial view.

B Lateral view.

Fig. 25.8 Menisci in the knee joint

Right tibial plateau, proximal view.

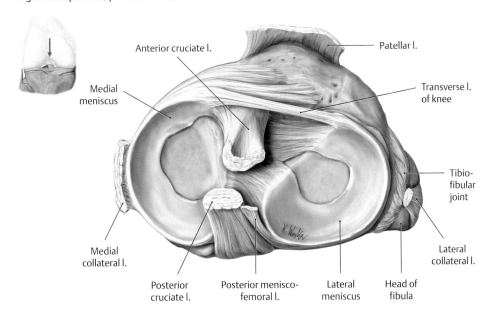

A Right tibial plateau with cruciate, patellar, and collateral ligaments divided.

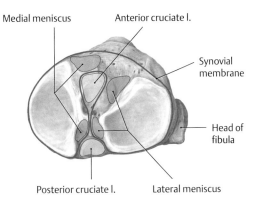

B Attachment sites of menisci and cruciate ligaments. Red line indicates the tibial attachment of the synovial membrane that covers the cruciate ligaments. The cruciate ligaments lie in the subsynovial connective tissue.

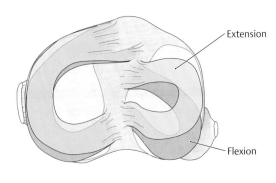
Fig. 25.9 Movements of the menisci

Right knee joint.

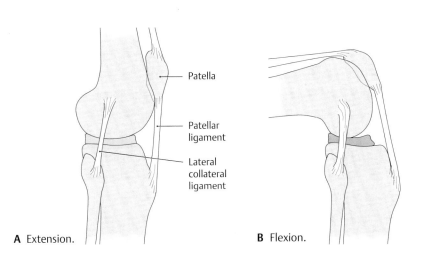

A Extension.

B Flexion.

C Tibial plateau, proximal view.

Cruciate Ligaments

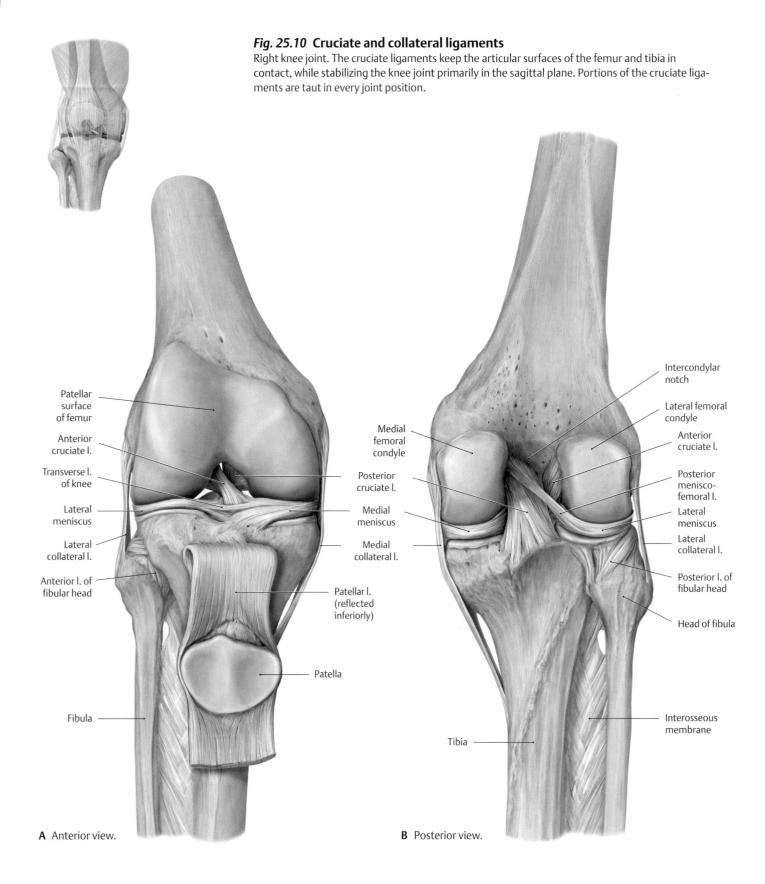

Fig. 25.10 **Cruciate and collateral ligaments**

Right knee joint. The cruciate ligaments keep the articular surfaces of the femur and tibia in contact, while stabilizing the knee joint primarily in the sagittal plane. Portions of the cruciate ligaments are taut in every joint position.

Patellar surface of femur

Anterior cruciate l.

Transverse l. of knee

Lateral meniscus

Lateral collateral l.

Anterior l. of fibular head

Fibula

Posterior cruciate l.

Medial meniscus

Medial collateral l.

Patellar l. (reflected inferiorly)

Patella

A Anterior view.

Intercondylar notch

Lateral femoral condyle

Anterior cruciate l.

Posterior menisco-femoral l.

Lateral meniscus

Lateral collateral l.

Posterior l. of fibular head

Head of fibula

Medial femoral condyle

Interosseous membrane

Tibia

B Posterior view.

Fig. 25.11 Right knee joint in flexion

Anterior view with joint capsule and patella removed.

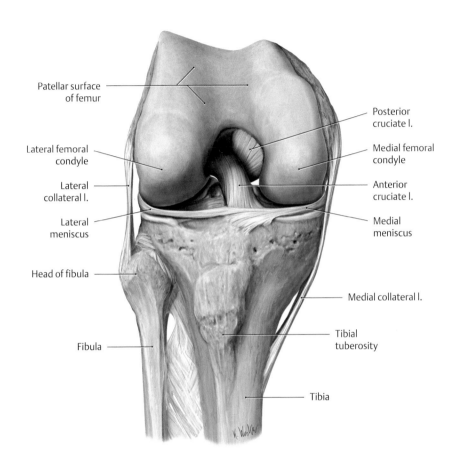

Patellar surface
of femur

Posterior
cruciate l.

Lateral femoral
condyle

Medial femoral
condyle

Lateral
collateral l.

Anterior
cruciate l.

Lateral
meniscus

Medial
meniscus

Head of fibula

Medial collateral l.

Fibula

Tibial
tuberosity

Tibia

Fig. 25.12 Cruciate and collateral ligaments in flexion and extension

Right knee, anterior view. Taut ligament fibers in red.

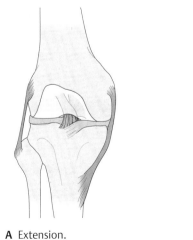

A Extension.

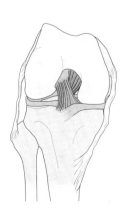

B Flexion.

25 Knee & Leg

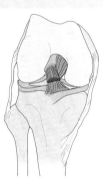
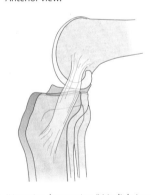
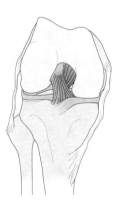

C Flexion and internal rotation.

Knee Joint Cavity

Fig. 25.13 Joint cavity

Right knee, lateral view. The joint cavity was demonstrated by injecting liquid plastic into the knee joint and later removing the capsule.

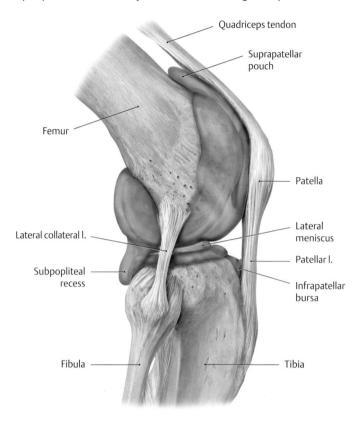

Quadriceps tendon

Suprapatellar pouch

Femur

Patella

Lateral collateral l.

Lateral meniscus

Subpopliteal recess

Patellar l.

Infrapatellar bursa

Fibula

Tibia

Fig. 25.15 Attachments of the joint capsule

Right knee joint, anterior view.

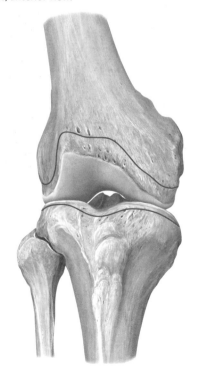

Fig. 25.14 Opened joint capsule

Right knee, anterior view with patella reflected downward.

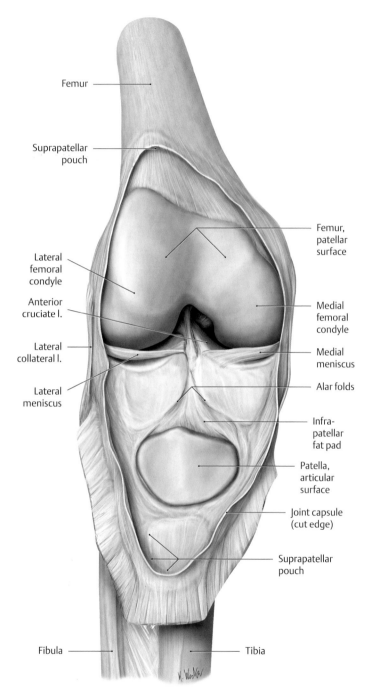

Femur

Suprapatellar pouch

Lateral femoral condyle

Anterior cruciate l.

Lateral collateral l.

Lateral meniscus

Femur, patellar surface

Medial femoral condyle

Medial meniscus

Alar folds

Infra-patellar fat pad

Patella, articular surface

Joint capsule (cut edge)

Suprapatellar pouch

Fibula

Tibia

K. Wesker

Fig. 25.16 Suprapatellar pouch during flexion

Right knee joint, medial view.

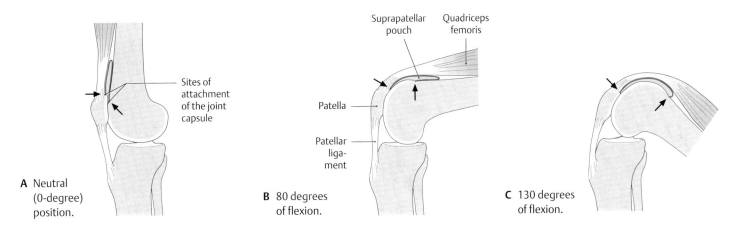

A Neutral (0-degree) position.

Sites of attachment of the joint capsule

Suprapatellar pouch

Quadriceps femoris

Patella

Patellar ligament

B 80 degrees of flexion.

C 130 degrees of flexion.

Fig. 25.17 Right knee joint: Midsagittal section

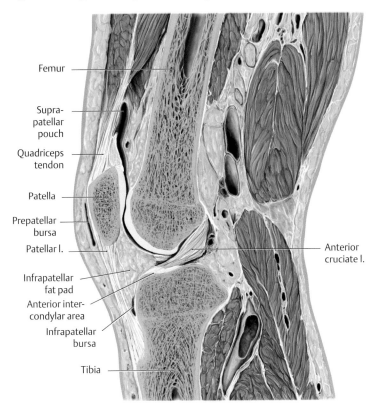

Femur

Suprapatellar pouch

Quadriceps tendon

Patella

Prepatellar bursa

Patellar l.

Infrapatellar fat pad

Anterior intercondylar area

Infrapatellar bursa

Tibia

Anterior cruciate l.

Fig. 25.18 MRI of knee joint

Sagittal T2-weighted MRI.

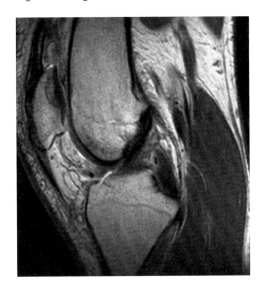

Muscles of the Leg: Anterior & Lateral Views

Fig. 25.19 Muscles of the leg: Anterior view

Right leg. Muscle origins (O) shown in red, insertions (I) in blue.

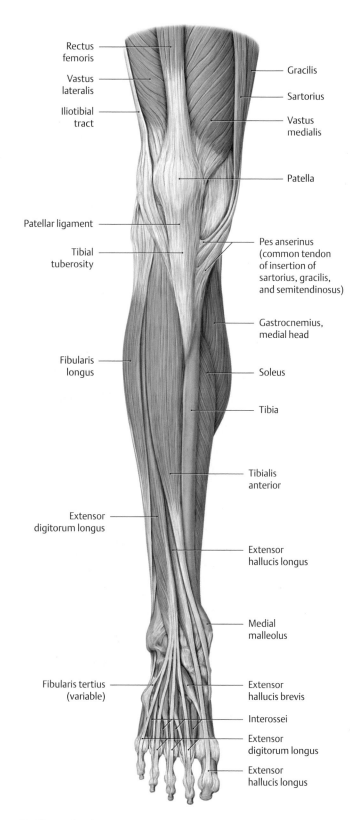

Rectus femoris
Vastus lateralis
Iliotibial tract
Gracilis
Sartorius
Vastus medialis
Patella
Patellar ligament
Tibial tuberosity
Pes anserinus (common tendon of insertion of sartorius, gracilis, and semitendinosus)
Gastrocnemius, medial head
Fibularis longus
Soleus
Tibia
Tibialis anterior
Extensor digitorum longus
Extensor hallucis longus
Medial malleolus
Fibularis tertius (variable)
Extensor hallucis brevis
Interossei
Extensor digitorum longus
Extensor hallucis longus

A All muscles shown.

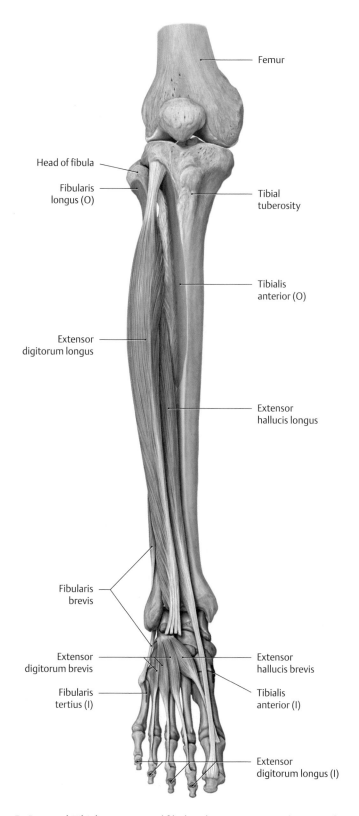

Femur
Head of fibula
Fibularis longus (O)
Tibial tuberosity
Tibialis anterior (O)
Extensor digitorum longus
Extensor hallucis longus
Fibularis brevis
Extensor digitorum brevis
Fibularis tertius (I)
Extensor hallucis brevis
Tibialis anterior (I)
Extensor digitorum longus (I)

B *Removed:* Tibialis anterior and fibularis longus; extensor digitorum longus tendons (distal portions). *Note:* The fibularis tertius is a division of the extensor digitorum longus.

Fig. 25.20 Muscles of the leg: Lateral view
Right leg.

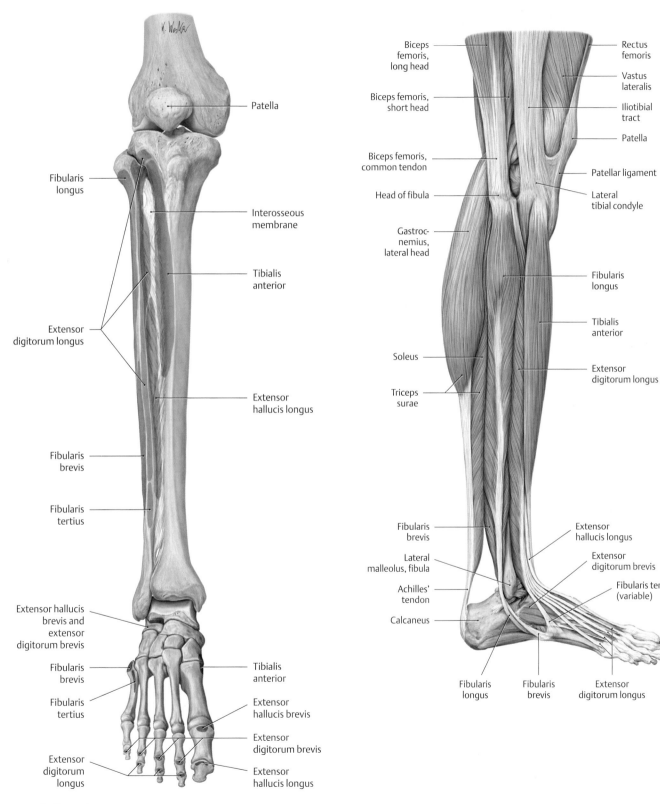

Patella

Fibularis longus

Interosseous membrane

Tibialis anterior

Extensor digitorum longus

Extensor hallucis longus

Fibularis brevis

Fibularis tertius

Extensor hallucis brevis and extensor digitorum brevis

Fibularis brevis

Tibialis anterior

Fibularis tertius

Extensor hallucis brevis

Extensor digitorum longus

Extensor digitorum brevis

Extensor hallucis longus

Biceps femoris, long head

Rectus femoris

Biceps femoris, short head

Vastus lateralis

Iliotibial tract

Patella

Biceps femoris, common tendon

Patellar ligament

Head of fibula

Lateral tibial condyle

Gastrocnemius, lateral head

Fibularis longus

Tibialis anterior

Extensor digitorum longus

Soleus

Triceps surae

Fibularis brevis

Extensor hallucis longus

Lateral malleolus, fibula

Extensor digitorum brevis

Achilles' tendon

Fibularis tertius (variable)

Calcaneus

Fibularis longus

Fibularis brevis

Extensor digitorum longus

C *Removed:* All muscles.

Muscles of the Leg: Posterior View

Fig. 25.21 **Muscles of the leg: Posterior view**
Right leg. Muscle origins (O) shown in red, insertions (I) in blue.

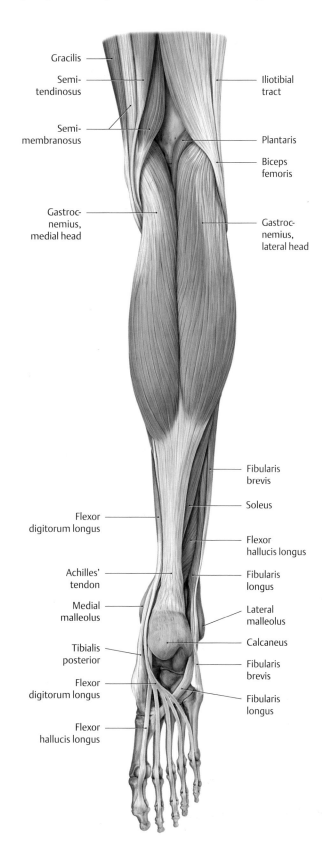

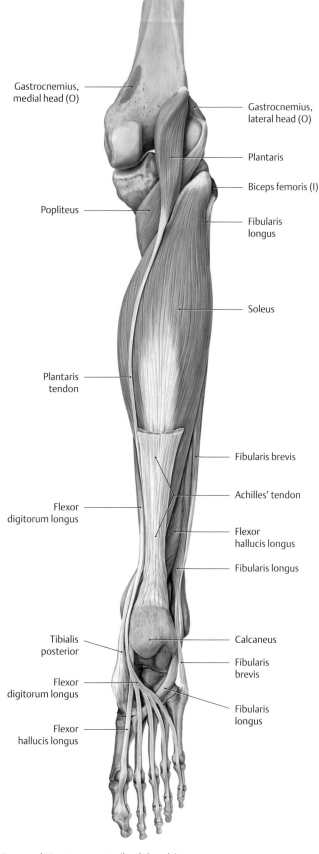

A *Note:* The bulge of the calf is produced mainly by the triceps surae (soleus and the two heads of the gastrocnemius).

B *Removed:* Gastrocnemius (both heads).

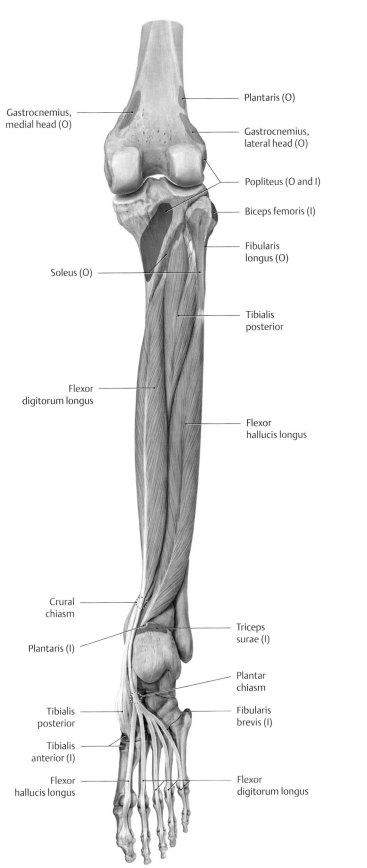

Gastrocnemius, medial head (O)

Plantaris (O)

Gastrocnemius, lateral head (O)

Popliteus (O and I)

Biceps femoris (I)

Fibularis longus (O)

Soleus (O)

Tibialis posterior

Flexor digitorum longus

Flexor hallucis longus

Crural chiasm

Triceps surae (I)

Plantaris (I)

Plantar chiasm

Tibialis posterior

Fibularis brevis (I)

Tibialis anterior (I)

Flexor hallucis longus

Flexor digitorum longus

C *Removed:* Triceps surae, plantaris, popliteus, and fibularis longus muscles.

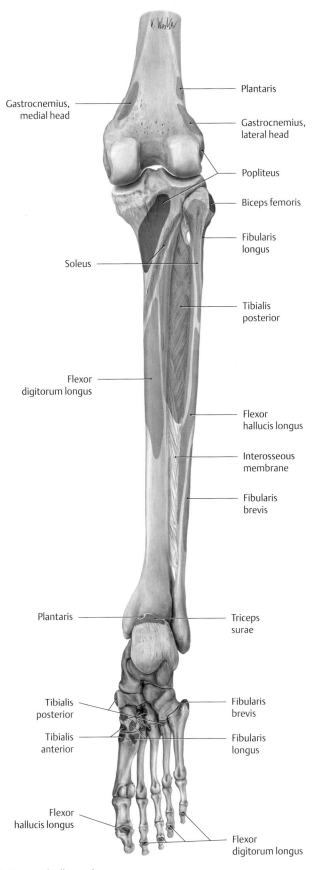

Gastrocnemius, medial head

Plantaris

Gastrocnemius, lateral head

Popliteus

Biceps femoris

Fibularis longus

Soleus

Tibialis posterior

Flexor digitorum longus

Flexor hallucis longus

Interosseous membrane

Fibularis brevis

Plantaris

Triceps surae

Tibialis posterior

Fibularis brevis

Tibialis anterior

Fibularis longus

Flexor hallucis longus

Flexor digitorum longus

D *Removed:* All muscles.

395

Muscle Facts (I)

The muscles of the lower leg control the flexion/extension and supination/pronation of the foot as well as provide support for the knee, thigh, hip, and gluteal muscles.

Fig. 25.22 **Lateral compartment**
Right leg and foot.

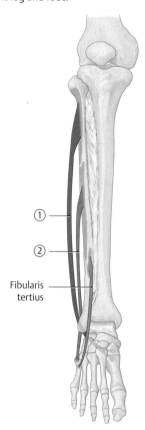

A Fibularis group, anterior view.

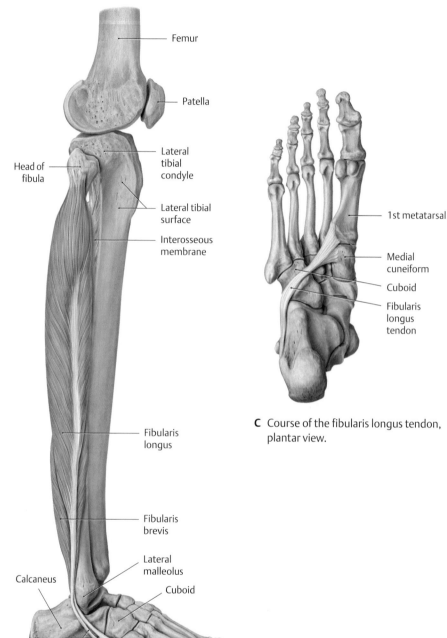

B Lateral compartment, right lateral view.

C Course of the fibularis longus tendon, plantar view.

Table 25.2	**Lateral compartment**			
Muscle	**Origin**	**Insertion**	**Innervation**	**Action**
① Fibularis longus	Fibula (head and proximal two thirds of the lateral surface, arising partly from the intermuscular septa)	Medial cuneiform (plantar side), 1st metatarsal (base)	Superficial fibular n. (L5, S1)	• Talocrural joint: plantar flexion • Subtalar joint: eversion (pronation) • Supports the transverse arch of the foot
② Fibularis brevis	Fibula (distal half of the lateral surface), intermuscular septa	5th metatarsal (tuberosity at the base, with an occasional division to the dorsal aponeurosis of the 5th toe)		• Talocrural joint: plantar flexion • Subtalar joint: eversion (pronation)

Fig. 25.23 **Anterior compartment**

Right leg, anterior view.

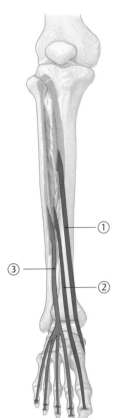

A Schematic.

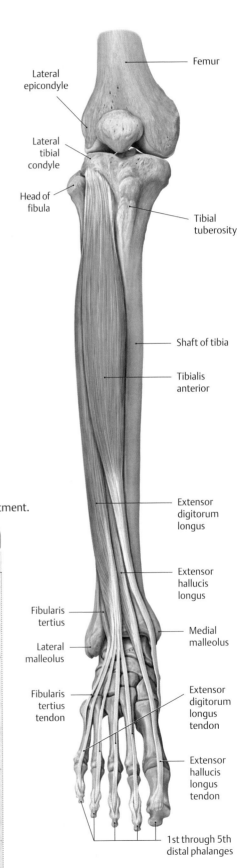

B Anterior compartment.

Table 25.3	**Anterior compartment**			
Muscle	**Origin**	**Insertion**	**Innervation**	**Action**
① Tibialis anterior	Tibia (upper two thirds of the lateral surface), interosseous membrane, and superficial crural fascia (highest part)	Medial cuneiform (medial and plantar surface), first metatarsal (medial base)	Deep fibular n. (L4, L5)	• Talocrural joint: dorsiflexion • Subtalar joint: inversion (supination)
② Extensor hallucis longus	Fibula (middle third of the medial surface) interosseous membrane	1st toe (at the dorsal aponeurosis and the base of its distal phalanx)	Deep fibular n. (L5)	• Talocrural joint: dorsiflexion • Subtalar joint: active in both eversion and inversion (pronation/supination), depending on the initial position of the foot • Extends the MTP and IP joints of the big toe
③ Extensor digitorum longus	Fibula (head and anterior border), tibia (lateral condyle), and interosseous membrane	2nd to 5th toes (at the dorsal aponeuroses and bases of the distal phalanges)	Deep fibular n. (L5, S1)	• Talocrural joint: dorsiflexion • Subtalar joint: eversion (pronation) • Extends the MTP and IP joints of the 2nd to 5th toes
Fibularis tertius (see Fig. 25.22A)	Distal fibula (anterior border)	5th metatarsal (base)	Deep fibular n. (L5, S1)	• Talocrural joint: dorsiflexion • Subtalar joint: eversion (pronation)
IP = interphalangeal; MTP = metatarsophalangeal.				

Muscle Facts (II)

The muscles of the posterior compartment are divided into two groups: the superficial and deep flexors. These groups are separated by the transverse intermuscular septum.

Fig. 25.24 **Superficial flexors**

Right leg, posterior view.

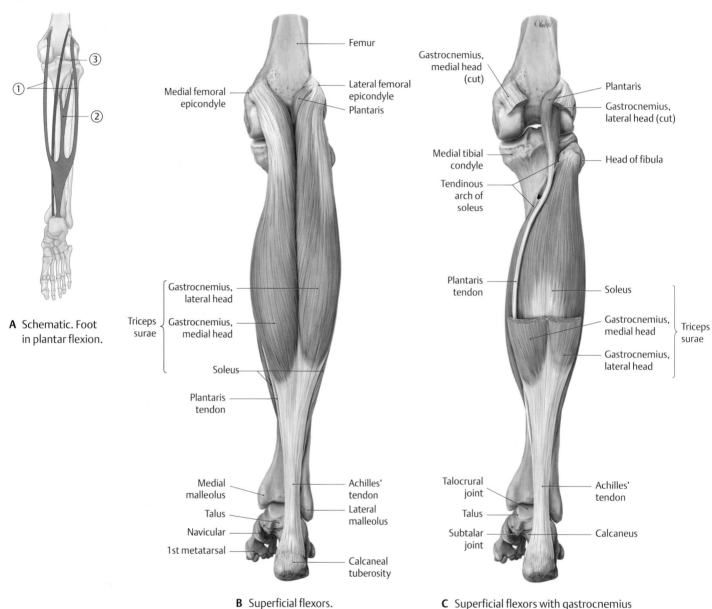

A Schematic. Foot in plantar flexion.

B Superficial flexors.

C Superficial flexors with gastrocnemius removed (portions of medial and lateral heads).

Table 25.4		Superficial flexors of the posterior compartment			
Muscle		**Origin**	**Insertion**	**Innervation**	**Action**
Triceps surae	① Gastrocnemius	Femur (medial and lateral epicondyles)	Calcaneal tuberosity via the Achilles' tendon	Tibial n. (S1, S2)	• Talocrural joint: plantar flexion • Knee joint: flexion (gastrocnemius)
	② Soleus	Fibula (head and neck, posterior surface), tibia (soleal line via a tendinous arch)			
③ Plantaris		Femur (lateral epicondyle, proximal to lateral head of gastrocnemius)			Negligible; may prevent compression of posterior leg musculature during knee flexion

Fig. 25.25 Deep flexors

Right leg with foot in plantar flexion, posterior view.

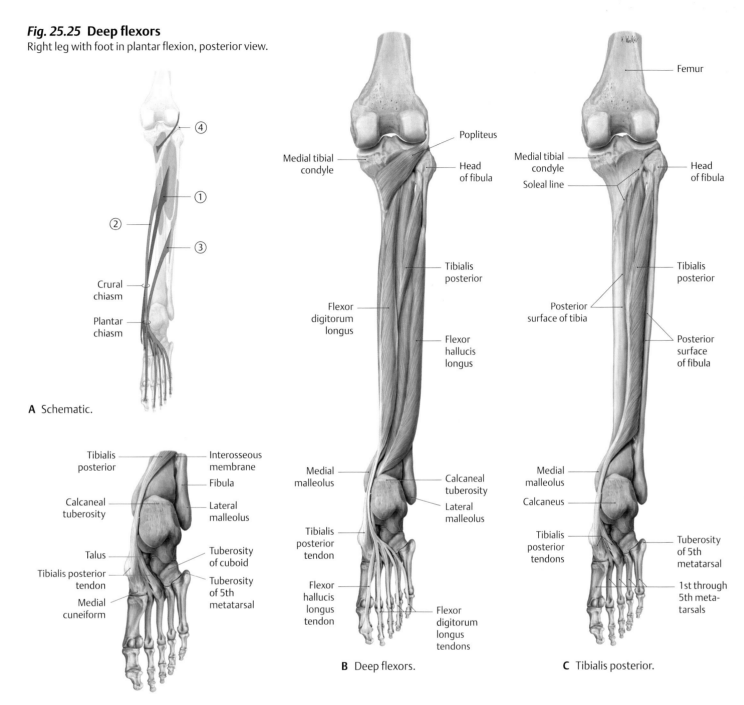

A Schematic.

B Deep flexors.

C Tibialis posterior.

D Insertion of the tibialis posterior.

Table 25.5		Deep flexors of the posterior compartment		
Muscle	**Origin**	**Insertion**	**Innervation**	**Action**
① Tibialis posterior	Interosseous membrane, adjacent borders of tibia and fibula	Navicular tuberosity; cuneiforms (medial, intermediate, and lateral); 2nd to 4th metatarsals (bases)	Tibial n. (L4, L5)	• Talocrural joint: plantar flexion • Subtalar joint: inversion (supination) • Supports the longitudinal and transverse arches
② Flexor digitorum longus	Tibia (middle third of posterior surface)	2nd to 5th distal phalanges (bases)	Tibial n. (L5–S2)	• Talocrural joint: plantar flexion • Subtalar joint: inversion (supination) • MTP and IP joints of the 2nd to 5th toes: plantar flexion
③ Flexor hallucis longus	Fibula (distal two thirds of posterior surface), adjacent interosseous membrane	1st distal phalanx (base)		• Talocrural joint: plantar flexion • Subtalar joint: inversion (supination) • MTP and IP joints of the 2nd to 5th toes: plantar flexion • Supports the medial longitudinal arch
④ Popliteus	Lateral femoral condyle, posterior horn of the lateral meniscus	Posterior tibial surface (above the origin at the soleus)	Tibial n. (L4–S1)	Knee joint: flexion and internal rotation (stabilizes the knee)
IP = interphalangeal; MTP = metatarsophalangeal.				

Bones of the Foot

Fig. 26.1 Subdivisions of the pedal skeleton

Right foot, dorsal view. Descriptive anatomy divides the skeletal elements of the foot into the tarsus, metatarsus, and forefoot (antetarsus). Functional and clinical criteria divide the pedal skeleton into hindfoot, midfoot, and forefoot.

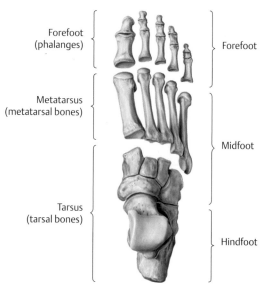

Fig. 26.2 Bones of the right foot

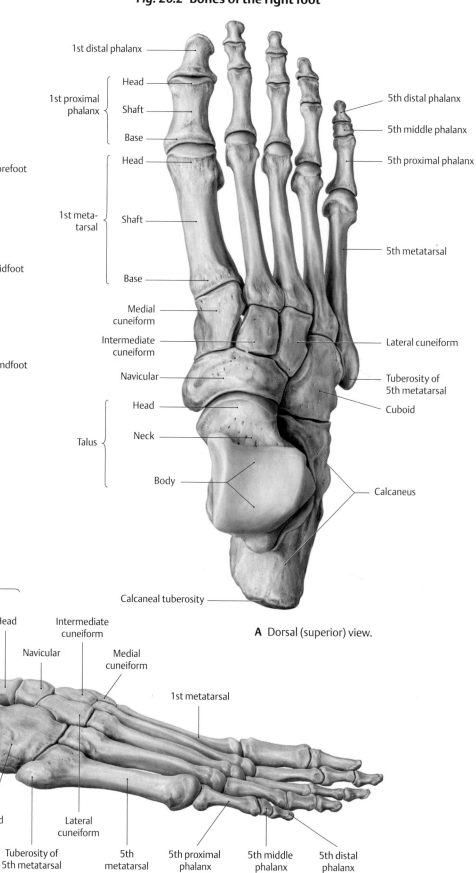

A Dorsal (superior) view.

B Lateral view.

400

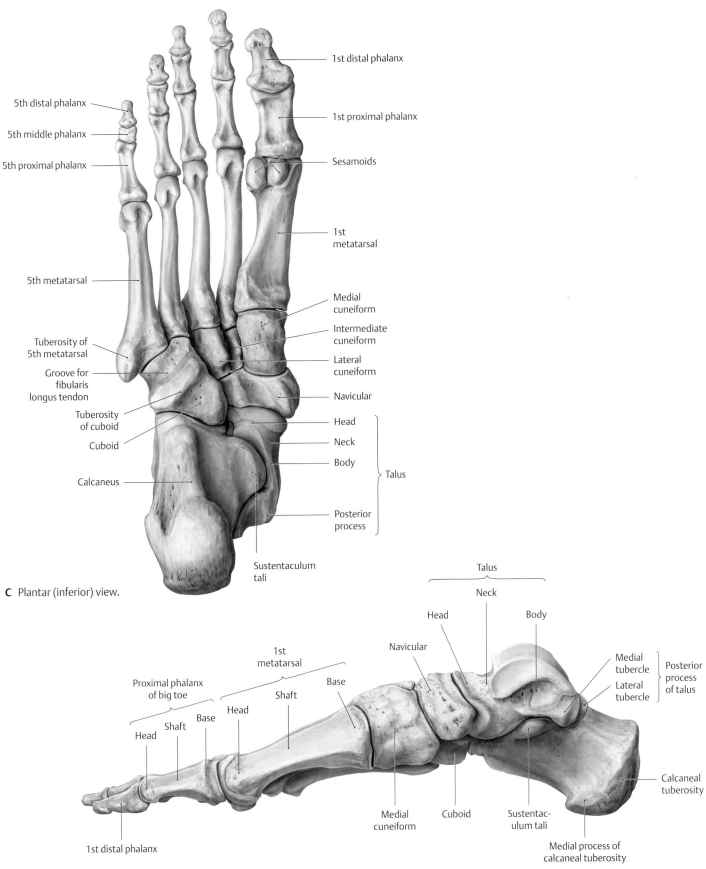

1st distal phalanx

5th distal phalanx

1st proximal phalanx

5th middle phalanx

5th proximal phalanx

Sesamoids

1st
metatarsal

5th metatarsal

Medial
cuneiform

Intermediate
cuneiform

Lateral
cuneiform

Tuberosity of
5th metatarsal

Groove for
fibularis
longus tendon

Navicular

Tuberosity
of cuboid

Head

Neck

Body

Talus

Cuboid

Calcaneus

Posterior
process

Sustentaculum
tali

C Plantar (inferior) view.

Talus

Neck

Head

Body

Navicular

Medial
tubercle

Posterior
process
of talus

1st
metatarsal

Lateral
tubercle

Proximal phalanx
of big toe

Base

Shaft

Head

Shaft

Base

Head

Calcaneal
tuberosity

Head

Shaft

Base

Medial
cuneiform

Cuboid

Sustentac-
ulum tali

1st distal phalanx

Medial process of
calcaneal tuberosity

D Medial view.

Joints of the Foot (I)

Handwritten annotations:

Plane Synovial Inversion/Eversion

Plane Synovial very little movement

Plane Synovial gliding

Hinge synovial Plantarflex/Dorsiflex.

Synovial ball & socket.

Plane Synovial Inversion/Eversion

condyloid synovial Flex/Extend, Abduct/Adduct.

Hinge Flex Extend

Hinge Flex/Extend

Subtalar (talocalcaneal) joint
Intercuneiform joints
Cuneocuboid joint
Tarsometatarsal joints

Talocrural (ankle) joint
Talonavicular joint
Calcaneocuboid joint
Tranverse tarsal joint
Cuneonavicular joint
Intermetatarsal joints
Metatarsophalangeal joints
Proximal interphalangeal joints

Distal interphalangeal joints

A Anterior view.

Plane of section

Fibula
Lateral malleolus
Interosseous talocalcanean ligament
Calcaneus
Talonavicular joint
Transverse tarsal joint
Calcaneo-cuboid joint
Cuboid
Intercuneiform joints
Tarsometatarsal joints (Lisfranc's joint line)
Abductor digiti minimi
Interossei
Proximal inter-phalangeal joints
5th middle phalanx
Distal inter-phalangeal joints

Tibia
Talocrural (ankle) joint
Medial malleolus
Talus
Navicular
Cuneonavicular joint
Intermediate cuneiform
Lateral cuneiform
Medial cuneiform
Abductor hallucis
1st metatarsal
1st metatarso-phalangeal joint
1st proximal phalanx
1st distal phalanx

B Superior view of coronal section.

Fig. 26.4 Proximal articular surfaces

Right foot, proximal view.

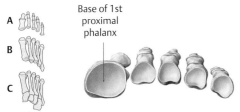

Base of 1st proximal phalanx

A Metatarsophalangeal joints.

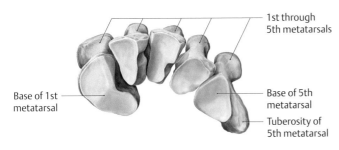

B Tarsometatarsal joints.

Base of 1st metatarsal

1st through 5th metatarsals

Base of 5th metatarsal

Tuberosity of 5th metatarsal

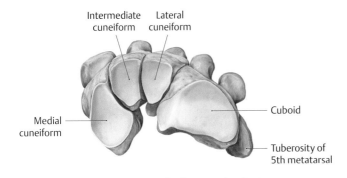

Intermediate cuneiform

Lateral cuneiform

Medial cuneiform

Cuboid

Tuberosity of 5th metatarsal

C Cuneonavicular and calcaneocuboid joints.

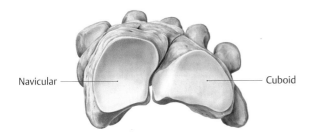

Navicular

Cuboid

D Talonavicular and calcaneocuboid joints.

Fig. 26.5 Distal articular surfaces

Right foot, distal view.

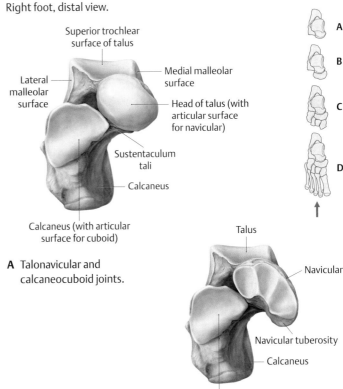

Superior trochlear surface of talus

Lateral malleolar surface

Medial malleolar surface

Head of talus (with articular surface for navicular)

Sustentaculum tali

Calcaneus

Calcaneus (with articular surface for cuboid)

A Talonavicular and calcaneocuboid joints.

Talus

Navicular

Navicular tuberosity

Calcaneus

Calcaneus (with articular surface for cuboid)

B Cuneonavicular and calcaneocuboid joints.

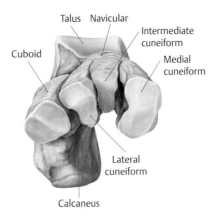

Talus Navicular

Cuboid

Intermediate cuneiform

Medial cuneiform

Lateral cuneiform

Calcaneus

C Tarsometatarsal joints.

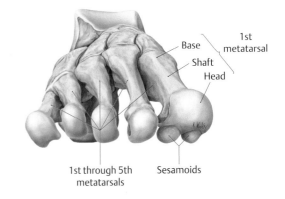

Base

Shaft

Head

1st metatarsal

1st through 5th metatarsals

Sesamoids

D Metatarsophalangeal joints.

Joints of the Foot (II)

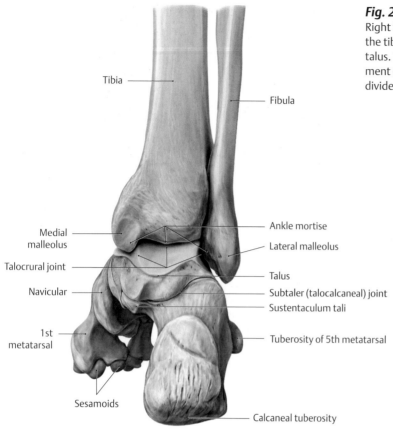

A Posterior view with foot in neutral (0-degree) position.

Fig. 26.6 Talocrural and subtalar joints

Right foot. The talocrural (ankle) joint is formed by the distal ends of the tibia and fibula (ankle mortise) articulating with the trochlea of the talus. The subtalar joint consists of an anterior and a posterior compartment (the talocalcanean and talocalcaneonavicular joints, respectively) divided by the interosseous talocalcanean ligament (see p. 409).

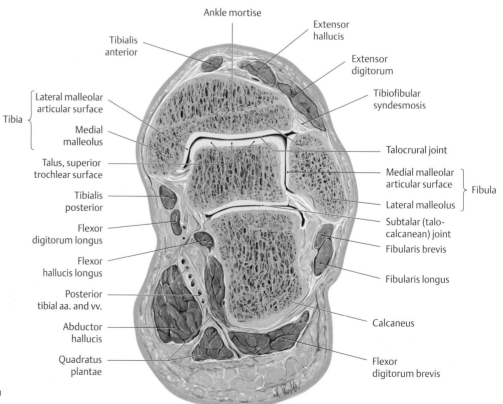

B Coronal section, proximal view. The talocrural joint is plantar flexed, and the subtalar joint has been sectioned through its posterior compartment.

Fig. 26.7 Talocrural and subtaler joints: Sagittal section
Right foot, medial view.

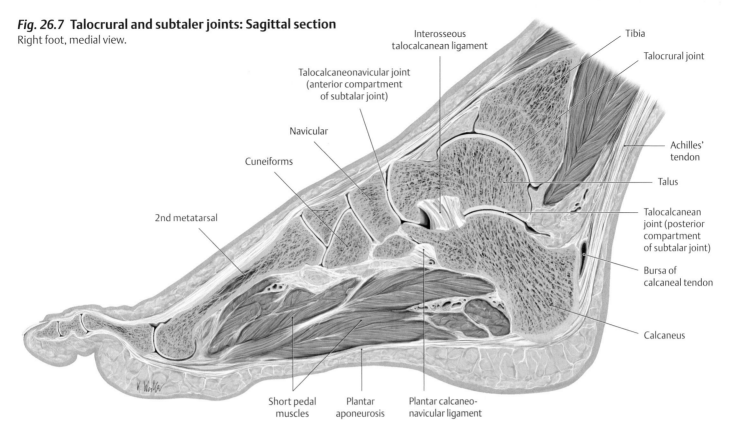

Interosseous talocalcanean ligament

Talocalcaneonavicular joint (anterior compartment of subtalar joint)

Navicular

Cuneiforms

2nd metatarsal

Tibia

Talocrural joint

Achilles' tendon

Talus

Talocalcanean joint (posterior compartment of subtalar joint)

Bursa of calcaneal tendon

Calcaneus

Short pedal muscles

Plantar aponeurosis

Plantar calcaneo-navicular ligament

Fig. 26.8 Talocrural joint
Right foot.

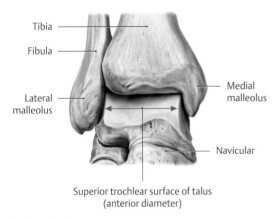

Tibia

Fibula

Lateral malleolus

Medial malleolus

Navicular

Superior trochlear surface of talus (anterior diameter)

A Anterior view.

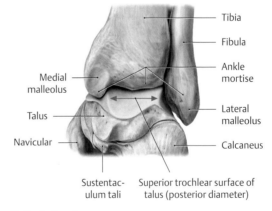

Medial malleolus

Talus

Navicular

Tibia

Fibula

Ankle mortise

Lateral malleolus

Calcaneus

Sustentac-ulum tali

Superior trochlear surface of talus (posterior diameter)

B Posterior view.

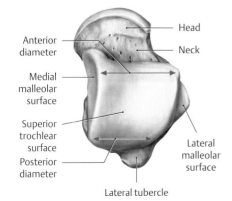

Head

Neck

Anterior diameter

Medial malleolar surface

Superior trochlear surface

Posterior diameter

Lateral malleolar surface

Lateral tubercle

C Proximal (superior) view of talus.

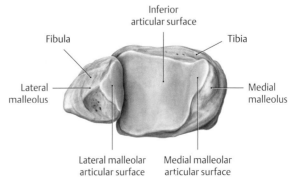

Inferior articular surface

Fibula

Lateral malleolus

Tibia

Medial malleolus

Lateral malleolar articular surface

Medial malleolar articular surface

D Distal (inferior) view of ankle mortise.

Joints of the Foot (III)

Fig. 26.9 Subtalar joint and ligaments

Right foot with opened subtalar joint. The subtalar joint consists of two distinct articulations separated by the interosseous talocalcanean liga- ment: the posterior compartment (talocalcanean joint) and the anterior compartment (talocalcaneonavicular joint).

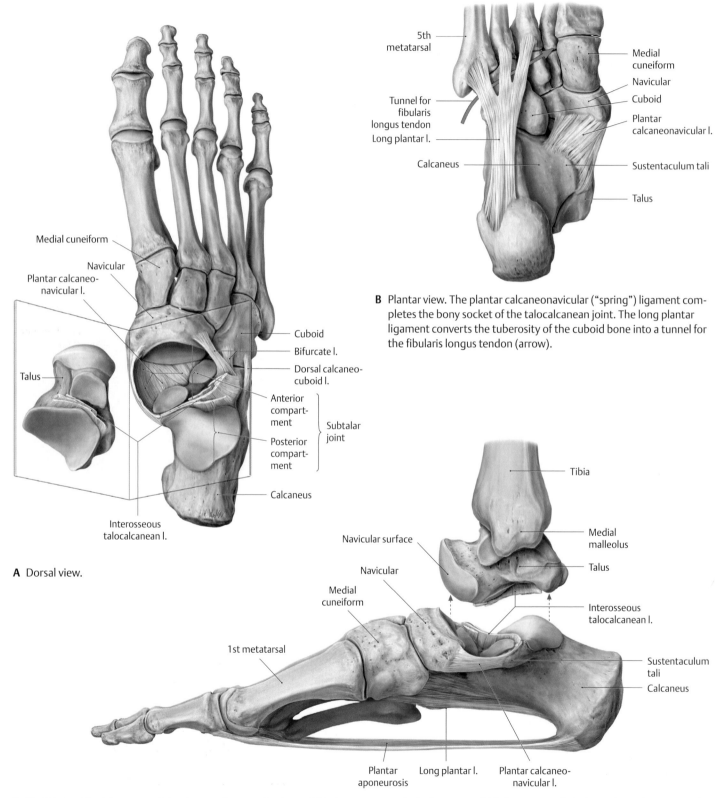

B Plantar view. The plantar calcaneonavicular ("spring") ligament completes the bony socket of the talocalcanean joint. The long plantar ligament converts the tuberosity of the cuboid bone into a tunnel for the fibularis longus tendon (arrow).

A Dorsal view.

C Medial view. The interosseous talocalcanean ligament has been divided and the talus displaced upward. Note the course of the plantar calcaneo- navicular ligament, which functions with the long plantar ligament and plantar aponeurosis to support the longitudinal arch of the foot.

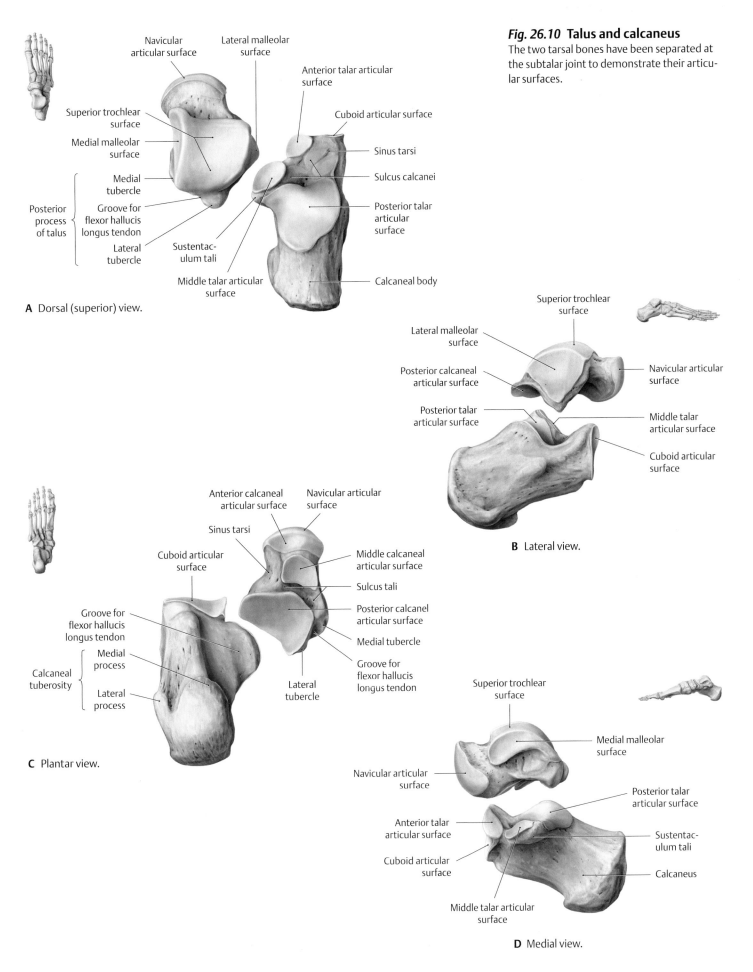

Fig. 26.10 Talus and calcaneus
The two tarsal bones have been separated at the subtalar joint to demonstrate their articular surfaces.

Navicular articular surface

Lateral malleolar surface

Anterior talar articular surface

Cuboid articular surface

Superior trochlear surface

Medial malleolar surface

Sinus tarsi

Sulcus calcanei

Medial tubercle

Posterior talar articular surface

Groove for flexor hallucis longus tendon

Posterior process of talus

Lateral tubercle

Sustentaculum tali

Middle talar articular surface

Calcaneal body

A Dorsal (superior) view.

Superior trochlear surface

Lateral malleolar surface

Posterior calcaneal articular surface

Navicular articular surface

Posterior talar articular surface

Middle talar articular surface

Cuboid articular surface

B Lateral view.

Anterior calcaneal articular surface

Navicular articular surface

Sinus tarsi

Cuboid articular surface

Middle calcaneal articular surface

Groove for flexor hallucis longus tendon

Sulcus tali

Posterior calcaneal articular surface

Medial process

Medial tubercle

Calcaneal tuberosity

Lateral process

Groove for flexor hallucis longus tendon

Lateral tubercle

C Plantar view.

Superior trochlear surface

Medial malleolar surface

Navicular articular surface

Posterior talar articular surface

Anterior talar articular surface

Sustentaculum tali

Cuboid articular surface

Calcaneus

Middle talar articular surface

D Medial view.

Ligaments of the Ankle & Foot

 The ligaments of the foot are classified as belonging to the talocrural joint, subtalar joint, metatarsus, forefoot, or sole of the foot. The medial and lateral collateral ligaments, along with the syndesmotic ligaments, are of major importance in the stabilization of the subtalar joint.

Fig. 26.11 Ligaments of the ankle and foot
Right foot. See p. 406 for inferior view.

Table 26.1	Ligaments of the talocrural joint		
Lateral ligaments*	Anterior talofibular l.		
	Posterior talofibular l.		
	Calcaneofibular l.		
Medial ligaments*	Deltoid l.		Anterior tibiotalar part
			Posterior tibiotalar part
			Tibionavicular part
			Tibiocalcanean part
Syndesmotic ligaments of the ankle mortise	Anterior tibiofibular l.		
	Posterior tibiofibular l.		
*The medial and lateral ligaments are also known as the medial and lateral collateral ligaments.			

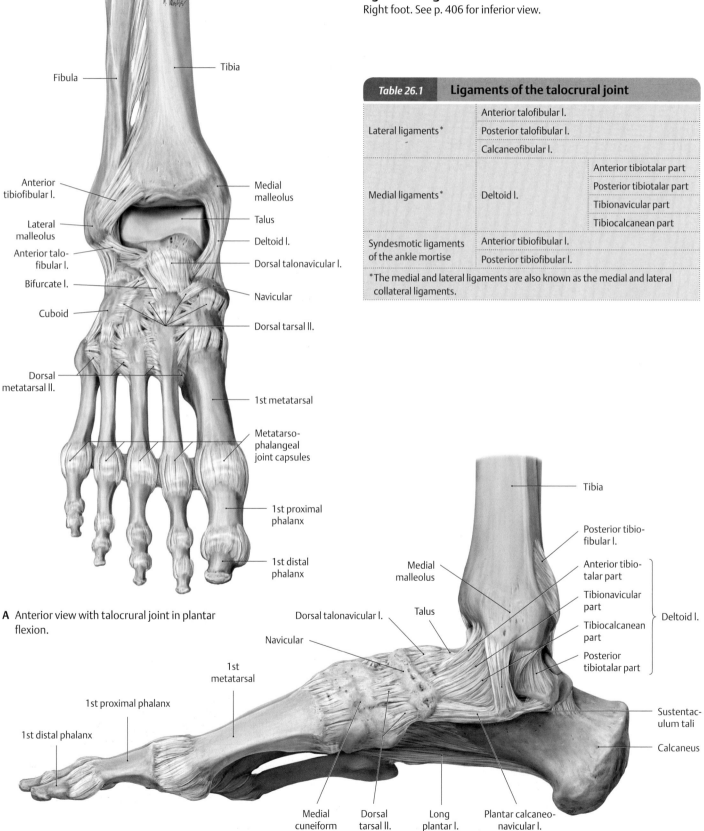

A Anterior view with talocrural joint in plantar flexion.

B Medial view.

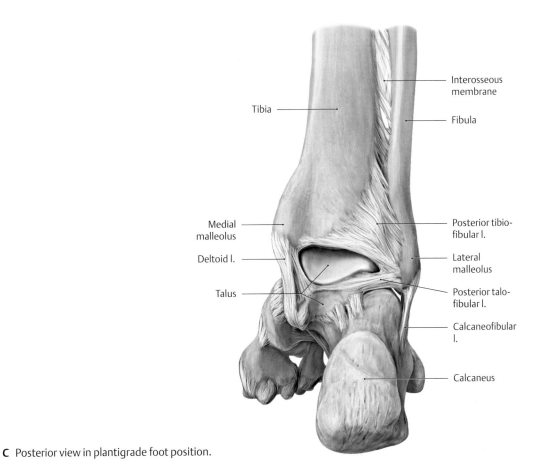

Tibia

Interosseous membrane

Fibula

Medial malleolus

Posterior tibio-fibular l.

Deltoid l.

Lateral malleolus

Talus

Posterior talo-fibular l.

Calcaneofibular l.

Calcaneus

C Posterior view in plantigrade foot position.

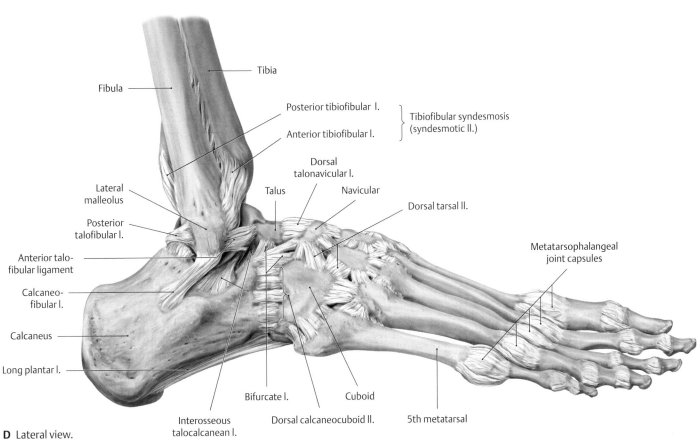

Fibula

Tibia

Posterior tibiofibular l.

Anterior tibiofibular l.

Tibiofibular syndesmosis (syndesmotic ll.)

Dorsal talonavicular l.

Talus

Navicular

Lateral malleolus

Dorsal tarsal ll.

Posterior talofibular l.

Anterior talo-fibular ligament

Metatarsophalangeal joint capsules

Calcaneo-fibular l.

Calcaneus

Long plantar l.

Bifurcate l.

Cuboid

Interosseous talocalcanean l.

Dorsal calcaneocuboid ll.

5th metatarsal

D Lateral view.

Plantar Vault & Arches of the Foot

Fig. 26.12 Plantar vault

Right foot. The forces of the foot are distributed among two lateral (fibular) and three medial (tibial) rays. The arrangement of these rays creates a longitudinal and a transverse arch in the sole of the foot, helping the foot absorb vertical loads.

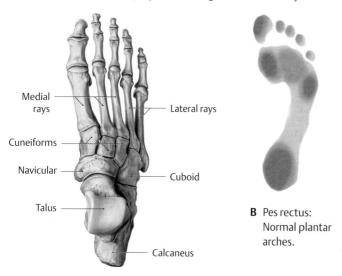

Medial rays

Lateral rays

Cuneiforms

Navicular

Cuboid

Talus

Calcaneus

A Plantar vault, superior view. Lateral rays in green, medial rays in red.

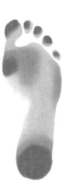

B Pes rectus: Normal plantar arches.

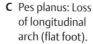

C Pes planus: Loss of longitudinal arch (flat foot).

D Pes cavus: Increased height of longitudinal arch.

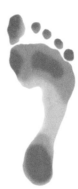

E Pes transverso-planus: Loss of transverse arch (splayfoot).

Fig. 26.13 Stabilizers of the transverse arch

Right foot. The transverse pedal arch is supported by both active and passive stabilizing structures (muscles and ligaments, respectively).

Note: The arch of the forefoot has only passive stabilizers, whereas the arches of the metatarsus and tarsus have only active stabilizers.

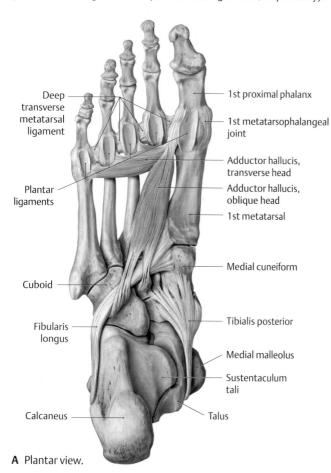

Deep transverse metatarsal ligament

1st proximal phalanx

1st metatarsophalangeal joint

Adductor hallucis, transverse head

Adductor hallucis, oblique head

1st metatarsal

Plantar ligaments

Medial cuneiform

Cuboid

Tibialis posterior

Fibularis longus

Medial malleolus

Sustentaculum tali

Calcaneus

Talus

A Plantar view.

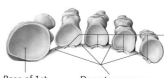

B Anterior arch (forefoot), proximal view.

Plantar ligament

Base of 1st proximal phalanx

Deep transverse metatarsal ligament

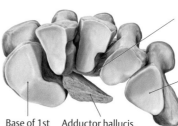

C Metatarsal arch, proximal view.

Base of 1st metatarsal

Adductor hallucis, oblique head

Adductor hallucis, transverse head

Base of 5th metatarsal

Intermediate cuneiform

Lateral cuneiform

Cuboid

D Tarsal region, proximal view.

Medial cuneiform

Tibialis posterior

Fibularis longus

Tuberosity of 5th metatarsal

Fig. 26.14 **Stabilizers of the longitudinal arch**

Right foot, medial view.

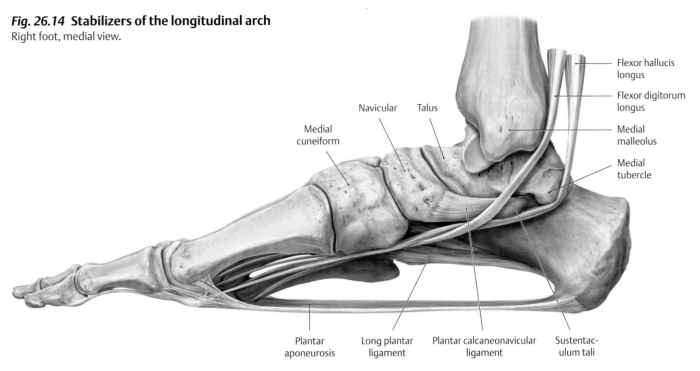

Flexor hallucis longus
Flexor digitorum longus
Medial malleolus
Medial tubercle
Navicular
Talus
Medial cuneiform
Plantar aponeurosis
Long plantar ligament
Plantar calcaneonavicular ligament
Sustentaculum tali

A Passive stabilizers of the longitudinal arch.

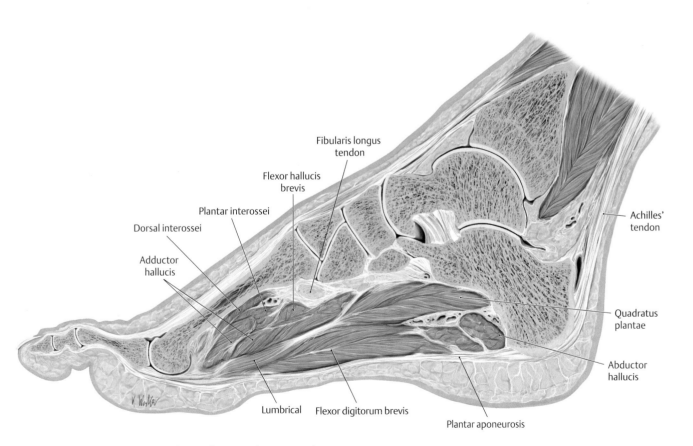

Fibularis longus tendon
Flexor hallucis brevis
Plantar interossei
Dorsal interossei
Adductor hallucis
Achilles' tendon
Quadratus plantae
Abductor hallucis
Lumbrical
Flexor digitorum brevis
Plantar aponeurosis

B Active stabilizers of the longitudinal arch. Sagittal section at the level of the second ray. The major active stabilizers of the foot are the abductor hallucis, flexor hallucis brevis, flexor digitorum brevis, quadratus plantae, and abductor digiti minimi.

Muscles of the Sole of the Foot

Fig. 26.15 Plantar aponeurosis
Right foot, plantar view. The plantar aponeurosis is a tough aponeurotic sheet, thickest at the center, that blends with the dorsal fascia (not shown) at the borders of the foot.

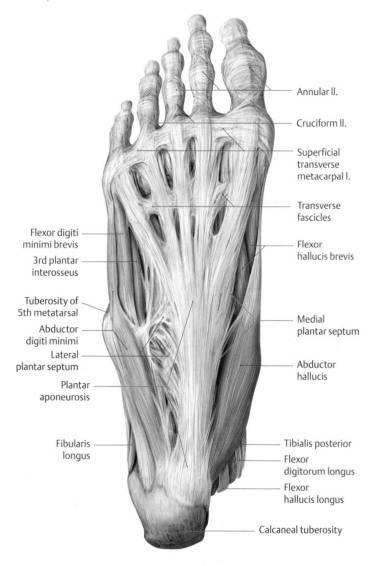

Annular ll.
Cruciform ll.
Superficial transverse metacarpal l.
Transverse fascicles
Flexor hallucis brevis
Medial plantar septum
Abductor hallucis
Tibialis posterior
Flexor digitorum longus
Flexor hallucis longus
Calcaneal tuberosity

Flexor digiti minimi brevis
3rd plantar interosseus
Tuberosity of 5th metatarsal
Abductor digiti minimi
Lateral plantar septum
Plantar aponeurosis
Fibularis longus

Fig. 26.16 Intrinsic muscles
Right foot, plantar view.

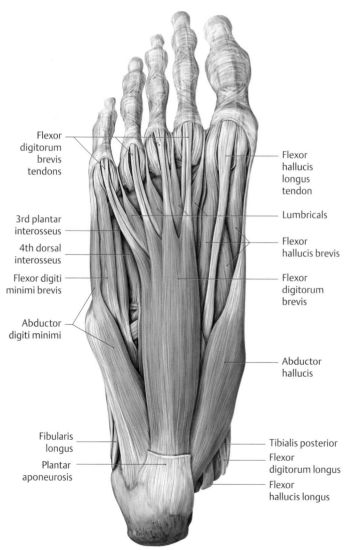

Flexor digitorum brevis tendons
3rd plantar interosseus
4th dorsal interosseus
Flexor digiti minimi brevis
Abductor digiti minimi
Fibularis longus
Plantar aponeurosis

Flexor hallucis longus tendon
Lumbricals
Flexor hallucis brevis
Flexor digitorum brevis
Abductor hallucis
Tibialis posterior
Flexor digitorum longus
Flexor hallucis longus

A Superficial (first) layer. *Removed:* Plantar aponeurosis, including the superficial transverse metacarpal ligament.

Lower Limb

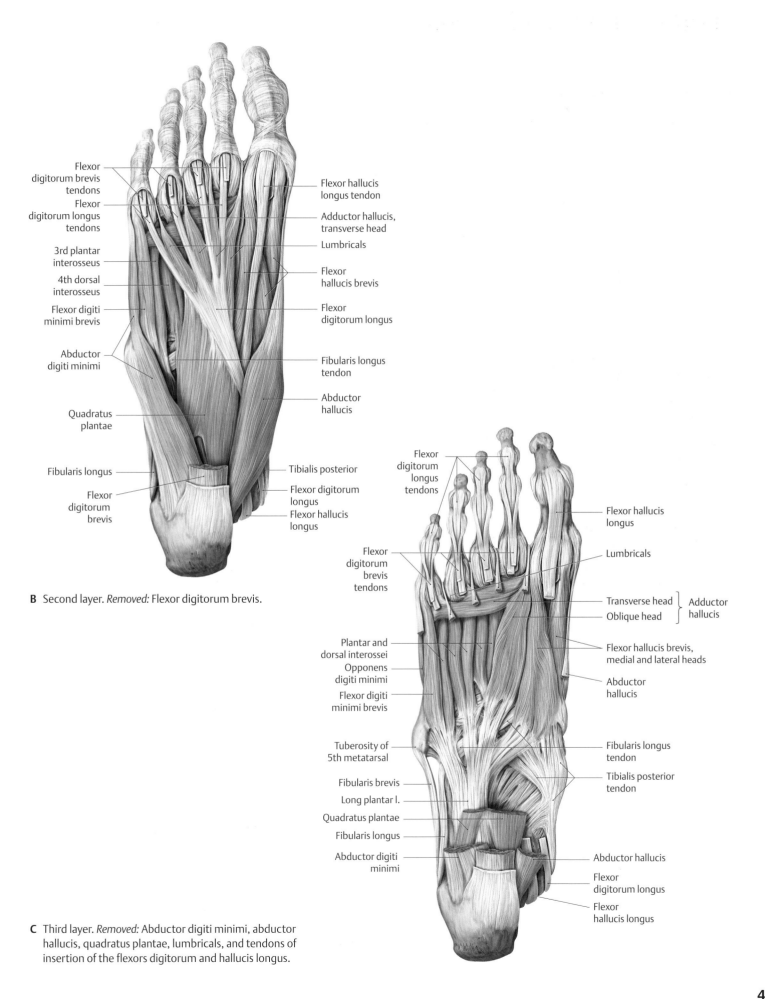

Flexor digitorum brevis tendons

Flexor digitorum longus tendons

3rd plantar interosseus

4th dorsal interosseus

Flexor digiti minimi brevis

Abductor digiti minimi

Quadratus plantae

Fibularis longus

Flexor digitorum brevis

Flexor hallucis longus tendon

Adductor hallucis, transverse head

Lumbricals

Flexor hallucis brevis

Flexor digitorum longus

Fibularis longus tendon

Abductor hallucis

Tibialis posterior

Flexor digitorum longus

Flexor hallucis longus

B Second layer. *Removed:* Flexor digitorum brevis.

Flexor digitorum longus tendons

Flexor digitorum brevis tendons

Plantar and dorsal interossei

Opponens digiti minimi

Flexor digiti minimi brevis

Tuberosity of 5th metatarsal

Fibularis brevis

Long plantar l.

Quadratus plantae

Fibularis longus

Abductor digiti minimi

Flexor hallucis longus

Lumbricals

Transverse head ⎱ Adductor
Oblique head ⎰ hallucis

Flexor hallucis brevis, medial and lateral heads

Abductor hallucis

Fibularis longus tendon

Tibialis posterior tendon

Abductor hallucis

Flexor digitorum longus

Flexor hallucis longus

C Third layer. *Removed:* Abductor digiti minimi, abductor hallucis, quadratus plantae, lumbricals, and tendons of insertion of the flexors digitorum and hallucis longus.

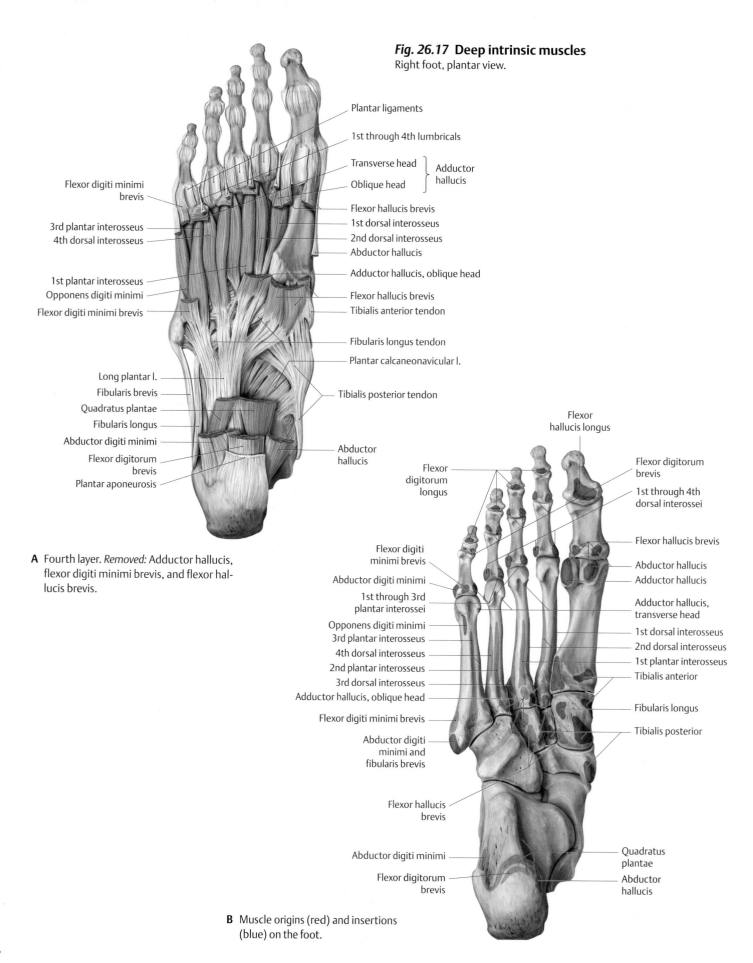

Muscles & Tendon Sheaths of the Foot

Fig. 26.17 Deep intrinsic muscles
Right foot, plantar view.

Plantar ligaments

1st through 4th lumbricals

Transverse head ⎱ Adductor
Oblique head ⎰ hallucis

Flexor digiti minimi brevis

3rd plantar interosseus
4th dorsal interosseus

1st plantar interosseus
Opponens digiti minimi
Flexor digiti minimi brevis

Flexor hallucis brevis
1st dorsal interosseus
2nd dorsal interosseus
Abductor hallucis
Adductor hallucis, oblique head
Flexor hallucis brevis
Tibialis anterior tendon

Fibularis longus tendon
Plantar calcaneonavicular l.

Long plantar l.
Fibularis brevis
Quadratus plantae
Fibularis longus
Abductor digiti minimi
Flexor digitorum brevis
Plantar aponeurosis

Tibialis posterior tendon

Abductor hallucis

A Fourth layer. *Removed:* Adductor hallucis, flexor digiti minimi brevis, and flexor hallucis brevis.

Flexor hallucis longus

Flexor digitorum longus

Flexor digiti minimi brevis
Abductor digiti minimi
1st through 3rd plantar interossei
Opponens digiti minimi
3rd plantar interosseus
4th dorsal interosseus
2nd plantar interosseus
3rd dorsal interosseus
Adductor hallucis, oblique head
Flexor digiti minimi brevis
Abductor digiti minimi and fibularis brevis

Flexor hallucis brevis

Abductor digiti minimi
Flexor digitorum brevis

Flexor digitorum brevis
1st through 4th dorsal interossei
Flexor hallucis brevis
Abductor hallucis
Adductor hallucis
Adductor hallucis, transverse head
1st dorsal interosseus
2nd dorsal interosseus
1st plantar interosseus
Tibialis anterior
Fibularis longus
Tibialis posterior

Quadratus plantae
Abductor hallucis

B Muscle origins (red) and insertions (blue) on the foot.

Fig. 26.18 Tendon sheaths and retinacula of the ankle

Right foot. The superior and inferior extensor retinacula retain the long extensor tendons, the fibularis retinacula hold the fibular muscle tendons in place, and the flexor retinaculum retains the long flexor tendons.

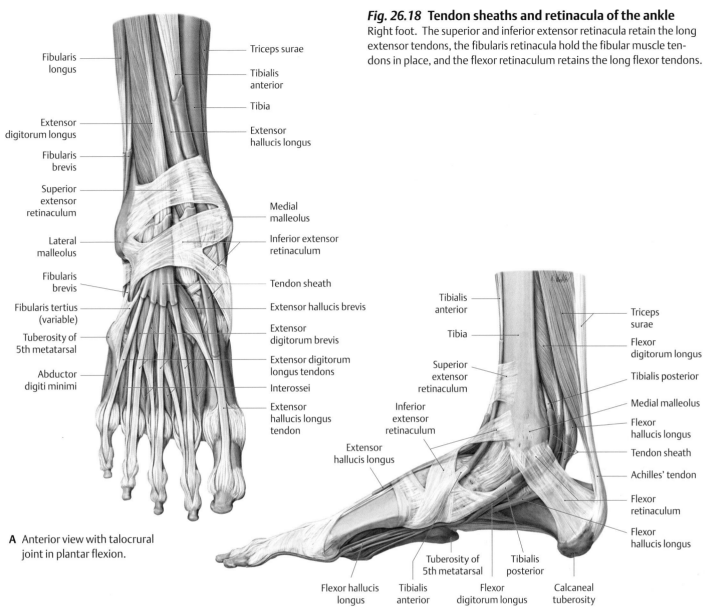

Fibularis longus

Triceps surae

Tibialis anterior

Tibia

Extensor digitorum longus

Extensor hallucis longus

Fibularis brevis

Superior extensor retinaculum

Medial malleolus

Lateral malleolus

Inferior extensor retinaculum

Fibularis brevis

Tendon sheath

Fibularis tertius (variable)

Extensor hallucis brevis

Tuberosity of 5th metatarsal

Extensor digitorum brevis

Abductor digiti minimi

Extensor digitorum longus tendons

Interossei

Extensor hallucis longus tendon

A Anterior view with talocrural joint in plantar flexion.

Tibialis anterior

Tibia

Superior extensor retinaculum

Inferior extensor retinaculum

Extensor hallucis longus

Triceps surae

Flexor digitorum longus

Tibialis posterior

Medial malleolus

Flexor hallucis longus

Tendon sheath

Achilles' tendon

Flexor retinaculum

Flexor hallucis longus

Flexor hallucis longus

Tibialis anterior

Tuberosity of 5th metatarsal

Flexor digitorum longus

Tibialis posterior

Calcaneal tuberosity

B Medial view.

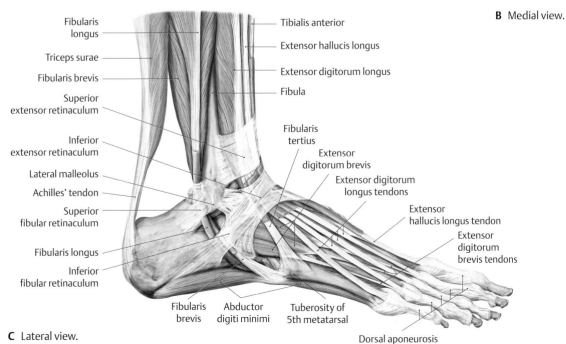

Fibularis longus

Tibialis anterior

Triceps surae

Extensor hallucis longus

Fibularis brevis

Extensor digitorum longus

Superior extensor retinaculum

Fibula

Inferior extensor retinaculum

Fibularis tertius

Lateral malleolus

Extensor digitorum brevis

Achilles' tendon

Extensor digitorum longus tendons

Superior fibular retinaculum

Extensor hallucis longus tendon

Fibularis longus

Extensor digitorum brevis tendons

Inferior fibular retinaculum

Fibularis brevis

Abductor digiti minimi

Tuberosity of 5th metatarsal

Dorsal aponeurosis

C Lateral view.

Muscle Facts (I)

 The dorsal surface (dorsum) of the foot contains only two muscles, the extensor digitorum brevis and the extensor hallucis brevis. The sole of the foot, however, is composed of four complex layers that maintain the arches of the foot.

***Fig. 26.19* Intrinsic muscles of the dorsum**
Right foot, dorsal view.

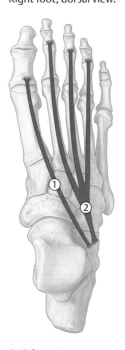

A Schematic.

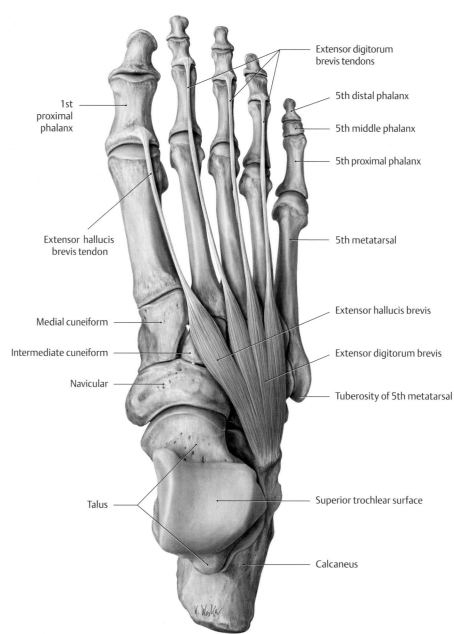

B Dorsal muscles of the foot.

Table 26.2		Intrinsic muscles of the dorsum			
Muscle	**Origin**	**Insertion**	**Innervation**	**Action**
① Extensor digitorum brevis	Calcaneus (dorsal surface)	2nd to 4th toes (at dorsal aponeuroses and bases of the middle phalanges)	Deep fibular n. (L5, S1)	Extension of the MTP and PIP joints of the 2nd to 4th toes
② Extensor hallucis brevis		1st toe (at dorsal aponeurosis and proximal phalanx)		Extension of the MTP joints of the 1st toe
MTP = metatarsophalangeal; PIP = proximal interphalangeal.				

Fig. 26.20 Superficial intrinsic muscles of the sole

Right foot, plantar view.

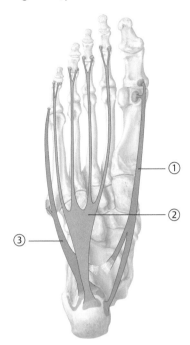

A First layer (schematic).

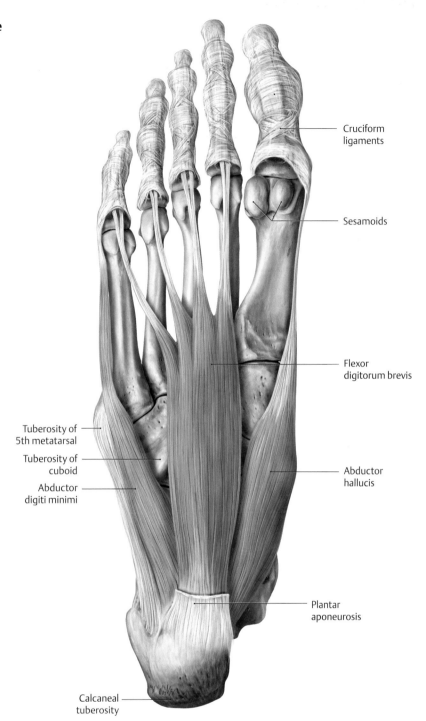

B Intrinsic muscles of the sole, first layer.

Table 26.3	Superficial intrinsic muscles of the sole			
Muscle	**Origin**	**Insertion**	**Innervation**	**Action**
① Abductor hallucis	Calcaneal tuberosity (medial process)	1st toe (base of proximal phalanx via the medial sesamoid)	Medial plantar n. (S1, S2)	• 1st MTP joint: flexion and abduction of the 1st toe • Supports the longitudinal arch
② Flexor digitorum brevis	Calcaneal tuberosity (medial tubercle), plantar aponeurosis	2nd to 5th toes (sides of middle phalanges)		• Flexes the MTP and PIP joints of the 2nd to 5th toes • Supports the longitudinal arch
③ Abductor digiti minimi		5th toe (base of proximal phalanx), 5th metatarsal (at tuberosity)	Lateral plantar n. (S1–S3)	• Flexes the MTP joint of the 5th toe • Abducts the 5th toe • Supports the longitudinal arch

MTP = metatarsophalangeal; PIP = proximal interphalangeal.

Muscle Facts (II)

Fig. 26.21 **Deep intrinsic muscles of the sole**
Right foot, plantar view.

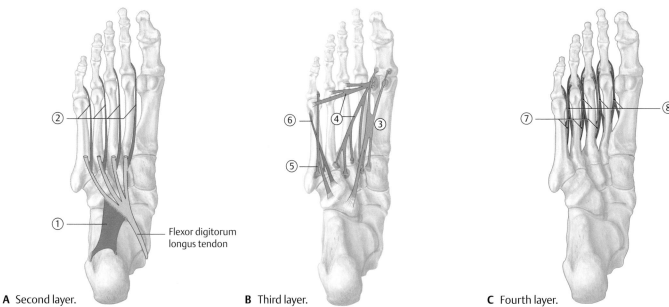

A Second layer. B Third layer. C Fourth layer.

Table 26.4	Deep intrinsic muscles of the sole			
Muscle	**Origin**	**Insertion**	**Innervation**	**Action**
① Quadratus plantae	Calcaneal tuberosity (medial and plantar borders on plantar side)	Flexor digitorum longus tendon (lateral border)	Lateral plantar n. (S1–S3)	Redirects and augments the pull of flexor digitorum longus
② Lumbricals (four muscles)	Flexor digitorum longus tendons (medial borders)	2nd to 5th toes (at dorsal aponeuroses)	1st lumbrical: medial plantar n. (S2, S3) 2nd and 4th lumbrical: lateral plantar n. (S2, S3)	• Flexes the MTP joints of 2nd to 5th toes • Extension of IP joints of 2nd to 5th toes • Adducts 2nd to 5th toes toward the big toe
③ Flexor hallucis brevis	Cuboid, lateral cuneiforms, and plantar calcaneocuboid ligament	1st toe (at base of proximal phalanx via medial and lateral sesamoids)	Medial head: medial plantar n. (S1, S2) Lateral head: lateral plantar n. (S1, S2)	• Flexes the first MTP joint • Supports the longitudinal arch
④ Adductor hallucis	Oblique head: 2nd to 4th metatarsals (at bases) Transverse head: MTPs of 3rd to 5th toes, deep transverse metatarsal ligament	1st proximal phalanx (at base, by a common tendon via the lateral sesamoid)	Lateral plantar n., deep branch (S2, S3)	• Flexes the first MTP joint • Adducts big toe • Transverse head: supports transverse arch • Oblique head: supports longitudinal arch
⑤ Flexor digiti minimi brevis	5th metatarsal (base), long plantar ligament	5th toe (base of proximal phalanx)	Lateral plantar n., superficial branch (S2, S3)	Flexes the MTP joint of the little toe
⑥ Opponens digiti minimi*	Long plantar ligament; fibularis longus (at plantar tendon sheath)	5th metatarsal		Pulls 5th metatarsal in plantar and medial direction
⑦ Plantar interossei (three muscles)	3rd to 5th metatarsals (medial border)	3rd to 5th toes (medial base of proximal phalanx)		• Flexes the MTP joints of 3rd to 5th toes • Extension of IP joints of 3rd to 5th toes • Adducts 3rd to 5th toes toward 2nd toe
⑧ Dorsal interossei (four muscles)	1st to 5th metatarsals (by two heads on opposing sides)	1st interosseus: 2nd proximal phalanx (medial base) 2nd to 4th interossei: 2nd to 4th proximal phalanges (lateral base), 2nd to 4th toes (at dorsal aponeuroses)	Lateral plantar n. (S2, S3)	• Flexes the MTP joints of 2nd to 4th toes • Extension of IP joints of 2nd to 4th toes • Abducts 3rd and 4th toes from 2nd toe
IP = interphalangeal; MTP = metatarsophalangeal. *May be absent.				

Fig. 26.22 Deep intrinsic muscles of the sole

Right foot, plantar view.

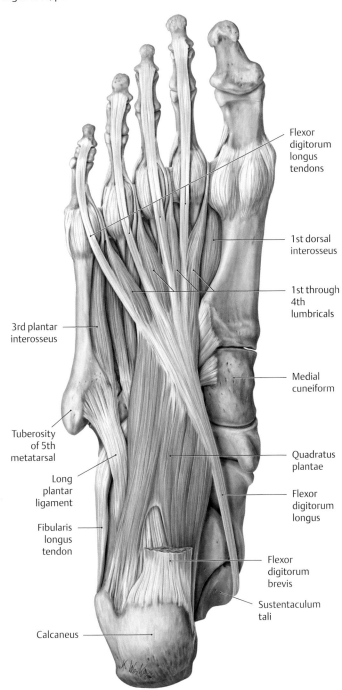

Flexor digitorum longus tendons

1st dorsal interosseus

1st through 4th lumbricals

3rd plantar interosseus

Medial cuneiform

Tuberosity of 5th metatarsal

Quadratus plantae

Long plantar ligament

Flexor digitorum longus

Fibularis longus tendon

Flexor digitorum brevis

Sustentaculum tali

Calcaneus

A Intrinsic muscles of the sole, second and fourth layers.

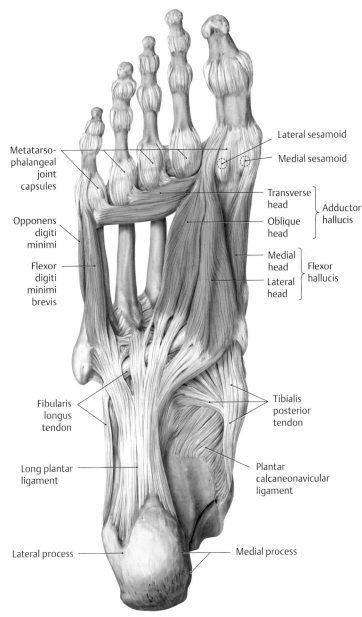

Metatarso-phalangeal joint capsules

Lateral sesamoid

Medial sesamoid

Opponens digiti minimi

Transverse head

Oblique head

Adductor hallucis

Flexor digiti minimi brevis

Medial head

Lateral head

Flexor hallucis

Fibularis longus tendon

Tibialis posterior tendon

Long plantar ligament

Plantar calcaneonavicular ligament

Lateral process

Medial process

B Intrinsic muscles of the sole, third layer.

Arteries of the Lower Limb

Fig. 27.1 Arteries of the lower limb

Right limb, anterior (**A**) and posterior (**B**) views.

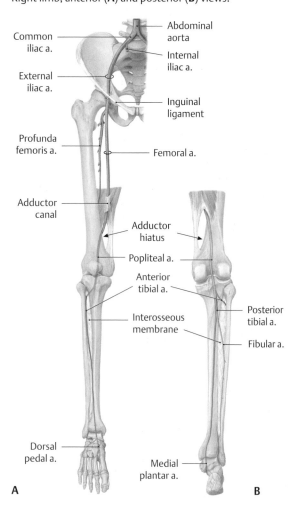

Common iliac a.

Abdominal aorta

Internal iliac a.

External iliac a.

Inguinal ligament

Profunda femoris a.

Femoral a.

Adductor canal

Adductor hiatus

Popliteal a.

Anterior tibial a.

Interosseous membrane

Posterior tibial a.

Fibular a.

Dorsal pedal a.

Medial plantar a.

A

B

Fig. 27.2 Arteries of the sole of the foot

Right foot, plantar view.

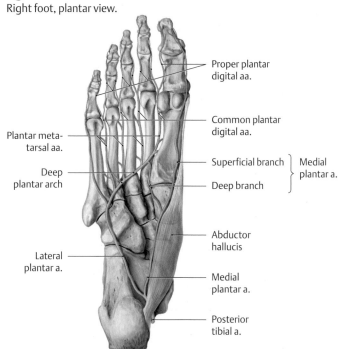

Proper plantar digital aa.

Common plantar digital aa.

Plantar meta-tarsal aa.

Superficial branch ⎫ Medial
Deep branch   ⎬ plantar a.

Deep plantar arch

Abductor hallucis

Lateral plantar a.

Medial plantar a.

Posterior tibial a.

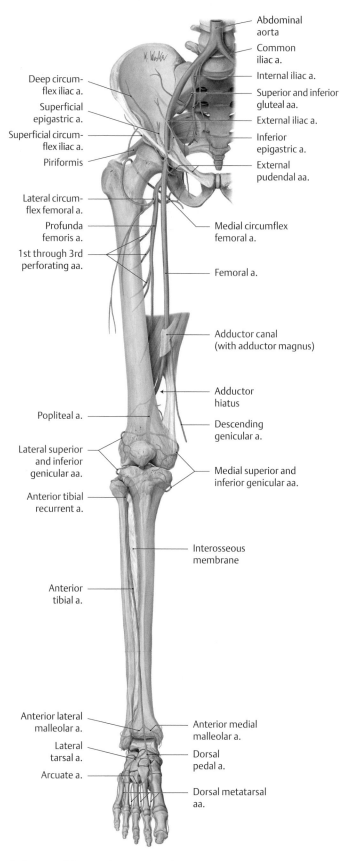

Deep circum-flex iliac a.

Superficial epigastric a.

Superficial circum-flex iliac a.

Piriformis

Lateral circum-flex femoral a.

Profunda femoris a.

1st through 3rd perforating aa.

Popliteal a.

Lateral superior and inferior genicular aa.

Anterior tibial recurrent a.

Anterior tibial a.

Anterior lateral malleolar a.

Lateral tarsal a.

Arcuate a.

Abdominal aorta

Common iliac a.

Internal iliac a.

Superior and inferior gluteal aa.

External iliac a.

Inferior epigastric a.

External pudendal aa.

Medial circumflex femoral a.

Femoral a.

Adductor canal (with adductor magnus)

Adductor hiatus

Descending genicular a.

Medial superior and inferior genicular aa.

Interosseous membrane

Anterior medial malleolar a.

Dorsal pedal a.

Dorsal metatarsal aa.

C Course of the arteries, anterior view.

Femoral head necrosis

Dislocation or fracture of the femoral head (e.g., in patients with osteoporosis) may disrupt the anastomoses between the foveal artery and the femoral neck vessels, resulting in femoral head necrosis.

Fig. 27.3 Arteries of the femoral head

Right hip joint, anterior view.

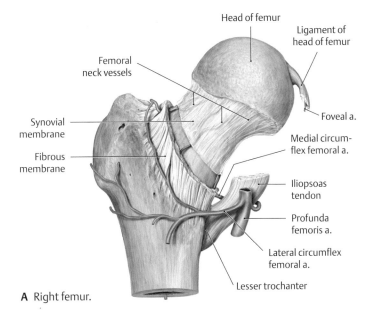

A Right femur.

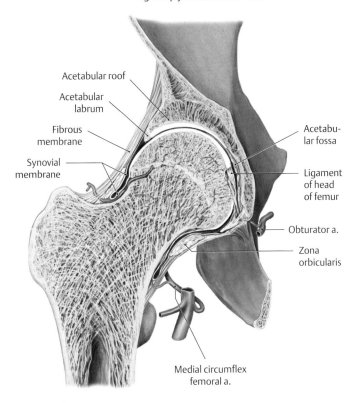

B Coronal section.

Fig. 27.4 Arteries of the thigh and leg

Right leg.

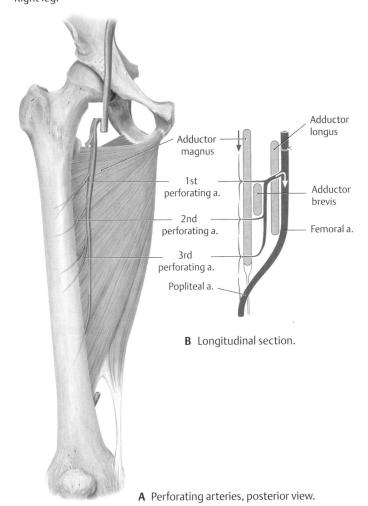

A Perforating arteries, posterior view.

B Longitudinal section.

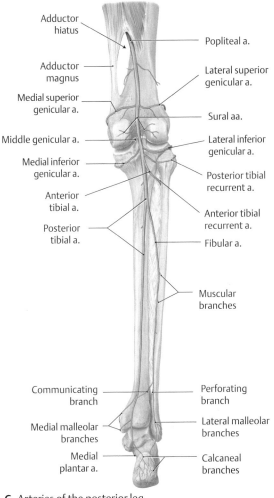

C Arteries of the posterior leg.

Veins & Lymphatics of the Lower Limb

Fig. 27.5 Veins of the lower limb
Right limb, anterior view.

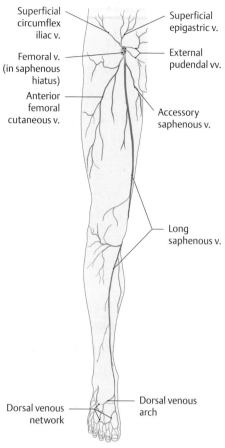

Superficial circumflex iliac v.

Femoral v. (in saphenous hiatus)

Anterior femoral cutaneous v.

Superficial epigastric v.

External pudendal vv.

Accessory saphenous v.

Long saphenous v.

Dorsal venous network

Dorsal venous arch

A Superficial (epifascial) veins.

Fig. 27.6 Veins of the sole of the foot
Right foot, plantar view.

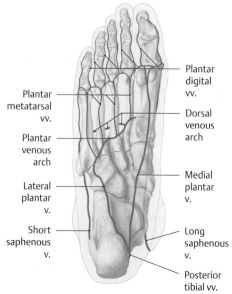

Plantar metatarsal vv.

Plantar venous arch

Lateral plantar v.

Short saphenous v.

Plantar digital vv.

Dorsal venous arch

Medial plantar v.

Long saphenous v.

Posterior tibial vv.

Inguinal ligament

Piriformis

Lateral circumflex femoral vv.

Deep femoral v.

Femoral v.

Adductor canal

Popliteal v.

Adductor hiatus

Anterior tibial vv.

Short saphenous v.

Dorsal venous network of the foot

External iliac v.

Medial circumflex femoral vv.

Long saphenous v.

Accessory saphenous v.

Adductor magnus

Genicular vv.

Long saphenous v.

B Deep veins.

Fig. 27.7 Veins of the leg
Right leg, posterior view.

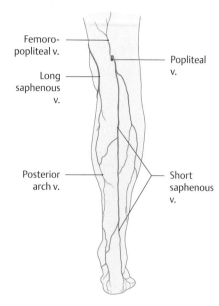

Femoro-popliteal v.

Long saphenous v.

Posterior arch v.

Popliteal v.

Short saphenous v.

A Superficial (epifascial) veins.

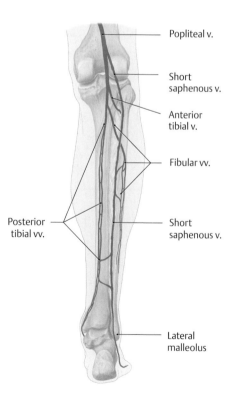

Popliteal v.

Short saphenous v.

Anterior tibial v.

Fibular vv.

Short saphenous v.

Posterior tibial vv.

Lateral malleolus

B Deep veins.

Fig. 27.8 Clinically important perforating veins

Right leg, medial view.

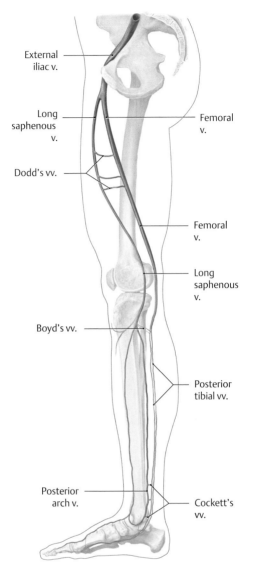

- External iliac v.
- Long saphenous v.
- Dodd's vv.
- Femoral v.
- Femoral v.
- Long saphenous v.
- Boyd's vv.
- Posterior tibial vv.
- Posterior arch v.
- Cockett's vv.

Fig. 27.9 Superficial lymphatics

Right limb. Arrows indicate the main directions of lymphatic drainage.

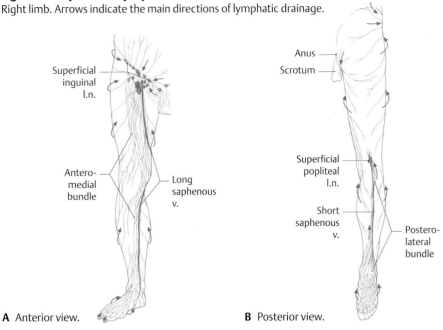

- Superficial inguinal l.n.
- Antero-medial bundle
- Long saphenous v.
- Anus
- Scrotum
- Superficial popliteal l.n.
- Short saphenous v.
- Postero-lateral bundle

A Anterior view.

B Posterior view.

Fig. 27.10 Lymph nodes and drainage

Right limb, anterior view.

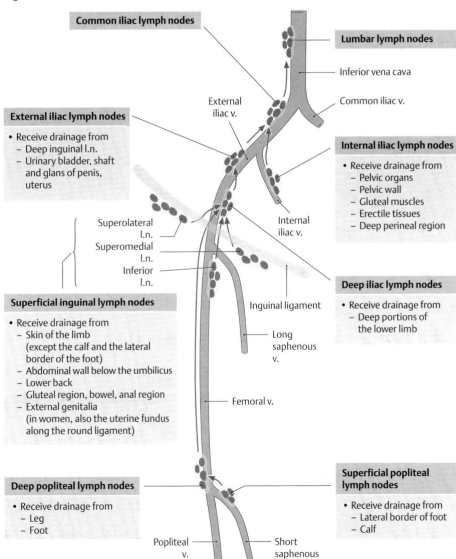

Common iliac lymph nodes

Lumbar lymph nodes

- Inferior vena cava
- Common iliac v.
- External iliac v.

External iliac lymph nodes

- Receive drainage from
  - Deep inguinal l.n.
  - Urinary bladder, shaft and glans of penis, uterus

Internal iliac lymph nodes

- Receive drainage from
  - Pelvic organs
  - Pelvic wall
  - Gluteal muscles
  - Erectile tissues
  - Deep perineal region

- Internal iliac v.

- Superolateral l.n.
- Superomedial l.n.
- Inferior l.n.

- Inguinal ligament

Deep iliac lymph nodes

- Receive drainage from
  - Deep portions of the lower limb

Superficial inguinal lymph nodes

- Receive drainage from
  - Skin of the limb (except the calf and the lateral border of the foot)
  - Abdominal wall below the umbilicus
  - Lower back
  - Gluteal region, bowel, anal region
  - External genitalia (in women, also the uterine fundus along the round ligament)

- Long saphenous v.

- Femoral v.

Deep popliteal lymph nodes

- Receive drainage from
  - Leg
  - Foot

Superficial popliteal lymph nodes

- Receive drainage from
  - Lateral border of foot
  - Calf

Popliteal v.

Short saphenous v.

Lumbosacral Plexus

 The lumbosacral plexus supplies sensory and motor innervation to the lower limb. It is formed by the anterior (ventral) rami of the lumbar and sacral spinal nerves, with contributions from the subcostal nerve (T12) and coccygeal nerve (Co1).

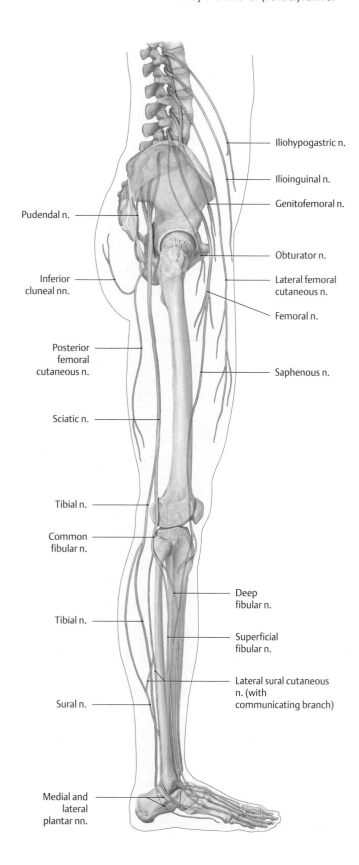

Iliohypogastric n.

Ilioinguinal n.

Genitofemoral n.

Pudendal n.

Obturator n.

Lateral femoral cutaneous n.

Inferior cluneal nn.

Femoral n.

Posterior femoral cutaneous n.

Saphenous n.

Sciatic n.

Tibial n.

Common fibular n.

Deep fibular n.

Tibial n.

Superficial fibular n.

Lateral sural cutaneous n. (with communicating branch)

Sural n.

Medial and lateral plantar nn.

Table 27.1	**Nerves of the lumbosacral plexus**		
Lumbar plexus			
Iliohypogastric n.		L1	
Ilioinguinal n.			p. 427
Genitofemoral n.		L1–L2	
Lateral femoral cutaneous n.		L2–L3	
Obturator n.		L2–L4	p. 428
Femoral n.			p. 429
Sacral plexus			
Superior gluteal n.		L4–S1	p. 431
Inferior gluteal n.		L5–S2	
Posterior femoral cutaneous n.		S1–S3	p. 430
Sciatic n.	Common fibular n.	L4–S2	p. 432
	Tibial n.	L4–S3	p. 433
Pudendal n.		S2–S4	pp. 194, 202

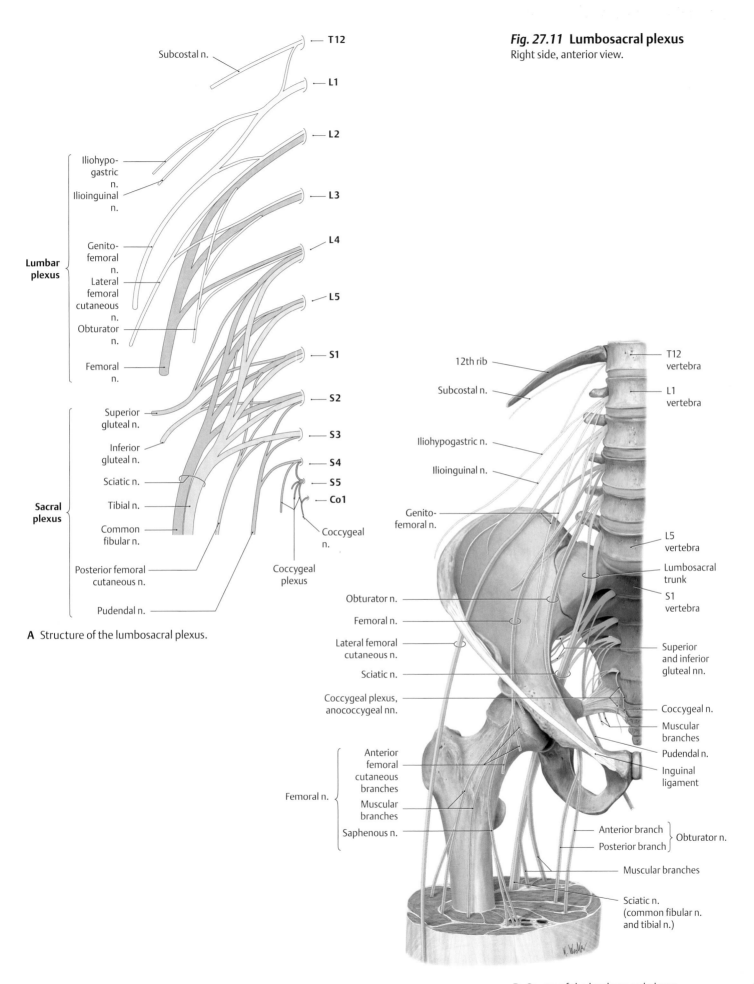

Fig. 27.11 Lumbosacral plexus
Right side, anterior view.

Subcostal n.

T12
L1
L2
L3
L4
L5
S1
S2
S3
S4
S5
Co1

Lumbar plexus

Iliohypo-gastric n.
Ilioinguinal n.
Genito-femoral n.
Lateral femoral cutaneous n.
Obturator n.
Femoral n.

Sacral plexus

Superior gluteal n.
Inferior gluteal n.
Sciatic n.
Tibial n.
Common fibular n.
Posterior femoral cutaneous n.
Pudendal n.

Coccygeal n.
Coccygeal plexus

A Structure of the lumbosacral plexus.

12th rib
Subcostal n.
Iliohypogastric n.
Ilioinguinal n.
Genito-femoral n.
Obturator n.
Femoral n.
Lateral femoral cutaneous n.
Sciatic n.
Coccygeal plexus, anococcygeal nn.

T12 vertebra
L1 vertebra
L5 vertebra
Lumbosacral trunk
S1 vertebra
Superior and inferior gluteal nn.
Coccygeal n.
Muscular branches
Pudendal n.
Inguinal ligament

Femoral n.
Anterior femoral cutaneous branches
Muscular branches
Saphenous n.

Anterior branch
Posterior branch } Obturator n.
Muscular branches
Sciatic n. (common fibular n. and tibial n.)

B Course of the lumbosacral plexus.

425

Nerves of the Lumbar Plexus

Table 27.2	Nerves of the lumbar plexus		
Nerve	**Level**	**Innervated muscle**	**Cutaneous branches**
Iliohypogastric n.	T12–L1	Transversus abdominis and internal oblique (inferior portions)	Anterior and lateral cutaneous branches
Ilioinguinal n.	L1		♂: Anterior scrotal nn. ♀: Anterior labial nn.
Genitofemoral n.	L1–L2	♂: Cremaster (genital branch)	Genital branch Femoral branch
Lateral femoral cutaneous n.	L2–L3	—	Lateral femoral cutaneous n.
Obturator n.	L2–L4	See p. 428	
Femoral n.	L2–L4	See p. 429	
Short, direct muscular branches	T12–L4	Psoas major Quadratus lumborum Iliacus Intertransversarii lumborum	—

Fig. 27.12 Sensory innervation of the inguinal region
Right male inguinal region, anterior view.

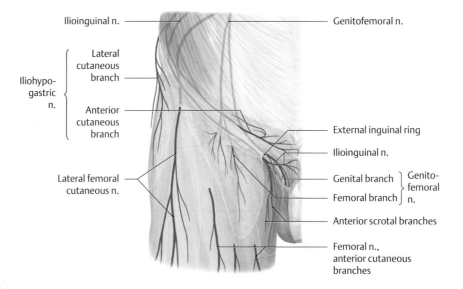

Fig. 27.13 **Nerves of the lumbar plexus**

Right side, anterior view with the anterior abdominal wall removed.

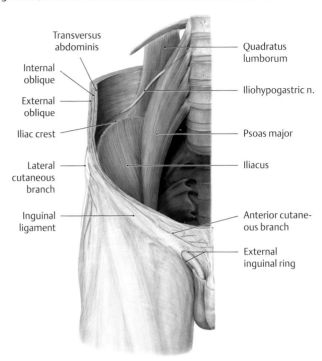

A Iliohypogastric nerve.

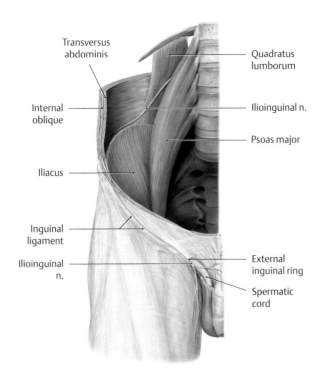

B Ilioinguinal nerve.

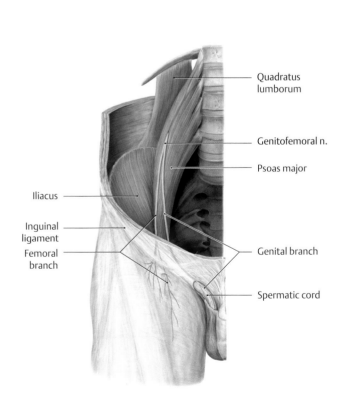

C Genitofemoral nerve.

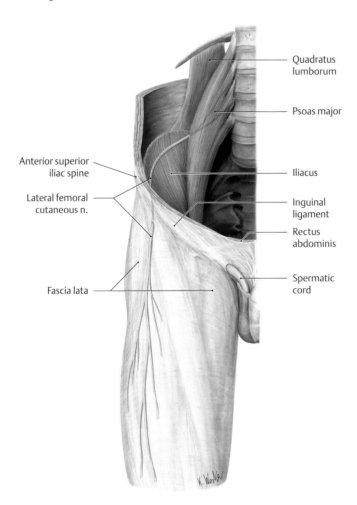

D Lateral femoral cutaneous nerve.

Nerves of the Lumbar Plexus: Obturator & Femoral Nerves

Fig. 27.14 Obturator nerve: Sensory distribution
Right leg, medial view.

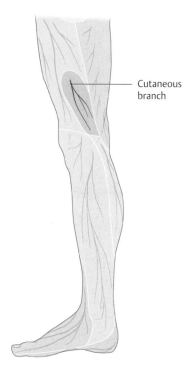

Cutaneous branch

Fig. 27.15 Obturator nerve
Right side, anterior view.

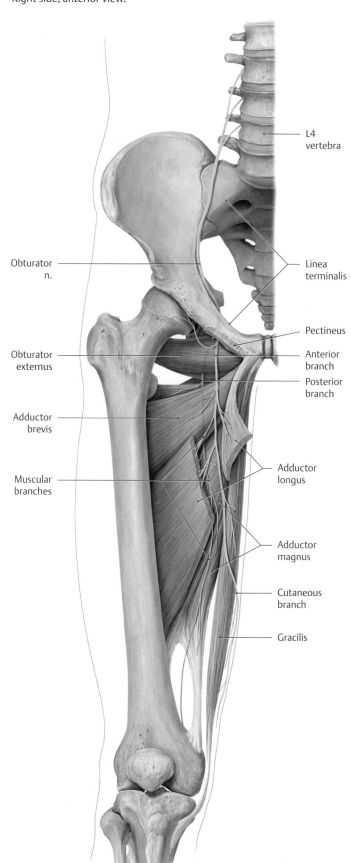

L4 vertebra

Obturator n.

Linea terminalis

Pectineus

Obturator externus

Anterior branch

Posterior branch

Adductor brevis

Muscular branches

Adductor longus

Adductor magnus

Cutaneous branch

Gracilis

Table 27.3	Obturator nerve (L2–L4)
Motor branches	**Innervated muscles**
Direct branch	Obturator externus
Anterior branch	Adductor longus
	Adductor brevis
	Gracilis
	Pectineus
Posterior branch	Adductor magnus
Sensory branches	
Cutaneous branch	

Fig. 27.16 Femoral nerve
Right side, anterior view.

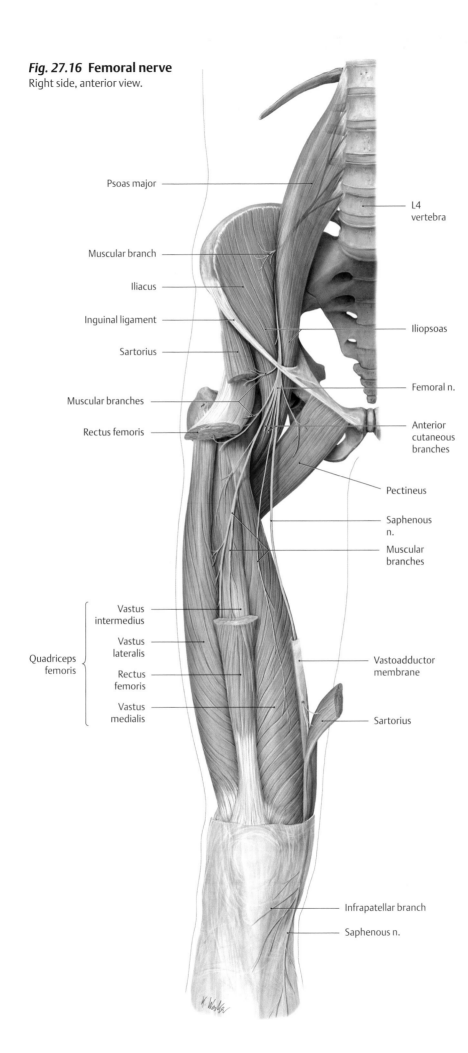

Psoas major

Muscular branch

Iliacus

Inguinal ligament

Sartorius

Muscular branches

Rectus femoris

L4 vertebra

Iliopsoas

Femoral n.

Anterior cutaneous branches

Pectineus

Saphenous n.

Muscular branches

Vastus intermedius

Vastus lateralis

Rectus femoris

Vastus medialis

Quadriceps femoris

Vastoadductor membrane

Sartorius

Infrapatellar branch

Saphenous n.

Fig. 27.17 Femoral nerve: Sensory distribution
Right limb, anterior view.

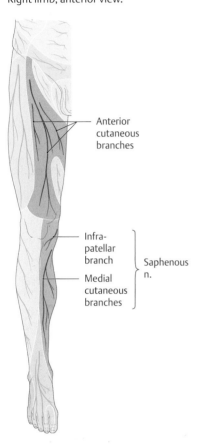

Anterior cutaneous branches

Infra-patellar branch

Medial cutaneous branches

Saphenous n.

Table 27.4	Femoral nerve (L2–L4)
Motor branches	**Innervated muscles**
Muscular branches	Iliopsoas
	Pectineus
	Sartorius
	Quadriceps femoris
Sensory branches	
Anterior cutaneous branch	
Saphenous n.	

Nerves of the Sacral Plexus

Table 27.5	Nerves of the sacral plexus				
Nerve		**Level**	**Innervated muscle**	**Cutaneous branches**	
Superior gluteal n.		L4–S1	Gluteus medius Gluteus minimus Tensor fasciae latae	—	
Inferior gluteal n.		L5–S2	Gluteus maximus	—	
Posterior femoral cutaneous n.		S1–S3	—	Posterior femoral cutaneous n.	Inferior cluneal nn.
					Perineal branches
Direct branches	N. of piriformis	S1–S2	Piriformis	—	
	N. of obturator internus	L5–S1	Obturator internus Gemelli	—	
	N. of quadratus femoris		Quadratus femoris	—	
Sciatic n.	Common fibular n.	L4–S2	See p. 432		
	Tibial n.	L4–S3	See p. 433		

Fig. 27.18 Sensory innervation of the gluteal region
Right limb, posterior view.

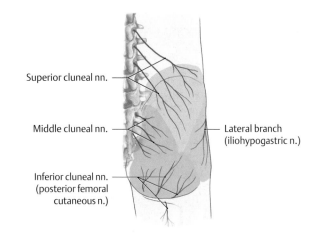

Fig. 27.19 Posterior femoral cutaneous nerve: Sensory distribution
Right limb, posterior view.

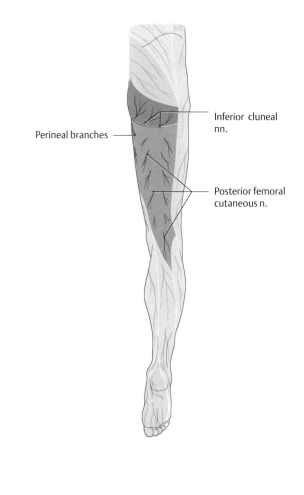

Fig. 27.20 Emerging sacral nerve
Horizontal section, superior view.

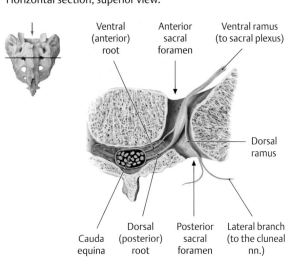

Fig. 27.21 Nerves of the sacral plexus
Right limb.

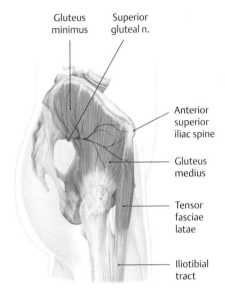

A Superior gluteal nerve. Lateral view.

Gluteus minimus

Superior gluteal n.

Anterior superior iliac spine

Gluteus medius

Tensor fasciae latae

Iliotibial tract

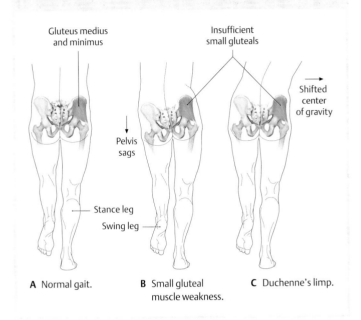
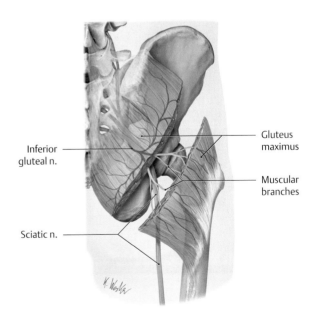

B Inferior gluteal nerve. Posterior view.

Inferior gluteal n.

Gluteus maximus

Muscular branches

Sciatic n.

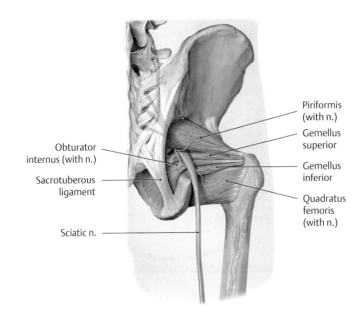

C Direct branches. Posterior view.

Obturator internus (with n.)

Sacrotuberous ligament

Sciatic n.

Piriformis (with n.)

Gemellus superior

Gemellus inferior

Quadratus femoris (with n.)

Nerves of the Sacral Plexus: Sciatic Nerve

 The sciatic nerve gives off several direct muscular branches before dividing into the tibial and common fibular nerves proximal to the popliteal fossa.

Fig. 27.22 Common fibular nerve: Sensory distribution

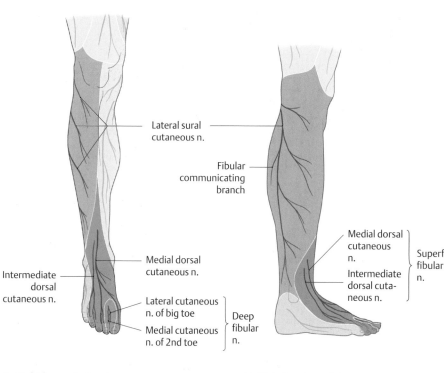

A Right leg, anterior view.

B Right leg, lateral view.

Fig. 27.23 Common fibular nerve
Right limb, lateral view.

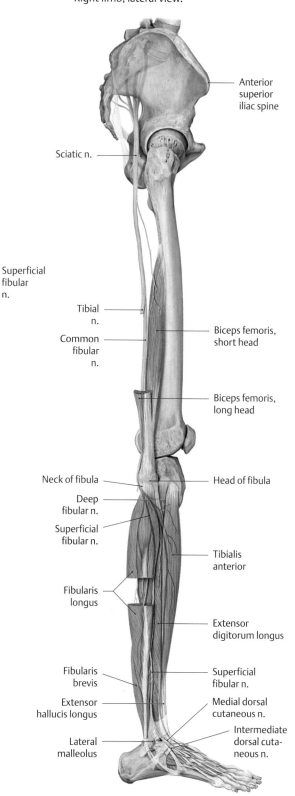

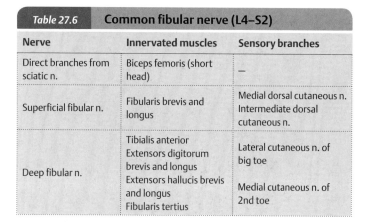

Table 27.6	Common fibular nerve (L4–S2)	
Nerve	**Innervated muscles**	**Sensory branches**
Direct branches from sciatic n.	Biceps femoris (short head)	—
Superficial fibular n.	Fibularis brevis and longus	Medial dorsal cutaneous n. Intermediate dorsal cutaneous n.
Deep fibular n.	Tibialis anterior Extensors digitorum brevis and longus Extensors hallucis brevis and longus Fibularis tertius	Lateral cutaneous n. of big toe Medial cutaneous n. of 2nd toe

Fig. 27.24 Tibial nerve
Right limb.

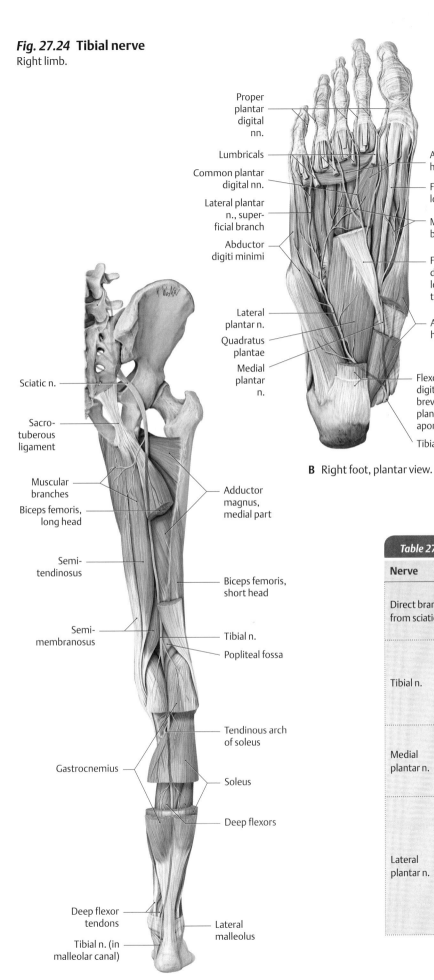

Proper plantar digital nn.

Lumbricals

Common plantar digital nn.

Lateral plantar n., superficial branch

Abductor digiti minimi

Lateral plantar n.

Quadratus plantae

Medial plantar n.

Adductor hallucis

Flexor hallucis longus tendon

Muscular branches

Flexor digitorum longus tendon

Abductor hallucis

Flexor digitorum brevis and plantar aponeurosis

Tibial n.

B Right foot, plantar view.

Sciatic n.

Sacro-tuberous ligament

Muscular branches

Biceps femoris, long head

Semi-tendinosus

Semi-membranosus

Adductor magnus, medial part

Biceps femoris, short head

Tibial n.

Popliteal fossa

Tendinous arch of soleus

Gastrocnemius

Soleus

Deep flexors

Deep flexor tendons

Lateral malleolus

Tibial n. (in malleolar canal)

A Posterior view.

Fig. 27.25 Tibial nerve: Sensory distribution
Right lower limb, posterior view.

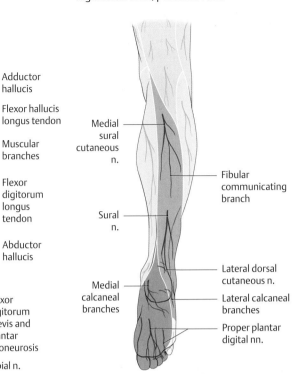

Medial sural cutaneous n.

Sural n.

Medial calcaneal branches

Fibular communicating branch

Lateral dorsal cutaneous n.

Lateral calcaneal branches

Proper plantar digital nn.

Table 27.7	Tibial nerve (L4–S3)	
Nerve	**Innervated muscles**	**Sensory branches**
Direct branches from sciatic n.	Semitendinosus Semimembranosus Biceps femoris (long head) Adductor magnus (medial part)	—
Tibial n.	Triceps surae Plantaris Popliteus Tibialis posterior Flexor digitorum longus Flexor hallucis longus	Medial sural cutaneous n. Medial and lateral calcaneal branches Lateral dorsal cutaneous n.
Medial plantar n.	Adductor hallucis Flexor digitorum brevis Flexor hallucis brevis (medial head) 1st and 2nd lumbricals	Proper plantar digital nn.
Lateral plantar n.	Flexor hallucis brevis (lateral head) Quadratus plantae Abductor digiti minimi Flexor digiti minimi brevis Opponens digiti minimi 3rd and 4th lumbricals 1st to 3rd plantar interossei 1st to 4th dorsal interossei Adductor hallucis	Proper plantar digital nn.

Superficial Nerves & Vessels of the Lower Limb

Fig. 27.26 **Cutaneous innervation: Anterior view**
Right limb.

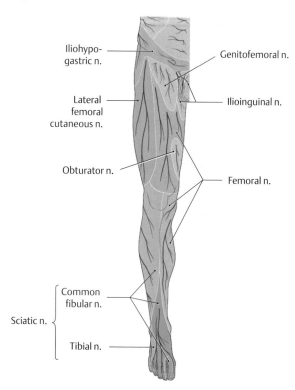

Iliohypo-
gastric n.

Genitofemoral n.

Lateral
femoral
cutaneous n.

Ilioinguinal n.

Obturator n.

Femoral n.

Common
fibular n.

Sciatic n.

Tibial n.

A Peripheral sensory cutaneous innervation.

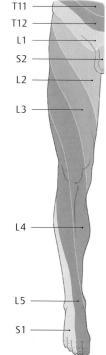

T11
T12
L1
S2
L2
L3
L4
L5
S1

B Segmental, radicular cutaneous
innervation (dermatomes).

Fig. 27.27 **Superficial cutaneous veins and nerves**
Right limb.

Inguinal ligament

Superficial
epigastric v.

Superficial
circumflex
iliac v.

Femoral a.
and v. (in
saphenous hiatus)

Lateral femoral
cutaneous n.

Ilioinguinal n.

External
inguinal ring

External
pudendal vv.

Accessory
saphenous v.

Femoral n.,
anterior femoral
cutaneous
branches

Long
saphenous v.

Fascia lata

Obturator n.

Saphenous n.,
infrapatellar
branch

Saphenous n.
(femoral n.)

Lateral sural
cutaneous n.
(common
fibular n.)

Long
saphenous v.

Superficial
fibular n.

Intermediate dorsal
cutaneous n.

Medial dorsal
cutaneous n.

Sural n.
(tibial n.)

Deep fibular
n.

A Anterior view.

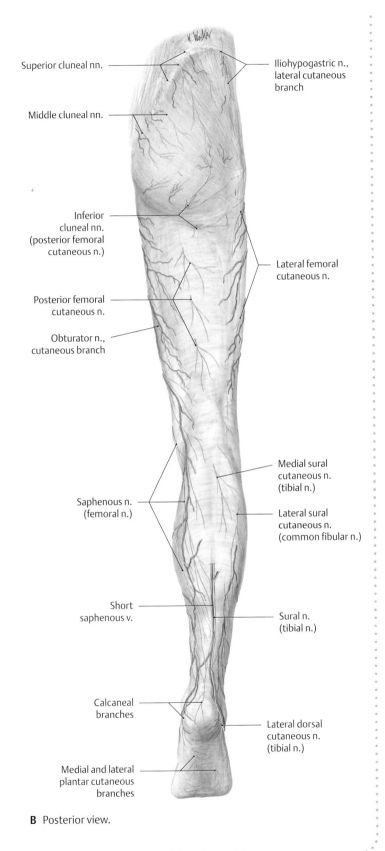

Superior cluneal nn.

Middle cluneal nn.

Inferior cluneal nn. (posterior femoral cutaneous n.)

Posterior femoral cutaneous n.

Obturator n., cutaneous branch

Iliohypogastric n., lateral cutaneous branch

Lateral femoral cutaneous n.

Saphenous n. (femoral n.)

Medial sural cutaneous n. (tibial n.)

Lateral sural cutaneous n. (common fibular n.)

Short saphenous v.

Sural n. (tibial n.)

Calcaneal branches

Lateral dorsal cutaneous n. (tibial n.)

Medial and lateral plantar cutaneous branches

B Posterior view.

Fig. 27.28 **Cutaneous innervation: Posterior view**
Right limb.

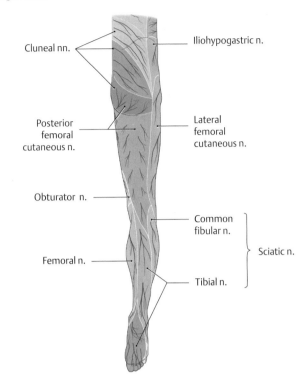

Cluneal nn.

Iliohypogastric n.

Posterior femoral cutaneous n.

Lateral femoral cutaneous n.

Obturator n.

Common fibular n.

Femoral n.

Tibial n.

Sciatic n.

A Peripheral sensory cutaneous innervation.

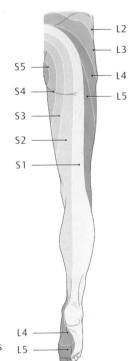

L2
L3
S5
L4
S4
L5
S3
S2
S1

L4
L5

B Segmental, radicular cutaneous innervation (dermatomes).

Topography of the Inguinal Region

Fig. 27.29 Superficial veins and lymph nodes
Right male inguinal region, anterior view. *Removed:* Cribriform fascia about the saphenous hiatus.

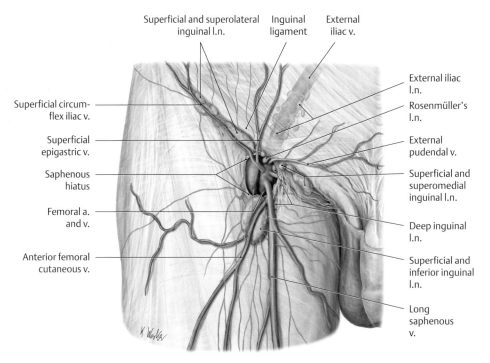

Superficial and superolateral inguinal l.n.

Inguinal ligament

External iliac v.

Superficial circumflex iliac v.

Superficial epigastric v.

Saphenous hiatus

Femoral a. and v.

Anterior femoral cutaneous v.

External iliac l.n.

Rosenmüller's l.n.

External pudendal v.

Superficial and superomedial inguinal l.n.

Deep inguinal l.n.

Superficial and inferior inguinal l.n.

Long saphenous v.

Fig. 27.30 Inguinal region
Right male inguinal region, anterior view.

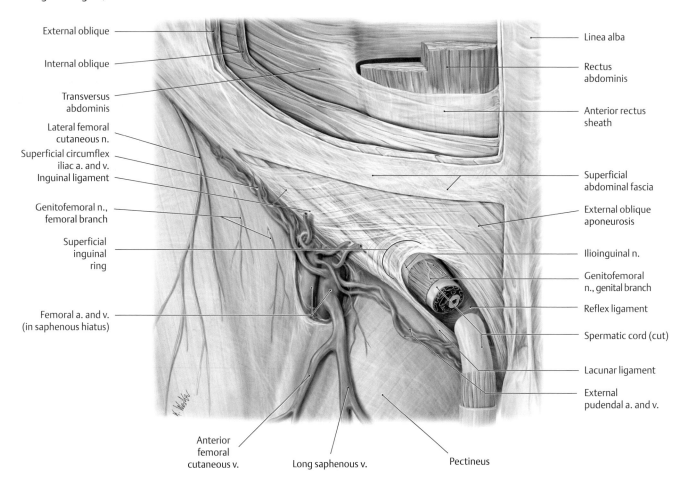

External oblique

Internal oblique

Transversus abdominis

Lateral femoral cutaneous n.

Superficial circumflex iliac a. and v.

Inguinal ligament

Genitofemoral n., femoral branch

Superficial inguinal ring

Femoral a. and v. (in saphenous hiatus)

Anterior femoral cutaneous v.

Long saphenous v.

Pectineus

Linea alba

Rectus abdominis

Anterior rectus sheath

Superficial abdominal fascia

External oblique aponeurosis

Ilioinguinal n.

Genitofemoral n., genital branch

Reflex ligament

Spermatic cord (cut)

Lacunar ligament

External pudendal a. and v.

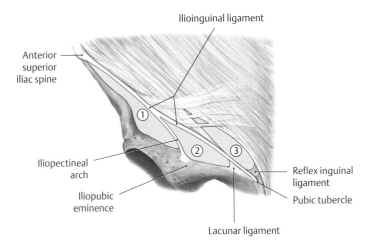

Table 27.8	Structures in the inguinal region		
Region	**Boundaries**	**Contents**	
① Lacuna musculorum	Anterior superior iliac spine Inguinal ligament Iliopectineal arch	Femoral n. Lateral femoral cutaneous n. Iliacus Psoas major	
② Lacuna vasorum	Inguinal ligament Iliopectineal arch Lacunar ligament	Femoral a. and v. Genitofemoral n. (femoral branch) Rosenmüller's lymph node	
③ External inguinal ring	Medial crus Lateral crus Reflex inguinal ligament	Ilioinguinal n. Genitofemoral n. (genital branch) Spermatic cord	

Fig. 27.31 Lacunae musculorum and vasorum
Right inguinal region, anterior view.

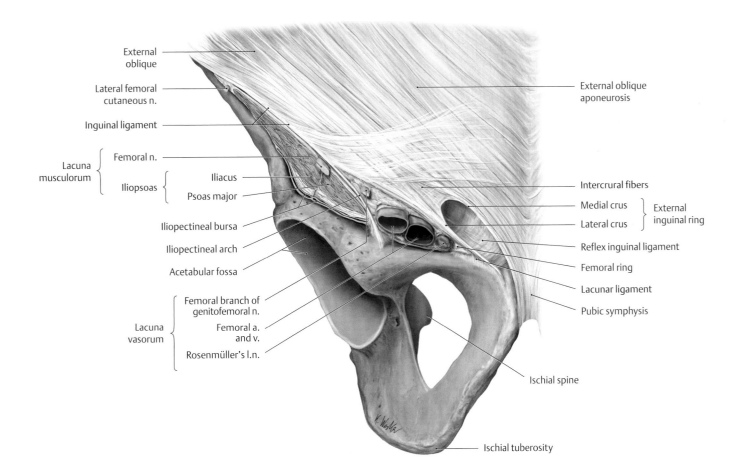

Topography of the Gluteal Region

Fig. 27.32 **Gluteal region**
Right gluteal region, posterior view.

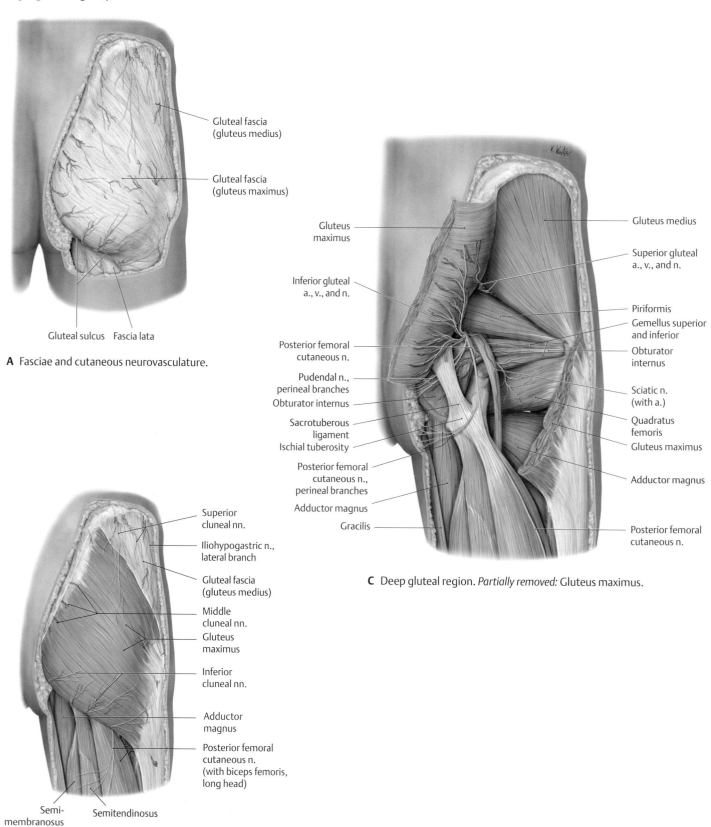

Gluteal fascia
(gluteus medius)

Gluteal fascia
(gluteus maximus)

Gluteal sulcus   Fascia lata

A Fasciae and cutaneous neurovasculature.

Gluteus
maximus

Inferior gluteal
a., v., and n.

Posterior femoral
cutaneous n.

Pudendal n.,
perineal branches

Obturator internus

Sacrotuberous
ligament

Ischial tuberosity

Posterior femoral
cutaneous n.,
perineal branches

Adductor magnus

Gracilis

Gluteus medius

Superior gluteal
a., v., and n.

Piriformis

Gemellus superior
and inferior

Obturator
internus

Sciatic n.
(with a.)

Quadratus
femoris

Gluteus maximus

Adductor magnus

Posterior femoral
cutaneous n.

C Deep gluteal region. *Partially removed:* Gluteus maximus.

Superior
cluneal nn.

Iliohypogastric n.,
lateral branch

Gluteal fascia
(gluteus medius)

Middle
cluneal nn.

Gluteus
maximus

Inferior
cluneal nn.

Adductor
magnus

Posterior femoral
cutaneous n.
(with biceps femoris,
long head)

Semi-
membranosus   Semitendinosus

B Gluteal region. *Removed:* Fascia lata.

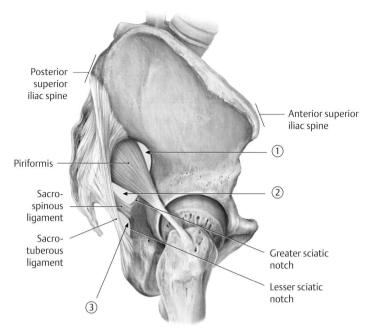

Posterior superior iliac spine

Anterior superior iliac spine

Piriformis

Sacro-spinous ligament

Sacro-tuberous ligament

①

②

③

Greater sciatic notch

Lesser sciatic notch

Table 27.9		Sciatic foramina	
Foramen		**Transmitted structures**	**Boundaries**
Greater sciatic foramen	① Suprapiriform portion	Superior gluteal a., v., and n.	Greater sciatic notch Sacrospinous ligament Sacrum
	② Infrapiriform portion	Inferior gluteal a., v., and n. Internal pudendal a. and v. Pudendal n. Sciatic n. Posterior femoral cutaneous n.	
③ Lesser sciatic foramen		Internal pudendal a. and v. Pudendal n. Obturator internus	Lesser sciatic notch Sacrospinous ligament Sacrotuberous ligament

Fig. 27.33 **Gluteal region and ischianal fossa**
Right gluteal region, posterior view.
Removed: Gluteus maximus and medius.

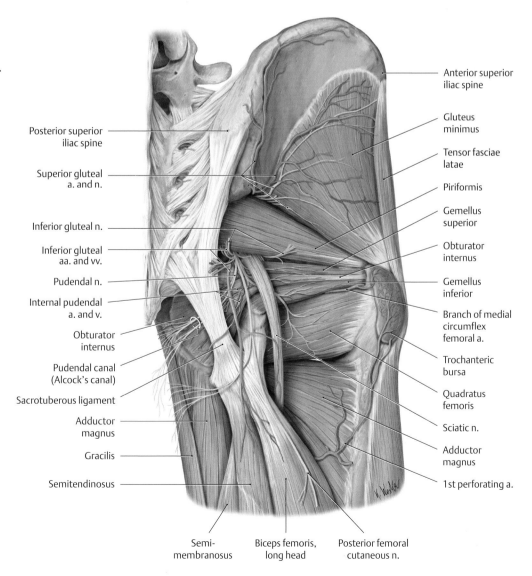

Posterior superior iliac spine

Superior gluteal a. and n.

Inferior gluteal n.

Inferior gluteal aa. and vv.

Pudendal n.

Internal pudendal a. and v.

Obturator internus

Pudendal canal (Alcock's canal)

Sacrotuberous ligament

Adductor magnus

Gracilis

Semitendinosus

Semi-membranosus

Biceps femoris, long head

Posterior femoral cutaneous n.

Anterior superior iliac spine

Gluteus minimus

Tensor fasciae latae

Piriformis

Gemellus superior

Obturator internus

Gemellus inferior

Branch of medial circumflex femoral a.

Trochanteric bursa

Quadratus femoris

Sciatic n.

Adductor magnus

1st perforating a.

Topography of the Anterior & Posterior Thigh

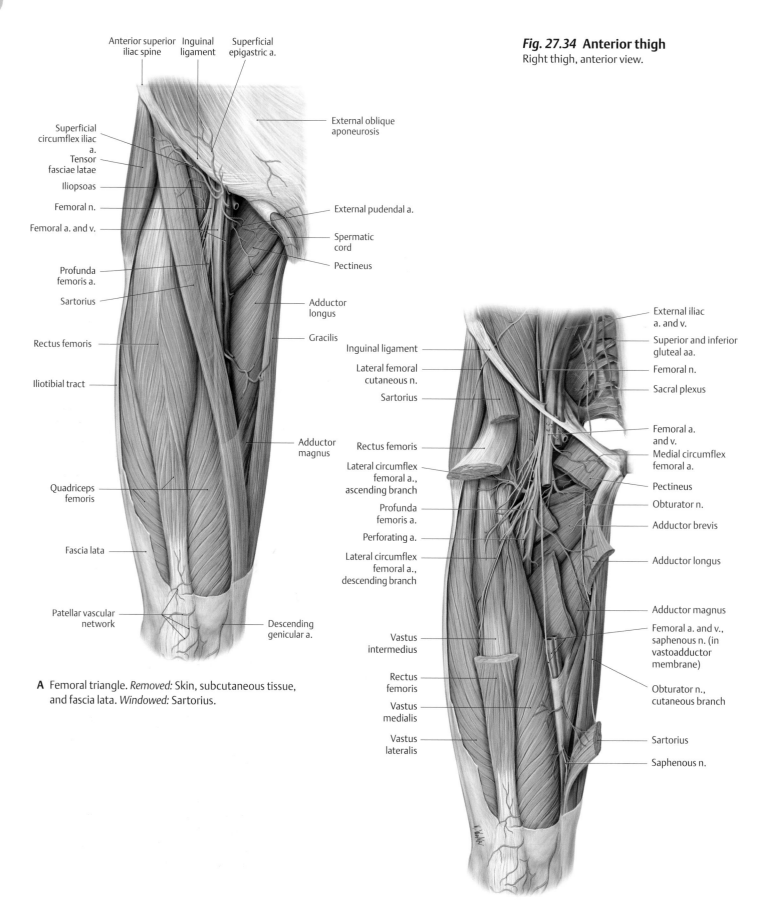

Fig. 27.34 Anterior thigh
Right thigh, anterior view.

Labels for figure A (Femoral triangle):
Anterior superior iliac spine
Inguinal ligament
Superficial epigastric a.
External oblique aponeurosis
Superficial circumflex iliac a.
Tensor fasciae latae
Iliopsoas
Femoral n.
Femoral a. and v.
External pudendal a.
Spermatic cord
Pectineus
Profunda femoris a.
Sartorius
Adductor longus
Gracilis
Rectus femoris
Iliotibial tract
Adductor magnus
Quadriceps femoris
Fascia lata
Patellar vascular network
Descending genicular a.

A Femoral triangle. *Removed:* Skin, subcutaneous tissue, and fascia lata. *Windowed:* Sartorius.

Labels for figure B (Neurovasculature):
Inguinal ligament
Lateral femoral cutaneous n.
Sartorius
Rectus femoris
Lateral circumflex femoral a., ascending branch
Profunda femoris a.
Perforating a.
Lateral circumflex femoral a., descending branch
Vastus intermedius
Rectus femoris
Vastus medialis
Vastus lateralis
External iliac a. and v.
Superior and inferior gluteal aa.
Femoral n.
Sacral plexus
Femoral a. and v.
Medial circumflex femoral a.
Pectineus
Obturator n.
Adductor brevis
Adductor longus
Adductor magnus
Femoral a. and v., saphenous n. (in vastoadductor membrane)
Obturator n., cutaneous branch
Sartorius
Saphenous n.

B Neurovasculature of the anterior thigh. *Removed:* Anterior abdominal wall. *Partially removed:* Sartorius, rectus femoris, adductor longus, and pectineus.

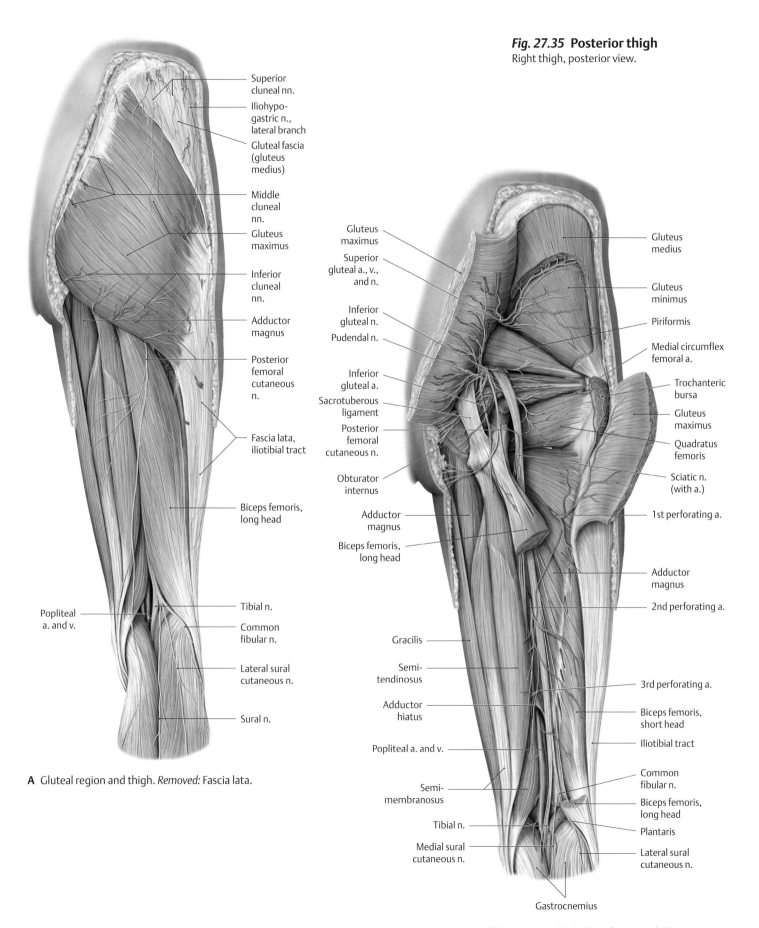

Fig. 27.35 Posterior thigh
Right thigh, posterior view.

Superior cluneal nn.

Iliohypogastric n., lateral branch

Gluteal fascia (gluteus medius)

Middle cluneal nn.

Gluteus maximus

Inferior cluneal nn.

Adductor magnus

Posterior femoral cutaneous n.

Fascia lata, iliotibial tract

Biceps femoris, long head

Popliteal a. and v.

Tibial n.

Common fibular n.

Lateral sural cutaneous n.

Sural n.

A Gluteal region and thigh. *Removed:* Fascia lata.

Gluteus maximus

Superior gluteal a., v., and n.

Inferior gluteal n.

Pudendal n.

Inferior gluteal a.

Sacrotuberous ligament

Posterior femoral cutaneous n.

Obturator internus

Adductor magnus

Biceps femoris, long head

Gracilis

Semi-tendinosus

Adductor hiatus

Popliteal a. and v.

Semi-membranosus

Tibial n.

Medial sural cutaneous n.

Gastrocnemius

Gluteus medius

Gluteus minimus

Piriformis

Medial circumflex femoral a.

Trochanteric bursa

Gluteus maximus

Quadratus femoris

Sciatic n. (with a.)

1st perforating a.

Adductor magnus

2nd perforating a.

3rd perforating a.

Biceps femoris, short head

Iliotibial tract

Common fibular n.

Biceps femoris, long head

Plantaris

Lateral sural cutaneous n.

B Neurovasculature of the posterior thigh. *Partially removed:* Gluteus maximus, gluteus medius, and biceps femoris. *Retracted:* Semimembranosus.

441

Topography of the Posterior & Medial Leg

Fig. 27.36 **Posterior compartment**
Right leg, posterior view.

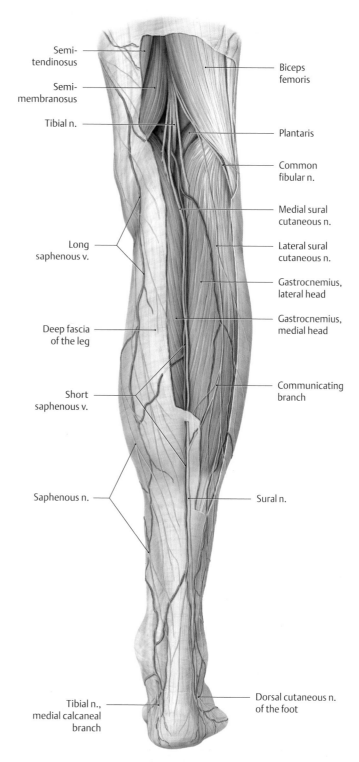

Semi-
tendinosus

Semi-
membranosus

Tibial n.

Long
saphenous v.

Deep fascia
of the leg

Short
saphenous v.

Saphenous n.

Tibial n.,
medial calcaneal
branch

Biceps
femoris

Plantaris

Common
fibular n.

Medial sural
cutaneous n.

Lateral sural
cutaneous n.

Gastrocnemius,
lateral head

Gastrocnemius,
medial head

Communicating
branch

Sural n.

Dorsal cutaneous n.
of the foot

A Superficial neurovascular structures.

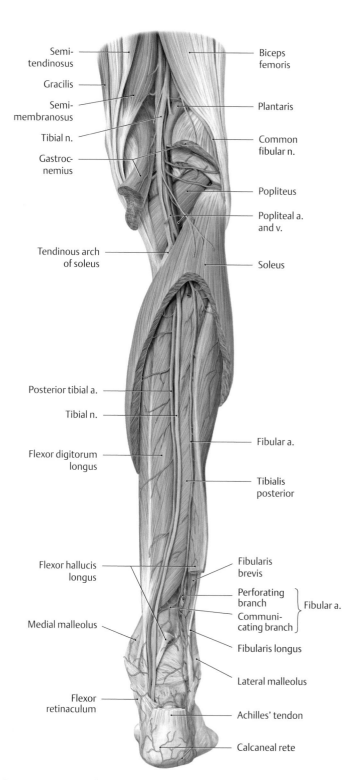

Semi-
tendinosus

Gracilis

Semi-
membranosus

Tibial n.

Gastroc-
nemius

Tendinous arch
of soleus

Posterior tibial a.

Tibial n.

Flexor digitorum
longus

Flexor hallucis
longus

Medial malleolus

Flexor
retinaculum

Biceps
femoris

Plantaris

Common
fibular n.

Popliteus

Popliteal a.
and v.

Soleus

Fibular a.

Tibialis
posterior

Fibularis
brevis

Perforating
branch

Communi-
cating branch

Fibular a.

Fibularis longus

Lateral malleolus

Achilles' tendon

Calcaneal rete

B Deep neurovascular structures.

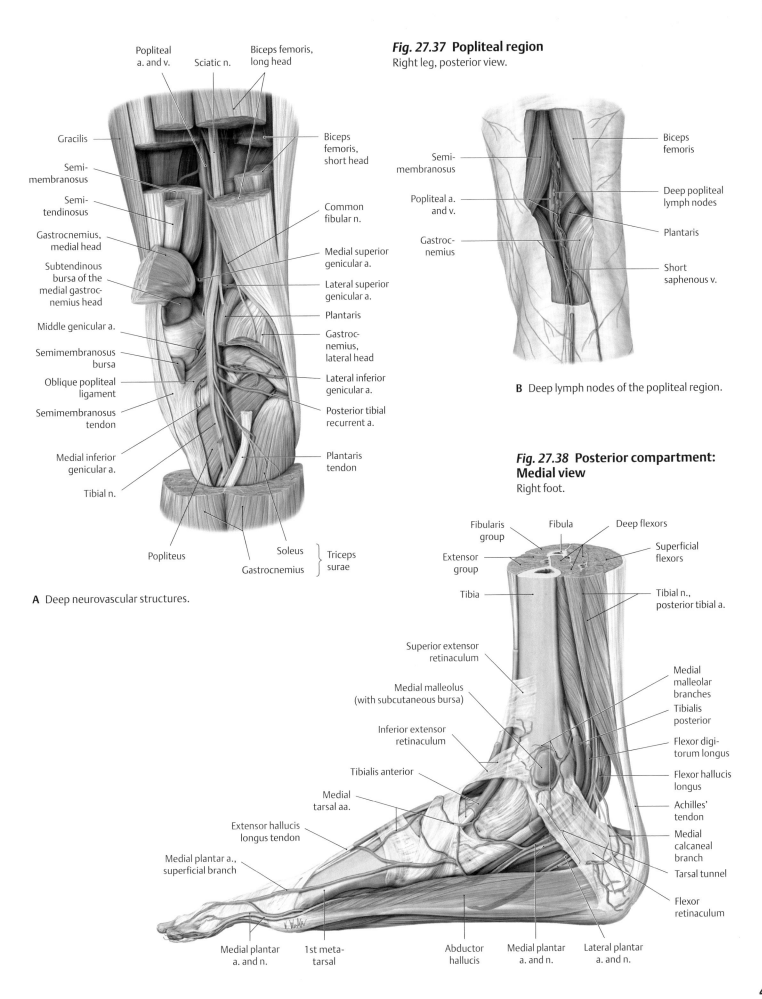

Fig. 27.37 Popliteal region
Right leg, posterior view.

Popliteal a. and v.

Sciatic n.

Biceps femoris, long head

Gracilis

Semi-membranosus

Semi-tendinosus

Gastrocnemius, medial head

Subtendinous bursa of the medial gastroc-nemius head

Middle genicular a.

Semimembranosus bursa

Oblique popliteal ligament

Semimembranosus tendon

Medial inferior genicular a.

Tibial n.

Biceps femoris, short head

Common fibular n.

Medial superior genicular a.

Lateral superior genicular a.

Plantaris

Gastroc-nemius, lateral head

Lateral inferior genicular a.

Posterior tibial recurrent a.

Plantaris tendon

Popliteus

Soleus

Gastrocnemius

Triceps surae

A Deep neurovascular structures.

Semi-membranosus

Popliteal a. and v.

Gastroc-nemius

Biceps femoris

Deep popliteal lymph nodes

Plantaris

Short saphenous v.

B Deep lymph nodes of the popliteal region.

Fig. 27.38 Posterior compartment: Medial view
Right foot.

Fibularis group

Fibula

Deep flexors

Extensor group

Superficial flexors

Tibia

Tibial n., posterior tibial a.

Superior extensor retinaculum

Medial malleolus (with subcutaneous bursa)

Inferior extensor retinaculum

Tibialis anterior

Medial tarsal aa.

Extensor hallucis longus tendon

Medial plantar a., superficial branch

Medial malleolar branches

Tibialis posterior

Flexor digi-torum longus

Flexor hallucis longus

Achilles' tendon

Medial calcaneal branch

Tarsal tunnel

Flexor retinaculum

Medial plantar a. and n.

1st meta-tarsal

Abductor hallucis

Medial plantar a. and n.

Lateral plantar a. and n.

Topography of the Lateral & Anterior Leg

Fig. 27.39 **Neurovasculature of the leg: Lateral view**

Right limb. *Removed:* Origins of the fibularis longus and extensor digitorum longus.

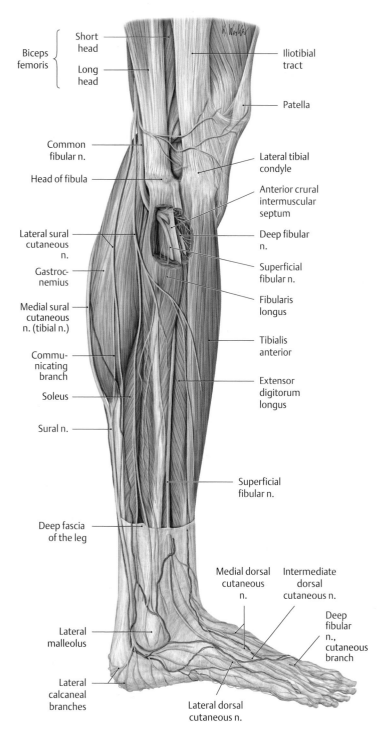

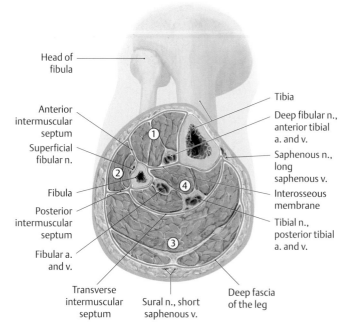

Table 27.10	Compartments of the leg		
Compartment		**Muscular contents**	**Neurovascular contents**
① Anterior compartment		Tibialis anterior	Deep fibular n. Anterior tibial a. and v.
		Extensor digitorum longus	
		Extensor hallucis longus	
		Fibularis tertius	
② Lateral compartment		Fibularis longus	Superficial fibular n.
		Fibularis brevis	
Posterior compartment	③ Superficial part	Triceps surae (gastrocnemius and soleus)	—
		Plantaris	
	④ Deep part	Tibialis posterior	Tibial n. Posterior tibial a. and v. Fibular a. and v.
		Flexor digitorum longus	
		Flexor hallucis longus	

Compartment syndrome

Muscle edema or hematoma can lead to a rise in tissue pressure in the compartments of the leg. Subsequent compression of neurovascular structures may cause ischemia and irreversible muscle and nerve damage. Patients with *anterior* compartment syndrome, the most common form, suffer excruciating pain and cannot dorsiflex the toes. Emergency incision of the fascia of the leg may be performed to relieve compression.

Fig. 27.40 Neurovasculature of the leg and foot: Anterior view

Right limb with foot in plantar flexion.

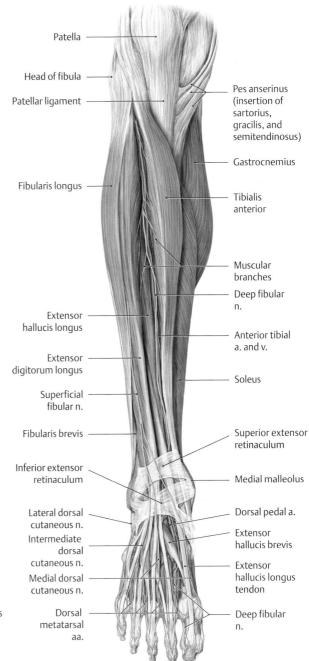

B Neurovasculature of the leg. *Removed:* Skin, subcutaneous tissue, and fasciae. *Retracted:* Tibialis anterior and extensor hallucis longus.

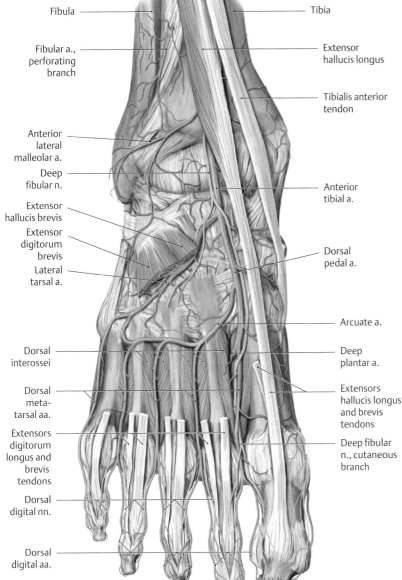

A Neurovasculature of the dorsum.

Topography of the Sole of the Foot

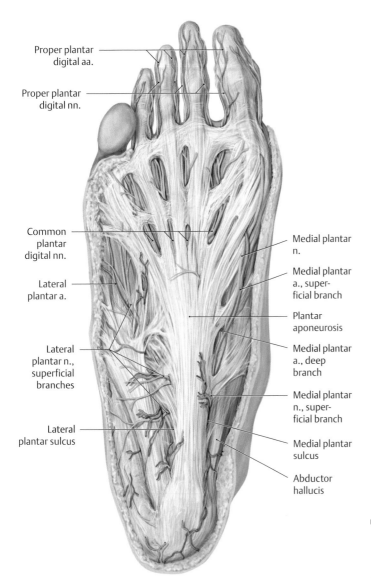

Proper plantar digital aa.

Proper plantar digital nn.

Common plantar digital nn.

Lateral plantar a.

Lateral plantar n., superficial branches

Lateral plantar sulcus

Medial plantar n.

Medial plantar a., superficial branch

Plantar aponeurosis

Medial plantar a., deep branch

Medial plantar n., superficial branch

Medial plantar sulcus

Abductor hallucis

A Superficial layer. *Removed:* Skin, subcutaneous tissue, and fascia.

Fig. 27.41 Neurovasculature of the foot: Sole
Right foot, plantar view.

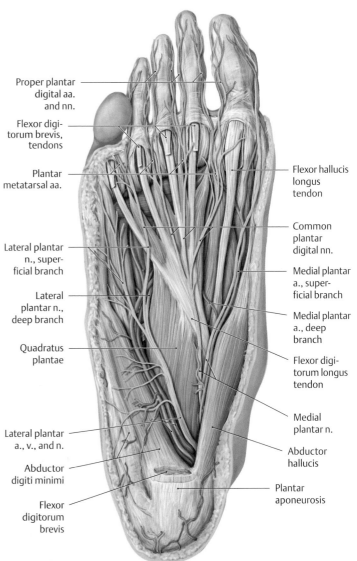

Proper plantar digital aa. and nn.

Flexor digitorum brevis, tendons

Plantar metatarsal aa.

Lateral plantar n., superficial branch

Lateral plantar n., deep branch

Quadratus plantae

Lateral plantar a., v., and n.

Abductor digiti minimi

Flexor digitorum brevis

Flexor hallucis longus tendon

Common plantar digital nn.

Medial plantar a., superficial branch

Medial plantar a., deep branch

Flexor digitorum longus tendon

Medial plantar n.

Abductor hallucis

Plantar aponeurosis

B Middle layer. *Removed:* Plantar aponeurosis and flexor digitorum brevis.

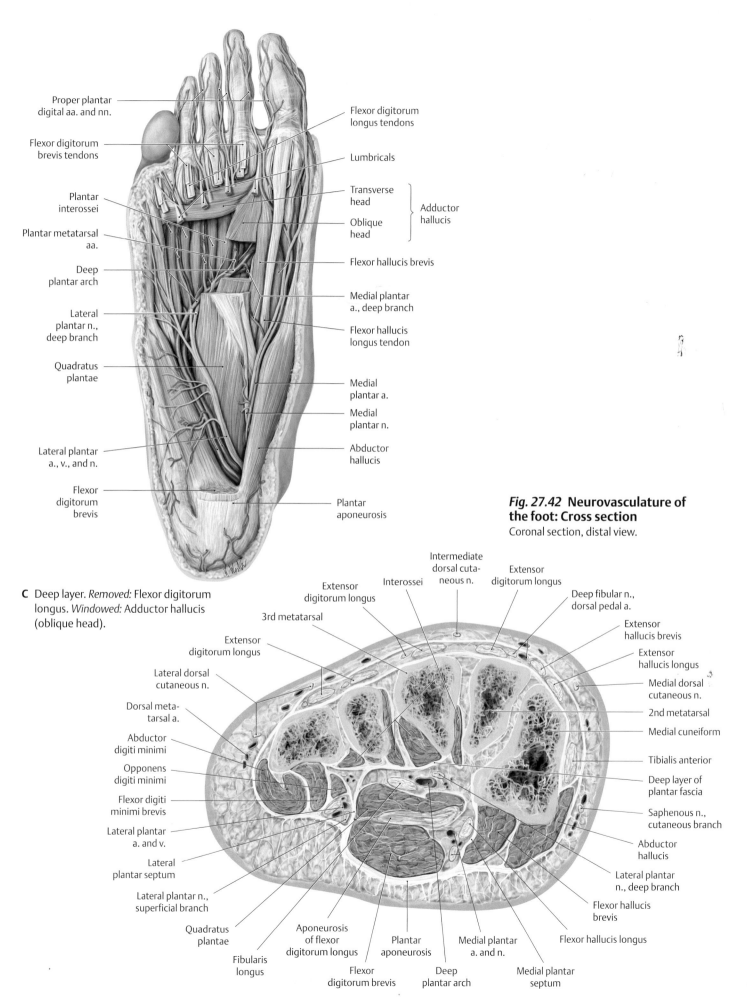

Proper plantar digital aa. and nn.

Flexor digitorum brevis tendons

Plantar interossei

Plantar metatarsal aa.

Deep plantar arch

Lateral plantar n., deep branch

Quadratus plantae

Lateral plantar a., v., and n.

Flexor digitorum brevis

Flexor digitorum longus tendons

Lumbricals

Transverse head ⎤
                  ⎥ Adductor hallucis
Oblique head   ⎦

Flexor hallucis brevis

Medial plantar a., deep branch

Flexor hallucis longus tendon

Medial plantar a.

Medial plantar n.

Abductor hallucis

Plantar aponeurosis

C Deep layer. *Removed:* Flexor digitorum longus. *Windowed:* Adductor hallucis (oblique head).

***Fig. 27.42* Neurovasculature of the foot: Cross section**
Coronal section, distal view.

Extensor digitorum longus

3rd metatarsal

Extensor digitorum longus

Lateral dorsal cutaneous n.

Dorsal metatarsal a.

Abductor digiti minimi

Opponens digiti minimi

Flexor digiti minimi brevis

Lateral plantar a. and v.

Lateral plantar septum

Lateral plantar n., superficial branch

Quadratus plantae

Aponeurosis of flexor digitorum longus

Fibularis longus

Flexor digitorum brevis

Plantar aponeurosis

Deep plantar arch

Medial plantar a. and n.

Medial plantar septum

Interossei

Intermediate dorsal cutaneous n.

Extensor digitorum longus

Deep fibular n., dorsal pedal a.

Extensor hallucis brevis

Extensor hallucis longus

Medial dorsal cutaneous n.

2nd metatarsal

Medial cuneiform

Tibialis anterior

Deep layer of plantar fascia

Saphenous n., cutaneous branch

Abductor hallucis

Lateral plantar n., deep branch

Flexor hallucis brevis

Flexor hallucis longus

Transverse Sections of the Thigh & Leg

***Fig. 27.43* Windowed dissection**
Right limb, posterior view.

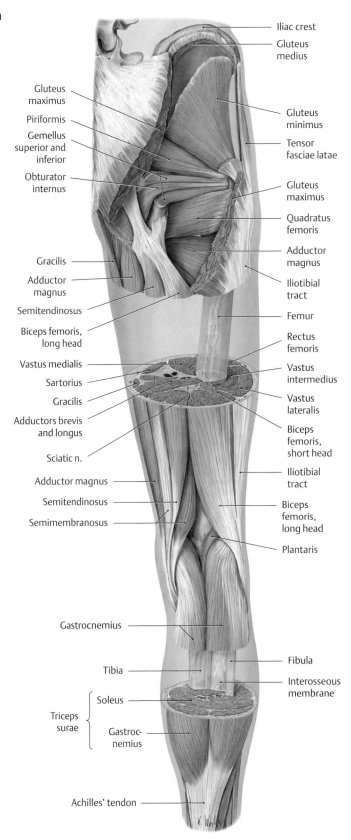

Gluteus maximus
Piriformis
Gemellus superior and inferior
Obturator internus
Gracilis
Adductor magnus
Semitendinosus
Biceps femoris, long head
Vastus medialis
Sartorius
Gracilis
Adductors brevis and longus
Sciatic n.
Adductor magnus
Semitendinosus
Semimembranosus
Gastrocnemius
Tibia
Soleus
Triceps surae
Gastrocnemius
Achilles' tendon

Iliac crest
Gluteus medius
Gluteus minimus
Tensor fasciae latae
Gluteus maximus
Quadratus femoris
Adductor magnus
Iliotibial tract
Femur
Rectus femoris
Vastus intermedius
Vastus lateralis
Biceps femoris, short head
Iliotibial tract
Biceps femoris, long head
Plantaris
Fibula
Interosseous membrane

Fig. 27.44 Transverse sections
Right limb, proximal (superior) view.

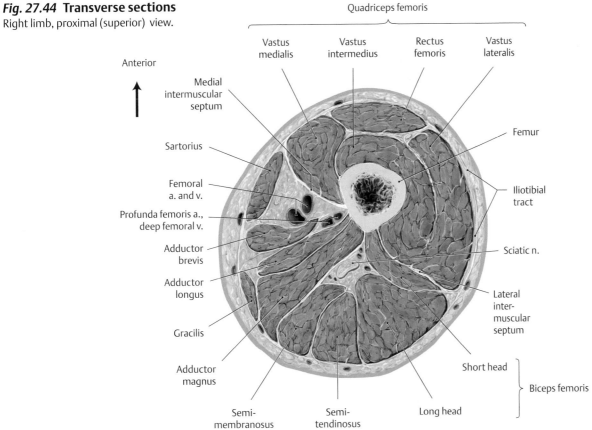

Quadriceps femoris

Vastus medialis

Vastus intermedius

Rectus femoris

Vastus lateralis

Anterior

Medial intermuscular septum

Sartorius

Femoral a. and v.

Profunda femoris a., deep femoral v.

Adductor brevis

Adductor longus

Gracilis

Adductor magnus

Femur

Iliotibial tract

Sciatic n.

Lateral intermuscular septum

Short head

Biceps femoris

Long head

Semi-membranosus

Semi-tendinosus

A Thigh (plane of section in Fig. 27.43).

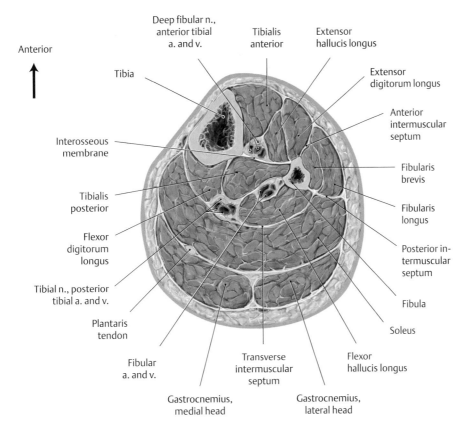

Deep fibular n., anterior tibial a. and v.

Tibialis anterior

Extensor hallucis longus

Anterior

Tibia

Interosseous membrane

Tibialis posterior

Flexor digitorum longus

Tibial n., posterior tibial a. and v.

Plantaris tendon

Fibular a. and v.

Gastrocnemius, medial head

Transverse intermuscular septum

Gastrocnemius, lateral head

Extensor digitorum longus

Anterior intermuscular septum

Fibularis brevis

Fibularis longus

Posterior intermuscular septum

Fibula

Soleus

Flexor hallucis longus

B Leg (plane of section in Fig. 27.43).

Surface Anatomy

Fig. 28.1 Lower limb: Anterior view

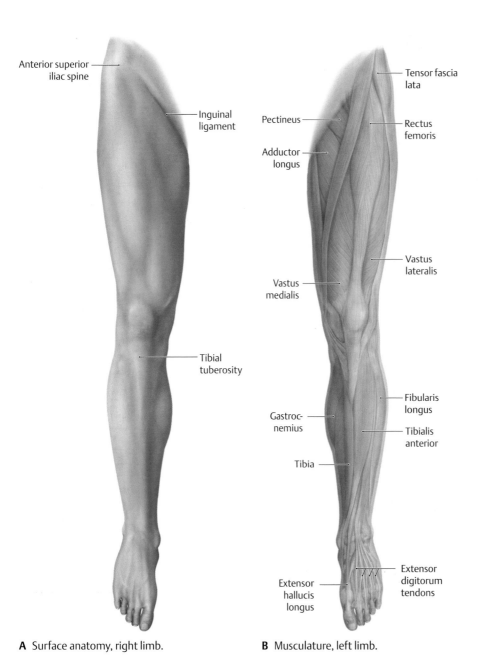

A Surface anatomy, right limb.

B Musculature, left limb.

Fig. 28.2 Palpable bony prominences
Right limb.

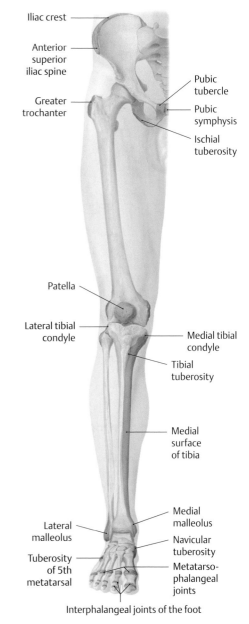

A Anterior view.

Q1: The hip joint is not directly palpable. How would you correctly locate the head of the femur based on surface anatomy?

Fig. 28.3 **Lower limb: Posterior view**

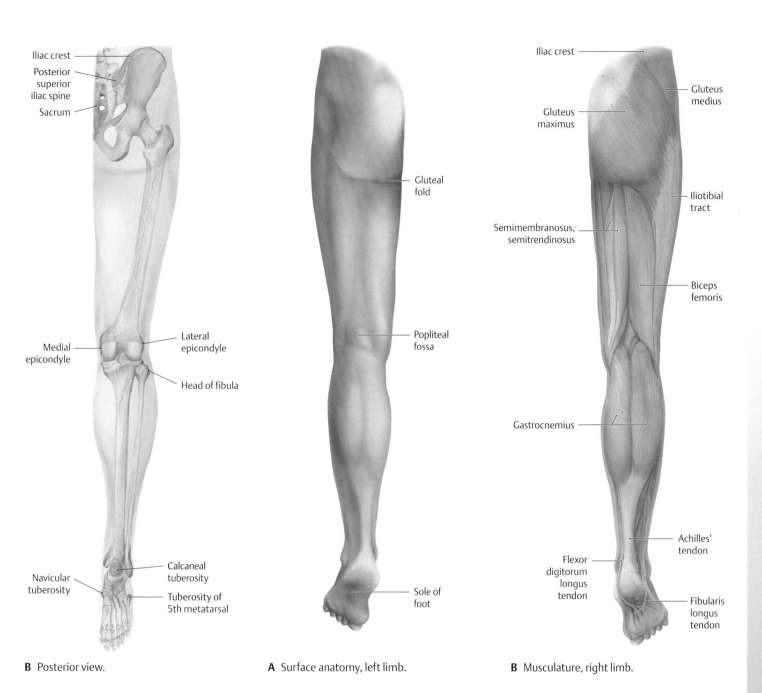

Iliac crest
Posterior superior iliac spine
Sacrum
Medial epicondyle
Lateral epicondyle
Head of fibula
Navicular tuberosity
Calcaneal tuberosity
Tuberosity of 5th metatarsal

B Posterior view.

Gluteal fold
Popliteal fossa
Sole of foot

A Surface anatomy, left limb.

Iliac crest
Gluteus medius
Gluteus maximus
Iliotibial tract
Semimembranosus, semitrendinosus
Biceps femoris
Gastrocnemius
Achilles' tendon
Flexor digitorum longus tendon
Fibularis longus tendon

B Musculature, right limb.

Q2: Which palpable landmarks would you use to locate the sciatic nerve (in the gluteal region), the common fibular nerve (at the knee), and the tibial nerve (at the ankle)?

See answers beginning on p. 626.

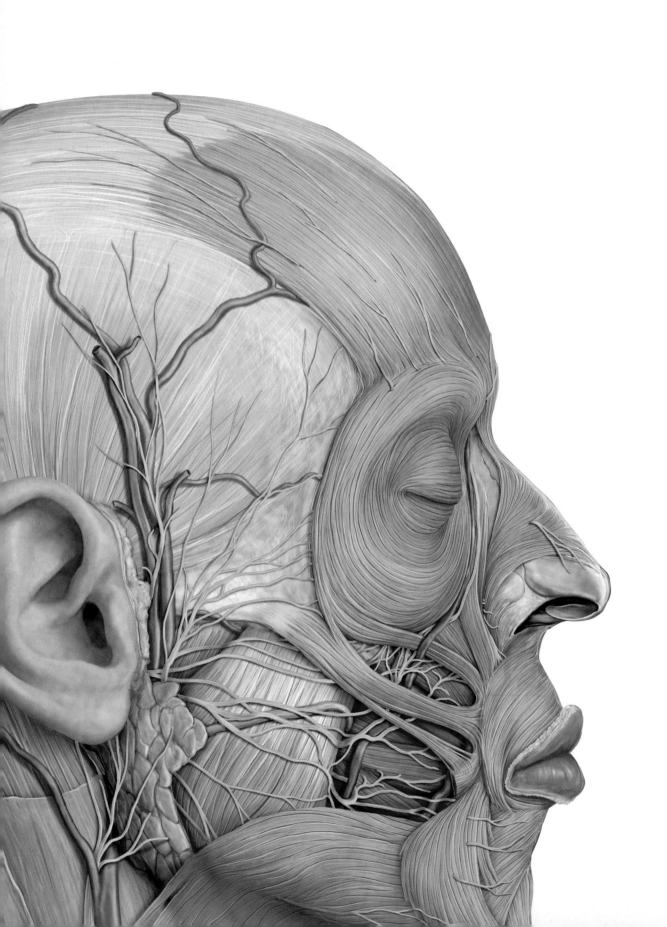

Head & Neck

Anterior & Lateral Skull

Fig. 29.1 Lateral skull
Left lateral view.

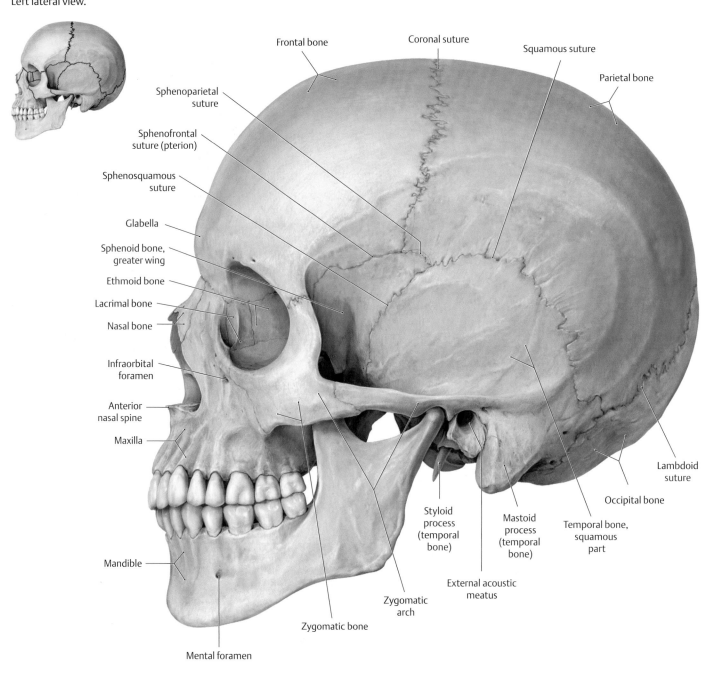

Frontal bone

Coronal suture

Squamous suture

Parietal bone

Sphenoparietal suture

Sphenofrontal suture (pterion)

Sphenosquamous suture

Glabella

Sphenoid bone, greater wing

Ethmoid bone

Lacrimal bone

Nasal bone

Infraorbital foramen

Anterior nasal spine

Maxilla

Mandible

Mental foramen

Zygomatic bone

Zygomatic arch

Styloid process (temporal bone)

Mastoid process (temporal bone)

External acoustic meatus

Temporal bone, squamous part

Occipital bone

Lambdoid suture

Table 29.1	Bones of the skull

The skull is subdivided into the neurocranium (gray) and viscerocranium (orange). The neurocranium protects the brain, while the viscerocranium houses and protects the facial regions.

Neurocranium	Viscerocranium	
• Ethmoid bone (cribriform plate)*	• Ethmoid bone	• Mandible
• Frontal bone	• Hyoid bone	• Maxilla
• Occipital bone	• Inferior nasal concha	• Nasal bone
• Parietal bone	• Lacrimal bone	• Palatine bone
• Sphenoid bone	• Sphenoid bone (pterygoid process)	
• Temporal bone (petrous and squamous parts)	• Temporal bone	
	• Vomer	

*Most of the ethmoid bone is in the viscerocranium; most of the sphenoid bone is in the neurocranium. The temporal bone is divided between the two.

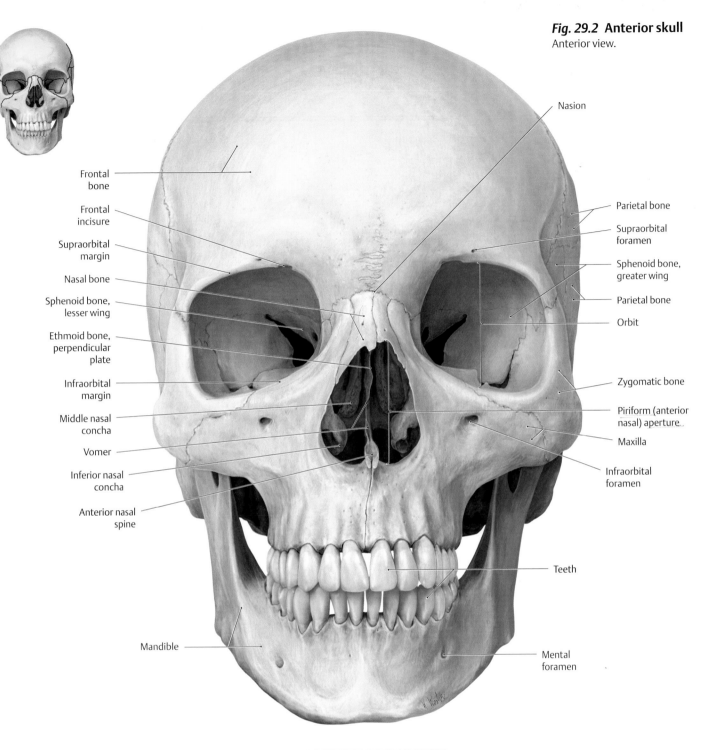

Fig. 29.2 Anterior skull
Anterior view.

Frontal bone

Frontal incisure

Supraorbital margin

Nasal bone

Sphenoid bone, lesser wing

Ethmoid bone, perpendicular plate

Infraorbital margin

Middle nasal concha

Vomer

Inferior nasal concha

Anterior nasal spine

Mandible

Nasion

Parietal bone

Supraorbital foramen

Sphenoid bone, greater wing

Parietal bone

Orbit

Zygomatic bone

Piriform (anterior nasal) aperture

Maxilla

Infraorbital foramen

Teeth

Mental foramen

Clinical

Fractures of the face

The framelike construction of the facial skeleton leads to characteristic patterns for fracture lines (classified as Le Fort I, II, and III fractures).

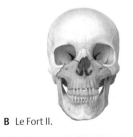

A Le Fort I.

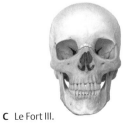

B Le Fort II.

C Le Fort III.

Posterior Skull & Calvaria

Fig. 29.3 **Posterior skull**
Posterior view.

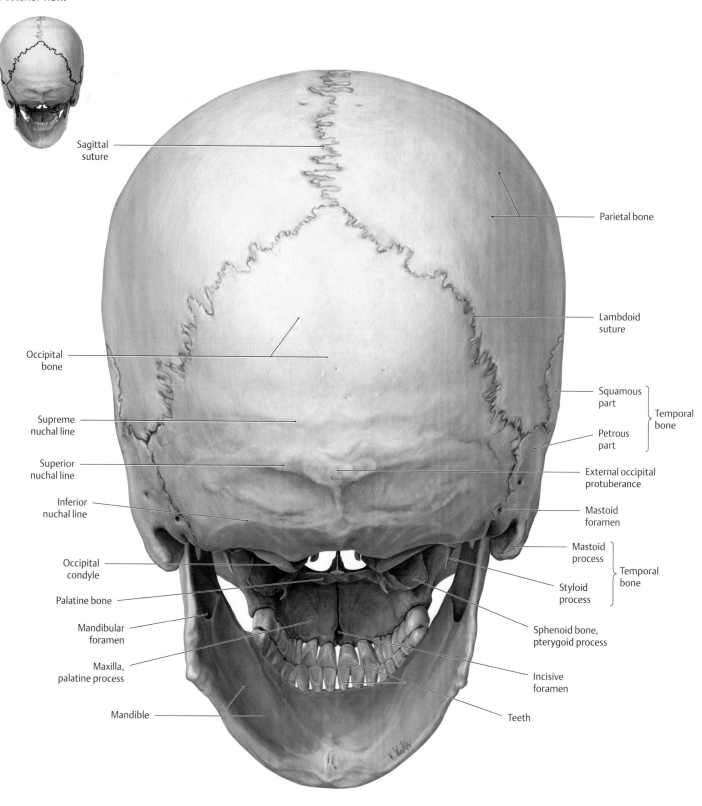

Sagittal suture

Parietal bone

Lambdoid suture

Occipital bone

Squamous part

Petrous part

Temporal bone

Supreme nuchal line

Superior nuchal line

External occipital protuberance

Inferior nuchal line

Mastoid foramen

Occipital condyle

Mastoid process

Palatine bone

Styloid process

Temporal bone

Mandibular foramen

Sphenoid bone, pterygoid process

Maxilla, palatine process

Incisive foramen

Mandible

Teeth

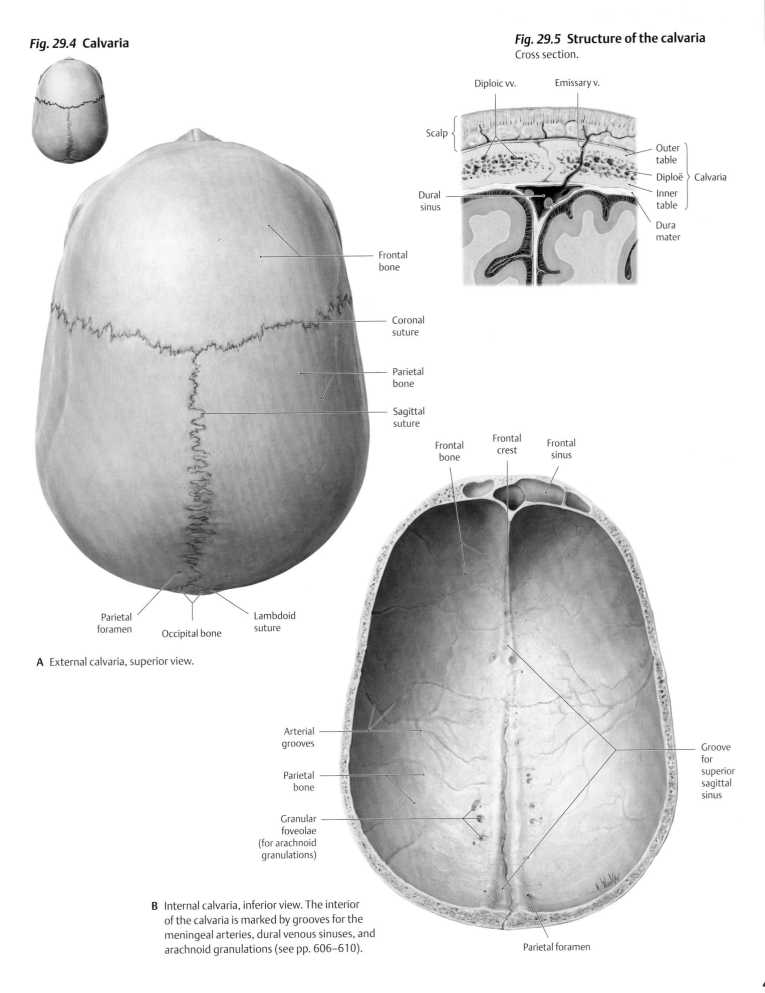

Fig. 29.4 Calvaria

Fig. 29.5 Structure of the calvaria
Cross section.

Diploic vv.   Emissary v.

Scalp

Outer table
Diploë ⟩ Calvaria
Inner table

Dural sinus

Dura mater

Frontal bone

Coronal suture

Parietal bone

Sagittal suture

Parietal foramen   Occipital bone   Lambdoid suture

A External calvaria, superior view.

Frontal bone   Frontal crest   Frontal sinus

Arterial grooves

Parietal bone

Granular foveolae (for arachnoid granulations)

Groove for superior sagittal sinus

Parietal foramen

B Internal calvaria, inferior view. The interior of the calvaria is marked by grooves for the meningeal arteries, dural venous sinuses, and arachnoid granulations (see pp. 606–610).

457

Base of the Skull

Fig. 29.6 **Base of the skull: Exterior**

Inferior view. *Revealed:* Foramina and canals for blood vessels
(see p. 490) and cranial nerves. *Note:* This view allows visual access
into the posterior region of the nasal cavity.

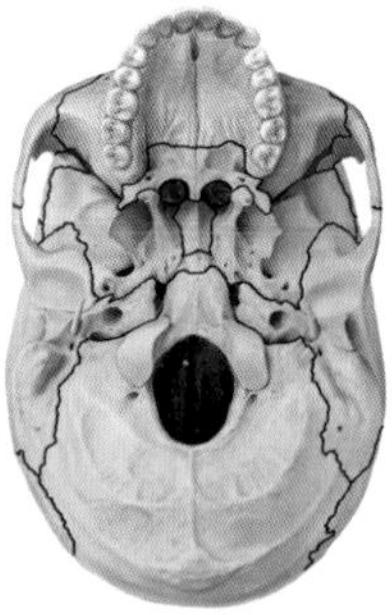

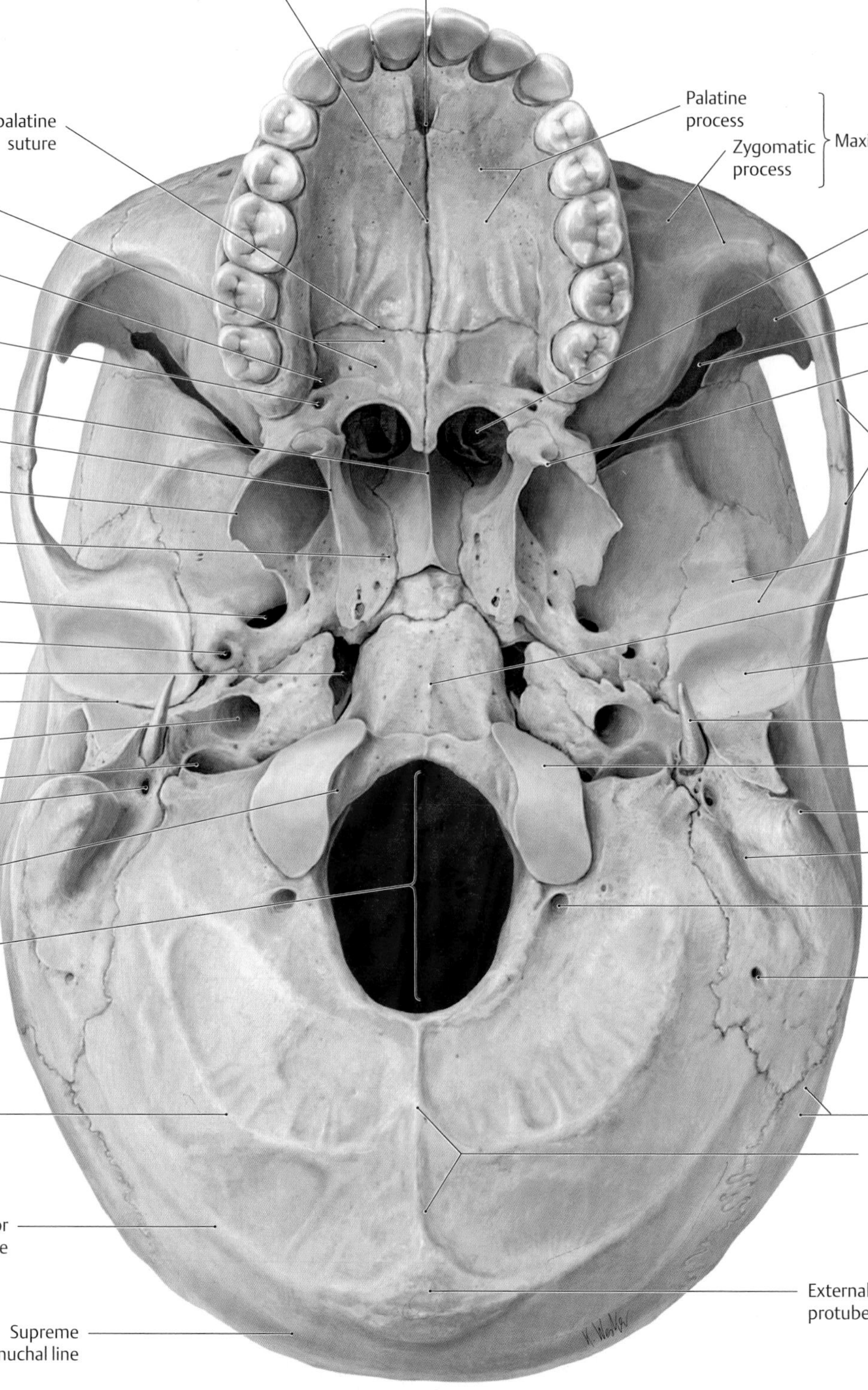

Fig. 29.7 Cranial fossae

The interior of the skull base consists of three successive fossae that become progressively deeper in the frontal-to-occipital direction.

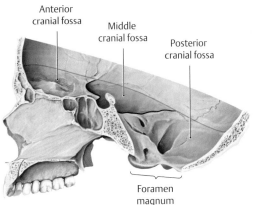

A Midsagittal section, left lateral view.

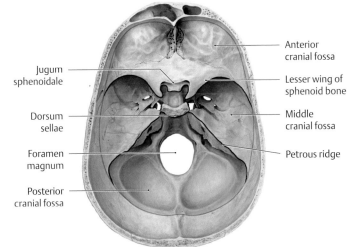

B Superior view of opened skull.

Fig. 29.8 Base of the skull: Interior

Superior view.

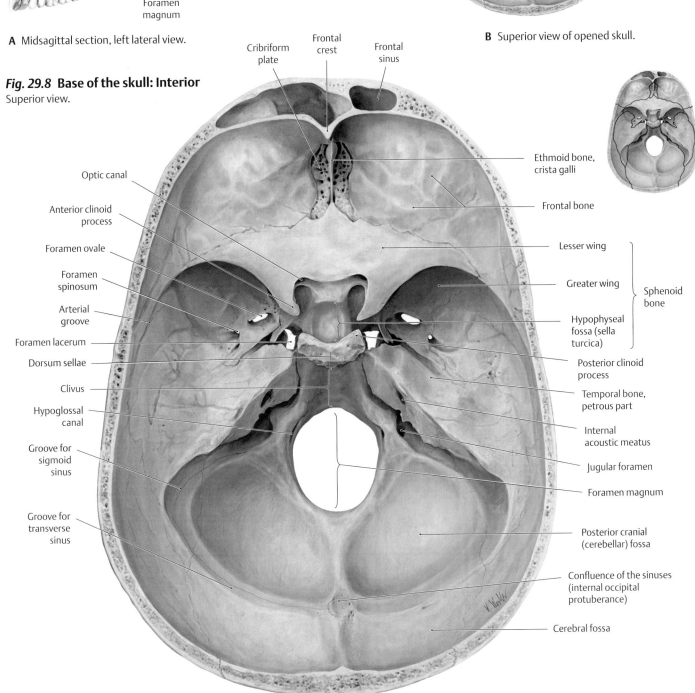

Ethmoid & Sphenoid Bones

The structurally complex ethmoid and sphenoid bones are shown here in isolation. The other bones of the skull are shown in their respective regions: orbit (see pp. 506–507), nasal cavity (see pp. 520–521), oral cavity (see pp. 538–539), and ear (see pp. 526–527).

Fig. 29.9 Ethmoid bone

The ethmoid bone is the central bone of the nose and paranasal air sinuses (see pp. 520–523).

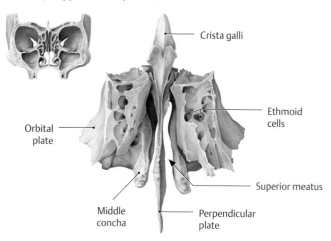

Labels: Crista galli, Ethmoid cells, Orbital plate, Superior meatus, Middle concha, Perpendicular plate

A Anterior view.

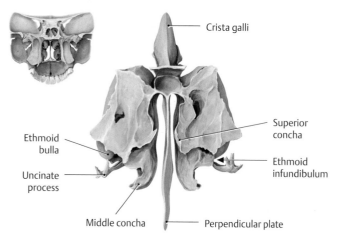

Labels: Crista galli, Superior concha, Ethmoid bulla, Ethmoid infundibulum, Uncinate process, Middle concha, Perpendicular plate

C Posterior view.

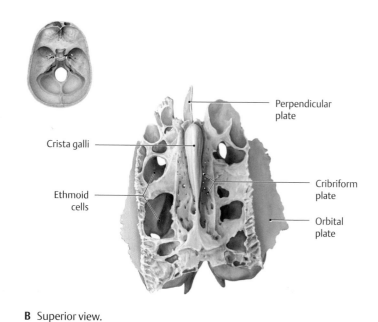

Labels: Perpendicular plate, Crista galli, Cribriform plate, Ethmoid cells, Orbital plate

B Superior view.

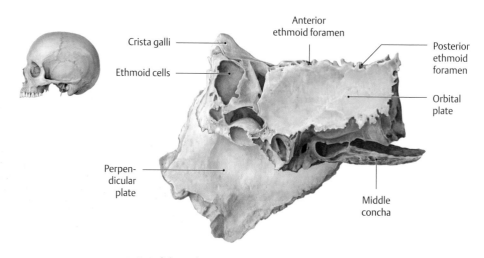

Labels: Anterior ethmoid foramen, Crista galli, Posterior ethmoid foramen, Ethmoid cells, Orbital plate, Perpendicular plate, Middle concha

D Left lateral view.

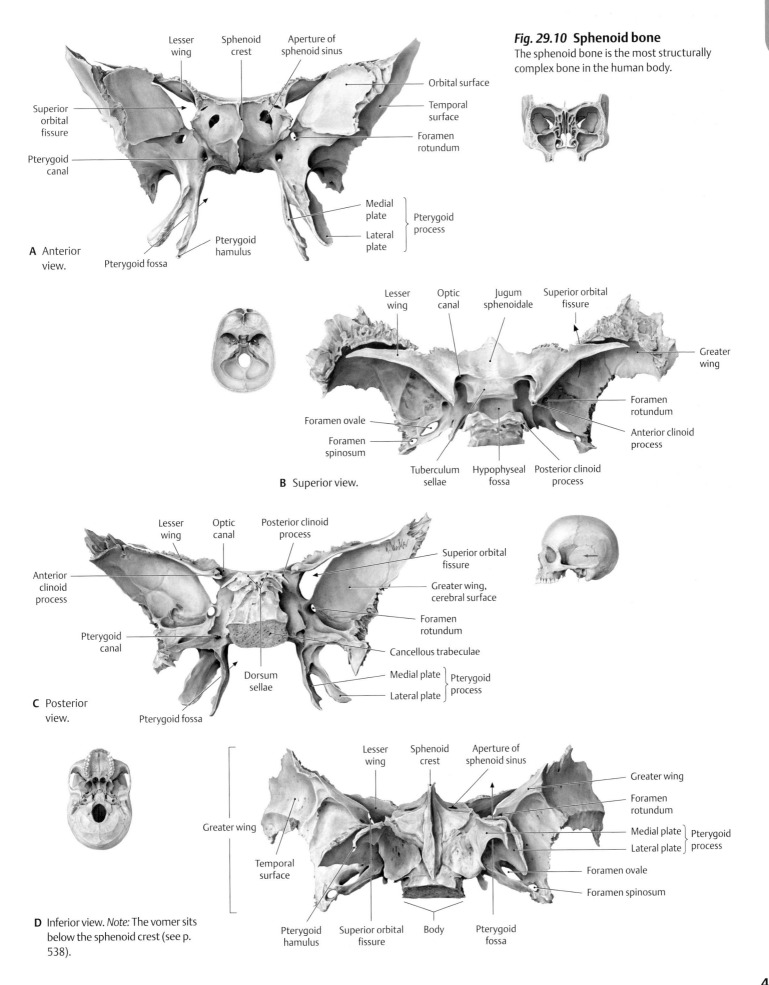

Fig. 29.10 Sphenoid bone
The sphenoid bone is the most structurally complex bone in the human body.

A Anterior view.

Lesser wing
Sphenoid crest
Aperture of sphenoid sinus
Orbital surface
Temporal surface
Foramen rotundum
Superior orbital fissure
Pterygoid canal
Medial plate
Lateral plate
Pterygoid process
Pterygoid fossa
Pterygoid hamulus

B Superior view.

Lesser wing
Optic canal
Jugum sphenoidale
Superior orbital fissure
Greater wing
Foramen ovale
Foramen rotundum
Anterior clinoid process
Foramen spinosum
Tuberculum sellae
Hypophyseal fossa
Posterior clinoid process

C Posterior view.

Lesser wing
Optic canal
Posterior clinoid process
Superior orbital fissure
Greater wing, cerebral surface
Foramen rotundum
Cancellous trabeculae
Medial plate
Lateral plate
Pterygoid process
Anterior clinoid process
Pterygoid canal
Dorsum sellae
Pterygoid fossa

D Inferior view. *Note:* The vomer sits below the sphenoid crest (see p. 538).

Lesser wing
Sphenoid crest
Aperture of sphenoid sinus
Greater wing
Foramen rotundum
Medial plate
Lateral plate
Pterygoid process
Foramen ovale
Foramen spinosum
Greater wing
Temporal surface
Pterygoid hamulus
Superior orbital fissure
Body
Pterygoid fossa

Muscles of Facial Expression & of Mastication

 The muscles of the skull and face are divided into two groups. The muscles of facial expression make up the superficial muscle layer in the face. The muscles of mastication are responsible for the movement of the mandible during mastication (chewing).

Fig. 30.1 Muscles of facial expression

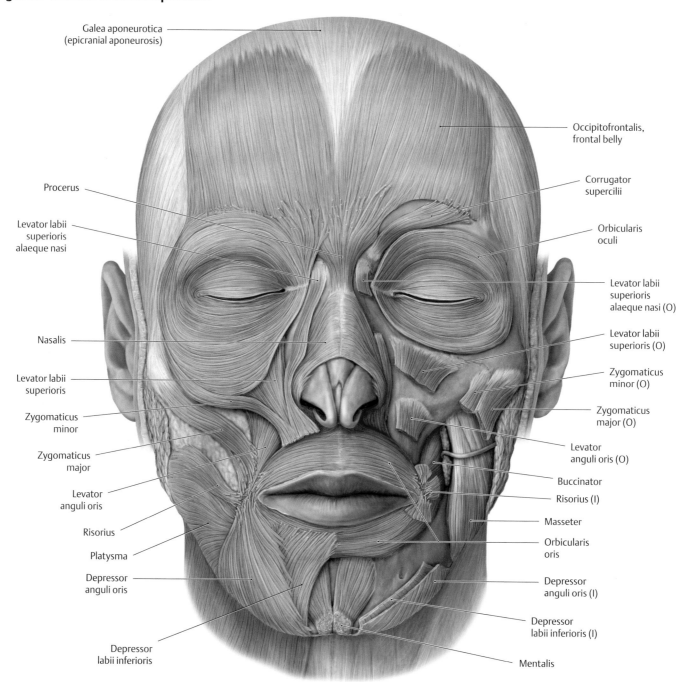

Galea aponeurotica (epicranial aponeurosis)

Occipitofrontalis, frontal belly

Procerus

Corrugator supercilii

Levator labii superioris alaeque nasi

Orbicularis oculi

Levator labii superioris alaeque nasi (O)

Nasalis

Levator labii superioris (O)

Levator labii superioris

Zygomaticus minor (O)

Zygomaticus minor

Zygomaticus major (O)

Zygomaticus major

Levator anguli oris (O)

Levator anguli oris

Buccinator

Risorius

Risorius (I)

Platysma

Masseter

Depressor anguli oris

Orbicularis oris

Depressor anguli oris (I)

Depressor labii inferioris (I)

Depressor labii inferioris

Mentalis

A Anterior view. Muscle origins (O) and insertions (I) indicated on left side of face.

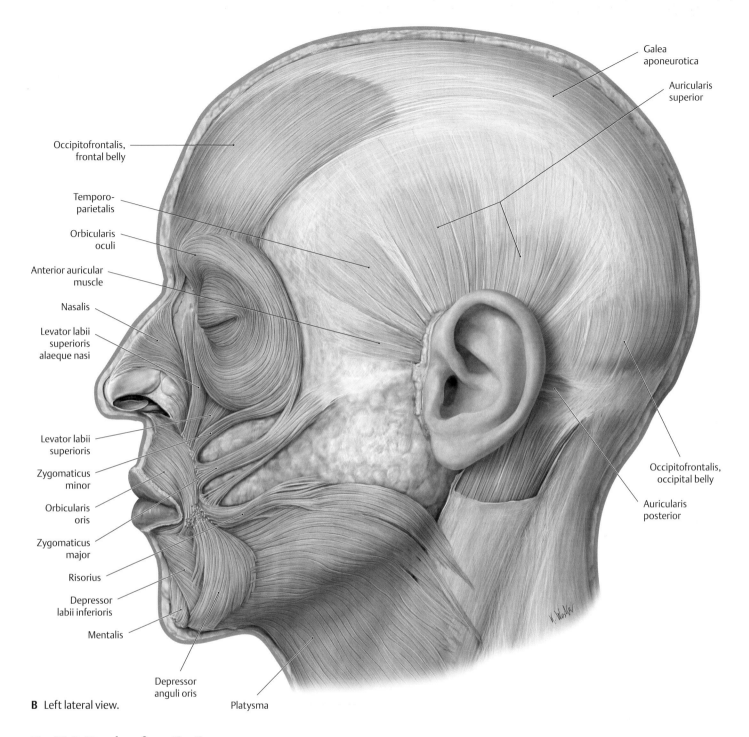

B Left lateral view.

Fig. 30.2 **Muscles of mastication**
Left lateral view.

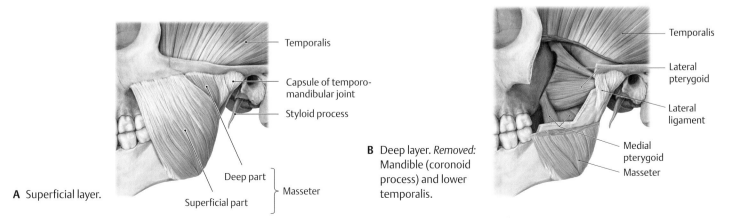

A Superficial layer.

B Deep layer. *Removed:* Mandible (coronoid process) and lower temporalis.

Muscle Origins & Insertions on the Skull

Fig. 30.3 Lateral skull: Origins and insertions

Left lateral view. Muscle origins (red), insertions (blue).
Note: There are generally no bony insertions for the
muscles of facial expression. These muscles insert into
skin and other muscles of facial expression.

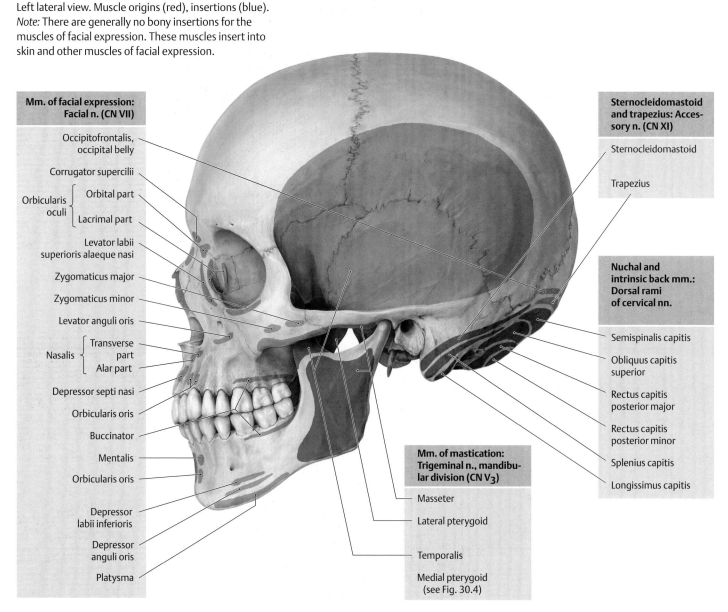

Mm. of facial expression:
Facial n. (CN VII)

Occipitofrontalis,
occipital belly

Corrugator supercilii

Orbicularis oculi — Orbital part

Lacrimal part

Levator labii
superioris alaeque nasi

Zygomaticus major

Zygomaticus minor

Levator anguli oris

Nasalis — Transverse part

Alar part

Depressor septi nasi

Orbicularis oris

Buccinator

Mentalis

Orbicularis oris

Depressor
labii inferioris

Depressor
anguli oris

Platysma

Sternocleidomastoid
and trapezius: Acces-
sory n. (CN XI)

Sternocleidomastoid

Trapezius

Nuchal and
intrinsic back mm.:
Dorsal rami
of cervical nn.

Semispinalis capitis

Obliquus capitis
superior

Rectus capitis
posterior major

Rectus capitis
posterior minor

Splenius capitis

Longissimus capitis

Mm. of mastication:
Trigeminal n., mandibu-
lar division (CN V₃)

Masseter

Lateral pterygoid

Temporalis

Medial pterygoid
(see Fig. 30.4)

Fig. 30.4 Mandible: Origins and insertions

Medial view of right hemimandible (inner surface).

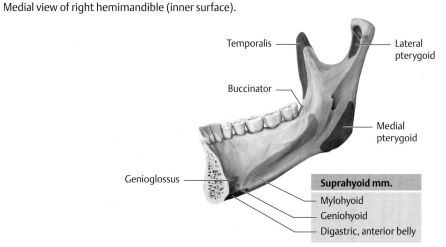

Temporalis

Lateral
pterygoid

Buccinator

Medial
pterygoid

Genioglossus

Suprahyoid mm.

Mylohyoid

Geniohyoid

Digastric, anterior belly

Fig. 30.5 Skull base: Origins and insertions

Inferior view of external skull.

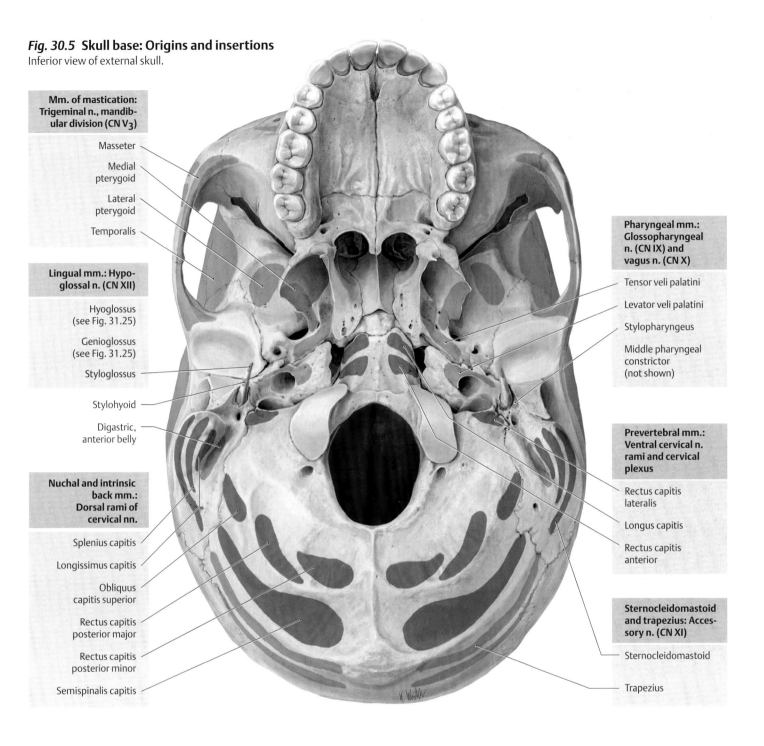

Mm. of mastication: Trigeminal n., mandibular division (CN V₃)

Masseter

Medial pterygoid

Lateral pterygoid

Temporalis

Lingual mm.: Hypoglossal n. (CN XII)

Hyoglossus (see Fig. 31.25)

Genioglossus (see Fig. 31.25)

Styloglossus

Stylohyoid

Digastric, anterior belly

Nuchal and intrinsic back mm.: Dorsal rami of cervical nn.

Splenius capitis

Longissimus capitis

Obliquus capitis superior

Rectus capitis posterior major

Rectus capitis posterior minor

Semispinalis capitis

Pharyngeal mm.: Glossopharyngeal n. (CN IX) and vagus n. (CN X)

Tensor veli palatini

Levator veli palatini

Stylopharyngeus

Middle pharyngeal constrictor (not shown)

Prevertebral mm.: Ventral cervical n. rami and cervical plexus

Rectus capitis lateralis

Longus capitis

Rectus capitis anterior

Sternocleidomastoid and trapezius: Accessory n. (CN XI)

Sternocleidomastoid

Trapezius

Fig. 30.6 Hyoid bone: Origins and insertions

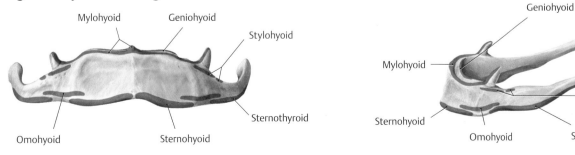

Mylohyoid

Geniohyoid

Stylohyoid

Omohyoid

Sternohyoid

Sternothyroid

A Anterior view.

Geniohyoid

Mylohyoid

Sternohyoid

Omohyoid

Stylohyoid

Sternothyroid

B Oblique left lateral view.

Muscle Facts (I)

The muscles of facial expression originate on bone and/or fascia, and insert into the subcutaneous tissue of the face. This allows them to produce their effects by pulling on the skin.

Fig. 30.7 Occipitofrontalis
Anterior view.

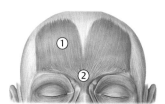

Fig. 30.8 Muscles of the palpebral fissure and nose
Anterior view.

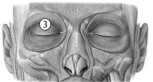

A Orbicularis oculi.

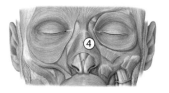

B Nasalis.

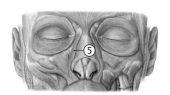

C Levator labii superioris alaeque nasi.

Fig. 30.9 Muscles of the ear
Left lateral view.

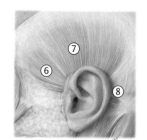

Table 30.1	Muscles of facial expression: Forehead, nose, and ear		
Muscle	**Origin**	**Insertion***	**Main action(s)***
Calvaria			
① Occipitofrontalis (frontal belly)	Epicranial aponeurosis	Skin and subcutaneous tissue of eyebrows and forehead	Elevates eyebrows, wrinkles skin of forehead
Palpebral fissure and nose			
② Procerus	Nasal bone, lateral nasal cartilage (upper part)	Skin of lower forehead between eyebrows	Pulls medial angle of eyebrows inferiorly, producing transverse wrinkles over bridge of nose
③ Orbicularis oculi	Medial orbital margin, medial palpebral ligament; lacrimal bone	Skin around margin of orbit, superior and inferior tarsal plates	Acts as orbital sphincter (closes eyelids) • Palpebral portion gently closes • Orbital portion tightly closes (as in winking)
④ Nasalis	Maxilla (superior region of canine ridge)	Nasal cartilages	Flares nostrils by drawing ala (side) of nose toward nasal septum
⑤ Levator labii superioris alaeque nasi	Maxilla (frontal process)	Alar cartilage of nose and upper lip	Elevates upper lip, opens nostril
Ear			
⑥ Anterior auricular muscles	Temporal fascia (anterior portion)	Helix of the ear	Pull ear superiorly and anteriorly
⑦ Superior auricular muscles	Epicranial aponeurosis on side of head	Upper portion of auricle	Elevate ear
⑧ Posterior auricular muscles	Mastoid process	Convexity of concha of ear	Pull ear superiorly and posteriorly

*There are no bony insertions for the muscles of facial expression.

**All muscles of facial expression are innervated by the facial nerve (CN VII) via temporal, zygomatic, buccal, mandibular, or cervical branches arising from the parotid plexus (see p. 478).

Fig. 30.10 Muscles of the mouth
Left lateral view.

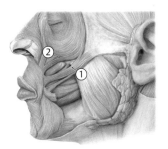

A Zygomaticus major and minor.

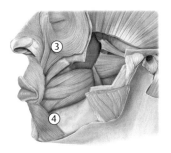

B Levator labii superioris and depressor labii inferioris.

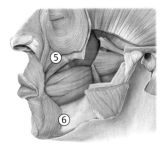

C Levator and depressor anguli oris.

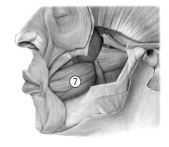

D Buccinator.

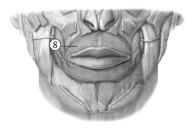

E Orbicularis oris, anterior view.

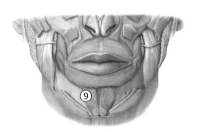

F Mentalis, anterior view.

Table 30.2	Muscles of facial expression: Mouth and neck		
Muscle	**Origin**	**Insertion***	**Main action(s)****
Mouth			
① Zygomaticus major	Zygomatic bone (lateral surface, posterior part)	Skin at corner of the mouth	Pulls corner of mouth superiorly and laterally
② Zygomaticus minor		Upper lip just medial to corner of the mouth	Pulls upper lip superiorly
Levator labii superioris alaeque nasi (see Fig. 30.8C)	Maxilla (frontal process)	Alar cartilage of nose and upper lip	Elevates upper lip, opens nostril
③ Levator labii superioris	Maxilla (frontal process) and infraorbital region	Skin of upper lip, alar cartilages of nose	Elevates upper lip, dilates nostril, raises angle of the mouth
④ Depressor labii inferioris	Mandible (anterior portion of oblique line)	Lower lip at midline; blends with muscle from opposite side	Pulls lower lip inferiorly and laterally
⑤ Levator anguli oris	Maxilla (below infraorbital foramen)	Skin at corner of the mouth	Raises angle of mouth, helps form nasolabial furrow
⑥ Depressor anguli oris	Mandible (oblique line below canine, premolar, and first molar teeth)	Skin at corner of the mouth; blends with orbicularis oris	Pulls angle of mouth inferiorly and laterally
⑦ Buccinator	Mandible, alveolar processes of maxilla and mandible, pterygo-mandibular raphe	Angle of mouth, orbicularis oris	Presses cheek against molar teeth, working with tongue to keep food between occlusal surfaces and out of oral vestibule; expels air from oral cavity/resists distension when blowing *Unilateral:* Draws mouth to one side
⑧ Orbicularis oris	Deep surface of skin Superiorly: maxilla (median plane) Inferiorly: mandible	Mucous membrane of lips	Acts as oral sphincter • Compresses and protrudes lips (e.g., when whistling, sucking, and kissing) • Resists distension (when blowing)
Risorius (see p. 462)	Fascia over masseter	Skin of corner of the mouth	Retracts corner of mouth as in grimacing
⑨ Mentalis	Mandible (incisive fossa)	Skin of chin	Elevates and protrudes lower lip
Neck			
Platysma (see p. 463)	Skin over lower neck and upper lateral thorax	Mandible (inferior border), skin over lower face, angle of mouth	Depresses and wrinkles skin of lower face and mouth; tenses skin of neck; aids in forced depression of the mandible

*There are no bony insertions for the muscles of facial expression.
**All muscles of facial expression are innervated by the facial nerve (CN VII) via temporal, zygomatic, buccal, mandibular, or cervical branches arising from its parotid plexus.

Muscle Facts (II)

The muscles of mastication are located at various depths in the parotid and infratemporal regions of the face. They attach to the mandible and receive their motor innervation from the mandibu-lar division of the trigeminal nerve (CN V₃). The muscles of the oral floor that aid in opening the mouth are found on p. 562.

Table 30.3	Muscles of mastication: Masseter and temporalis			
Muscle	**Origin**	**Insertion**	**Innervation**	**Action**
① Masseter	Superficial part: zygomatic arch (anterior two thirds)	Mandibular angle (masseteric tuberosity)	Mandibular n. (CN V₃) via masseteric n.	Elevates (adducts) and protrudes mandible
	Deep part: zygomatic arch (posterior one third)			
② Temporalis	Temporal fossa (inferior temporal line)	Coronoid process of mandible (apex and medial surface)	Mandibular n. (CN V₃) via deep temporal nn.	*Vertical fibers:* Elevate (adduct) mandible *Horizontal fibers:* Retract (retrude) mandible *Unilateral:* Lateral movement of mandible (chewing)

Fig. 30.11 Masseter muscle
Left lateral view.

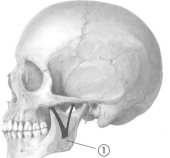

A Schematic.

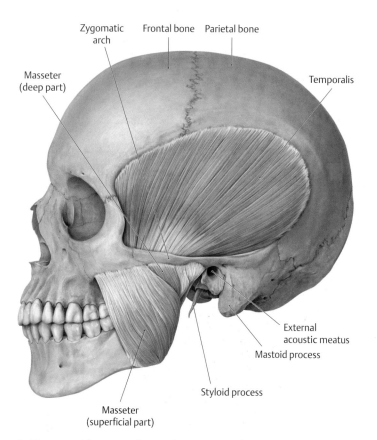

B Masseter with temporalis muscle.

Fig. 30.12 Temporalis muscle
Left lateral view.

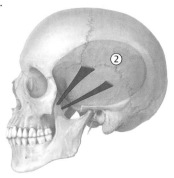

A Schematic.

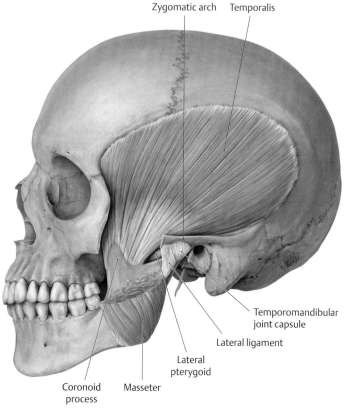

B Temporalis muscle. *Removed:* Masseter and zygomatic arch.

Table 30.4		Muscles of mastication: Pterygoid muscles			
Muscle		Origin	Insertion	Innervation	Action
Lateral pterygoid	③ Superior head	Greater wing of sphenoid bone (infratemporal crest)	Temporomandibular joint (articular disk)	Mandibular n. (CN V₃) via lateral pterygoid n.	*Bilateral:* Protrudes mandible (pulls articular disk forward) *Unilateral:* Lateral movements of mandible (chewing)
	④ Inferior head	Lateral pterygoid plate (lateral surface)	Mandible (condylar process)		
Medial pterygoid	⑤ Superficial head	Maxilla (tuberosity)	Pterygoid tuberosity on medial surface of the mandibular angle	Mandibular n. (CN V₃) via medial pterygoid n.	Elevates (adducts) mandible
	⑥ Deep head	Medial surface of lateral pterygoid plate and pterygoid fossa			

Fig. 30.13 Lateral pterygoid muscle
Left lateral view.

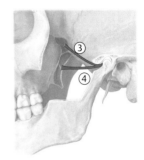

A Schematic.

B Left lateral pterygoid muscle. *Removed:* Coronoid process of mandible.

Labels: Zygomatic arch (cut); Superior head, Inferior head (Lateral pterygoid); Articular disk; Condylar head; Styloid process; Coronoid process (cut)

Fig. 30.14 Medial pterygoid muscle
Left lateral view.

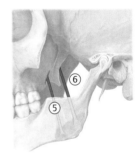

A Schematic.

B Left medial pterygoid muscle. *Removed:* Coronoid process of mandible.

Labels: Pterygoid process, lateral plate; Medial pterygoid (superficial head); Medial pterygoid (deep head); Mandibular angle

Fig. 30.15 Masticatory muscle sling
Oblique posterior view.

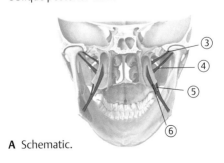

A Schematic.

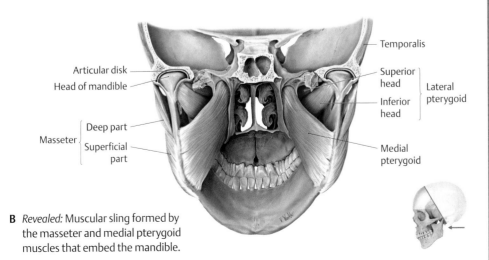

B *Revealed:* Muscular sling formed by the masseter and medial pterygoid muscles that embed the mandible.

Labels: Articular disk; Head of mandible; Masseter — Deep part, Superficial part; Temporalis; Superior head, Inferior head (Lateral pterygoid); Medial pterygoid

Cranial Nerves: Overview

Fig. 31.1 **Cranial nerves**

Inferior (basal) view. The 12 pairs of cranial nerves (CN) are numbered according to the order of their emergence from the brainstem. *Note:* The sensory and motor fibers of the cranial nerves enter and exit the brainstem at the same sites (in contrast to spinal nerves, whose sensory and motor fibers enter and leave through posterior and anterior roots, respectively).

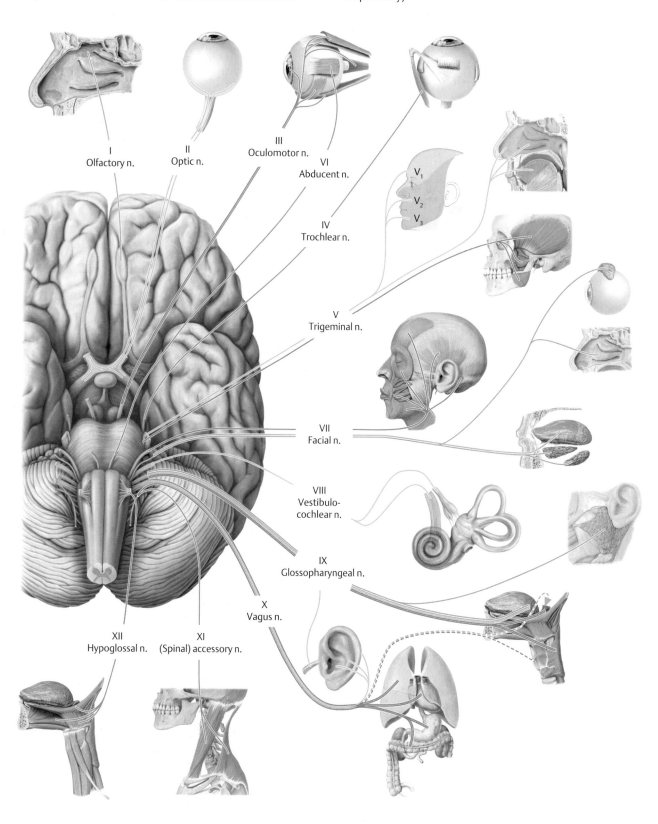

I Olfactory n.

II Optic n.

III Oculomotor n.

VI Abducent n.

IV Trochlear n.

V Trigeminal n.

VII Facial n.

VIII Vestibulo-cochlear n.

IX Glossopharyngeal n.

X Vagus n.

XI (Spinal) accessory n.

XII Hypoglossal n.

V_1

V_2

V_3

The cranial nerves contain both afferent (sensory) and efferent (motor) axons that belong to either the somatic or the autonomic (visceral) nervous system (see pp. 622–623). The somatic fibers allow interaction with the environment, whereas the visceral fibers regulate the autonomic activity of internal organs. In addi- tion to the general fiber types, the cranial nerves may contain special fiber types associated with particular structures (e.g., auditory apparatus and taste buds). The cranial nerve fibers originate or terminate at specific nuclei, which are similarly classified as either general or special, somatic or visceral, and afferent or efferent.

Table 31.1 Classification of cranial nerve fibers and nuclei

This color coding is used in subsequent chapters to indicate fiber and nuclei classifications.

Fiber type	Example	Fiber type	Example
General somatic efferent (somatomotor function)	Innervate skeletal muscles	General somatic afferent (somatic sensation)	Conduct impulses from skin, skeletal muscle spindles
General visceral efferent (visceromotor function)	Innervate smooth muscle of the viscera, intraocular muscles, heart, salivary glands, etc.	Special somatic afferent	Conduct impulses from retina, auditory and vestibular apparatuses
Special visceral efferent	Innervate skeletal and cardiac muscle derived from branchial arches	General visceral afferent (visceral sensation)	Conduct impulses from viscera, blood vessels
		Special visceral afferent	Conduct impulses from taste buds, olfactory mucosa

Fig. 31.2 Cranial nerve nuclei

The sensory and motor fibers of cranial nerves III to XII originate and terminate in the brainstem at specific nuclei.

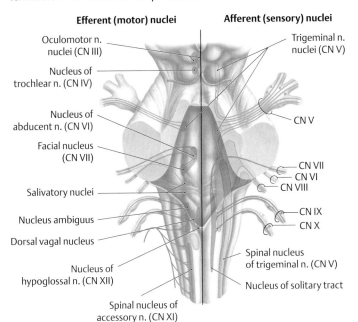

Efferent (motor) nuclei
- Oculomotor n. nuclei (CN III)
- Nucleus of trochlear n. (CN IV)
- Nucleus of abducent n. (CN VI)
- Facial nucleus (CN VII)
- Salivatory nuclei
- Nucleus ambiguus
- Dorsal vagal nucleus
- Nucleus of hypoglossal n. (CN XII)
- Spinal nucleus of accessory n. (CN XI)

Afferent (sensory) nuclei
- Trigeminal n. nuclei (CN V)
- CN V
- CN VII
- CN VI
- CN VIII
- CN IX
- CN X
- Spinal nucleus of trigeminal n. (CN V)
- Nucleus of solitary tract

A Posterior view with the cerebellum removed.

Table 31.2 Cranial nerves

Cranial nerve	Origin	Functional fiber types
CN I: Olfactory n.	Telencephalon*	
CN II: Optic n.	Diencephalon*	
CN III: Oculomotor n.	Mesencephalon	
CN IV: Trochlear n.		
CN V: Trigeminal n.	Pons	
CN VI: Abducent n.		
CN VII: Facial n.		
CN VIII: Vestibulocochlear n.		
CN IX: Glossopharyngeal n.	Medulla oblongata	
CN X: Vagus n.		
CN XI: Accessory n.		
CN XII: Hypoglossal n.		

* The olfactory and optic nerves are extensions of the brain rather than true nerves; they are therefore not associated with nuclei in the brainstem.

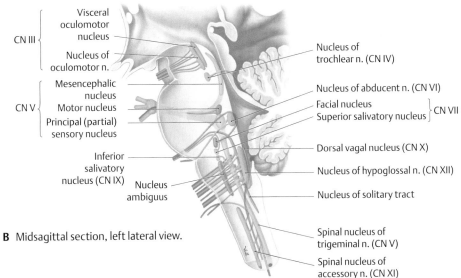

CN III
- Visceral oculomotor nucleus
- Nucleus of oculomotor n.

CN V
- Mesencephalic nucleus
- Motor nucleus
- Principal (partial) sensory nucleus

- Inferior salivatory nucleus (CN IX)
- Nucleus ambiguus

- Nucleus of trochlear n. (CN IV)
- Nucleus of abducent n. (CN VI)
- Facial nucleus
- Superior salivatory nucleus } CN VII
- Dorsal vagal nucleus (CN X)
- Nucleus of hypoglossal n. (CN XII)
- Nucleus of solitary tract
- Spinal nucleus of trigeminal n. (CN V)
- Spinal nucleus of accessory n. (CN XI)

B Midsagittal section, left lateral view.

CN I & II: Olfactory & Optic Nerves

The olfactory and optic nerves are not true peripheral nerves, but extensions (tracts) of the telencephalon and diencephalon, respectively. They are therefore not associated with cranial nerve nuclei in the brainstem.

Fig. 31.3 Olfactory nerve (CN I)

Fiber bundles in the olfactory mucosa pass from the nasal cavity through the cribriform plate of the ethmoid bone into the anterior cranial fossa, where they synapse in the olfactory bulb. Axons from second-order afferent neurons in the olfactory bulb pass through the olfactory tract and medial or lateral olfactory stria, terminating in the cerebral cortex of the prepiriform area, in the amygdala, or in neighboring areas. See p. 617 for the mechanisms of smell.

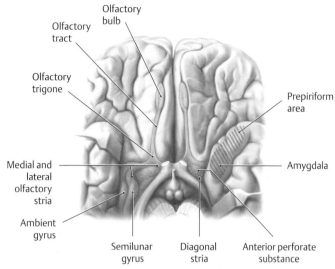

A Olfactory bulb and tract, inferior view. *Note:* The amygdala and prepiriform area are deep to the basal surface of the brain.

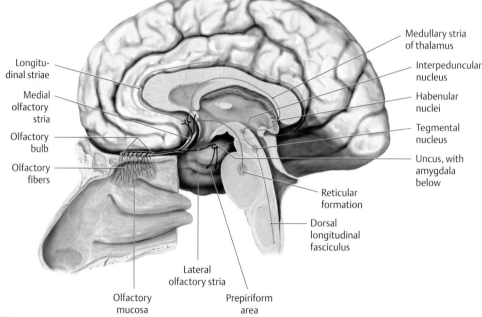

B Course of the olfactory nerve. Parasagittal section, viewed from left side.

C Olfactory fibers. Portion of left nasal septum and lateral wall of right nasal cavity, left lateral view.

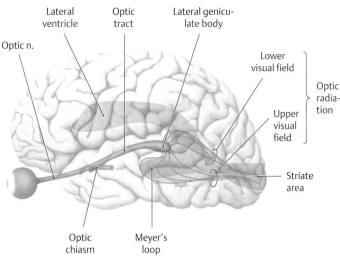

A Optic nerve in the geniculate visual pathway, left lateral view.

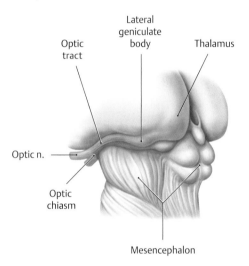

B Termination of the optic tract, left posterolateral view of the brainstem. The optic nerve contains the axons of retinal ganglion cells, which terminate mainly in the lateral geniculate body of the diencephalon and in the mesencephalon (superior colliculus).

Fig. 31.4 **Optic nerve (CN II)**

The optic nerve passes from the eyeball through the optic canal into the middle cranial fossa. The two optic nerves join below the base of the diencephalon to form the optic chiasm, before dividing into the two optic tracts. Each of these tracts divides into a lateral and medial root. Many retinal cell ganglion axons cross the midline to the contralateral side of the brain in the optic chiasm. See p. 619 for the mechanisms of sight.

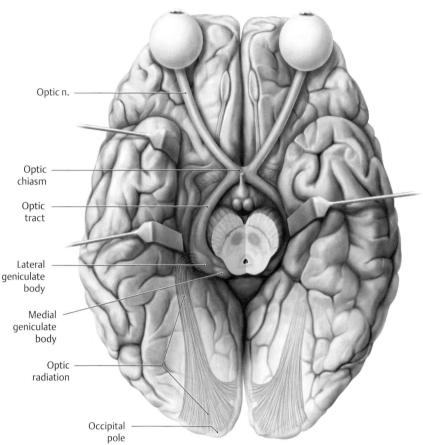

C Course of the optic nerve, inferior (basal) view.

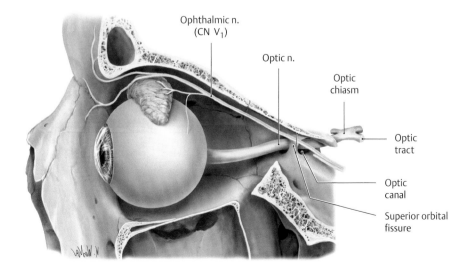

D Optic nerve in the left orbit, lateral view. The optic nerve exits the orbit via the optic canal. *Note:* The other cranial nerves entering the orbit do so via the superior orbital fissure.

CN III, IV & VI: Oculomotor, Trochlear & Abducent Nerves

Cranial nerves III, IV, and VI innervate the extraocular muscles (see p. 509). Of the three, only the oculomotor nerve (CN III) contains both somatic and visceral efferent fibers; it is also the only

cranial nerve of the extraocular muscles to innervate multiple extra- and intraocular muscles.

Fig. 31.5 Nuclei of the oculomotor, trochlear, and abducent nerves

The trochlear nerve (CN IV) is the only cranial nerve in which all the fibers cross to the opposite side. It is also the only cranial nerve to

emerge from the dorsal side of the brainstem and, consequently, has the longest intradural (intracranial) course of any cranial nerve.

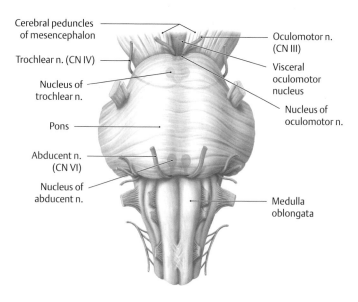

A Emergence of the cranial nerves of the extraocular muscles. Anterior view of the brainstem.

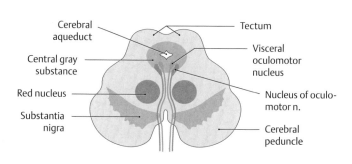

B Oculomotor nerve nuclei. Transverse section, superior view.

Table 31.3	Cranial nerves of the extraocular muscles			
Course*	Fibers	Nuclei	Function	Effects of nerve injury
Oculomotor nerve (CN III)				
Runs anteriorly from mesencephalon	Somatic efferent	Oculomotor nucleus	Innervates: • Levator palpebrae superioris • Superior, medial, and inferior rectus • Inferior oblique	Complete oculomotor palsy (paralysis of extra- and intraocular muscles): • Ptosis (drooping of eyelid) • Downward and lateral gaze deviation • Diplopia (double vision) • Mydriasis (pupil dilation) • Accommodation difficulties (ciliary paralysis)
	Visceral efferent	Visceral oculomotor (Edinger-Westphal) nucleus	Synapse with neurons in ciliary ganglia. Innervates: • Pupillary sphincter • Ciliary muscle	
Trochlear nerve (CN IV)				
Emerges from posterior surface of brainstem near midline, courses anteriorly around the cerebral peduncle	Somatic efferent	Nucleus of the trochlear n.	Innervates: • Superior oblique	• Diplopia • Affected eye is higher and deviated medially (dominance of inferior oblique)
Abducent nerve (CN VI)				
Follows a long extradural path**	Somatic efferent	Nucleus of the abducent n.	Innervates: • Lateral rectus	• Diplopia • Affected eye is deviated superiorly

* All three nerves enter the orbit through the superior orbital fissure; CN III and CN VI pass through the common tendinous ring of the extraocular muscles.
** The abducent nerve follows an extradural course; abducent nerve palsy may therefore develop in association with meningitis and subarachnoid hemorrhage.

Note: The oculomotor nerve supplies parasympathetic innervation to the intraocular muscles and somatic motor innervation to most of the extraocular muscles (also the levator palpebrae superioris). Its parasympathetic fibers synapse in the ciliary ganglion. *Note:* Oculomotor nerve palsy may affect exclusively the parasympathetic or somatic fibers, or both concurrently.

Fig. 31.6 Course of the nerves innervating the extraocular muscles
Right orbit.

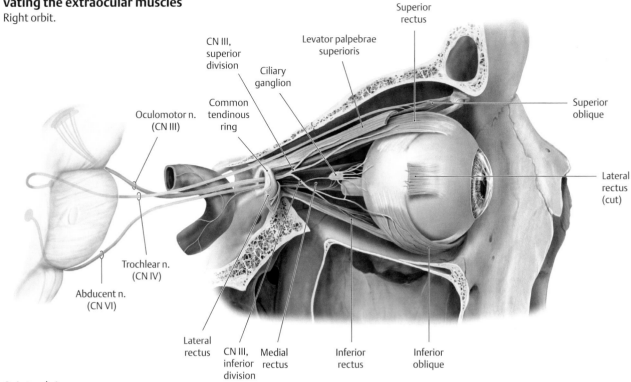

A Lateral view.

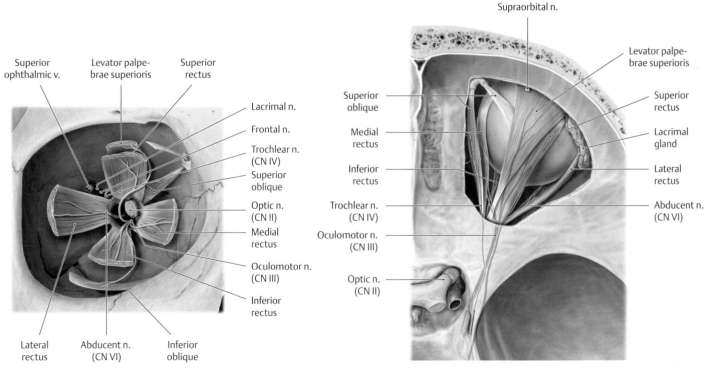

B Anterior view. CN II exits the orbit via the optic canal, which lies medial to the superior orbital fissure (site of emergence of CN III, IV, and VI).

C Superior view of the opened orbit. Note the relationship between the optic canal and the superior orbital fissure.

CN V: Trigeminal Nerve

 The trigeminal nerve, the sensory nerve of the head, has three somatic afferent nuclei: the mesencephalic nucleus, which receives proprioceptive fibers from the muscles of mastication; the principal (pontine) sensory nucleus, which chiefly mediates touch; and the spinal nucleus, which mediates pain and temperature sensation. The motor nucleus supplies motor innervation to the muscles of mastication.

Fig. 31.7 Trigeminal nerve nuclei

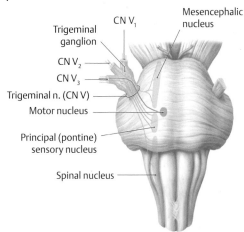

A Anterior view of the brainstem.

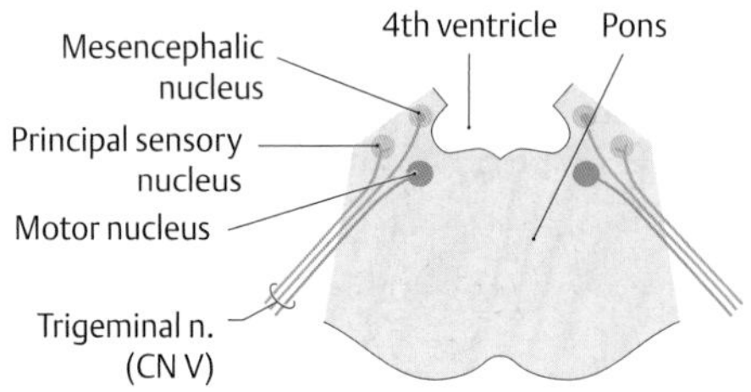

B Cross section through the pons, superior view.

Fig. 31.8 Divisions of the trigeminal nerve (CN V)

Right lateral view.

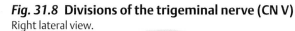
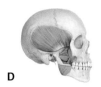

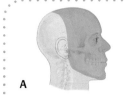
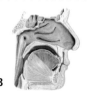

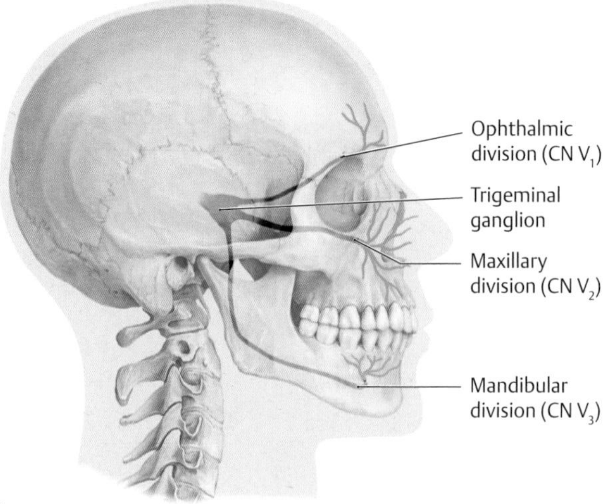

A	**B**	**C**	**D**

Table 31.4   Trigeminal nerve (CN V)

Course	Fibers	Nuclei	Function	Effects of nerve injury
Exits from the middle cranial fossa. **Ophthalmic division (CN V₁):** Enters orbit through superior orbital fissure **Maxillary division (CN V₂):** Enters pterygopalatine fossa through foramen rotundum **Mandibular division (CN V₃):** Passes through foramen ovale to inferior surface of base of the skull	Somatic afferent	• Principal (pontine) sensory nucleus of the trigeminal n. • Mesencephalic nucleus of the trigeminal n. • Spinal nucleus of the trigeminal n.	Innervates: • Facial skin (**A**) • Nasopharyngeal mucosa (**B**) • Tongue (anterior two thirds) (**C**) Involved in the corneal reflex (reflex closure of eyelid)	• Sensory loss (traumatic nerve lesions) • Herpes zoster ophthalmicus (varicella-zoster virus); herpes zoster of the face
	Special visceral efferent	Motor nucleus of the trigeminal n.	Innervates (via CN V₃): • Muscles of mastication (temporalis, masseter, medial and lateral pterygoids (**D**)) • Oral floor muscles (mylohyoid, anterior digastric) • Tensor tympani • Tensor veli palatini	
	Visceral efferent pathway*	• Lacrimal n. (CN V₁) conveys parasympathetic fibers from CN VII along the zygomatic n. (CN V₂) to the lacrimal gland • Lingual n. (CN V₃) conveys parasympathetic fibers from CN VII (via the chorda tympani) to the submandibular and sublingual glands • Auriculotemporal n. (CN V₃) conveys parasympathetic fibers from CN IX to the parotid gland	
	Visceral afferent pathway*	Gustatory (taste) fibers from CN VII (via chorda tympani) travel with the lingual n. (CN V₃) to the anterior two thirds of the tongue	

* Fibers of certain cranial nerves adhere to divisions or branches of the trigeminal nerve, by which they travel to their destination.

Fig. 31.9 **Course of the trigeminal nerve divisions**

Right lateral view.

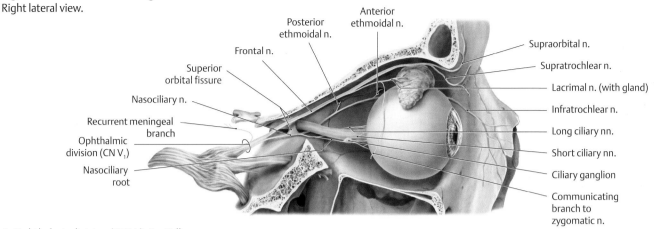

A Ophthalmic division (CN V₁). Partially opened right orbit.

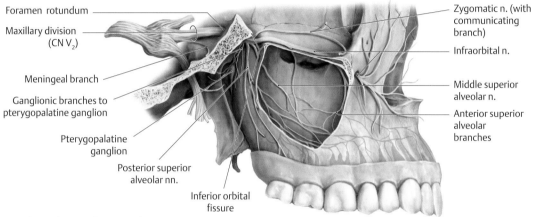

B Maxillary division (CN V₂). Partially opened right maxillary sinus with the zygomatic arch removed.

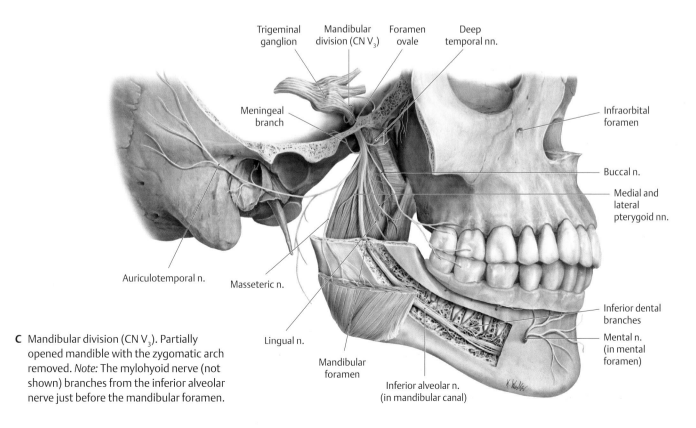

C Mandibular division (CN V₃). Partially opened mandible with the zygomatic arch removed. *Note:* The mylohyoid nerve (not shown) branches from the inferior alveolar nerve just before the mandibular foramen.

CN VII: Facial Nerve

The facial nerve mainly conveys special visceral efferent (branchiogenic) fibers from the facial nerve nucleus to the muscles of facial expression. The other visceral efferent (para-sympathetic) fibers from the superior salivatory nucleus are grouped with the visceral afferent (gustatory) fibers to form the nervus intermedius.

***Fig. 31.10* Facial nerve nuclei**

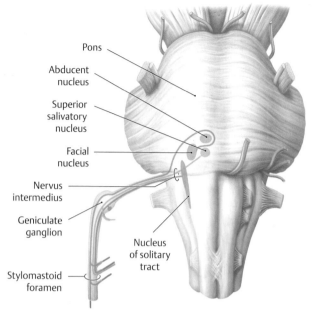

A Anterior view of the brainstem.

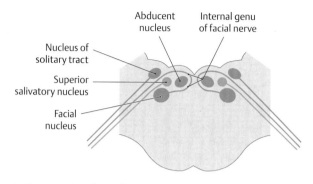

B Cross section through the pons, superior view.

***Fig. 31.11* Branches of the facial nerve**
Right lateral view.

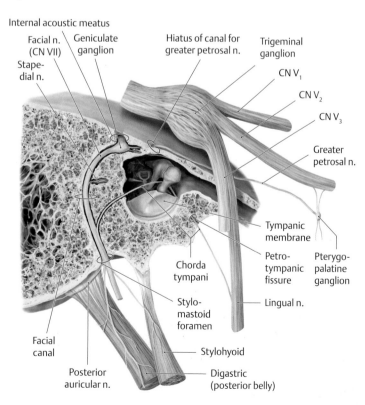

A Facial nerve in the temporal bone.

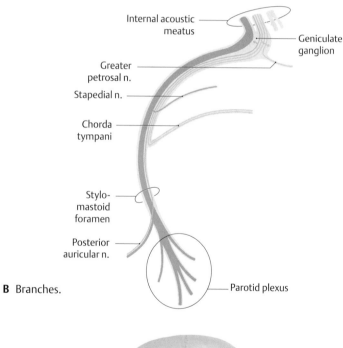

B Branches.

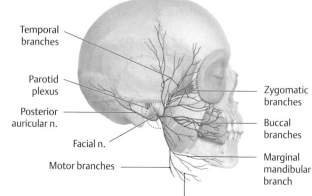

C Parotid plexus.

Table 31.5	Facial nerve (CN VII)				
Course	**Fibers**	**Nuclei**	**Function**		**Effects of nerve injury**
Emerges in the cerebellopontine angle between the pons and olive; passes through the internal acoustic meatus into the temporal bone (petrous part), where it divides into: • Greater petrosal nerve • Stapedial nerve • Chorda tympani Certain visceral efferent fibers pass through the stylomastoid foramen to the skull base, forming the intraparotid plexus	Special visceral efferent	Facial nucleus	Innervate: • Muscles of facial expression • Stylohyoid • Digastric (posterior belly) • Stapedius		Peripheral facial nerve injury: paralysis of muscles of facial expression on affected side Associated disturbances of taste, lacrimation, salivation, etc.
	Visceral efferent (para-sympathetic)*	Superior salivatory nucleus	Synapse with neurons in the pterygopalatine or submandibular ganglion. Innervate: • Lacrimal gland • Small glands of nasal mucosa, hard and soft palate • Submandibular gland • Sublingual gland • Small salivary glands of tongue (dorsum)		
	Special visceral afferent*	Nucleus of the solitary tract	Peripheral processes of fibers from geniculate ganglion form the chorda tympani (gustatory fibers from tongue)		
	Somatic afferent		Sensory fibers from the auricle, skin of the auditory canal, and outer surface of the tympanic membrane travel via CN VII to the principal sensory nucleus of the trigeminal nerve		

* Grouped to form nervus intermedius, which aggregates with the visceral efferent fibers from the facial nerve nucleus.

Fig. 31.12 Course of the facial nerve

Right lateral view. Visceral efferent (parasympathetic) and special visceral afferent (taste) fibers shown in black.

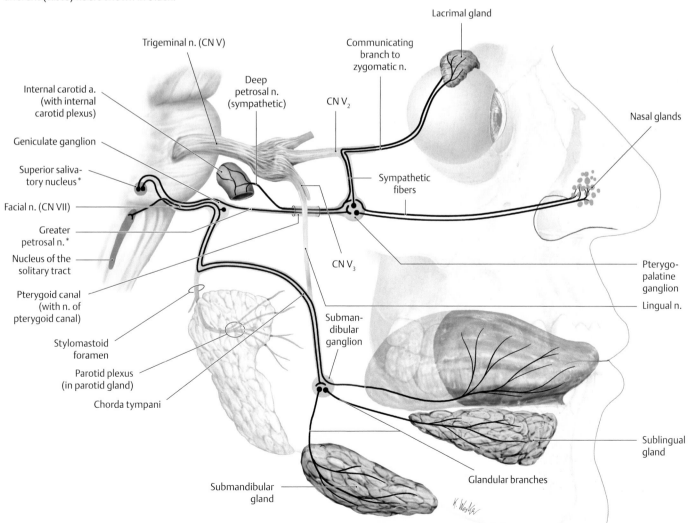

*Parasympathetic

CN VIII: Vestibulocochlear Nerve

The vestibulochochlear nerve is a special somatic afferent nerve that consists of two roots. The vestibular root transmits impulses from the vestibular apparatus (balance, see p. 618); the cochlear root transmits impulses from the auditory apparatus (hearing, see p. 616).

Fig. 31.13 **Vestibulocochlear nerve: Vestibular part**

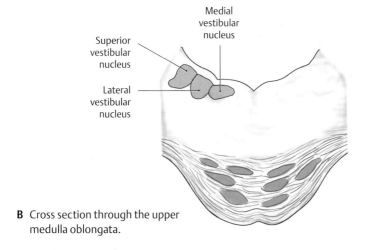

A Anterior view of the medulla oblongata and pons with cerebellum.

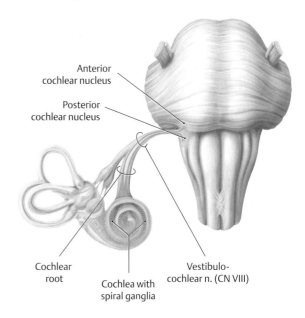

Fig. 31.14 **Vestibulocochlear nerve: Cochlear part**

A Anterior view of the medulla oblongata and pons.

B Cross section through the upper medulla oblongata.

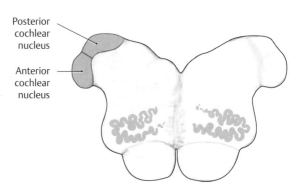

B Cross section through the upper medulla oblongata.

Table 31.6	Vestibulocochlear nerve (CN VIII)				
Part	Course	Fibers	Nuclei	Function	Effects of nerve injury
Vestibular part	Pass from the inner ear through the internal acoustic meatus to the cerebellopontine angle, where they enter the brain	Special somatic afferent	Superior, lateral, medial, and inferior vestibular nuclei	Peripheral processes from the semicircular canals, saccule, and utricle pass to the vestibular ganglion and then to the four vestibular nuclei	Dizziness
Cochlear part			Anterior and posterior cochlear nuclei	Peripheral processes beginning at the hair cells of the organ of Corti pass to the spiral ganglion and then to the two cochlear nuclei	Hearing loss

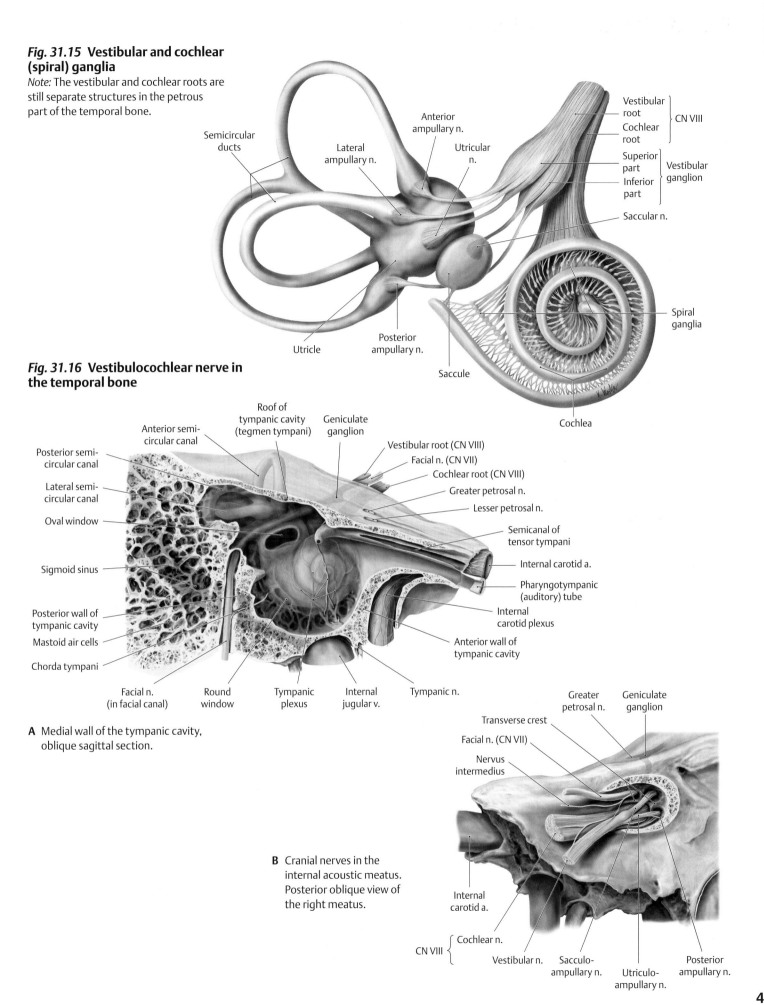

Fig. 31.15 Vestibular and cochlear (spiral) ganglia

Note: The vestibular and cochlear roots are still separate structures in the petrous part of the temporal bone.

Semicircular ducts

Anterior ampullary n.

Lateral ampullary n.

Utricular n.

Vestibular root
Cochlear root
} CN VIII

Superior part
Inferior part
} Vestibular ganglion

Saccular n.

Spiral ganglia

Utricle

Posterior ampullary n.

Saccule

Cochlea

Fig. 31.16 Vestibulocochlear nerve in the temporal bone

Anterior semi-circular canal

Roof of tympanic cavity (tegmen tympani)

Geniculate ganglion

Vestibular root (CN VIII)

Facial n. (CN VII)

Cochlear root (CN VIII)

Greater petrosal n.

Lesser petrosal n.

Semicanal of tensor tympani

Internal carotid a.

Pharyngotympanic (auditory) tube

Internal carotid plexus

Anterior wall of tympanic cavity

Posterior semi-circular canal

Lateral semi-circular canal

Oval window

Sigmoid sinus

Posterior wall of tympanic cavity

Mastoid air cells

Chorda tympani

Facial n. (in facial canal)

Round window

Tympanic plexus

Internal jugular v.

Tympanic n.

A Medial wall of the tympanic cavity, oblique sagittal section.

B Cranial nerves in the internal acoustic meatus. Posterior oblique view of the right meatus.

Greater petrosal n.

Geniculate ganglion

Transverse crest

Facial n. (CN VII)

Nervus intermedius

Internal carotid a.

CN VIII {
Cochlear n.
Vestibular n.

Sacculo-ampullary n.

Utriculo-ampullary n.

Posterior ampullary n.

CN IX: Glossopharyngeal Nerve

Fig. 31.17 **Glossopharyngeal nerve nuclei**

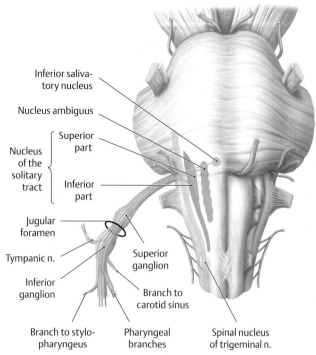

A Anterior view of the medulla oblongata.

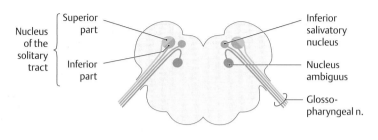

B Cross section through the medulla oblongata, superior view. *Not shown:* Nuclei of the trigeminal nerve.

Fig. 31.18 **Course of the glossopharyngeal nerve**

Left lateral view. *Note:* Fibers from the vagus nerve (CN X) combine with fibers from CN IX to form the pharyngeal plexus and supply the carotid sinus.

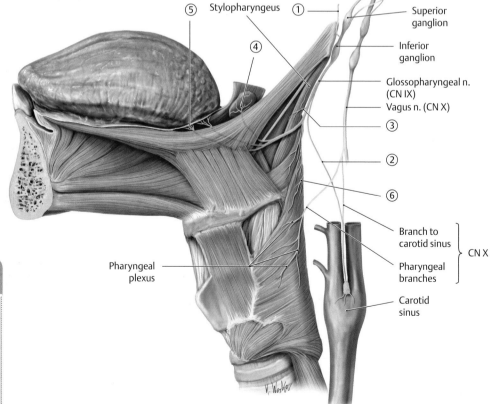

Table 31.7	Glossopharyngeal nerve branches
①	Tympanic n.
②	Branch to carotid sinus
③	Branch to stylopharyngeus muscle
④	Tonsillar branches
⑤	Lingual branches
⑥	Pharyngeal branches

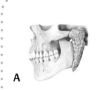   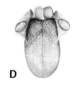 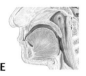 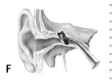

A   B   C   D   E   F

Table 31.8	Glossopharyngeal nerve (CN IX)			
Course	Fibers	Nuclei	Function	Effects of nerve injury
Emerges from the medulla oblongata; leaves cranial cavity through the jugular foramen	Visceral efferent (parasympathetic)	Inferior salivatory nucleus	Parasympathetic presynaptic fibers are sent to the otic ganglion; postsynaptic fibers are distributed to • Parotid gland (**A**) • Buccal gland • Labial gland	Isolated lesions of CN IX are rare. Lesions are generally accompanied by lesions of CN X and CN XI (cranial part), as all three emerge jointly from the jugular foramen and are susceptible to injury in basal skull fractures.
	Special visceral efferent (branchiogenic)	Nucleus ambiguus	Innervate: • Constrictor muscles of the pharynx (pharyngeal branches join with the vagus nerve to form the pharyngeal plexus) • Stylopharyngeus	
	Visceral afferent	Nucleus of the solitary tract (inferior part)	Receive sensory information from • Chemoreceptors in the carotid body (**B**) • Pressure receptors in the carotid sinus	
	Special visceral afferent	Nucleus of the solitary tract (superior part)	Receives sensory information from the posterior third of the tongue (via the inferior ganglion) (**C**)	
	Somatic afferent	Spinal nucleus of trigeminal nerve	Peripheral processes of the intracranial superior ganglion or the extracranial inferior ganglion arise from • Tongue, soft palate, pharyngeal mucosa, and tonsils (**D,E**) • Mucosa of the tympanic cavity, internal surface of the tympanic membrane, pharyngotympanic tube (tympanic plexus) (**F**) • Skin of the external ear and auditory canal (blends with the vagus nerve)	

Fig. 31.19 Glossopharyngeal nerve in the tympanic cavity

Left anterolateral view. The tympanic nerve contains visceral efferent (presynaptic parasympathetic) fibers for the otic ganglion, as well as somatic afferent fibers for the tympanic cavity and pharyngotympanic tube. It joins with sympathetic fibers from the internal carotid plexus (via the caroticotympanic nerve) to form the tympanic plexus.

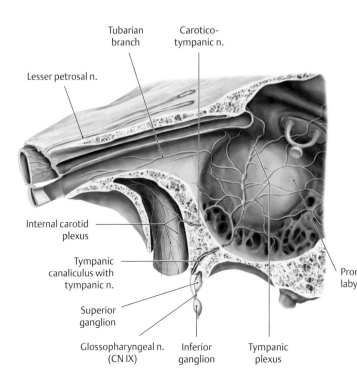

Fig. 31.20 Visceral efferent (parasympathetic) fibers of CN IX

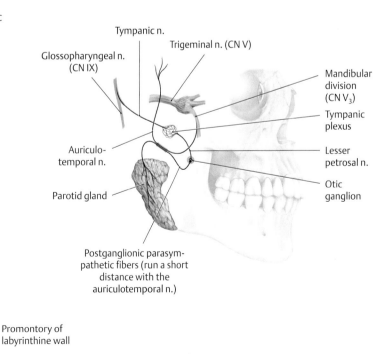

CN X: Vagus Nerve

Fig. 31.21 **Vagus nerve nuclei**

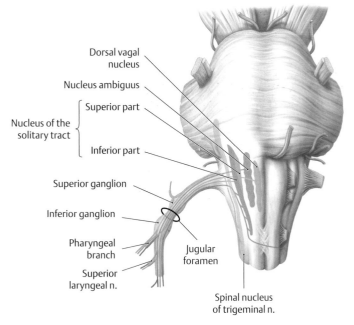

Dorsal vagal nucleus

Nucleus ambiguus

Nucleus of the solitary tract
- Superior part
- Inferior part

Superior ganglion

Inferior ganglion

Pharyngeal branch

Jugular foramen

Superior laryngeal n.

Spinal nucleus of trigeminal n.

A Anterior view of the medulla oblongata.

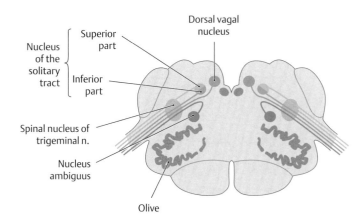

Nucleus of the solitary tract
- Superior part
- Inferior part

Dorsal vagal nucleus

Spinal nucleus of trigeminal n.

Nucleus ambiguus

Olive

B Cross section through the medulla oblongata, superior view.

Table 31.9	Vagus nerve (CN X)			
Course	**Fibers**	**Nuclei**	**Function**	**Effects of nerve injury**
Emerges from the medulla oblongata; leaves the cranial cavity through the jugular foramen. CN X has the most extensive distribution of all the cranial nerves (vagus = "vagabond"), consisting of cranial, cervical, thoracic (see p. 91), and abdominal (see p. 237) parts.	Special visceral efferent (branchio-genic)	Nucleus ambiguus	Innervate: • Pharyngeal muscles (via pharyngeal plexus with CN IX) • Muscles of the soft palate • Laryngeal muscles (superior laryngeal n. supplies the cricothyroid; inferior laryngeal n. supplies all other laryngeal muscles)	The recurrent laryngeal nerve supplies visceromotor innervation to the only muscle abducting the vocal cords, the posterior cricoarytenoid. Unilateral destruction of this nerve leads to hoarseness; bilateral destruction leads to respiratory distress (dyspnea).
	Visceral efferent (parasympa-thetic)	Dorsal vagal nucleus	Synapse in prevertebral or intramural ganglia. Innervate smooth muscle and glands of • Thoracic viscera (**A**) • Abdominal viscera (**A**)	
	Somatic afferent	Spinal nucleus of trigeminal nerve	Superior (jugular) ganglion receives peripheral fibers from • Dura in posterior cranial fossa (**C**) • Skin of ear (**D**), external auditory canal (**E**)	
	Special visceral afferent	Nucleus of solitary tract (superior part)	Inferior nodose ganglion receives peripheral processes from • Taste buds on the epiglottis (**F**)	
	Visceral afferent	Nucleus of solitary tract (inferior part)	Inferior ganglion receives peripheral processes from • Mucosa of lower pharynx at its esophageal junction (**G**) • Laryngeal mucosa above (superior laryngeal n.) and below (inferior laryngeal n.) the vocal fold (**G**) • Pressure receptors in the aortic arch (**B**) • Chemoreceptors in the para-aortic body (**B**) • Thoracic and abdominal viscera (**A**)	

Fig. 31.22 Course of the vagus nerve

The vagus nerve gives off four major branches in the neck. The inferior laryngeal nerves are the terminal branches of the recurrent laryngeal nerves. *Note:* The left recurrent laryngeal nerve winds around the aortic arch, while the right nerve winds around the subclavian artery.

Table 31.10	Vagus nerve branches in the neck
①	Pharyngeal branches
②	Superior laryngeal n.
③R	Right recurrent laryngeal n.
③L	Left recurrent laryngeal n.
④	Cervical cardiac branches

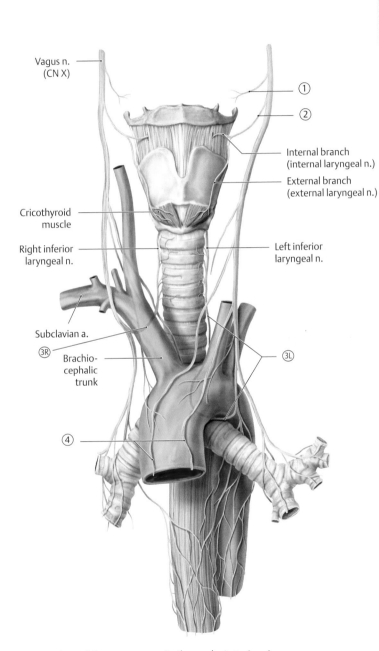

A Branches of the vagus nerve in the neck. Anterior view.

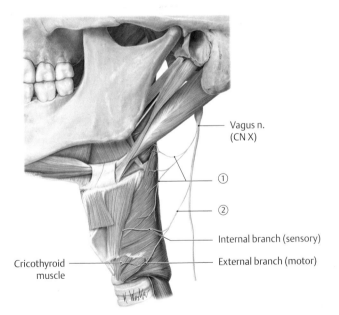

B Innervation of the pharyngeal and laryngeal muscles. Left lateral view.

CN XI & XII: Accessory & Hypoglossal Nerves

The traditional "cranial root" of the accessory nerve (CN XI) is now considered a part of the vagus nerve (CN X) that travels with the spinal root for a short distance before splitting. The cranial fibers are distributed via the vagus nerve while the spinal root fibers continue on as the (spinal) accessory nerve (CN XI).

Fig. 31.23 Accessory nerve
Posterior view of the brainstem with the cerebellum removed. *Note:* For didactic reasons, the muscles are displayed from the right side.

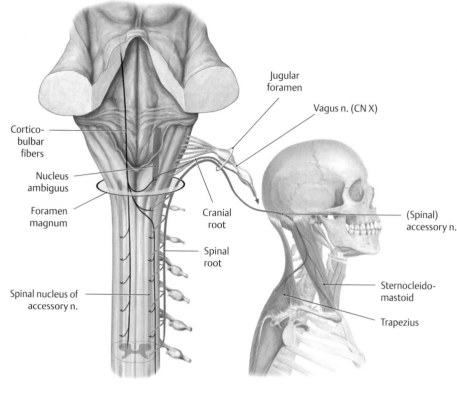

Fig. 31.24 Accessory nerve lesions
Lesion of the right accessory nerve.

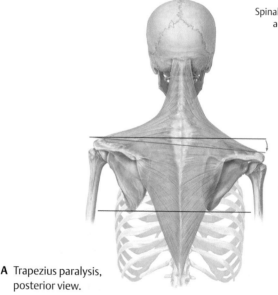

A Trapezius paralysis, posterior view.

B Sternocleidomastoid paralysis, right anterolateral view.

Table 31.11	(Spinal) accessory nerve (CN XI)			
Course	**Fibers**	**Nuclei**	**Function**	**Effects of nerve injury**
The spinal root emerges from the spinal cord (at the level of C1–C5/6), passes superiorly, and enters the skull through the foramen magnum, where it joins with the cranial root from the medulla oblongata. Both roots leave the skull through the jugular foramen. Within the jugular foramen, fibers from the cranial root pass to the vagus nerve (internal branch). The spinal portion descends to the nuchal region as the external branch.	Special visceral efferent	Nucleus ambiguus (caudal part)	Join CN X and are distributed with the recurrent laryngeal nerve. Innervate: • All laryngeal muscles (except cricothyroid)	*Trapezius paralysis:* drooping of shoulder on affected side and difficulty raising arm above horizontal plane. This paralysis is a concern during neck operations (e.g., lymph node biopsies). An injury of the accessory nerve will not result in complete trapezius paralysis (the muscle is also innervated by segments C3 and C4/5). *Sternocleidomastoid paralysis:* torticollis (wry neck, i.e., difficulty turning head). Unilateral lesions cause flaccid paralysis (the muscle is supplied exclusively by the accessory nerve). Bilateral lesions make it difficult to hold the head upright.
	Somatic efferent	Spinal nucleus of accessory n.	Form the external branch of the accessory nerve. Innervate: • Trapezius • Sternocleidomastoid	

Fig. 31.25 Hypoglossal nerve

Posterior view of the brainstem with the cerebellum removed. *Note:* C1, which innervates the thyrohyoid and geniohyoid, runs briefly with the hypoglossal nerve.

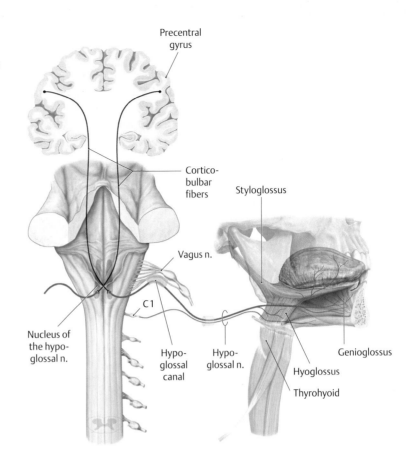

Fig. 31.26 Hypoglossal nerve nuclei

Note: The nucleus of the hypoglossal nerve is innervated by cortical neurons from the contralateral side.

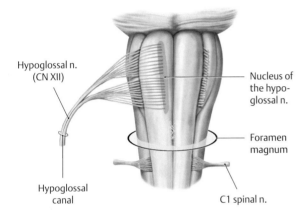

A Anterior view.

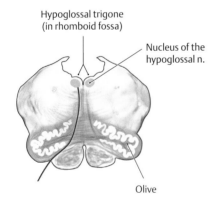

B Cross section through the medulla oblongata.

Fig. 31.27 Hypoglossal nerve lesions

Superior view.

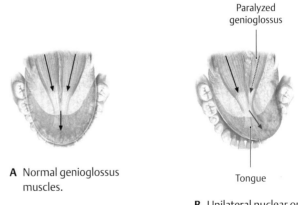

A Normal genioglossus muscles.

B Unilateral nuclear or peripheral lesion.

Table 31.12	**Hypoglossal nerve (CN XII)**				
Course	**Fibers**	**Nuclei**	**Function**		**Effects of nerve injury**
Emerges from the medulla oblongata, leaves the cranial cavity through the hypoglossal canal, and descends laterally to the vagus nerve. CN XII enters the root of the tongue above the hyoid bone.	Somatic efferent	Nucleus of the hypoglossal n.	Innervates: • Intrinsic and extrinsic muscles of the tongue (except the palatoglossus, supplied by CN X)		Central hypoglossal paralysis (supranuclear): tongue deviates *away* from the side of the lesion Nuclear or peripheral paralysis: tongue deviates *toward* the affected side (due to preponderance of muscle on healthy side) Flaccid paralysis: both nuclei injured; tongue cannot be protruded

Innervation of the Face

Fig. 32.1 Motor innervation of the face

Left lateral view. Five branches of the facial nerve (CN VII) provide motor innervation to the muscles of facial expression. The mandibular division of the trigeminal nerve (CN V$_3$) supplies motor innervation to the muscles of mastication.

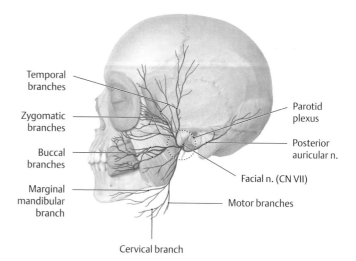

A Motor innervation of the muscles of facial expression.

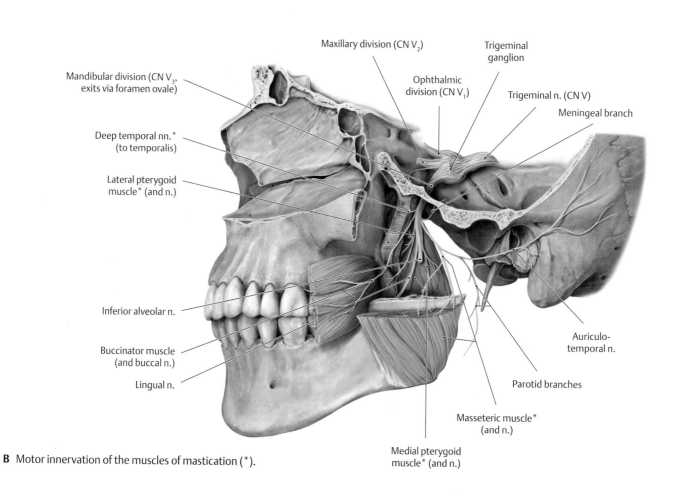

B Motor innervation of the muscles of mastication (*).

Fig. 32.2 Sensory innervation of the face

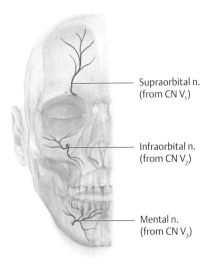

Supraorbital n. (from CN V₁)

Infraorbital n. (from CN V₂)

Mental n. (from CN V₃)

A Sensory branches of the trigeminal nerve, anterior view. The sensory branches of the three divisions emerge from the supraorbital, infraorbital, and mental foramina, respectively.

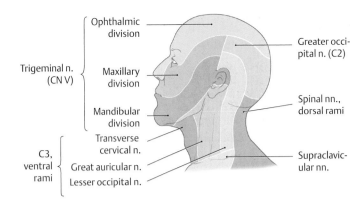

Ophthalmic division

Greater occipital n. (C2)

Trigeminal n. (CN V)

Maxillary division

Mandibular division

Spinal nn., dorsal rami

Transverse cervical n.

C3, ventral rami

Great auricular n.

Lesser occipital n.

Supraclavicular nn.

B Sensory innervation of the head and neck, left lateral view. The occiput and nuchal regions are supplied by the dorsal rami (blue) of the spinal nerves (the greater occipital nerve is the dorsal ramus of C2).

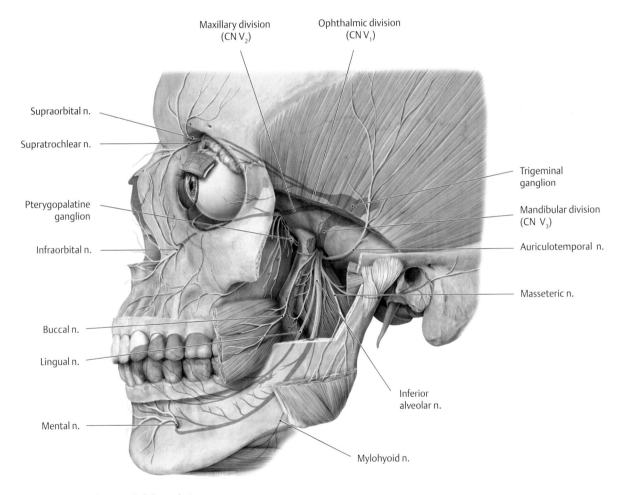

Maxillary division (CN V₂)

Ophthalmic division (CN V₁)

Supraorbital n.

Supratrochlear n.

Pterygopalatine ganglion

Infraorbital n.

Buccal n.

Lingual n.

Mental n.

Trigeminal ganglion

Mandibular division (CN V₃)

Auriculotemporal n.

Masseteric n.

Inferior alveolar n.

Mylohyoid n.

C Divisions of the trigeminal nerve, left lateral view.

Arteries of the Head & Neck

The head and neck are supplied by branches of the common carotid artery. The common carotid splits at the carotid bifurcation into two branches: the internal and external carotid arteries. The internal carotid chiefly supplies the brain (p. 606), although its branches anastomose with the external carotid in the orbit and nasal septum. The external carotid is the major supplier of structures of the head and neck.

Fig. 32.3 Internal carotid artery

Left lateral view. The most important extra-cerebral branch of the internal carotid artery is the ophthalmic artery, which supplies the upper nasal septum (p. 524) and the orbit (p. 512). See pp. 608–609 for arteries of the brain.

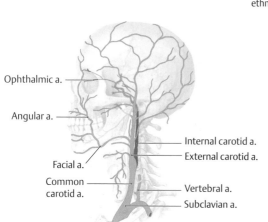

A Schematic.

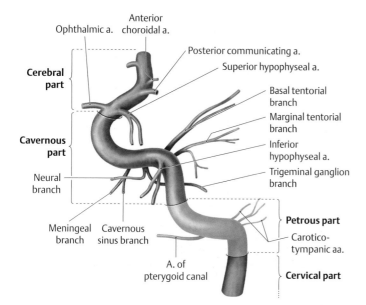

C Course of the internal carotid artery.

B Parts and branches of the internal carotid artery.

Carotid artery atherosclerosis

The carotid artery is often affected by atherosclerosis, a hardening of arterial walls due to plaque formation. The examiner can determine the status of the arteries using ultrasound. *Note:* The absence of atherosclerosis in the carotid artery does not preclude coronary heart disease or atherosclerotic changes in other locations.

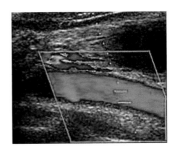

A Common carotid artery with "normal" flow.

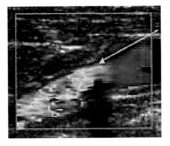

B Calcified plaque in the carotid bulb.

Fig. 32.4 External carotid artery: Overview

Left lateral view.

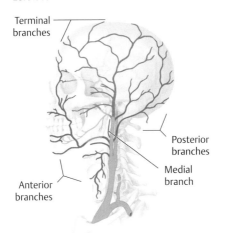

Terminal branches

Posterior branches

Medial branch

Anterior branches

A Schematic of the external carotid artery.

Table 32.1	Branches of the external carotid artery
Group	**Artery**
Anterior (p. 492)	Superior thyroid a.
	Lingual a.
	Facial a.
Medial (p. 492)	Ascending pharyngeal a.
Posterior (p. 493)	Occipital a.
	Posterior auricular a.
Terminal (p. 494)	Maxillary a.
	Superficial temporal a.

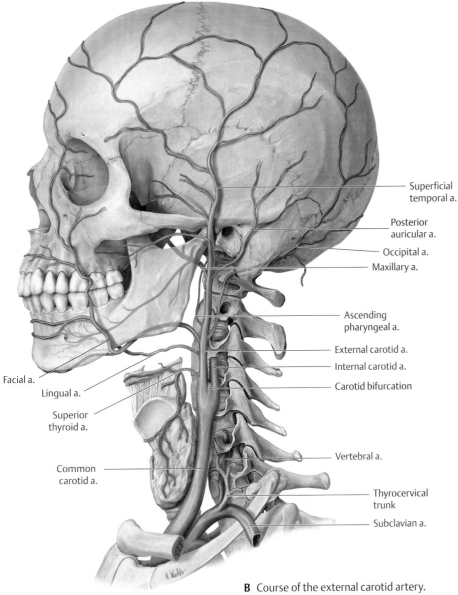

Superficial temporal a.

Posterior auricular a.

Occipital a.

Maxillary a.

Ascending pharyngeal a.

External carotid a.

Internal carotid a.

Carotid bifurcation

Vertebral a.

Thyrocervical trunk

Subclavian a.

Facial a.

Lingual a.

Superior thyroid a.

Common carotid a.

B Course of the external carotid artery.

External Carotid Artery: Anterior, Medial & Posterior Branches

Fig. 32.5 **Anterior and medial branches**

Left lateral view. The arteries of the anterior aspect supply the anterior structures of the head and neck, including the orbit (p. 510), ear (p. 534), larynx (p. 575), pharynx (p. 556), and oral cavity. *Note:* The angular artery anastomoses with the dorsal nasal artery of the internal carotid (via the ophthalmic artery).

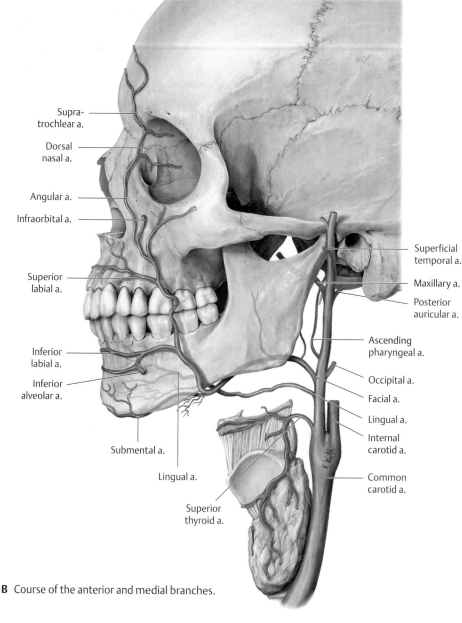

Supra-trochlear a.

Dorsal nasal a.

Angular a.

Infraorbital a.

Superior labial a.

Inferior labial a.

Inferior alveolar a.

Submental a.

Lingual a.

Superior thyroid a.

Superficial temporal a.

Maxillary a.

Posterior auricular a.

Ascending pharyngeal a.

Occipital a.

Facial a.

Lingual a.

Internal carotid a.

Common carotid a.

B Course of the anterior and medial branches.

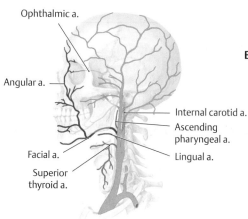

Ophthalmic a.

Angular a.

Facial a.

Superior thyroid a.

Internal carotid a.

Ascending pharyngeal a.

Lingual a.

A Arteries of the anterior and medial branches. The copious blood supply to the face makes facial injuries bleed profusely, but heal quickly. There are extensive anastomoses between branches of the external carotid, and between the external carotid artery and branches of the ophthalmic artery.

Fig. 32.6 Posterior branches

Left lateral view. The posterior branches of the external carotid artery supply the ear (p. 534), posterior skull (p. 499), and posterior neck muscles (p. 585).

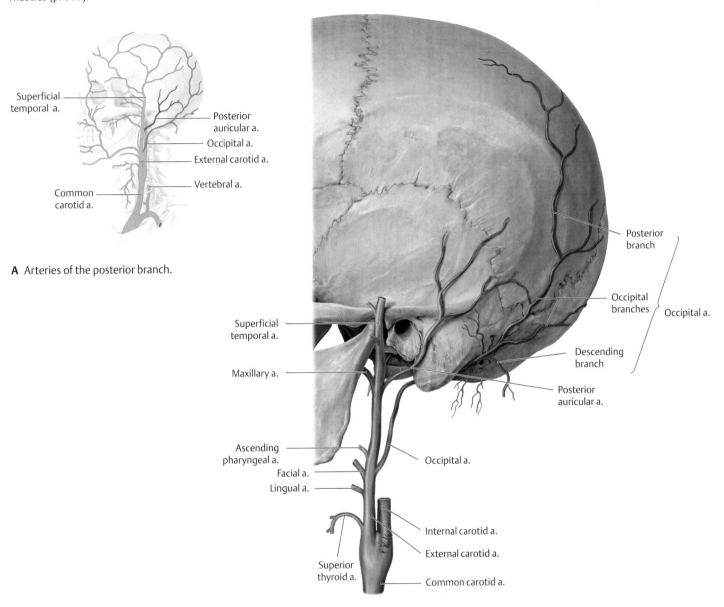

A Arteries of the posterior branch.

B Course of the posterior branches.

Table 32.2		Anterior, medial, and posterior branches of the external carotid artery
Branch	**Artery**	**Divisions and distribution**
Anterior branch	Superior thyroid a.	Glandular branch (to thyroid gland); superior laryngeal a.; sternocleidomastoid branch
	Lingual a.	Dorsal lingual branches (to base of tongue, epiglottis); sublingual a. (to sublingual gland, tongue, oral floor, oral cavity)
	Facial a.	Ascending palatine a. (to pharyngeal wall, soft palate, pharyngotympanic tube); tonsillar branch (to palatine tonsils); submental a. (to oral floor, submandibular gland); labial aa.; angular a. (to nasal root)
Medial branch	Ascending pharyngeal a.	Pharyngeal branches; interior tympanic a. (to mucosa of inner ear); posterior meningeal a.
Posterior branches	Occipital a.	Occipital branches; descending branch (to posterior neck muscles)
	Posterior auricular a.	Stylomastoid a. (to facial nerve in facial canal); posterior tympanic a.; auricular branch; occipital branch; parotid branch
For terminal branches, see Table 32.3.		

External Carotid Artery: Terminal Branches

The terminal branches of the external carotid artery consist of two major arteries: superficial temporal and maxillary. The superficial temporal artery supplies the lateral skull. The maxillary artery is a major artery for internal structures of the face.

Fig. 32.7 Superficial temporal artery

Left lateral view. Inflammation of the superficial temporal artery due to temporal arteritis can cause severe headaches. The course of the frontal branch of the artery can often be seen superficially under the skin of elderly patients.

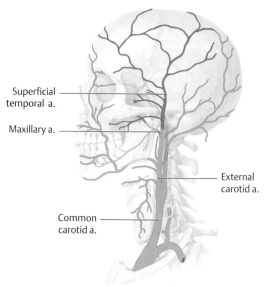

A Arteries of the terminal branch.

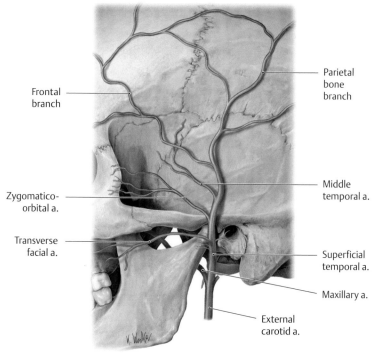

B Course of the superficial temporal artery.

Table 32.3	Terminal branches of the external carotid artery			
Branch	**Artery**		**Divisions and distribution**	
Terminal branches	Superficial temporal a.		Transverse facial a. (to soft tissues below the zygomatic arch); frontal branches; parietal branches; zygomatico-orbital a. (to lateral orbital wall)	
	Maxillary a.	Mandibular part	Inferior alveolar a. (to mandible, teeth, gingiva); middle meningeal a.; deep auricular a. (to temporomandibular joint, external auditory canal); anterior tympanic a.	
		Pterygoid part	Masseteric a.; deep temporal branches; pterygoid branches; buccal a.	
		Pterygopalatine part	Posterosuperior alveolar a. (to maxillary molars, maxillary sinus, gingiva); infraorbital a. (to maxillary alveoli)	
			Descending palatine a.	Greater palatine a. (to hard palate)
				Lesser palatine a. (to soft palate, palatine tonsil, pharyngeal wall)
			Sphenopalatine a.	Lateral posterior nasal aa. (to lateral wall of nasal cavity, conchae)
				Posterior septal branches (to nasal septum)

Fig. 32.8 Maxillary artery

Left lateral view. The maxillary artery consists of three parts: mandibular (blue), pterygoid (green), and pterygopalatine (yellow).

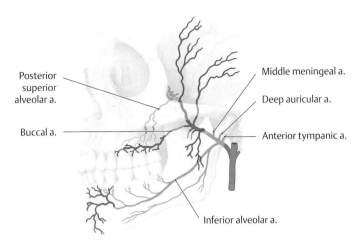

Posterior superior alveolar a.

Buccal a.

Middle meningeal a.

Deep auricular a.

Anterior tympanic a.

Inferior alveolar a.

A Divisions of the maxillary artery.

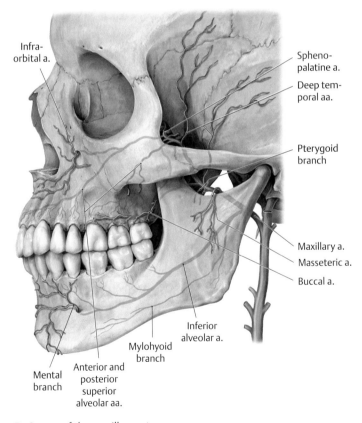

Infra-orbital a.

Spheno-palatine a.

Deep temporal aa.

Pterygoid branch

Maxillary a.

Masseteric a.

Buccal a.

Inferior alveolar a.

Mylohyoid branch

Mental branch

Anterior and posterior superior alveolar aa.

B Course of the maxillary artery.

Middle meningeal artery

The middle meningeal artery supplies the meninges and overlying calvaria. Rupture of the artery (generally due to head trauma) results in an epidural hematoma.

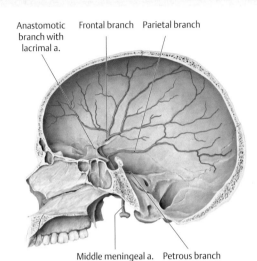

Anastomotic branch with lacrimal a.

Frontal branch

Parietal branch

Middle meningeal a.

Petrous branch

A Right middle meningeal artery, medial view of opened skull.

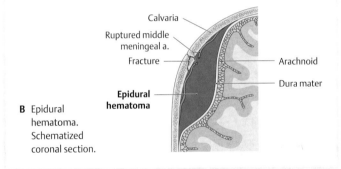

Calvaria

Ruptured middle meningeal a.

Fracture

Epidural hematoma

Arachnoid

Dura mater

B Epidural hematoma. Schematized coronal section.

Sphenopalatine artery

The sphenopalatine artery supplies the wall of the nasal cavity. Excessive nasopharyngeal bleeding from the branches of the sphenopalatine artery may necessitate ligation of the maxillary artery in the pterygopalatine fossa.

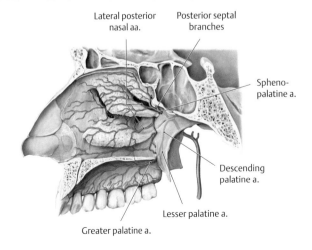

Lateral posterior nasal aa.

Posterior septal branches

Spheno-palatine a.

Descending palatine a.

Lesser palatine a.

Greater palatine a.

C Lateral wall of nasal cavity, left lateral view.

Veins of the Head & Neck

Fig. 32.9 Veins of the head and neck

Left lateral view. The veins of the head and neck drain into the brachiocephalic vein. *Note:* The left and right brachiocephalic veins are not symmetrical.

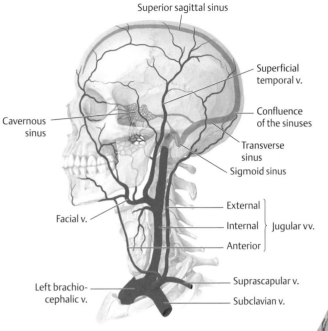

A Principal veins of the head and neck.

Table 32.4	Principal superficial veins	
Vein	**Region drained**	**Location**
Internal jugular v.	Interior of skull (including brain)	Within carotid sheath
External jugular v.	Superficial head	Within superficial cervical fascia
Anterior jugular v.	Neck, portions of head	

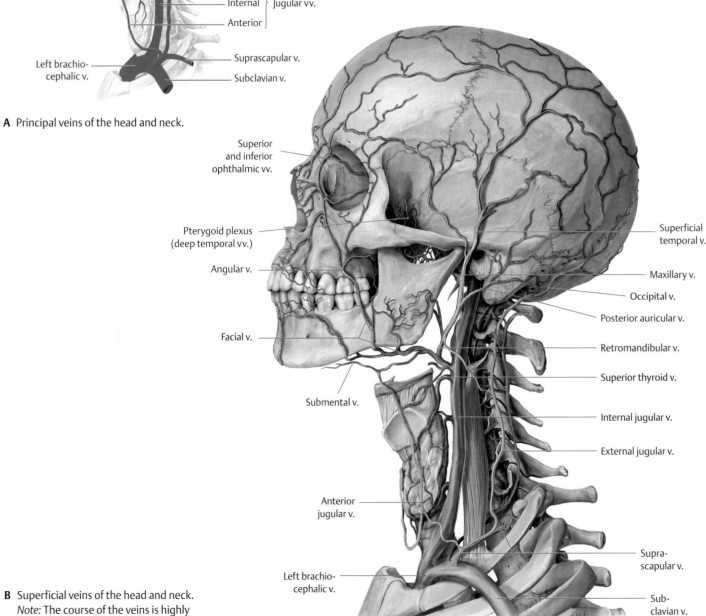

B Superficial veins of the head and neck.
Note: The course of the veins is highly variable.

Fig. 32.10 Deep veins of the head

Left lateral view. *Removed:* Upper ramus, condylar and coronoid processes of mandible. The pterygoid plexus is a venous network situated between the mandibular ramus and the muscles of mastication. The cavernous sinus connects branches of the facial vein to the sigmoid sinuses.

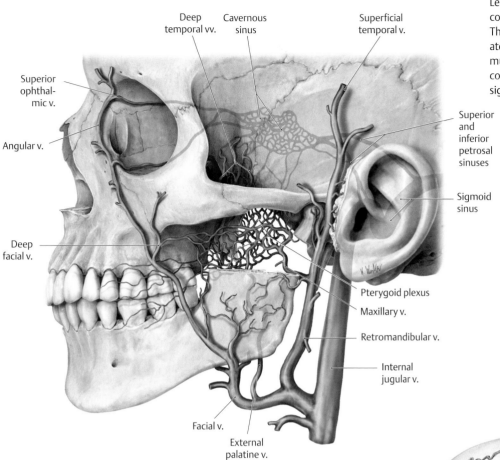

Fig. 32.11 Veins of the occiput

Posterior view. The superficial veins of the occiput communicate with the dural venous sinuses via emissary veins that drain to diploic veins (calvaria, p. 457). *Note:* The external vertebral venous plexus traverses the entire length of the spine (p. 611).

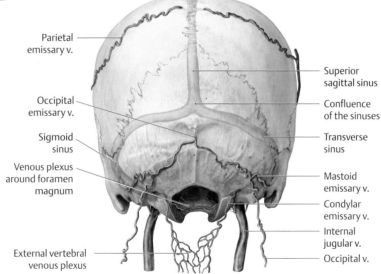

Table 32.5	Venous anastomoses	
The extensive venous anastomoses in this region provide routes for the spread of infections.		
Extracranial vein	**Connecting vein**	**Venous sinus**
Angular v.	Superior and inferior ophthalmic vv.	Cavernous sinus*
Vv. of palatine tonsil	Pterygoid plexus; inferior ophthalmic v.	
Superficial temporal v.	Parietal emissary vv.	Superior sagittal sinus
Occipital v.	Occipital emissary v.	Transverse sinus, confluence of the sinuses
Posterior auricular v.	Mastoid emissary v.	Sigmoid sinus
External vertebral venous plexus	Condylar emissary v.	
*Deep spread of bacterial infection from the facial region may result in cavernous sinus thrombosis.		

Topography of the Superficial Face

***Fig. 32.12* Superficial neurovasculature of the face**

Anterior view. *Removed:* Skin and fatty subcutaneous tissue; muscles of facial expression (left side).

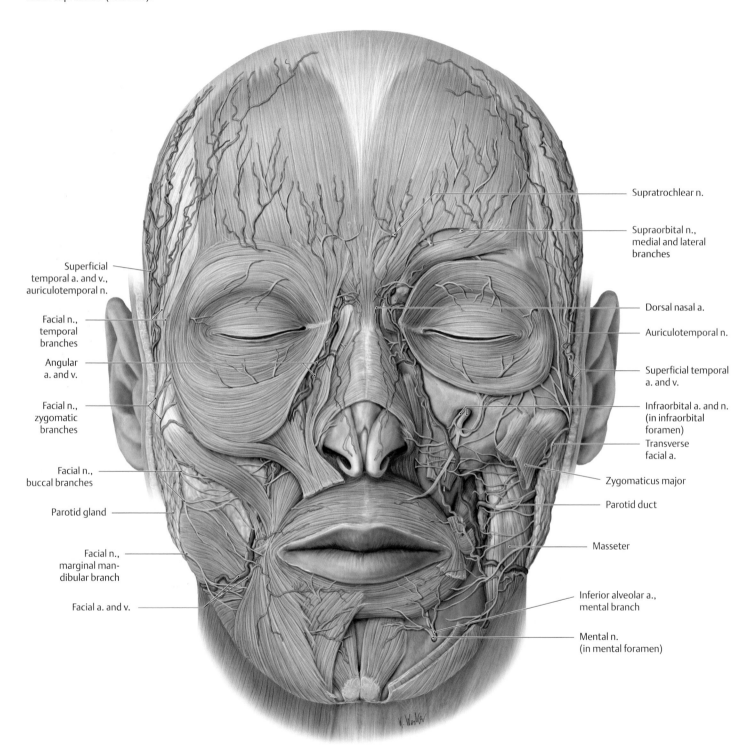

Supratrochlear n.

Supraorbital n., medial and lateral branches

Superficial temporal a. and v., auriculotemporal n.

Facial n., temporal branches

Angular a. and v.

Facial n., zygomatic branches

Facial n., buccal branches

Parotid gland

Facial n., marginal mandibular branch

Facial a. and v.

Dorsal nasal a.

Auriculotemporal n.

Superficial temporal a. and v.

Infraorbital a. and n. (in infraorbital foramen)

Transverse facial a.

Zygomaticus major

Parotid duct

Masseter

Inferior alveolar a., mental branch

Mental n. (in mental foramen)

Fig. 32.13 **Superficial neurovasculature of the head**
Left lateral view.

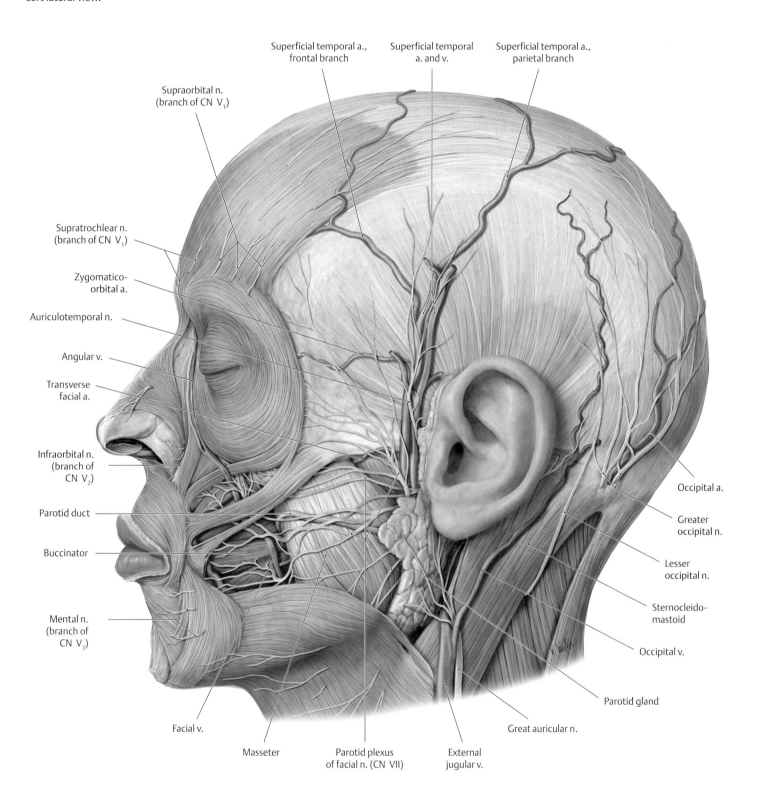

Superficial temporal a., frontal branch

Superficial temporal a. and v.

Superficial temporal a., parietal branch

Supraorbital n. (branch of CN V₁)

Supratrochlear n. (branch of CN V₁)

Zygomatico- orbital a.

Auriculotemporal n.

Angular v.

Transverse facial a.

Infraorbital n. (branch of CN V₂)

Parotid duct

Buccinator

Mental n. (branch of CN V₃)

Occipital a.

Greater occipital n.

Lesser occipital n.

Sternocleido- mastoid

Occipital v.

Parotid gland

Facial v.

Masseter

Parotid plexus of facial n. (CN VII)

External jugular v.

Great auricular n.

Topography of the Parotid Region & Temporal Fossa

Fig. 32.14 **Parotid region**
Left lateral view. *Removed:* Parotid gland, sternocleidomastoid, and veins of the head. *Revealed:* Parotid bed and carotid triangle.

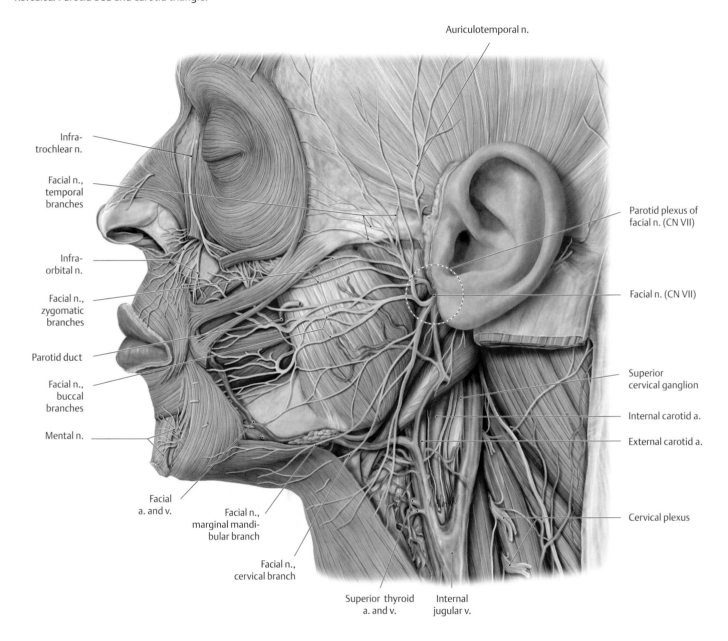

Auriculotemporal n.

Infra-trochlear n.

Facial n., temporal branches

Infra-orbital n.

Facial n., zygomatic branches

Parotid duct

Facial n., buccal branches

Mental n.

Parotid plexus of facial n. (CN VII)

Facial n. (CN VII)

Superior cervical ganglion

Internal carotid a.

External carotid a.

Cervical plexus

Facial a. and v.

Facial n., marginal mandibular branch

Facial n., cervical branch

Superior thyroid a. and v.

Internal jugular v.

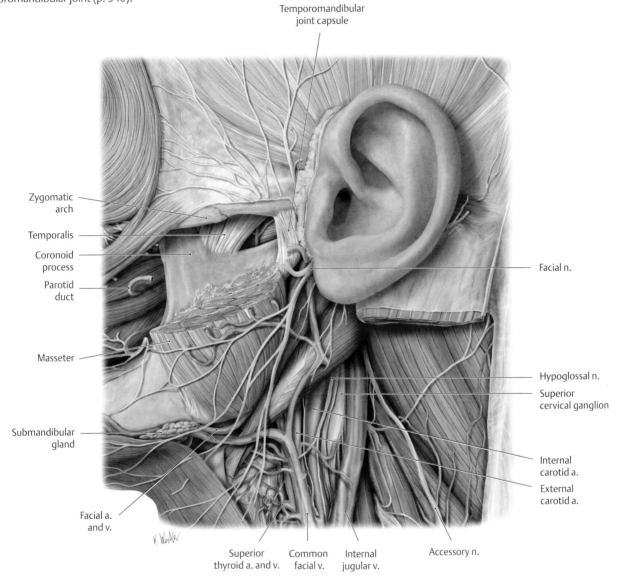

Fig. 32.15 **Temporal fossa**
Left lateral view. *Removed:* Sternocleidomastoid and masseter. *Revealed:* Temporal fossa and temporomandibular joint (p. 540).

Temporomandibular joint capsule

Zygomatic arch

Temporalis

Coronoid process

Parotid duct

Masseter

Submandibular gland

Facial a. and v.

Facial n.

Hypoglossal n.

Superior cervical ganglion

Internal carotid a.

External carotid a.

Superior thyroid a. and v.

Common facial v.

Internal jugular v.

Accessory n.

Topography of the Infratemporal Fossa

Fig. 32.16 Infratemporal fossa: Superficial layer

Left lateral view. *Removed:* Ramus of mandible. *Note:* The mylohyoid nerve (see p. 547) branches from the inferior alveolar nerve just before the mandibular foramen.

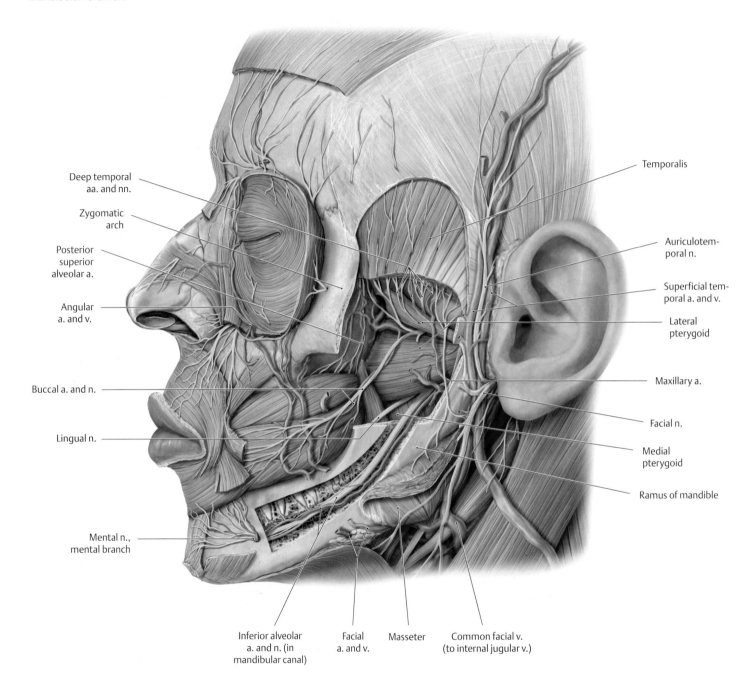

Deep temporal aa. and nn.

Zygomatic arch

Posterior superior alveolar a.

Angular a. and v.

Buccal a. and n.

Lingual n.

Mental n., mental branch

Temporalis

Auriculotemporal n.

Superficial temporal a. and v.

Lateral pterygoid

Maxillary a.

Facial n.

Medial pterygoid

Ramus of mandible

Inferior alveolar a. and n. (in mandibular canal)

Facial a. and v.

Masseter

Common facial v. (to internal jugular v.)

Fig. 32.17 Deep layer

Left lateral view. *Removed:* Lateral pterygoid muscle (both heads). *Revealed:* Deep infratemporal fossa and mandibular nerve as it enters the mandibular canal via the foramen ovale in the roof of the fossa.

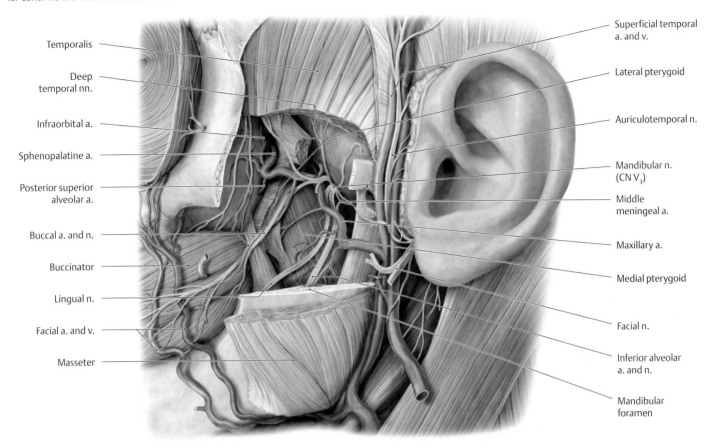

Temporalis

Deep temporal nn.

Infraorbital a.

Sphenopalatine a.

Posterior superior alveolar a.

Buccal a. and n.

Buccinator

Lingual n.

Facial a. and v.

Masseter

Superficial temporal a. and v.

Lateral pterygoid

Auriculotemporal n.

Mandibular n. (CN V₃)

Middle meningeal a.

Maxillary a.

Medial pterygoid

Facial n.

Inferior alveolar a. and n.

Mandibular foramen

Fig. 32.18 Mandibular nerve (CN V₃) in the infratemporal fossa

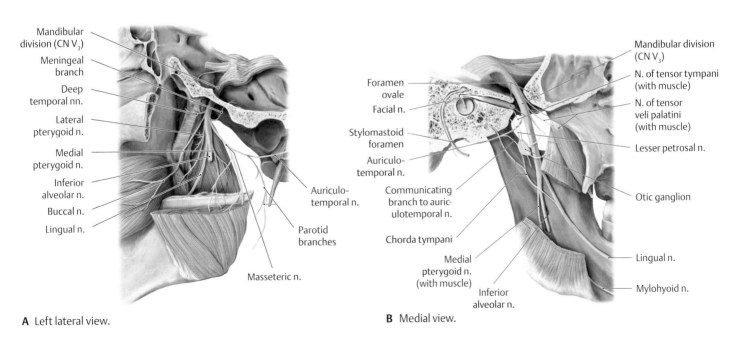

Mandibular division (CN V₃)

Meningeal branch

Deep temporal nn.

Lateral pterygoid n.

Medial pterygoid n.

Inferior alveolar n.

Buccal n.

Lingual n.

Auriculo-temporal n.

Parotid branches

Masseteric n.

A Left lateral view.

Foramen ovale

Facial n.

Stylomastoid foramen

Auriculo-temporal n.

Communicating branch to auriculotemporal n.

Chorda tympani

Medial pterygoid n. (with muscle)

Inferior alveolar n.

Mandibular division (CN V₃)

N. of tensor tympani (with muscle)

N. of tensor veli palatini (with muscle)

Lesser petrosal n.

Otic ganglion

Lingual n.

Mylohyoid n.

B Medial view.

Topography of the Pterygopalatine Fossa

The pterygopalatine fossa is a small pyramidal space just inferior to the apex of the orbit. It is continuous with the infratemporal fossa, with no clear line of demarcation between them. The pterygopalatine fossa is a crossroads for neurovascular structures traveling between the middle cranial fossa, orbit, nasal cavity, and oral cavity.

Table 32.6	**Borders of the pterygopalatine fossa**		
Direction	**Boundaries**	**Direction**	**Boundaries**
Superior	Sphenoid bone (greater wing), junction with inferior orbital fissure	Posterior	Pterygoid process (lateral plate)
Anterior	Maxillary tuberosity	Lateral	Communicates with the infratemporal fossa via the pterygomaxillary fissure
Medial	Palatine bone (perpendicular plate)	Inferior	None; opens into the retropharyngeal space

Fig. 32.19 **Arteries in the pterygopalatine fossa**
Left lateral view into area. The maxillary artery passes over the lateral pterygoid in the infratemporal fossa (see Fig. 32.16) and enters the pterygopalatine fossa through the pterygomaxillary fissure.

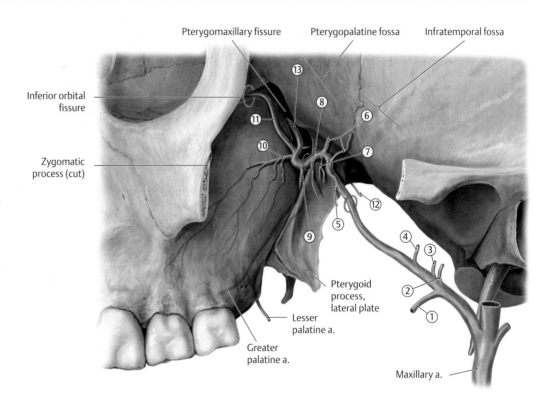

Table 32.7	**Branches of the maxillary artery**		
Part	**Artery**		**Distribution**
Mandibular part	① Inferior alveolar a.		Mandible, teeth, gingiva
	② Anterior tympanic a.		Tympanic cavity
	③ Deep auricular a.		Temporomandibular joint, external auditory canal
	④ Middle meningeal a.		Calvaria, dura, anterior and middle cranial fossae
Pterygoid part	⑤ Masseteric a.		Masseter muscle
	⑥ Deep temporal aa.		Temporalis muscle
	⑦ Pterygoid branches		Pterygoid muscles
	⑧ Buccal a.		Buccal mucosa
Pterygopalatine part	⑨ Descending palatine a.	Greater palatine a.	Hard palate
		Lesser palatine a.	Soft palate, palatine tonsil, pharyngeal wall
	⑩ Posterosuperior alveolar a.		Maxillary molars, maxillary sinus, gingiva
	⑪ Infraorbital a.		Maxillary alveoli
	⑫ A. of pterygoid canal		
	⑬ Sphenopalatine a.	Lateral posterior nasal aa.	Lateral wall of nasal cavity, choanae
		Posterior septal branches	Nasal septum

The maxillary division of the trigeminal nerve (CN V$_2$, see p. 477) passes from the middle cranial fossa through the foramen rotundum into the pterygopalatine fossa. The parasympathetic pterygopalatine ganglion receives presynaptic fibers from the greater petrosal nerve (the parasympathetic root of the nervus intermedius branch of the facial nerve). The preganglionic fibers of the pterygopalatine ganglion synapse with ganglion cells that innervate the lacrimal, small palatal, and small nasal glands. The sympathetic fibers of the deep petrosal nerve (sympathetic root) and sensory fibers of the maxillary nerve (sensory root) pass through the pterygopalatine ganglion without synapsing.

Fig. 32.20 Nerves in the pterygopalatine fossa
Left lateral view.

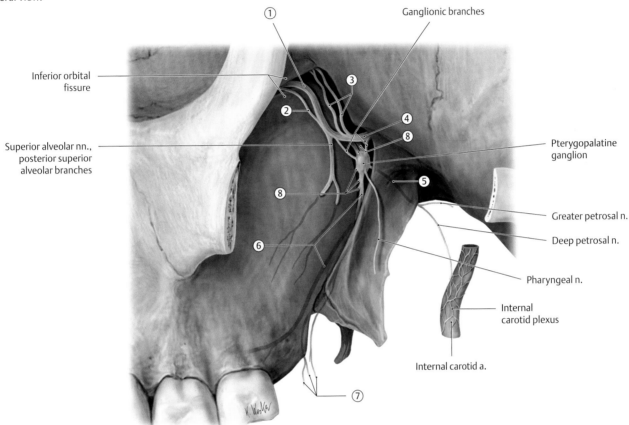

Table 32.8	Passage of neurovascular structures into pterygopalatine fossa		
Origin of structures	**Passageway**	**Transmitted nerves**	**Transmitted vessels**
Orbit	Inferior orbital fissure	① Infraorbital n.	Infraorbital a. (and accompanying vv.)
		② Zygomatic n.	Inferior ophthalmic v.
		③ Orbital branches (from CN V$_2$)	
Middle cranial fossa	Foramen rotundum	④ Maxillary n. (CN V$_2$)	
Base of skull	Pterygoid canal	⑤ N. of pterygoid canal (greater and deep petrosal nn.)	A. of pterygoid canal (with accompanying vv.)
Palate	Greater palatine canal	⑥ Greater palatine n.	Descending palatine a.
			Greater palatine a.
	Lesser palatine canals	⑦ Lesser palatine nn.	Lesser palatine aa. (terminal branches of descending palatine a.)
Nasal cavity	Sphenopalatine foramen	⑧ Medial and lateral posterior superior and posterior inferior nasal branches (from nasopalatine n., CN V$_2$)	Sphenopalatine a. (with accompanying vv.)

Bones of the Orbit

Fig. 33.1 Bones of the orbit

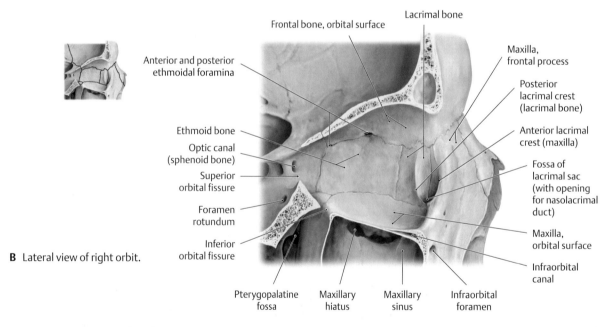

Supraorbital foramen

Frontal bone, orbital surface

Zygomatico-orbital foramen

Superior orbital fissure

Zygomatic bone

Inferior orbital fissure

Infraorbital groove

Frontal incisure

Posterior ethmoidal foramen

Anterior ethmoidal foramen

Optic canal (sphenoid bone)

Nasal bone

Maxilla, frontal process

Lacrimal bone

Ethmoid bone, orbital plate

A Anterior view.

Maxilla, orbital surface · Infraorbital foramen

Frontal bone, orbital surface · Lacrimal bone

Anterior and posterior ethmoidal foramina

Ethmoid bone

Optic canal (sphenoid bone)

Superior orbital fissure

Foramen rotundum

Inferior orbital fissure

Maxilla, frontal process

Posterior lacrimal crest (lacrimal bone)

Anterior lacrimal crest (maxilla)

Fossa of lacrimal sac (with opening for nasolacrimal duct)

Maxilla, orbital surface

Infraorbital canal

B Lateral view of right orbit.

Pterygopalatine fossa · Maxillary hiatus · Maxillary sinus · Infraorbital foramen

Table 33.1	Openings in the orbit for neurovascular structures		
Opening*	**Nerves**		**Vessels**
Optic canal	Optic n. (CN II)		Ophthalmic a.
Superior orbital fissure	Oculomotor n. (CN III) Trochlear n. (CN IV) Abducent n. (CN VI)	Trigeminal n., ophthalmic division (CN V$_1$) • Lacrimal n. • Frontal n. • Nasociliary n.	Superior ophthalmic v.
Inferior orbital fissure	Infraorbital n. (CN V$_2$) Zygomatic n. (CN V$_2$)		Infraorbital a. and v., inferior ophthalmic v.
Infraorbital canal	Infraorbital n. (CN V$_2$), a., and v.		
Supraorbital foramen	Supraorbital n. (lateral branch)		Supraorbital a.
Frontal incisure	Supraorbital n. (medial branch)		Supratrochlear a.
Anterior ethmoidal foramen	Anterior ethmoidal n., a., and v.		
Posterior ethmoidal foramen	Posterior ethmoidal n., a., and v.		
* The nasolacrimal canal transmits the nasolacrimal duct.			

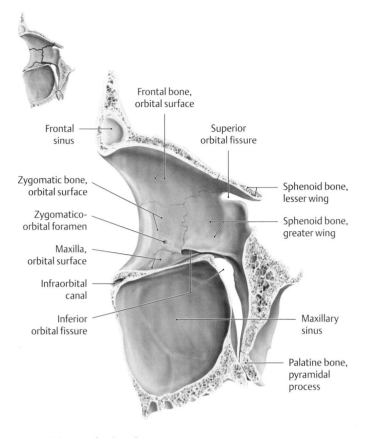

Frontal bone, orbital surface

Superior orbital fissure

Frontal sinus

Zygomatic bone, orbital surface

Zygomatico-orbital foramen

Maxilla, orbital surface

Infraorbital canal

Inferior orbital fissure

Sphenoid bone, lesser wing

Sphenoid bone, greater wing

Maxillary sinus

Palatine bone, pyramidal process

C Medial view of right orbit.

Table 33.2	Structures surrounding the orbit
Direction	**Bordering structure**
Superior	Frontal sinus
	Anterior cranial fossa
Medial	Ethmoid sinus
Inferior	Maxillary sinus
Certain deeper structures also have a clinically important relationship to the orbit:	
Sphenoid sinus	Hypophysis (pituitary)
Middle cranial fossa	Cavernous sinus
Optic chiasm	Pterygopalatine fossa

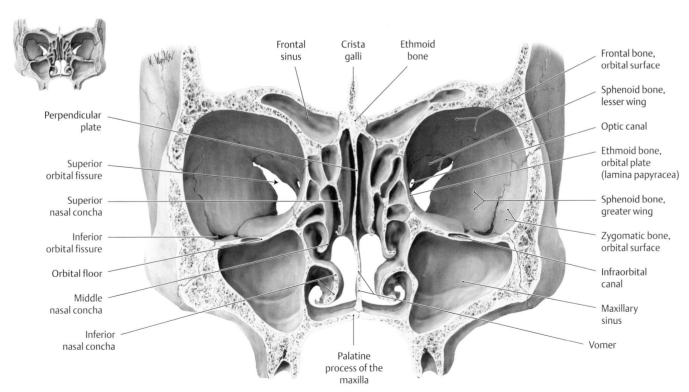

Frontal sinus

Crista galli

Ethmoid bone

Frontal bone, orbital surface

Sphenoid bone, lesser wing

Optic canal

Ethmoid bone, orbital plate (lamina papyracea)

Sphenoid bone, greater wing

Zygomatic bone, orbital surface

Infraorbital canal

Maxillary sinus

Vomer

Perpendicular plate

Superior orbital fissure

Superior nasal concha

Inferior orbital fissure

Orbital floor

Middle nasal concha

Inferior nasal concha

Palatine process of the maxilla

D Coronal section, anterior view.

Muscles of the Orbit

Fig. 33.2 Extraocular muscles

Right eye, superior view (except **A**). The eyeball is moved by six extrinsic muscles: four rectus (superior, inferior, medial, and lateral) and two oblique (superior and inferior).

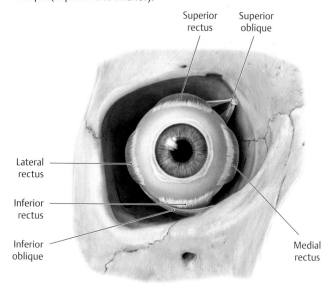

A Anterior view.

B Superior view of opened orbit.

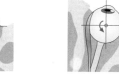 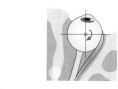

C Superior rectus.   **D** Medial rectus.   **E** Inferior rectus.   **F** Lateral rectus.   **G** Superior oblique.   **H** Inferior oblique.

Table 33.3	**Extraocular muscles**					

Muscle	Origin	Insertion	Primary action (red)	Secondary action (blue)	Innervation
Superior rectus	Common tendinous ring (common annular tendon)	Sclera of the eye	Elevation	Adduction and medial rotation	Oculomotor n. (CN III), superior branch
Medial rectus			Adduction	—	Oculomotor n. (CN III), inferior branch
Inferior rectus			Depression	Adduction and lateral rotation	
Lateral rectus			Abduction	—	Abducent n. (CN VI)
Superior oblique	Sphenoid bone*		Depression and abduction	Medial rotation	Trochlear n. (CN IV)
Inferior oblique	Medial orbital margin		Elevation and abduction	Lateral rotation	Oculomotor n. (CN III), inferior branch

* The tendon of insertion of the superior oblique passes through a tendinous loop (trochlea) attached to the superomedial orbital margin.

Fig. 33.3 Cardinal directions of gaze

There are six cardinal directions of gaze, all of which are tested during clinical evaluation of ocular motility. *Note:* Each gaze requires activation of two different muscles (not a muscle pair) and therefore two cranial nerves.

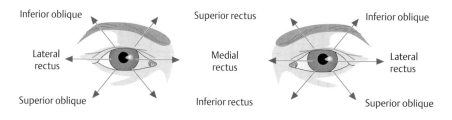

Fig. 33.4 Innervation of the extraocular muscles

Right eye, lateral view with the temporal wall of the orbit removed.

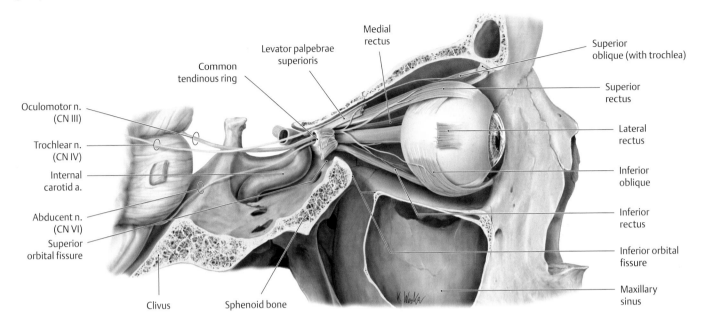

Levator palpebrae superioris

Common tendinous ring

Medial rectus

Superior oblique (with trochlea)

Superior rectus

Oculomotor n. (CN III)

Trochlear n. (CN IV)

Internal carotid a.

Abducent n. (CN VI)

Superior orbital fissure

Lateral rectus

Inferior oblique

Inferior rectus

Inferior orbital fissure

Maxillary sinus

Clivus

Sphenoid bone

✳ *Clinical*

Oculomotor palsies

Oculomotor palsies may result from a lesion involving an eye muscle or its associated cranial nerve (at the nucleus or along the course of the nerve). If one extraocular muscle is weak or paralyzed, deviation of the eye will be noted.

Impairment of the coordinated actions of the extraocular muscles may cause the visual axis of one eye to deviate from its normal position. The patient will therefore perceive a double image (diplopia).

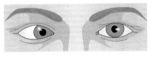

A Abducent nerve palsy. *Disabled:* Lateral rectus.

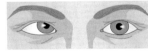

B Trochlear nerve palsy. *Disabled:* Superior oblique.

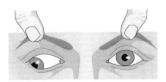

C Complete oculomotor palsy. *Disabled:* Superior, inferior, and medial recti and inferior oblique.

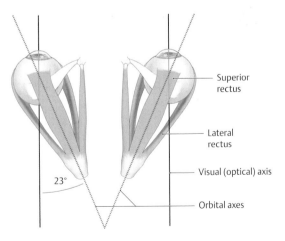

Superior rectus

Lateral rectus

Visual (optical) axis

Orbital axes

23°

D Normal visual and orbital axes.

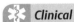

Neurovasculature of the Orbit

Fig. 33.5 **Veins of the orbit**

Lateral view of the right orbit. *Removed:* Lateral orbital wall. *Opened:* Maxillary sinus.

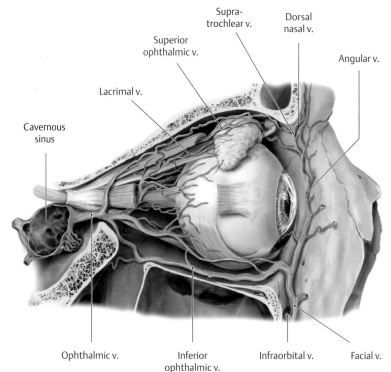

Supra-trochlear v.

Dorsal nasal v.

Superior ophthalmic v.

Angular v.

Lacrimal v.

Cavernous sinus

Ophthalmic v.

Inferior ophthalmic v.

Infraorbital v.

Facial v.

Fig. 33.6 **Arteries of the orbit**

Superior view of the right orbit. *Opened:* Optic canal and orbital roof.

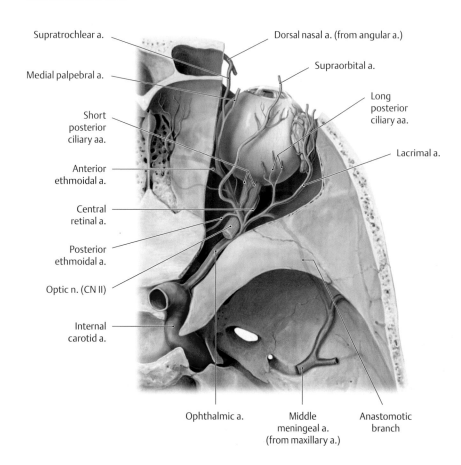

Supratrochlear a.

Dorsal nasal a. (from angular a.)

Medial palpebral a.

Supraorbital a.

Short posterior ciliary aa.

Long posterior ciliary aa.

Anterior ethmoidal a.

Lacrimal a.

Central retinal a.

Posterior ethmoidal a.

Optic n. (CN II)

Internal carotid a.

Ophthalmic a.

Middle meningeal a. (from maxillary a.)

Anastomotic branch

Fig. 33.7 Innervation of the orbit

Lateral view of the right orbit. *Removed:* Temporal bony wall.

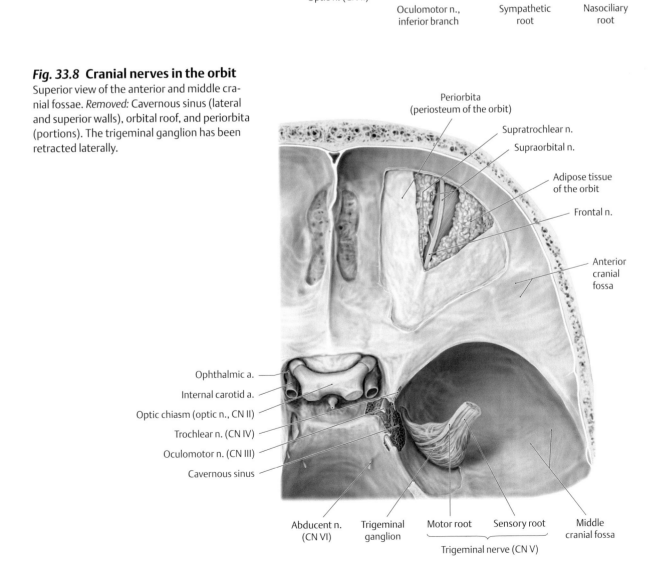

Trochlear n. (CN IV)

Ophthalmic division (CN V₁)

Trigeminal n. (CN V)

Trigeminal ganglion

Oculomotor n. (CN III)

Internal carotid a. with internal carotid plexus

Oculomotor n., superior branch

Frontal n.

Lacrimal n. (with gland)

Supraorbital n.

Infra-trochlear n.

Long ciliary nn.

Naso-ciliary n.

Short ciliary nn.

Ciliary ganglion

Parasym-pathetic root

Mandibular division (CN V₃)

Maxillary division (CN V₂)

Abducent n. (CN VI)

Optic n. (CN II)

Oculomotor n., inferior branch

Sympathetic root

Nasociliary root

Fig. 33.8 Cranial nerves in the orbit

Superior view of the anterior and middle cranial fossae. *Removed:* Cavernous sinus (lateral and superior walls), orbital roof, and periorbita (portions). The trigeminal ganglion has been retracted laterally.

Periorbita (periosteum of the orbit)

Supratrochlear n.

Supraorbital n.

Adipose tissue of the orbit

Frontal n.

Anterior cranial fossa

Ophthalmic a.

Internal carotid a.

Optic chiasm (optic n., CN II)

Trochlear n. (CN IV)

Oculomotor n. (CN III)

Cavernous sinus

Abducent n. (CN VI)

Trigeminal ganglion

Motor root   Sensory root

Middle cranial fossa

Trigeminal nerve (CN V)

Topography of the Orbit

Fig. 33.9 **Neurovascular structures of the orbit**

Anterior view. *Right side:* Orbicularis oculi removed. *Left side:* Orbital septum partially removed.

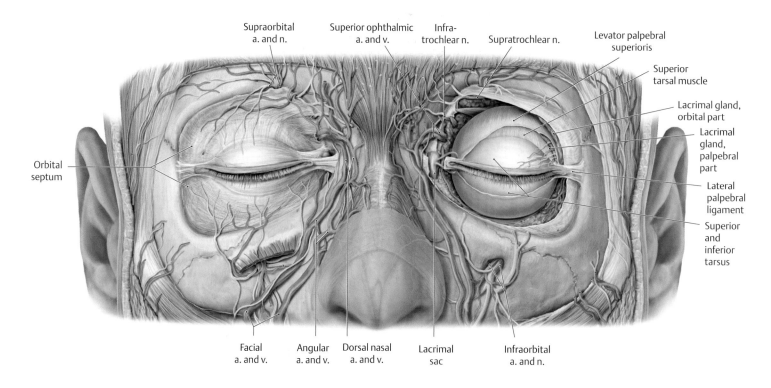

Labels (clockwise from top): Supraorbital a. and n. · Superior ophthalmic a. and v. · Infra-trochlear n. · Supratrochlear n. · Levator palpebral superioris · Superior tarsal muscle · Lacrimal gland, orbital part · Lacrimal gland, palpebral part · Lateral palpebral ligament · Superior and inferior tarsus · Infraorbital a. and n. · Lacrimal sac · Dorsal nasal a. and v. · Angular a. and v. · Facial a. and v. · Orbital septum

Fig. 33.10 **Passage of neurovascular structures through the orbit**

Anterior view. *Removed:* Orbital contents. *Note:* The optic nerve and ophthalmic artery travel in the optic canal. The remaining structures pass through the superior orbital fissure.

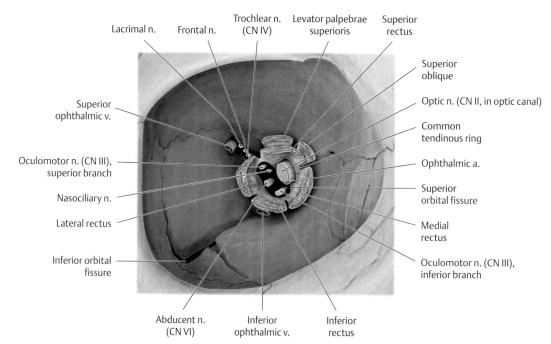

Labels: Lacrimal n. · Frontal n. · Trochlear n. (CN IV) · Levator palpebrae superioris · Superior rectus · Superior oblique · Optic n. (CN II, in optic canal) · Common tendinous ring · Ophthalmic a. · Superior orbital fissure · Medial rectus · Oculomotor n. (CN III), inferior branch · Inferior rectus · Inferior ophthalmic v. · Abducent n. (CN VI) · Inferior orbital fissure · Lateral rectus · Nasociliary n. · Oculomotor n. (CN III), superior branch · Superior ophthalmic v.

Fig. 33.11 **Neurovascular contents of the orbit**
Superior view. *Removed:* Bony roof of orbit, peritorbita, and
retro-orbital fat.

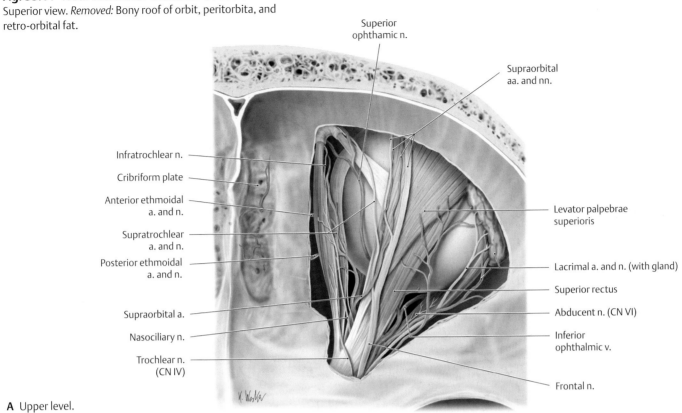

Superior
ophthamic n.

Supraorbital
aa. and nn.

Infratrochlear n.

Cribriform plate

Anterior ethmoidal
a. and n.

Supratrochlear
a. and n.

Posterior ethmoidal
a. and n.

Levator palpebrae
superioris

Lacrimal a. and n. (with gland)

Superior rectus

Supraorbital a.

Nasociliary n.

Trochlear n.
(CN IV)

Abducent n. (CN VI)

Inferior
ophthalmic v.

Frontal n.

A Upper level.

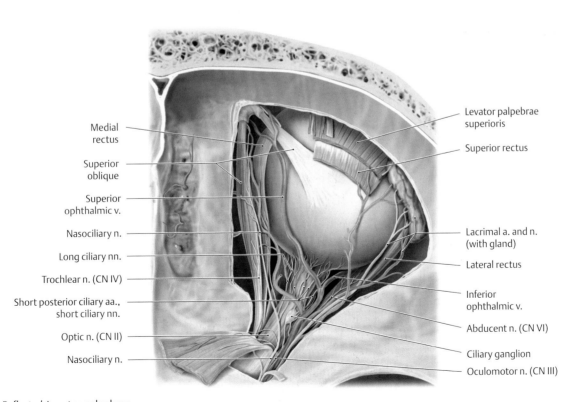

Levator palpebrae
superioris

Superior rectus

Medial
rectus

Superior
oblique

Superior
ophthalmic v.

Nasociliary n.

Long ciliary nn.

Trochlear n. (CN IV)

Short posterior ciliary aa.,
short ciliary nn.

Optic n. (CN II)

Nasociliary n.

Lacrimal a. and n.
(with gland)

Lateral rectus

Inferior
ophthalmic v.

Abducent n. (CN VI)

Ciliary ganglion

Oculomotor n. (CN III)

B Middle level. *Reflected:* Levator palpebrae
superioris and superior rectus. *Revealed:*
Optic nerve.

Fig. 33.12 **Topography of the orbit**
Sagittal section through the right orbit, medial view.

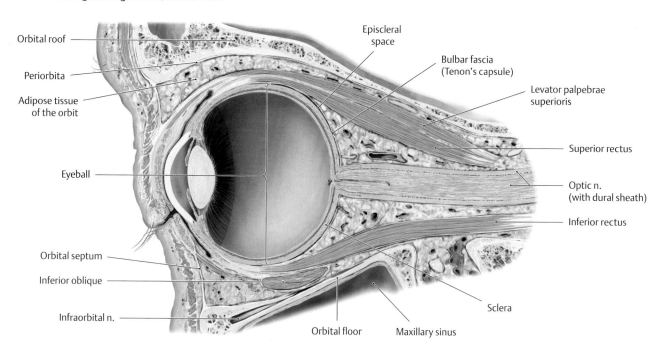

Orbital roof

Periorbita

Adipose tissue
of the orbit

Eyeball

Orbital septum

Inferior oblique

Infraorbital n.

Episcleral
space

Bulbar fascia
(Tenon's capsule)

Levator palpebrae
superioris

Superior rectus

Optic n.
(with dural sheath)

Inferior rectus

Sclera

Orbital floor

Maxillary sinus

Fig. 33.13 **Eyelids and conjuctiva**
Sagittal section through the anterior orbital cavity.

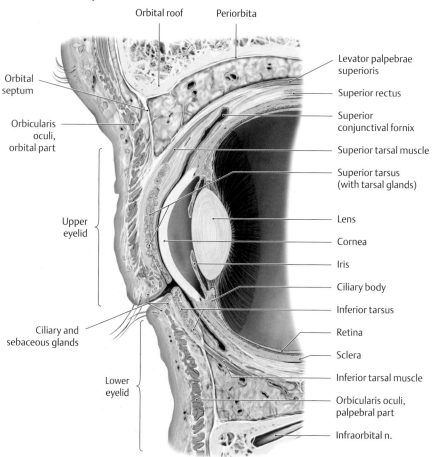

Orbital roof

Periorbita

Orbital
septum

Orbicularis
oculi,
orbital part

Upper
eyelid

Ciliary and
sebaceous glands

Lower
eyelid

Levator palpebrae
superioris

Superior rectus

Superior
conjunctival fornix

Superior tarsal muscle

Superior tarsus
(with tarsal glands)

Lens

Cornea

Iris

Ciliary body

Inferior tarsus

Retina

Sclera

Inferior tarsal muscle

Orbicularis oculi,
palpebral part

Infraorbital n.

Fig. 33.14 Lacrimal apparatus

Right eye, anterior view. *Removed:* Orbital septum (partial). *Divided:*
Levator palpebrae superioris (tendon of insertion).

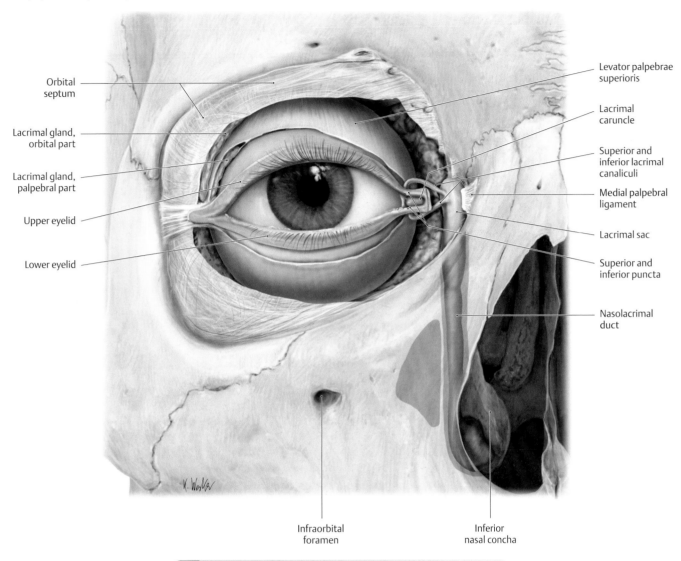

Labels (left): Orbital septum · Lacrimal gland, orbital part · Lacrimal gland, palpebral part · Upper eyelid · Lower eyelid

Labels (right): Levator palpebrae superioris · Lacrimal caruncle · Superior and inferior lacrimal canaliculi · Medial palpebral ligament · Lacrimal sac · Superior and inferior puncta · Nasolacrimal duct

Labels (bottom): Infraorbital foramen · Inferior nasal concha

---

Clinical

Lacrimal drainage

Perimenopausal women are frequently subject to chronically dry eyes
(*keratoconjunctivitis sicca*), due to insufficient tear production by the
lacrimal gland. Acute inflammation of the lacrimal gland (due to bacteria)
is less common and characterized by intense inflammation and extreme
tenderness to palpation. The upper eyelid shows a characteristic S-curve.

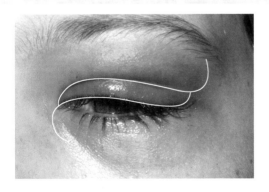

Eyeball

Fig. 33.15 **Structure of the eyeball**

Transverse section through right eyeball, superior view. *Note:* The orbital axis (running along the optic nerve through the optic disk) deviates from the optical axis (running down the center of the eye to the fovea centralis) by 23 degrees.

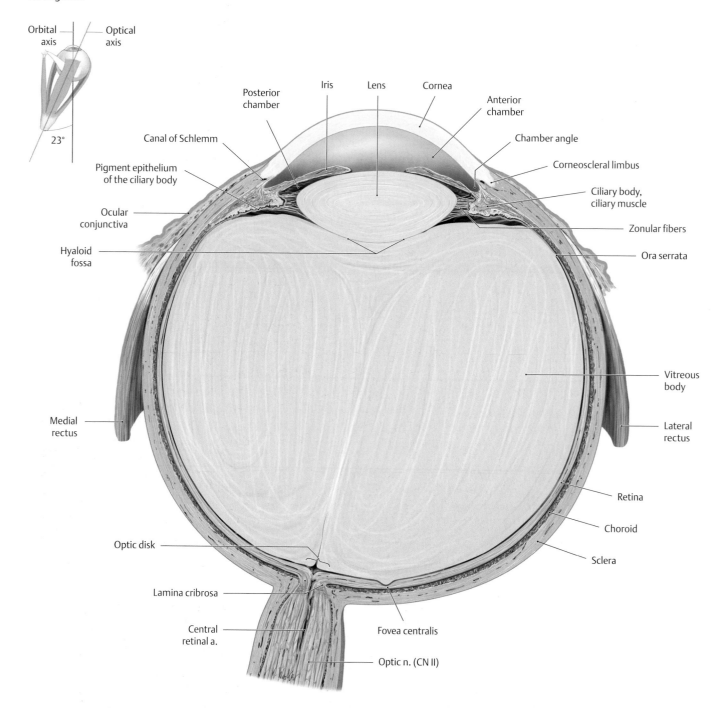

Orbital axis — Optical axis

23°

Iris   Lens   Cornea

Posterior chamber

Anterior chamber

Canal of Schlemm

Chamber angle

Corneoscleral limbus

Pigment epithelium of the ciliary body

Ciliary body, ciliary muscle

Ocular conjunctiva

Zonular fibers

Hyaloid fossa

Ora serrata

Vitreous body

Medial rectus

Lateral rectus

Retina

Choroid

Optic disk

Sclera

Lamina cribrosa

Central retinal a.

Fovea centralis

Optic n. (CN II)

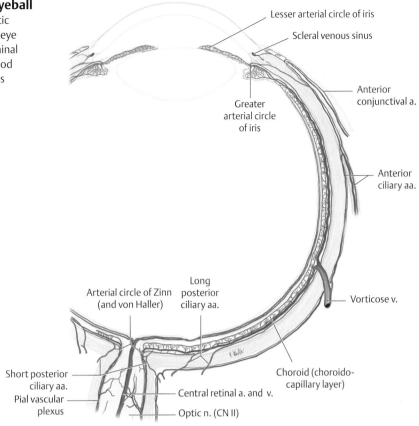

Fig. 33.16 Blood vessels of the eyeball

Transverse section at the level of the optic nerve, superior view. The arteries of the eye arise from the ophthalmic artery, a terminal branch of the internal carotid artery. Blood is drained by four to eight vorticose veins that open into the superior and inferior ophthalmic veins.

Lesser arterial circle of iris

Scleral venous sinus

Anterior conjunctival a.

Greater arterial circle of iris

Anterior ciliary aa.

Arterial circle of Zinn (and von Haller)

Long posterior ciliary aa.

Vorticose v.

Short posterior ciliary aa.

Pial vascular plexus

Central retinal a. and v.

Optic n. (CN II)

Choroid (choroido-capillary layer)

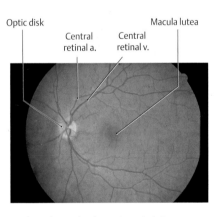

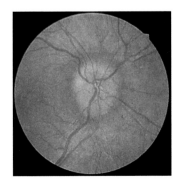

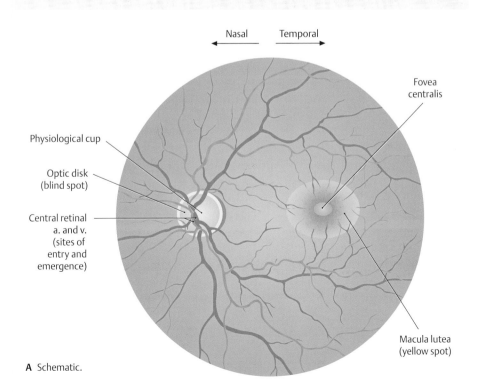

Clinical

Optic fundus

The optic fundus is the only place in the body where capillaries can be examined directly. Examination of the optic fundus permits observation of vascular changes that may be caused by high blood pressure or diabetes. Examination of the optic disk is important in determining intracranial pressure and diagnosing multiple sclerosis.

Nasal   Temporal

Optic disk

Central retinal a.

Central retinal v.

Macula lutea

B Normal optic fundus in the ophthalmoscopic examination.

Fovea centralis

Physiological cup

Optic disk (blind spot)

Central retinal a. and v. (sites of entry and emergence)

Macula lutea (yellow spot)

A Schematic.

C High intracranial pressure; the edges of the optic disk appear less sharp.

Cornea, Iris & Lens

Fig. 33.17 **Cornea, iris, and lens**
Transverse section through the anterior segment of the eye. Anterosuperior view.

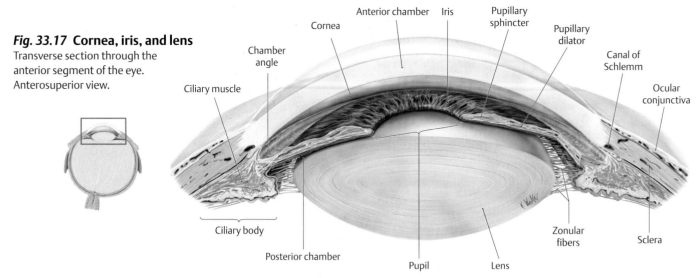

Fig. 33.18 **Iris**
Transverse section through the anterior segment of the eye. Anterosuperior view.

✳ *Clinical*

Glaucoma

Aqueous humor produced in the posterior chamber passes through the pupil into the anterior chamber. It seeps through the spaces of the trabecular meshwork into the canal of Schlemm and enters the venous sinus of the sclera before passing into the episcleral veins. Obstruction of aqueous humor drainage causes an increase in intraocular pressure (glaucoma), which constricts the optic nerve in the lamina cribrosa. This constriction eventually leads to blindness. The most common glaucoma (approximately 90% of cases) is chronic (open-angle) glaucoma. The more rare acute glaucoma is characterized by red eye, strong headache and/or eye pain, nausea, dilated episcleral veins, and edema of the cornea.

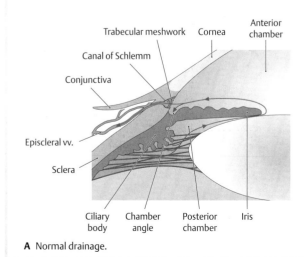

A Normal drainage.

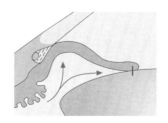

B Chronic (open-angle) glaucoma. Drainage through the trabecular meshwork is impaired.

C Acute (angle-closure) glaucoma. The chamber angle is obstructed by iris tissue. Aqueous fluid cannot drain into the anterior chamber, which pushes portions of the iris upward, blocking the chamber angle.

Fig. 33.19 Pupil

Pupil size is regulated by two intraocular muscles of the iris: the pupillary sphincter, which narrows the pupil (parasympathetic innervation), and the pupillary dilator, which enlarges it (sympathetic innervation).

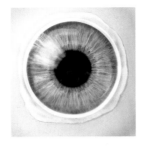 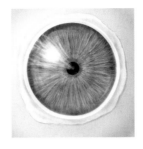 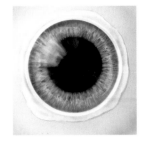

A Normal pupil size.

B Maximum constriction (miosis).

C Maximum dilation (mydriasis).

Fig. 33.20 Lens and ciliary body

Posterior view. The curvature of the lens is regulated by the muscle fibers of the annular ciliary body.

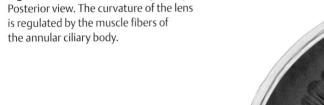

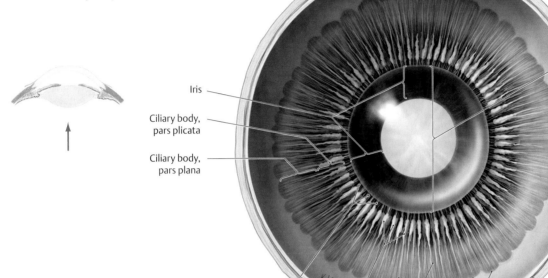

Fig. 33.21 Light refraction by the lens

Transverse section, superior view. In the normal (emmetropic) eye, light rays are refracted by the lens (and cornea) to a focal point on the retinal surface (fovea centralis). Tensing of the zonular fibers, with ciliary muscle relaxation, flattens the lens in response to parallel rays arriving from a distant source (far vision). Contraction of the ciliary muscle, with zonular fiber relaxation, causes the lens to assume a more rounded shape (near vision).

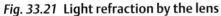

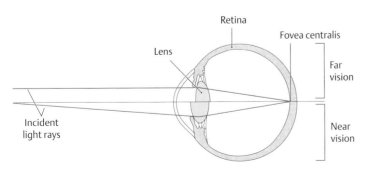

A Normal dynamics of the lens.

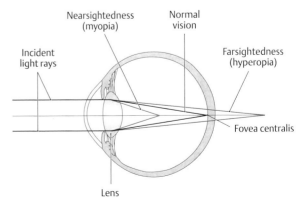

B Abnormal lens dynamics.

Bones of the Nasal Cavity

Fig. 34.1 **Skeleton of the nose**

The skeleton of the nose is composed of an upper bony portion and a lower cartilaginous portion. The proximal portions of the nostrils (alae) are composed of connective tissue with small embedded pieces of cartilage.

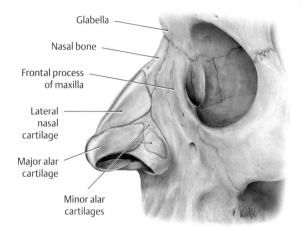

A Left lateral view.

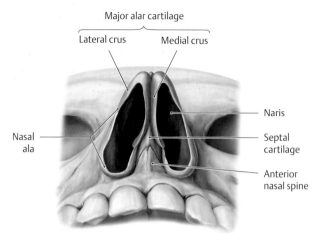

B Inferior view.

Fig. 34.2 **Bones of the nasal cavity**

The left and right nasal cavities are flanked by lateral walls and separated by the nasal septum. Air enters the nasal cavity through the anterior nasal aperture and travels through three passages: the superior, middle, and inferior meatuses (arrows). These passages are separated by the superior, middle, and inferior conchae. Air leaves the nose through the choanae, entering the nasopharynx.

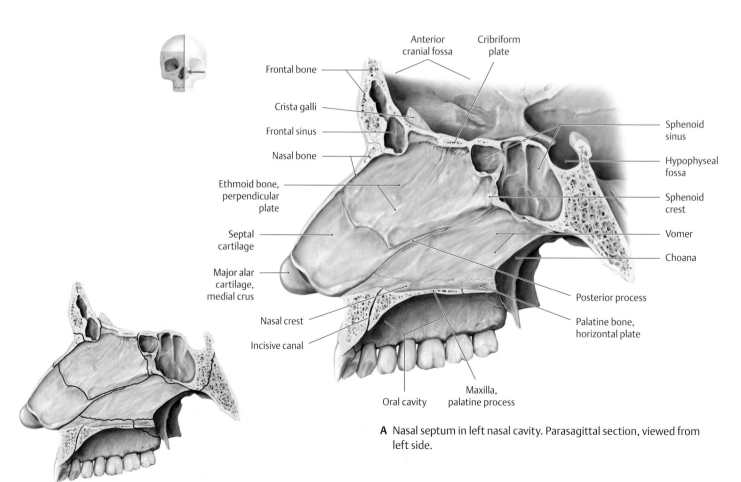

A Nasal septum in left nasal cavity. Parasagittal section, viewed from left side.

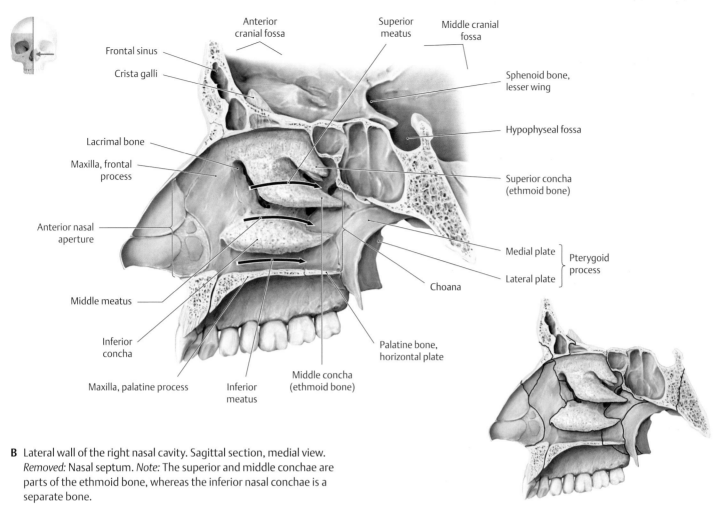

B Lateral wall of the right nasal cavity. Sagittal section, medial view. *Removed:* Nasal septum. *Note:* The superior and middle conchae are parts of the ethmoid bone, whereas the inferior nasal conchae is a separate bone.

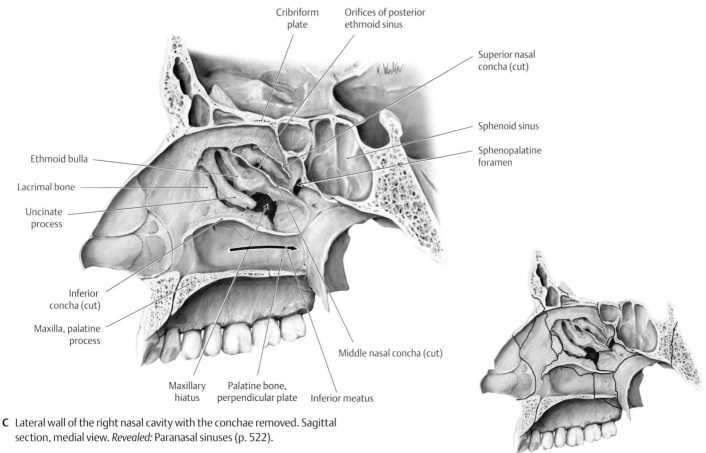

C Lateral wall of the right nasal cavity with the conchae removed. Sagittal section, medial view. *Revealed:* Paranasal sinuses (p. 522).

Paranasal Air Sinuses

Fig. 34.3 Location of the paranasal sinuses

The paranasal sinuses (frontal, ethmoid, maxillary, and sphenoid) are air-filled cavities that reduce the weight of the skull.

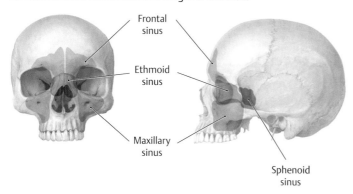

A Anterior view.   **B** Left lateral view.

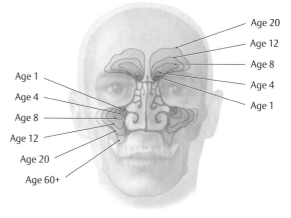

C Pneumatization of the sinuses. The frontal and maxillary sinuses develop gradually over the course of cranial growth.

Table 34.1	Opening of nasal structures into the nose	
Nasal passage	**Sinuses/duct**	
Sphenoethmoid recess	Sphenoid sinus (blue)	
Superior meatus	Posterior ethmoid sinus (green)	
Middle meatus	Anterior and middle ethmoid sinus (green)	
	Frontal sinus (yellow)	
	Maxillary sinus (orange)	
Inferior meatus	Nasolacrimal duct (red)	

Fig. 34.4 Paranasal sinuses

Mucosal secretions from the sinuses and nasolacrimal duct open into the nose.

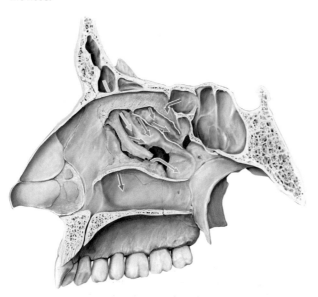

A Openings of the paranasal sinuses and nasolacrimal duct. Sagittal section, medial view of the right nasal cavity.

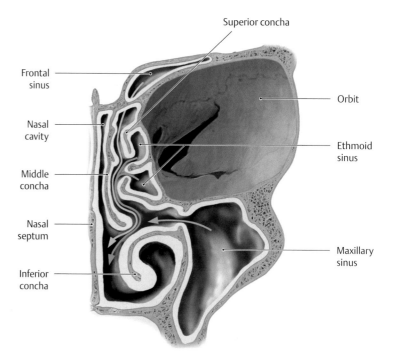

B Paranasal sinuses and osteomeatal unit in the left nasal cavity. Coronal section, anterior view.

Fig. 34.5 **Bony structure of the paranasal sinuses**
Coronal section, anterior view.

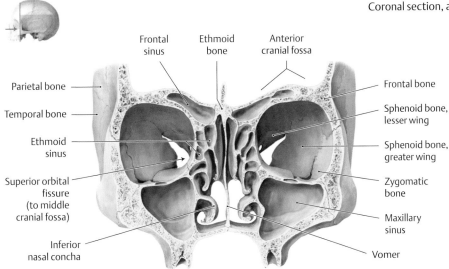

Frontal sinus — **Ethmoid bone** — **Anterior cranial fossa**

Parietal bone

Temporal bone

Ethmoid sinus

Superior orbital fissure (to middle cranial fossa)

Inferior nasal concha

Frontal bone

Sphenoid bone, lesser wing

Sphenoid bone, greater wing

Zygomatic bone

Maxillary sinus

Vomer

A Bones of the paranasal sinuses.

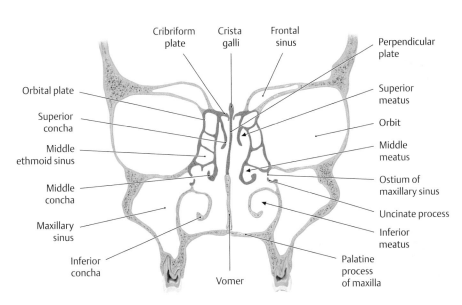

Cribriform plate — Crista galli — Frontal sinus — Perpendicular plate

Orbital plate

Superior concha

Middle ethmoid sinus

Middle concha

Maxillary sinus

Inferior concha

Superior meatus

Orbit

Middle meatus

Ostium of maxillary sinus

Uncinate process

Inferior meatus

Palatine process of maxilla

Vomer

B Ethmoid bone (red) in the paranasal sinuses.

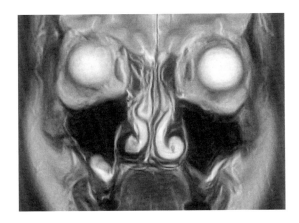

C MRI through the paranasal sinuses.

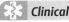

Clinical

Deviated septum

The normal position of the nasal septum creates two roughly symmetrical nasal cavities. Extreme lateral deviation of the septum may result in obstruction of the nasal passages. This may be corrected by removing portions of the cartilage (septoplasty).

Sinusitis

When the mucosa in the ethmoid sinuses becomes swollen due to inflammation (*sinusitis*), it blocks the flow of secretions from the frontal and maxillary sinuses in the osteomeatal unit (see Fig. 34.4). This may cause microorganisms to become trapped, causing secondary inflammations. In patients with chronic sinusitis, the narrow sites can be surgically widened to establish more effective drainage routes.

Neurovasculature of the Nasal Cavity

Fig. 34.6 **Nasal septum**

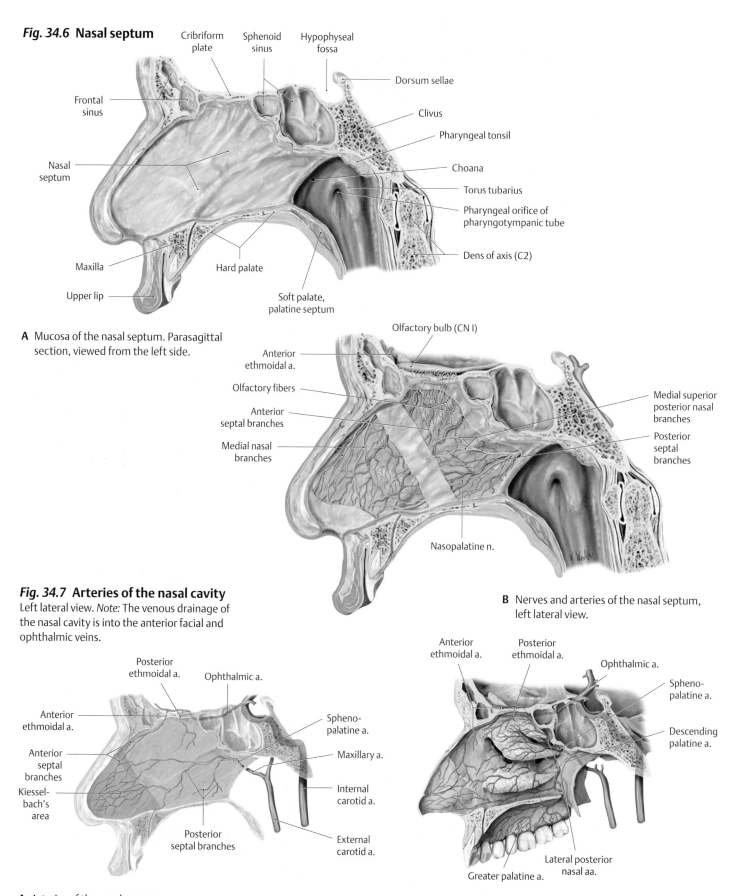

A Mucosa of the nasal septum. Parasagittal section, viewed from the left side.

B Nerves and arteries of the nasal septum, left lateral view.

Fig. 34.7 **Arteries of the nasal cavity**

Left lateral view. *Note:* The venous drainage of the nasal cavity is into the anterior facial and ophthalmic veins.

A Arteries of the nasal septum.

B Arteries of the right lateral nasal wall.

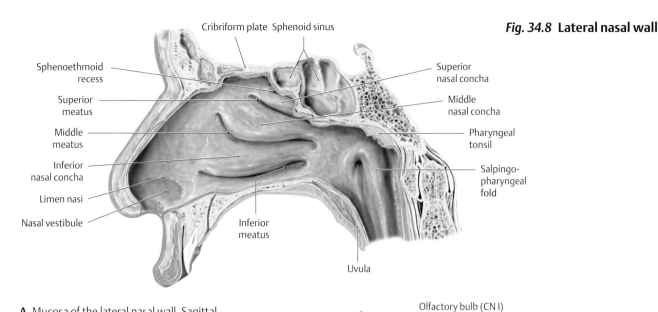

Fig. 34.8 **Lateral nasal wall**

Cribriform plate Sphenoid sinus

Sphenoethmoid recess

Superior meatus

Middle meatus

Inferior nasal concha

Limen nasi

Nasal vestibule

Superior nasal concha

Middle nasal concha

Pharyngeal tonsil

Salpingo-pharyngeal fold

Inferior meatus

Uvula

A Mucosa of the lateral nasal wall. Sagittal section, viewed from the left side.

Olfactory bulb (CN I)

Olfactory fibers, posterior ethmoidal a.

Anterior ethmoidal a.

Inferior posterior nasal branches, lateral posterior nasal aa.

Pterygopalatine ganglion

Descending palatine a., greater and lesser palatine nn.

Greater palatine a. and n.

B Nerves and arteries of the lateral nasal wall, left lateral view.

Clinical

Nosebleeds

Vascular supply to the nasal cavity arises from both the internal and external carotid arteries. The anterior part of the nasal septum contains a very vascularized region referred to as Kiesselbach's area. This area is the most common site of significant nosebleeds.

Fig. 34.9 **Nerves of the nasal cavity**

Left lateral view.

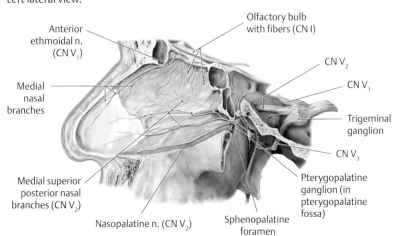

Anterior ethmoidal n. (CN V₁)

Olfactory bulb with fibers (CN I)

CN V₂

CN V₁

Trigeminal ganglion

CN V₃

Medial nasal branches

Medial superior posterior nasal branches (CN V₂)

Nasopalatine n. (CN V₂)

Sphenopalatine foramen

Pterygopalatine ganglion (in pterygopalatine fossa)

A Nerves of the nasal septum.

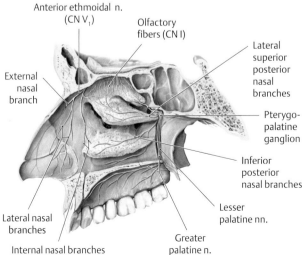

Anterior ethmoidal n. (CN V₁)

Olfactory fibers (CN I)

External nasal branch

Lateral superior posterior nasal branches

Pterygo-palatine ganglion

Inferior posterior nasal branches

Lesser palatine nn.

Greater palatine n.

Lateral nasal branches

Internal nasal branches

B Nerves of the lateral nasal wall.

Temporal Bone

Fig. 35.1 **Temporal bone**
Left bone. The temporal bone consists of three major parts: squamous, petrous, and tympanic (see Fig. 35.2).

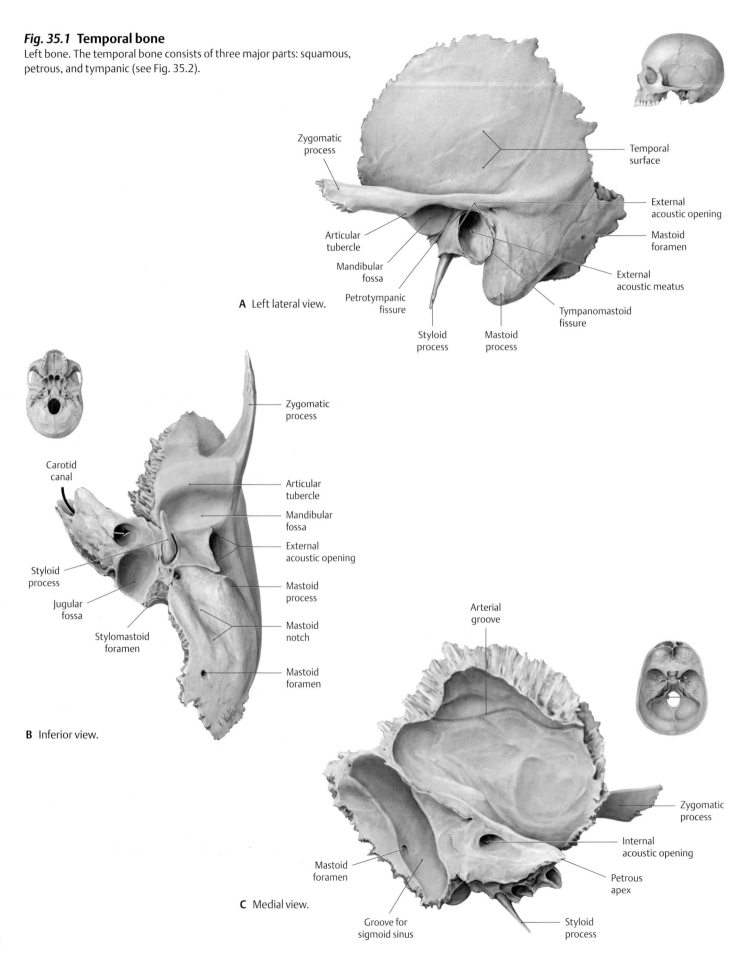

A Left lateral view.

Zygomatic process

Temporal surface

External acoustic opening

Mastoid foramen

External acoustic meatus

Tympanomastoid fissure

Articular tubercle

Mandibular fossa

Petrotympanic fissure

Styloid process

Mastoid process

B Inferior view.

Carotid canal

Zygomatic process

Articular tubercle

Mandibular fossa

External acoustic opening

Mastoid process

Mastoid notch

Mastoid foramen

Styloid process

Jugular fossa

Stylomastoid foramen

C Medial view.

Arterial groove

Zygomatic process

Internal acoustic opening

Petrous apex

Mastoid foramen

Groove for sigmoid sinus

Styloid process

Fig. 35.2 Parts of the temporal bone

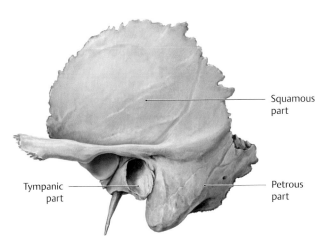

Squamous part

Tympanic part

Petrous part

A Left lateral view.

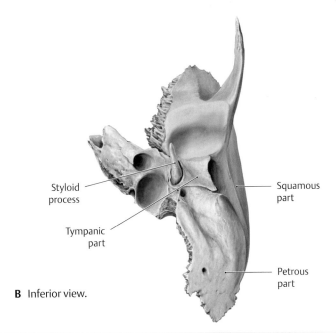

Styloid process

Squamous part

Tympanic part

Petrous part

B Inferior view.

⚕ Clinical

Structures in the temporal bone

The mastoid process contains mastoid air cells that communicate with the middle ear; the middle ear in turn communicates with the nasopharynx via the pharyngotympanic (auditory) tube. Bacteria may use this pathway to move from the nasopharynx into the middle ear. In severe cases, bacteria may pass from the mastoid air cells into the cranial cavity, causing meningitis.

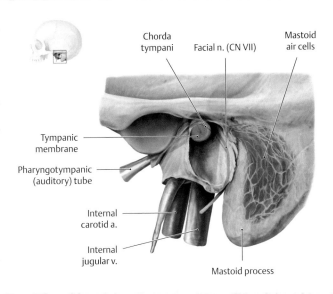

Chorda tympani

Facial n. (CN VII)

Mastoid air cells

Tympanic membrane

Pharyngotympanic (auditory) tube

Internal carotid a.

Internal jugular v.

Mastoid process

Irrigation of the auditory canal with warm (44°C) or cool (30°C) water can induce a thermal current in the endolymph of the semicircular canal, causing the patient to manifest vestibular nystagmus (jerky eye movements, vestibulo-ocular reflex). This caloric testing is important in the diagnosis of unexplained vertigo. The patient must be oriented so that the semicircular canal of interest lies in the vertical plane.

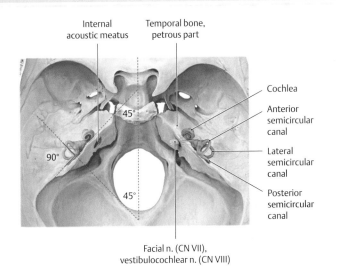

Internal acoustic meatus

Temporal bone, petrous part

Cochlea

Anterior semicircular canal

Lateral semicircular canal

Posterior semicircular canal

45°

90°

45°

Facial n. (CN VII), vestibulocochlear n. (CN VIII)

The petrous portion of the temporal bone contains the middle and inner ear as well as the tympanic membrane. The bony semicircular canals are oriented at an approximately 45-degree angle from the coronal, transverse, and sagittal planes.

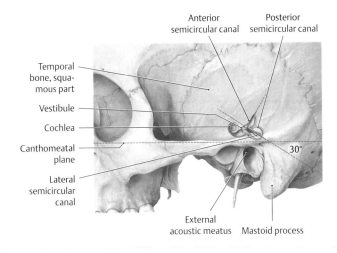

Anterior semicircular canal

Posterior semicircular canal

Temporal bone, squamous part

Vestibule

Cochlea

Canthomeatal plane

Lateral semicircular canal

30°

External acoustic meatus

Mastoid process

External Ear & Auditory Canal

The auditory apparatus is divided into three main parts: external, middle, and inner ear. The external and middle ear are part of the sound conduction apparatus, and the inner ear is the actual organ of hearing (see p. 619). The inner ear also contains the vestibular apparatus, the organ of balance (see p. 618).

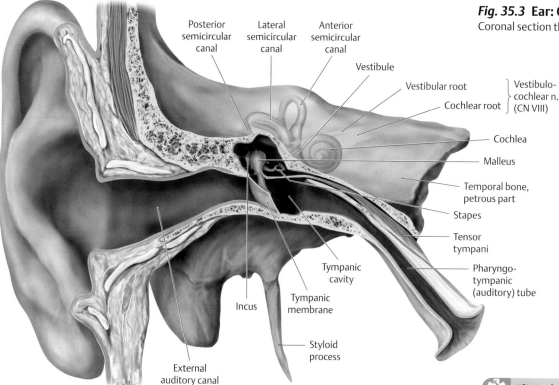

Fig. 35.3 **Ear: Overview**
Coronal section through right ear, anterior view.

Posterior semicircular canal · Lateral semicircular canal · Anterior semicircular canal · Vestibule · Vestibular root · Cochlear root · Vestibulo-cochlear n. (CN VIII) · Cochlea · Malleus · Temporal bone, petrous part · Stapes · Tensor tympani · Pharyngo-tympanic (auditory) tube · Tympanic cavity · Tympanic membrane · Incus · Styloid process · External auditory canal

Fig. 35.4 **External auditory canal**
Coronal section through right ear, anterior view. The tympanic membrane separates the external auditory canal from the tympanic cavity (middle ear). The outer third of the auditory canal is cartilaginous, and the inner two thirds are osseous (tympanic part of temporal bone).

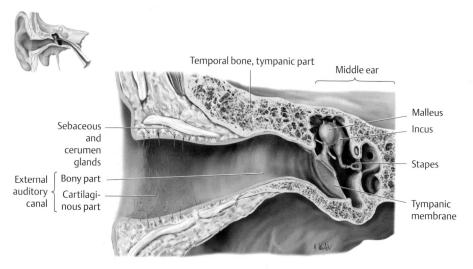

Temporal bone, tympanic part · Middle ear · Malleus · Incus · Stapes · Tympanic membrane · Sebaceous and cerumen glands · External auditory canal { Bony part · Cartilaginous part }

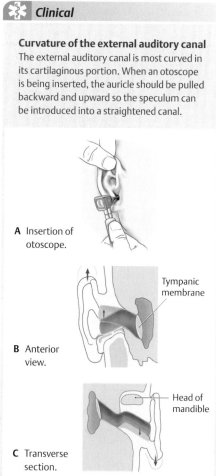

Clinical

Curvature of the external auditory canal
The external auditory canal is most curved in its cartilaginous portion. When an otoscope is being inserted, the auricle should be pulled backward and upward so the speculum can be introduced into a straightened canal.

A Insertion of otoscope.

B Anterior view. — Tympanic membrane

C Transverse section. — Head of mandible

Fig. 35.5 Structure of the auricle

The auricle of the ear encloses a cartilaginous framework that forms a funnel-shaped receptor for acoustic vibrations. The muscles of the auricle are considered muscles of facial expression, although they are vestigial in humans.

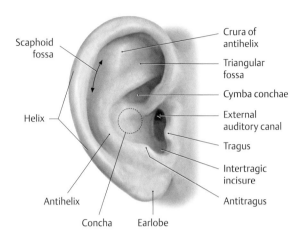

A Right auricle, right lateral view.

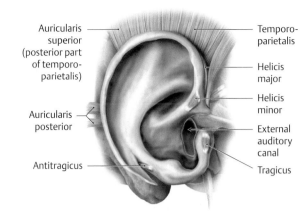

B Cartilage and muscles of the auricle, right lateral view.

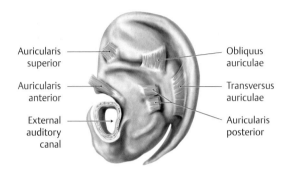

C Cartilage and muscles of the auricle, medial view of posterior surface.

Fig. 35.6 Arteries of the auricle

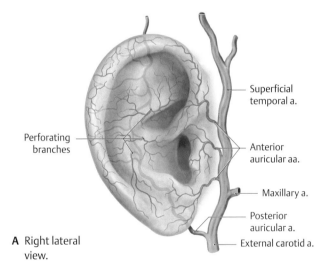

A Right lateral view.

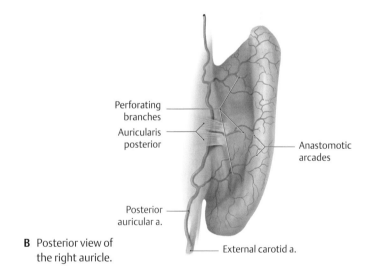

B Posterior view of the right auricle.

Fig. 35.7 Innervation of the auricle

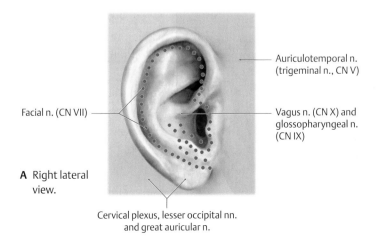

A Right lateral view.

Cervical plexus, lesser occipital nn. and great auricular n.

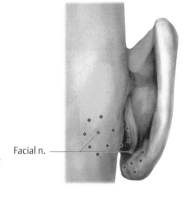

B Posterior view of the right auricle.

Facial n.

529

Middle Ear: Tympanic Cavity

Fig. 35.8 Middle ear

Right petrous bone, superior view. The tympanic cavity of the middle ear communicates anteriorly with the pharynx via the pharyngotympanic (auditory) tube and posteriorly with the mastoid air cells.

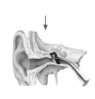

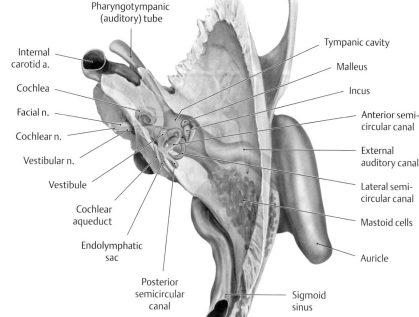

Fig. 35.9 Tympanic cavity and pharyngotympanic tube

Medial view of opened tympanic cavity.

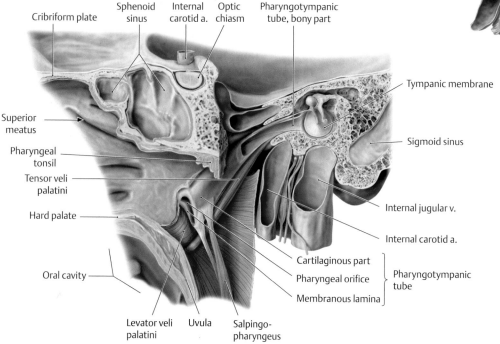

Table 35.1	Boundaries of the tympanic cavity

During chronic suppurative otitis media (inflammation of the middle ear), pathogenic bacteria may spread to adjacent regions.

Direction	Wall	Anatomical boundary	Neighboring structures	Infection
Anterior	Carotid	Opening to pharyngotympanic tube	Carotid canal	
Lateral	Membranous	Tympanic membrane	External ear	
Superior	Tegmental	Tegmen tympani	Middle cranial fossa	Meningitis, cerebral abscess (especially of temporal lobe)
Medial	Labyrinthine	Promontory overlying basal turn of cochlea	Inner ear	
			CSF space (via petrous apex)	Abducent paralysis, trigeminal nerve irritation, visual disturbances (Gradenigo's syndrome)
Inferior	Jugular	Temporal bone, tympanic part	Bulb of jugular vein	
			Sigmoid sinus	Sinus thrombosis
Posterior	Mastoid	Aditus to mastoid antrum	Air cells of mastoid process	Mastoiditis
			Facial nerve canal	Facial paralysis

CSF = cerebrospinal fluid.

Fig. 35.10 Tympanic cavity

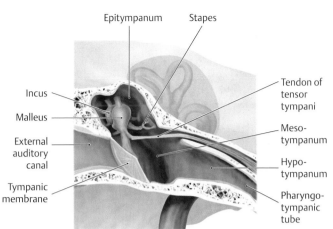

Epitympanum
Stapes
Incus
Malleus
External auditory canal
Tympanic membrane
Tendon of tensor tympani
Meso-tympanum
Hypo-tympanum
Pharyngo-tympanic tube

A Levels of the tympanic cavity. Anterior view. The tympanic cavity is divided into three levels: epi-, meso-, and hypotympanum.

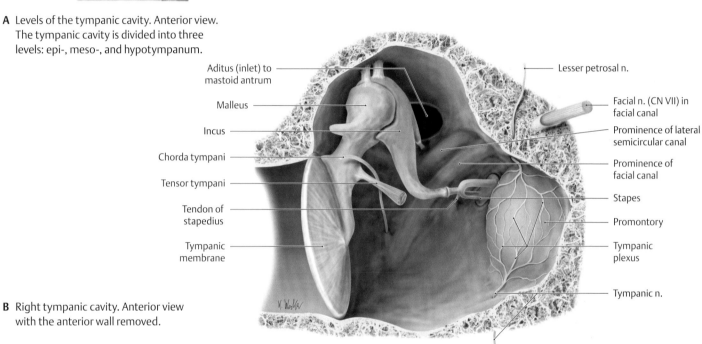

Aditus (inlet) to mastoid antrum
Malleus
Incus
Chorda tympani
Tensor tympani
Tendon of stapedius
Tympanic membrane
Lesser petrosal n.
Facial n. (CN VII) in facial canal
Prominence of lateral semicircular canal
Prominence of facial canal
Stapes
Promontory
Tympanic plexus
Tympanic n.

B Right tympanic cavity. Anterior view with the anterior wall removed.

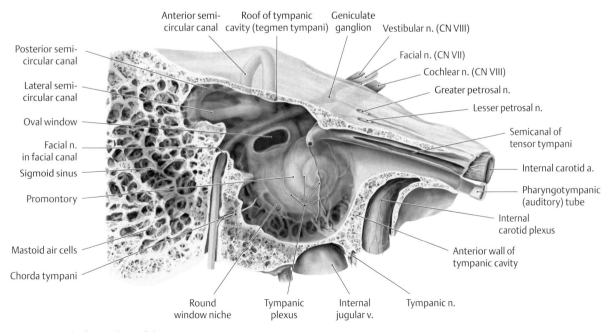

Anterior semi-circular canal
Roof of tympanic cavity (tegmen tympani)
Geniculate ganglion
Vestibular n. (CN VIII)
Facial n. (CN VII)
Cochlear n. (CN VIII)
Greater petrosal n.
Lesser petrosal n.
Semicanal of tensor tympani
Internal carotid a.
Pharyngotympanic (auditory) tube
Internal carotid plexus
Anterior wall of tympanic cavity
Tympanic n.
Posterior semi-circular canal
Lateral semi-circular canal
Oval window
Facial n. in facial canal
Sigmoid sinus
Promontory
Mastoid air cells
Chorda tympani
Round window niche
Tympanic plexus
Internal jugular v.

C Anatomical relationships of the tympanic cavity. Oblique sagittal section showing the medial wall.

531

Middle Ear: Ossicular Chain & Tympanic Membrane

Fig. 35.11 **Auditory ossicles**

Left ear. The ossicular chain consists of three small bones that establish an articular connection between the tympanic membrane and the oval window.

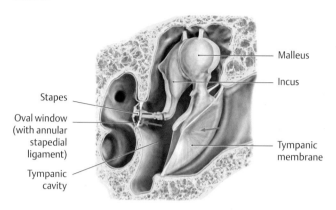

A Auditory ossicles in the middle ear. Anterior view of the left ear.

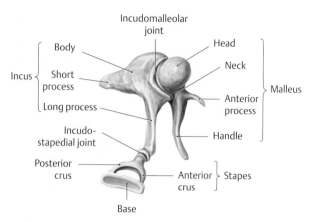

B Bones of the ossicular chain. Medial view of the left ossicular chain.

Fig. 35.12 **Malleus ("hammer")**

Left ear.

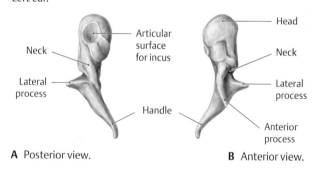

A Posterior view. **B** Anterior view.

Fig. 35.13 **Incus ("anvil")**

Left ear.

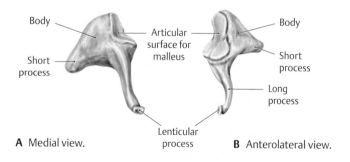

A Medial view. **B** Anterolateral view.

Fig. 35.14 **Stapes ("stirrup")**

Left ear.

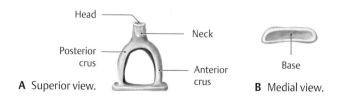

A Superior view. **B** Medial view.

Fig. 35.15 **Tympanic membrane**

Right tympanic membrane. The tympanic membrane is divided into four quadrants: anterosuperior (I), anteroinferior (II), posteroinferior (III), and posterosuperior (IV).

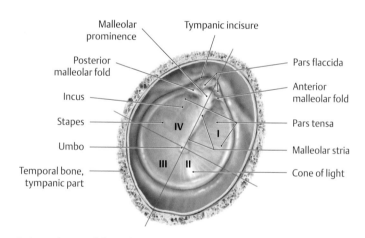

A Lateral view of the right tympanic membrane.

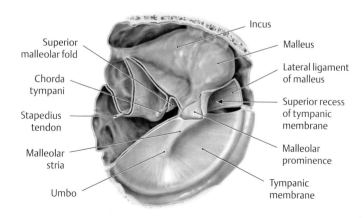

B Mucosal lining of the tympanic cavity. Posterolateral view with the tympanic membrane partially removed.

Fig. 35.16 Ossicular chain in the tympanic cavity

Lateral view of the right ear. *Revealed:* Ligaments of the ossicular chain and muscles of the middle ear (stapedius and tensor tympani).

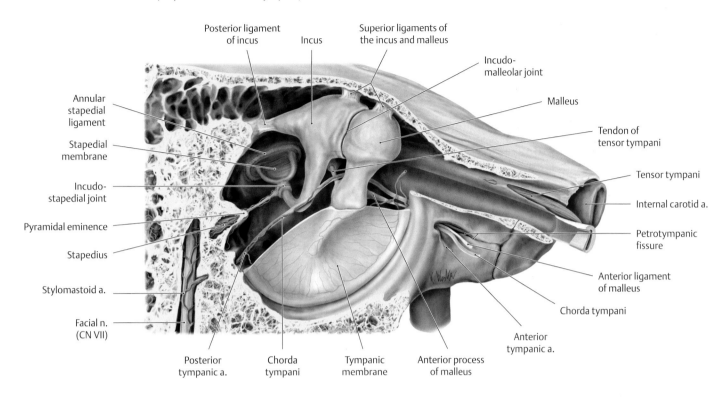

 Clinical

Ossicular chain in hearing

Sound waves funneled into the external auditory canal set the tympanic membrane into vibration. The ossicular chain transmits the vibrations to the oval window, which communicates them to the fluid column of the inner ear. Sound waves in fluid meet with higher impedance; they must therefore be amplified in the middle ear. The difference in surface area between the tympanic membrane and the oval window increases the sound pressure 17-fold. A total amplification factor of 22 is achieved through the lever action of the ossicular chain. If the ossicular chain fails to transform the sound pressure between the tympanic membrane and the footplate of the stapes, the patient will experience conductive hearing loss of magnitude 20 dB. See p. 619 for hearing.

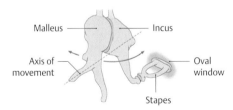

A Vibration of the tympanic membrane causes a rocking movement in the ossicular chain. The mechanical advantage of the lever action of the ossicular chain amplifies the sound waves by a factor of 1.3.

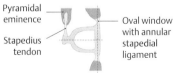

B The stapes in its normal position lies in the plane of the oval window.

C Rocking of the ossicular chain causes the stapes to tilt. The movement of the stapes base against the membrane of the oval window (stapedial membrane) induces corresponding waves in the fluid column of the inner ear.

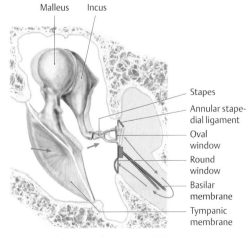

D Propagation of sound waves by the ossicular chain.

Arteries of the Middle Ear

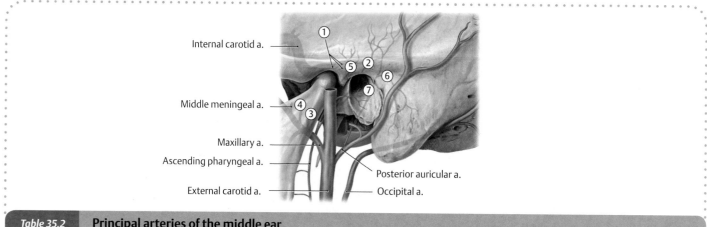

Internal carotid a.

Middle meningeal a.

Maxillary a.

Ascending pharyngeal a.

External carotid a.

Posterior auricular a.

Occipital a.

Table 35.2	Principal arteries of the middle ear		
Origin	**Artery**		**Distribution**
Internal carotid a.	① Caroticotympanic aa.		Tympanic cavity (anterior wall), pharyngotympanic (auditory) tube
External carotid a.	Ascending pharyngeal a. (medial branch)	② Inferior tympanic a.	Tympanic cavity (floor), promontory
	Maxillary a. (terminal branch)	③ Deep auricular a.	Tympanic cavity (floor), tympanic membrane
		④ Anterior tympanic a.	Tympanic membrane, mastoid antrum, malleus, incus
	Middle meningeal a.	⑤ Superior tympanic a.	Tympanic cavity (roof), tensor tympani, stapes
	Posterior auricular a. (posterior branch) Stylomastoid a.	⑥ Stylomastoid a.	Tympanic cavity (posterior wall), mastoid air cells, stapedius muscle, stapes
		⑦ Posterior tympanic a.	Chorda tympani, tympanic membrane, malleus

Fig. 35.17 Arteries of the middle ear: Ossicular chain and tympanic membrane

Medial view of the right tympanic membrane. With inflammation, the arteries of the tympanic membrane may become so dilated that their course can be observed (as shown here).

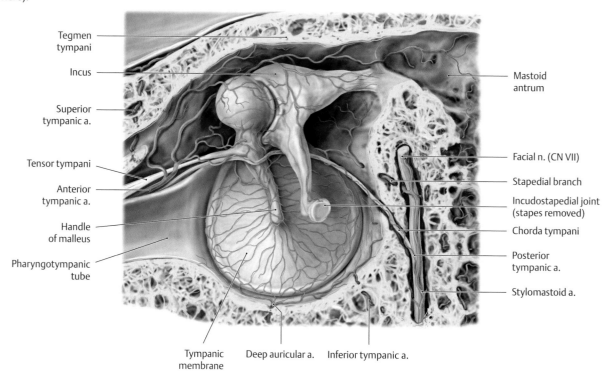

Tegmen tympani

Incus

Superior tympanic a.

Tensor tympani

Anterior tympanic a.

Handle of malleus

Pharyngotympanic tube

Mastoid antrum

Facial n. (CN VII)

Stapedial branch

Incudostapedial joint (stapes removed)

Chorda tympani

Posterior tympanic a.

Stylomastoid a.

Tympanic membrane

Deep auricular a.

Inferior tympanic a.

Fig. 35.18 Arteries of the middle ear: Tympanic cavity

Right petrous bone, anterior view. *Removed:* Malleus, incus, portions of chorda tympani, and anterior tympanic artery.

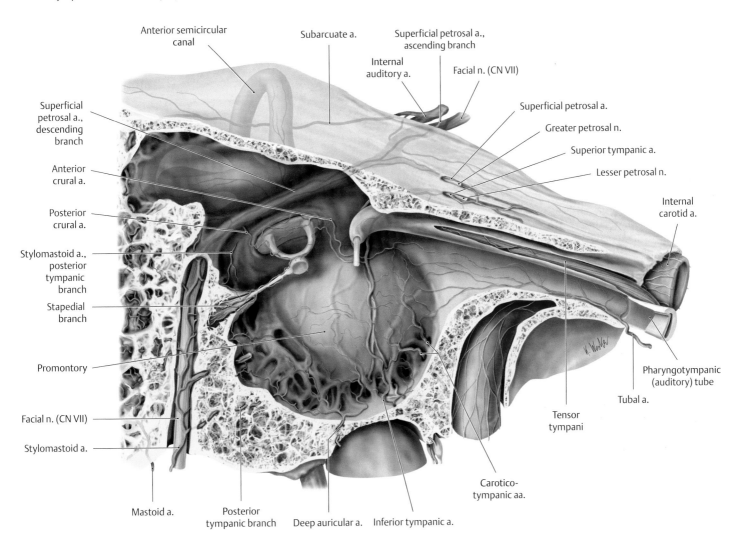

Labels (clockwise from top):
Anterior semicircular canal — Subarcuate a. — Superficial petrosal a., ascending branch — Internal auditory a. — Facial n. (CN VII) — Superficial petrosal a. — Greater petrosal n. — Superior tympanic a. — Lesser petrosal n. — Internal carotid a. — Pharyngotympanic (auditory) tube — Tubal a. — Tensor tympani — Carotico-tympanic aa. — Inferior tympanic a. — Deep auricular a. — Posterior tympanic branch — Mastoid a. — Stylomastoid a. — Facial n. (CN VII) — Promontory — Stapedial branch — Stylomastoid a., posterior tympanic branch — Posterior crural a. — Anterior crural a. — Superficial petrosal a., descending branch

Inner Ear

The inner ear consists of the vestibular apparatus (for balance) and the auditory apparatus (for hearing). Both are formed by a membranous labyrinth filled with endolymph floating within a bony labyrinth filled with perilymph and embedded in the petrous part of the temporal bone.

Fig. 35.19 Vestibular apparatus

Right lateral view.

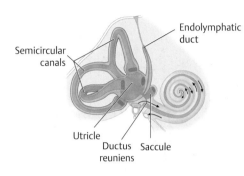

A Schematic. Ampullary crests and maculae of utricle and saccule shown in red.

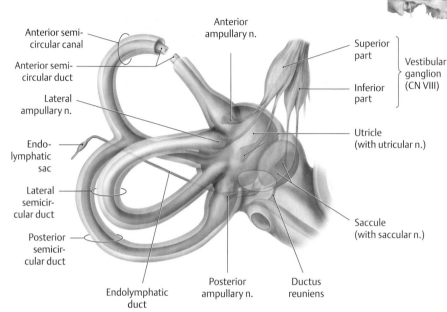

B Structure of the vestibular apparatus.

Fig. 35.20 Auditory apparatus

The cochlear labyrinth and its bony shell form the cochlea, which contains the sensory epithelium of the auditory apparatus (organ of Corti).

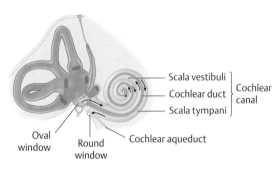

A Schematic.

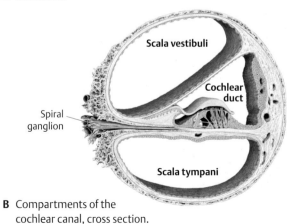

B Compartments of the cochlear canal, cross section.

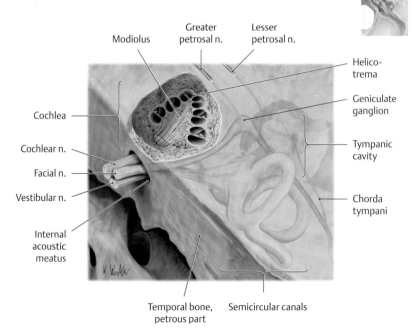

C Location of the cochlea. Superior view of the petrous part of the temporal bone with the cochlea sectioned transversely. The bony canal of the cochlea (spiral canal) makes 2.5 turns around its bony axis (modiolus).

Fig. 35.21 Innervation of the membranous labyrinth

Right ear, anterior view. The vestibulocochlear nerve (CN VIII; see p. 480) transmits afferent impulses from the inner ear to the brainstem through the internal acoustic meatus. The vestibulocochlear nerve is divided into the vestibular and cochlear nerves. *Note:* The sensory organs in the semicircular canals respond to angular acceleration, and the macular organs respond to horizontal and vertical linear acceleration.

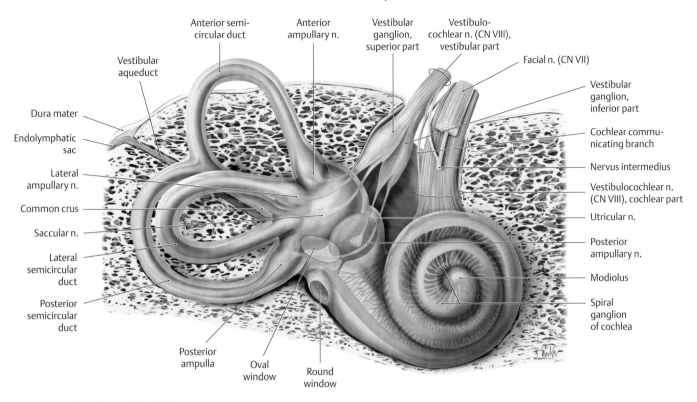

Fig. 35.22 Blood vessels of the inner ear

Right anterior view. The labyrinth receives its blood supply from the internal auditory artery, a branch of the anteroinferior cerebellar artery (see p. 608).

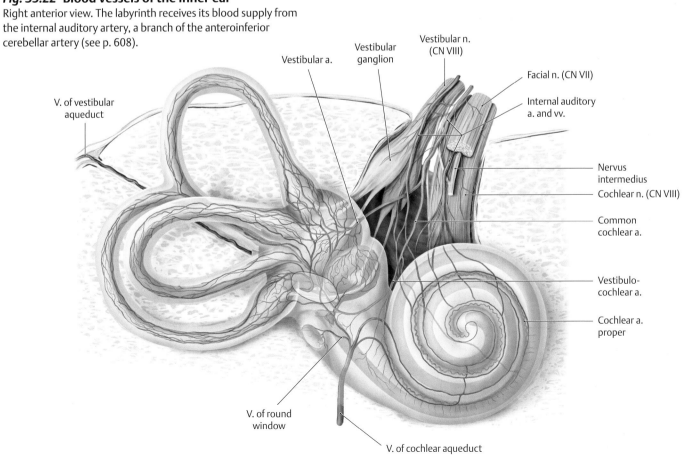

Bones of the Oral Cavity

 The floor of the nasal cavity (the maxilla and palatine bone) forms the roof of the oral cavity, the hard palate. The two horizontal processes of the maxilla (the palatine processes) grow together during development, eventually fusing at the median palatine suture. Failure to fuse results in a cleft palate.

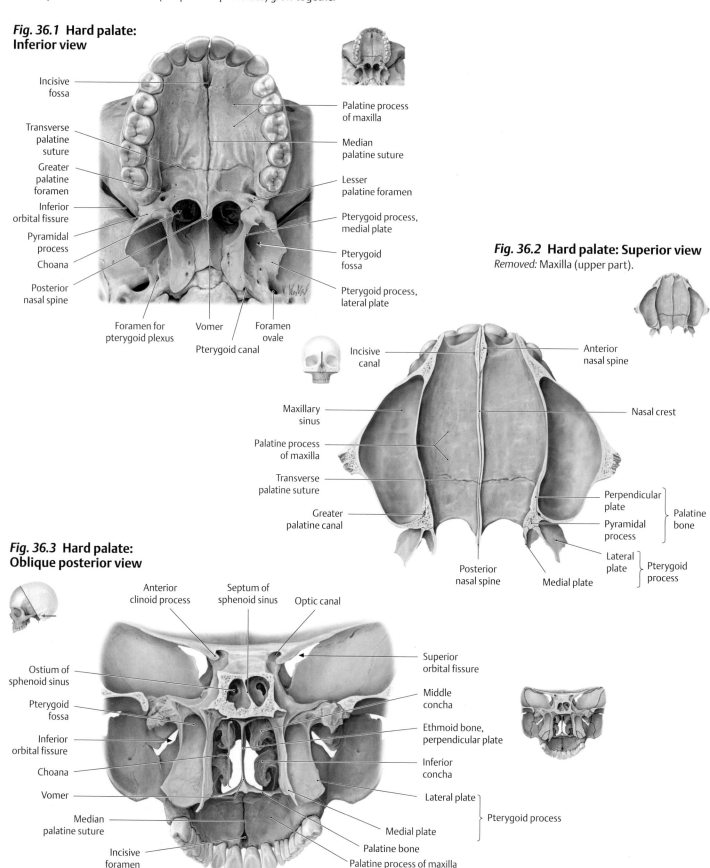

Fig. 36.1 Hard palate: Inferior view

Incisive fossa
Transverse palatine suture
Greater palatine foramen
Inferior orbital fissure
Pyramidal process
Choana
Posterior nasal spine
Foramen for pterygoid plexus
Vomer
Pterygoid canal
Foramen ovale
Palatine process of maxilla
Median palatine suture
Lesser palatine foramen
Pterygoid process, medial plate
Pterygoid fossa
Pterygoid process, lateral plate

Fig. 36.2 Hard palate: Superior view
Removed: Maxilla (upper part).

Incisive canal
Maxillary sinus
Palatine process of maxilla
Transverse palatine suture
Greater palatine canal
Anterior nasal spine
Nasal crest
Perpendicular plate
Pyramidal process
Lateral plate
Posterior nasal spine
Medial plate
Palatine bone
Pterygoid process

Fig. 36.3 Hard palate: Oblique posterior view

Anterior clinoid process
Septum of sphenoid sinus
Optic canal
Ostium of sphenoid sinus
Pterygoid fossa
Inferior orbital fissure
Choana
Vomer
Median palatine suture
Incisive foramen
Superior orbital fissure
Middle concha
Ethmoid bone, perpendicular plate
Inferior concha
Lateral plate
Medial plate
Pterygoid process
Palatine bone
Palatine process of maxilla

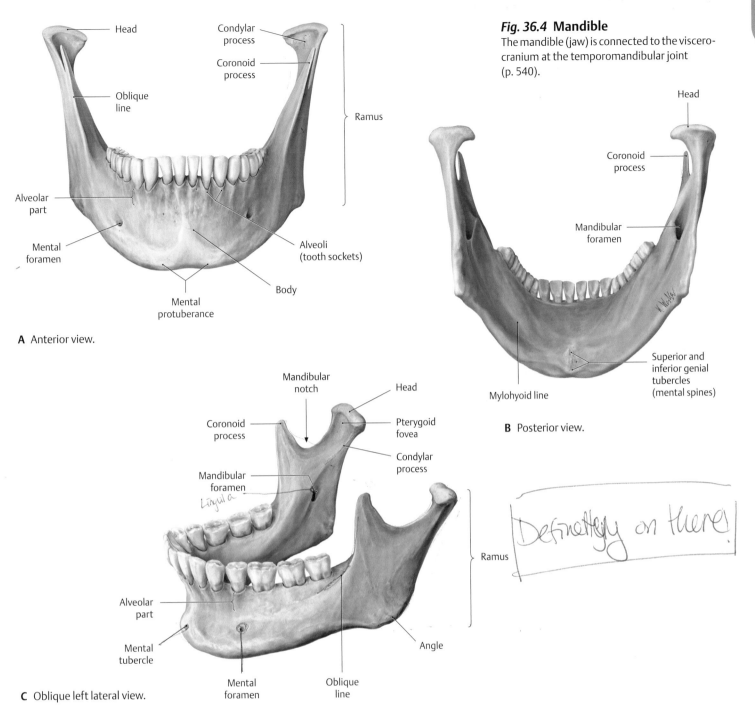

Fig. 36.4 Mandible

The mandible (jaw) is connected to the viscero-cranium at the temporomandibular joint (p. 540).

A Anterior view.

B Posterior view.

C Oblique left lateral view.

Fig. 36.5 Hyoid bone

The hyoid bone is suspended in the neck by muscles between the floor of the mouth and the larynx. Although not listed among the cranial bones, the hyoid bone gives attachment to the muscles of the oral floor. The greater horn and body of the hyoid are palpable in the neck.

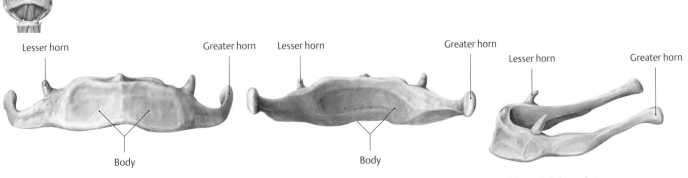

A Anterior view.

B Posterior view.

C Oblique left lateral view.

Temporomandibular Joint

Fig. 36.6 Temporomandibular joint
The head of the mandible articulates with the mandibular fossa in the temporomandibular joint.

Articular tubercle
Mandibular fossa
Articular disk
Head of mandible

Head of mandible

Pterygoid fovea
Coronoid process
Neck of mandible

Neck of mandible
Lingula
Mandibular foramen
Mylohyoid groove

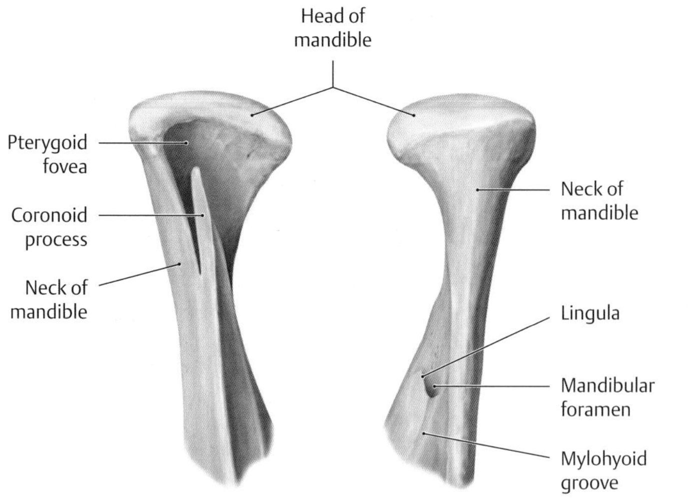

B Head of mandible, anterior view.

C Head of mandible, posterior view.

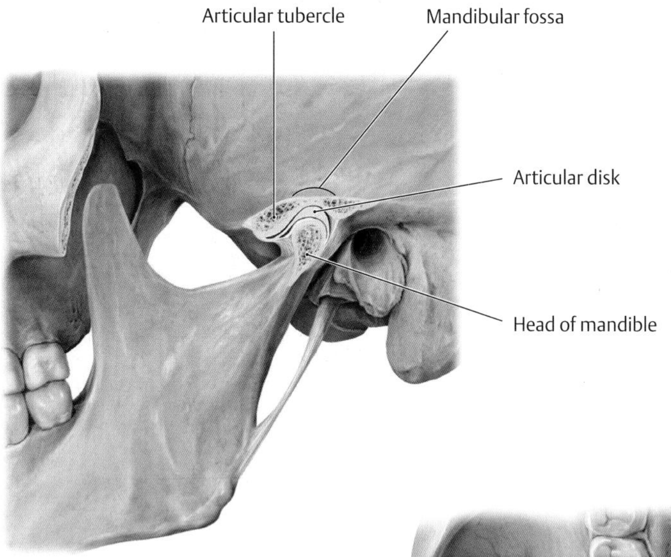

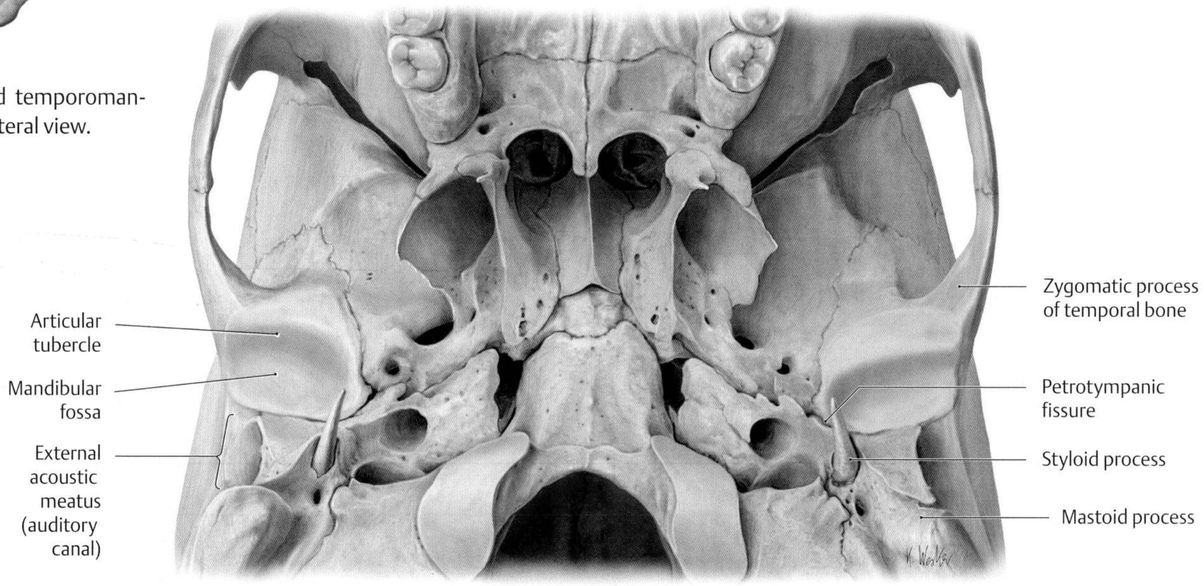

A Sagittally sectioned temporomandibular joint, left lateral view.

Articular tubercle
Mandibular fossa
External acoustic meatus (auditory canal)

Zygomatic process of temporal bone
Petrotympanic fissure
Styloid process
Mastoid process

D Mandibular fossa of the temporomandibular joint, inferior view.

Fig. 36.7 Ligaments of the temporomandibular joint

Pterygoid process, lateral plate

Joint capsule
Lateral ligament
Stylomandibular ligament

Pterygospinous ligament
Spheno-mandibular ligament
Stylomandibular ligament
Pterygoid process, medial plate

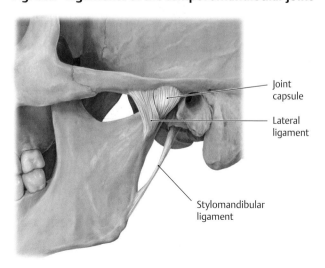

A Lateral view of the left temporomandibular joint.

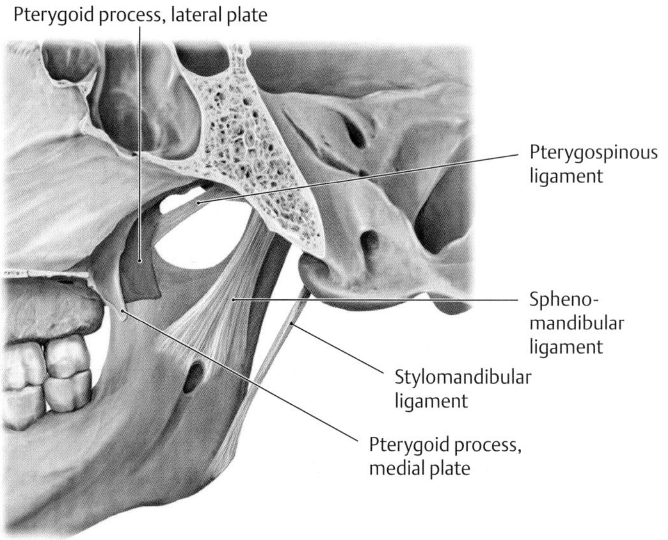

B Medial view of the right temporomandibular joint.

Fig. 36.8 Movement of the temporomandibular joint

Left lateral view. Up to 15 degrees of abduction, the head of the mandible remains in the mandibular fossa. Past 15 degrees, the head of the mandible glides forward onto the articular tubercle.

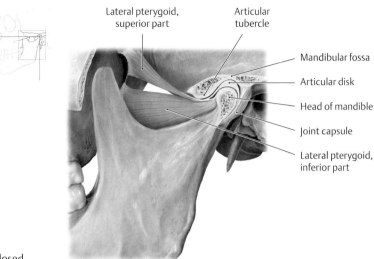

Lateral pterygoid, superior part

Articular tubercle

Mandibular fossa

Articular disk

Head of mandible

Joint capsule

Lateral pterygoid, inferior part

A Mouth closed.

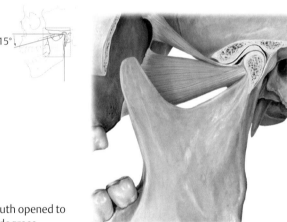

15°

B Mouth opened to 15 degrees.

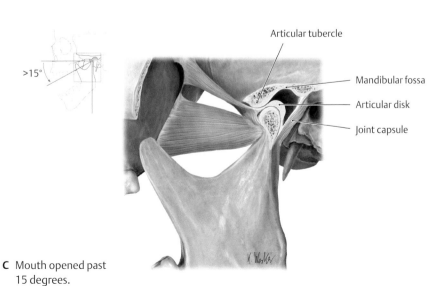

Articular tubercle

Mandibular fossa

Articular disk

Joint capsule

>15°

C Mouth opened past 15 degrees.

K. Wesker

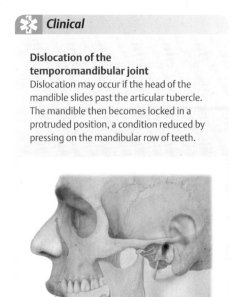
Fig. 36.9 Innervation of the temporomandibular joint capsule

Superior view.

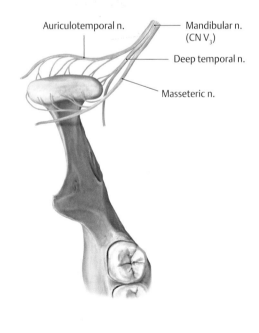

Auriculotemporal n.

Mandibular n. (CN V₃)

Deep temporal n.

Masseteric n.

Teeth

Fig. 36.10 Structure of a tooth

Each tooth consists of hard tissue (enamel, dentin, cementum) and soft tissue (dental pulp) arranged into a crown, neck (cervix), and root.

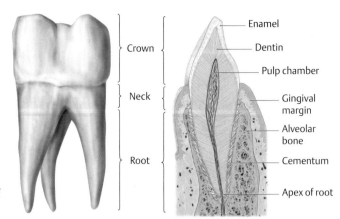

A Principal parts of a tooth (molar).

B Histology of a tooth (mandibular incisor).

Fig. 36.11 Permanent teeth

Each half of the maxilla and mandible contains a set of three anterior teeth (two incisors, one canine) and five posterior (postcanine) teeth (two premolars, three molars).

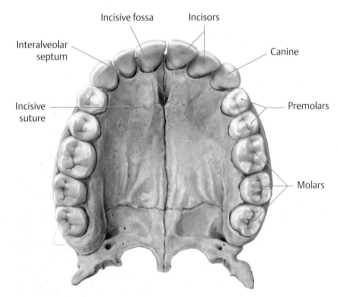

A Maxillary teeth. Inferior view of the maxilla.

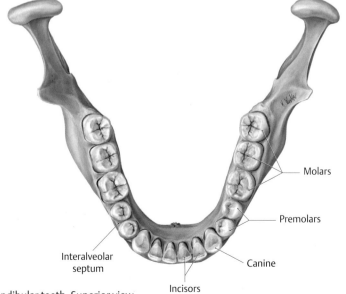

B Mandibular teeth. Superior view of the mandible.

Fig. 36.12 Tooth surfaces

The top of the tooth is known as the occlusal surface.

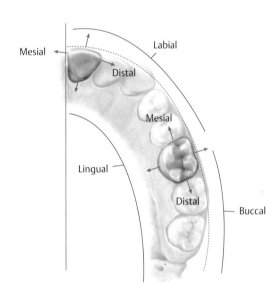

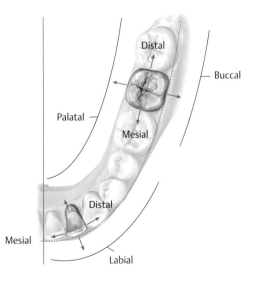

Fig. 36.13 Coding of the teeth

In the United States, the 32 permanent teeth are numbered sequentially (not assigned to quadrants). *Note:* The 20 deciduous (baby) teeth are coded A to J (upper arch), and K to T in a similar clockwise fashion. The third upper right molar is 1; the second upper right premolar is A.

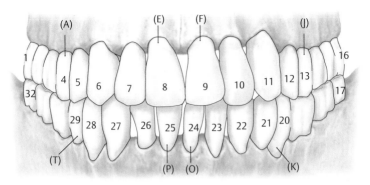

Fig. 36.14 Dental panoramic tomogram

The dental panoramic tomogram (DPT) is a survey radiograph that allows preliminary assessment of the temporomandibular joints, maxillary sinuses, maxillomandibular bone, and dental status (carious lesions, location of wisdom teeth, etc.). *DPT courtesy of Dr. U. J. Rother, Director of the Department of Diagnostic Radiology, Center for Dentistry and Oromaxillofacial Surgery, Eppendorf University Medical Center, Hamburg, Germany.*

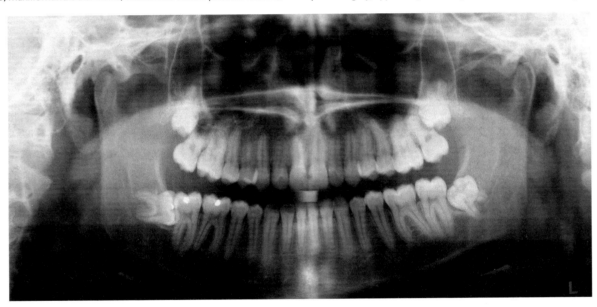

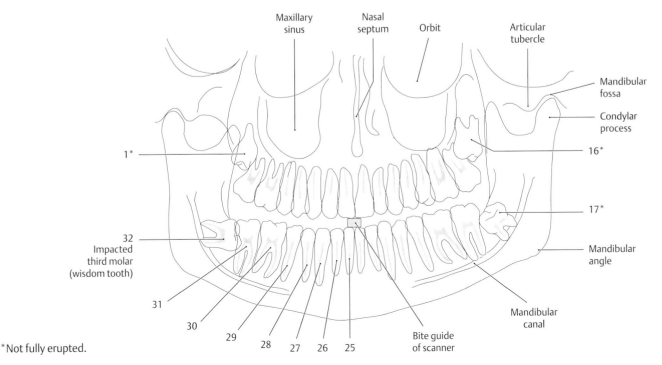

*Not fully erupted.

Oral Cavity Muscle Facts

Fig. 36.15 **Muscles of the oral floor**
See pp. 562–563 for the infrahyoid muscles.

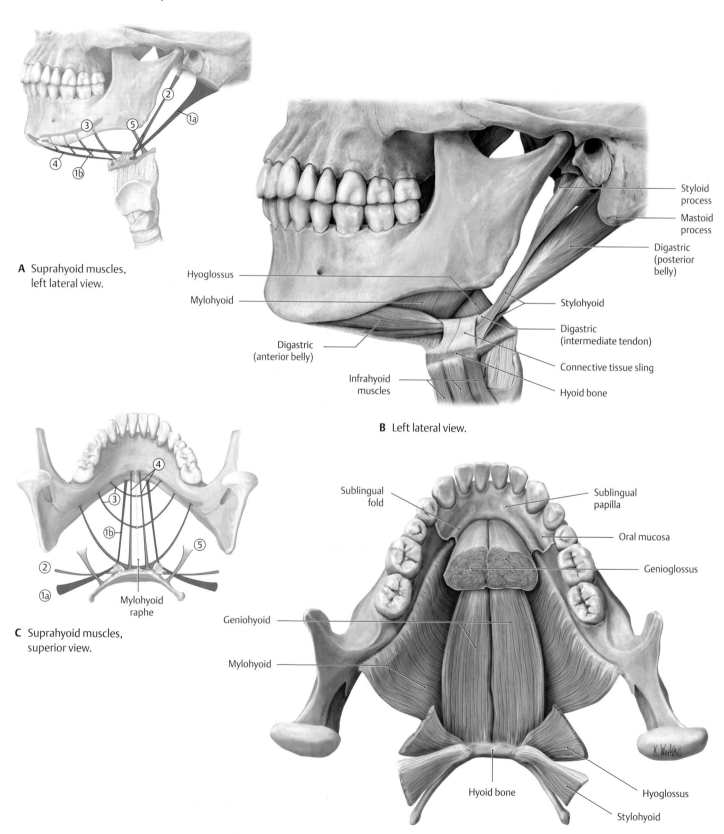

A Suprahyoid muscles, left lateral view.

Hyoglossus

Mylohyoid

Digastric (anterior belly)

Infrahyoid muscles

Styloid process

Mastoid process

Digastric (posterior belly)

Stylohyoid

Digastric (intermediate tendon)

Connective tissue sling

Hyoid bone

B Left lateral view.

Mylohyoid raphe

C Suprahyoid muscles, superior view.

Sublingual fold

Geniohyoid

Mylohyoid

Hyoid bone

Sublingual papilla

Oral mucosa

Genioglossus

Hyoglossus

Stylohyoid

D Superior view of the mandible and hyoid bone.

Table 36.1	Suprahyoid muscles					
Muscle		**Origin**	**Insertion**		**Innervation**	**Action**
① Digastric	ⓘa Anterior belly	Mandible (digastric fossa)	Hyoid bone (body)	Via an intermediate tendon with a fibrous loop	Mylohyoid n. (from CN V_3)	Elevates hyoid bone (during swallowing), assists in opening mandible
	ⓘb Posterior belly	Temporal bone (mastoid notch, medial to mastoid process)			Facial n. (CN VII)	
② Stylohyoid		Temporal bone (styloid process)		Via a split tendon		
③ Mylohyoid		Mandible (mylohyoid line)		Via median tendon of insertion (mylohyoid raphe)	Mylohyoid n. (from CN V_3)	Tightens and elevates oral floor, draws hyoid bone forward (during swallowing), assists in opening mandible and moving it side to side (mastication)
④ Geniohyoid		Mandible (inferior mental spine)		Body of hyoid bone	Ventral ramus of C1 via hypoglossal n. (CN XII)	Draws hyoid bone forward (during swallowing), assists in opening mandible
⑤ Hyoglossus		Hyoid bone (superior border of greater cornu)	Sides of tongue		Hypoglossal n. (CN XII)	Depresses the tongue

***Fig. 36.16* Muscles of the soft palate**
Inferior view. The soft palate forms the posterior boundary of the oral cavity, separating it from the oropharynx.

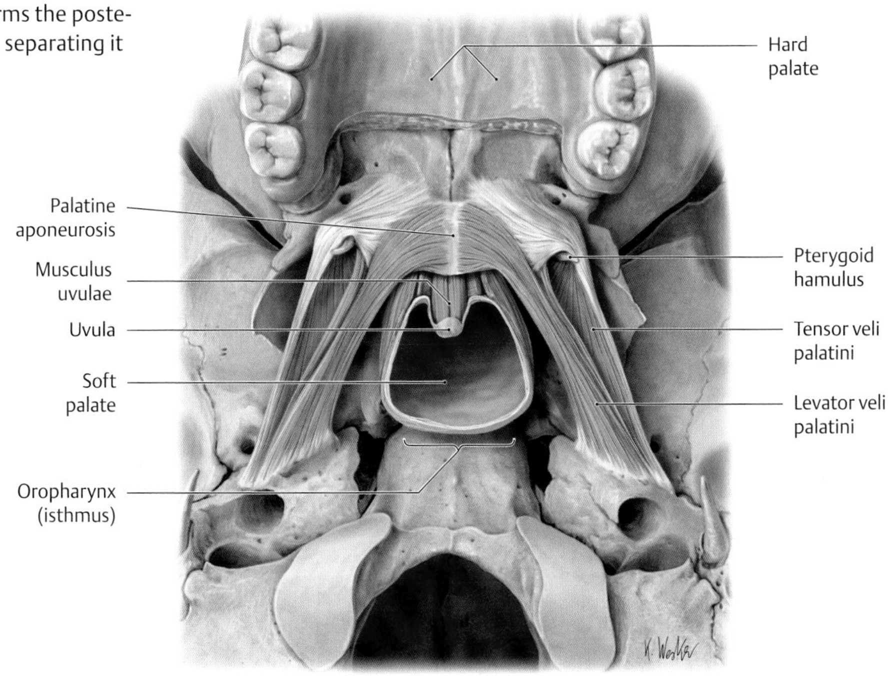

Table 36.2	Muscles of the soft palate			
Muscle	**Origin**	**Insertion**	**Innervation**	**Action**
Tensor veli palatini	Medial pterygoid plate (scaphoid fossa); sphenoid bone (spine); cartilage of pharyngotympanic tube	Palatine aponeurosis	Medial pterygoid n. (CN V_3 via otic ganglion)	Tightens soft palate; opens inlet to pharyngotympanic tube (during swallowing, yawning)
Levator veli palatini	Cartilage of pharyngotympanic tube; temporal bone (petrous part)		Accessory n. (CN XI, cranial part) via pharyngeal plexus (vagus n., CN X)	Raises soft palate to horizontal position
Musculus uvulae	Uvula (mucosa)	Palatine aponeurosis; posterior nasal spine		Shortens and raises uvula
Palatoglossus*	Tongue (side)	Palatine aponeurosis		Elevates tongue (posterior portion); pulls soft palate onto tongue
Palatopharyngeus*				Tightens soft palate; during swallowing pulls pharyngeal walls superiorly, anteriorly, and medially

*See pp. 548, 555.

Innervation of the Oral Cavity

Fig. 36.17 Trigeminal nerve in the oral cavity
Right lateral view.

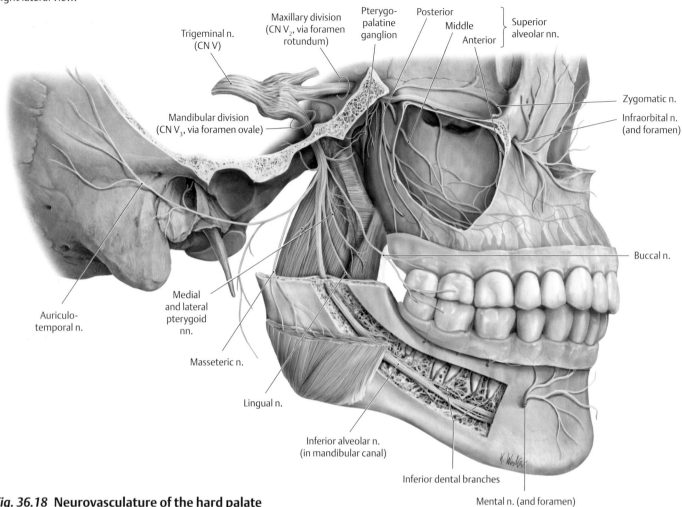

Fig. 36.18 Neurovasculature of the hard palate
Inferior view. The hard palate receives sensory innervation primarily from terminal branches of the maxillary division of the trigeminal nerve (CN V₂). The arteries of the hard palate arise from the maxillary artery.

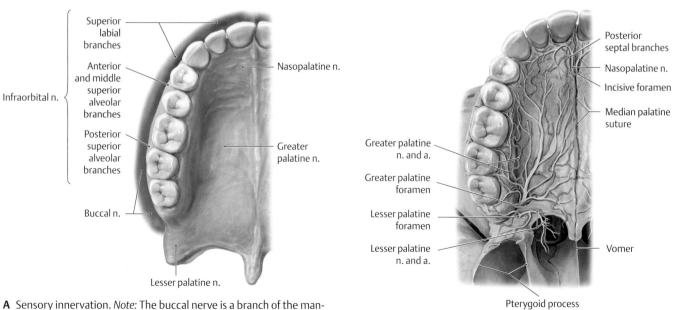

A Sensory innervation. *Note:* The buccal nerve is a branch of the mandibular division (CN V₃).

B Nerves and arteries.

The muscles of the oral floor have a complex nerve supply with contributions from the trigeminal nerve (CN V₃), facial nerve (CN VII), and C1 spinal nerve via the hypoglossal nerve (CN XII).

Fig. 36.19 Innervation of the oral floor muscles

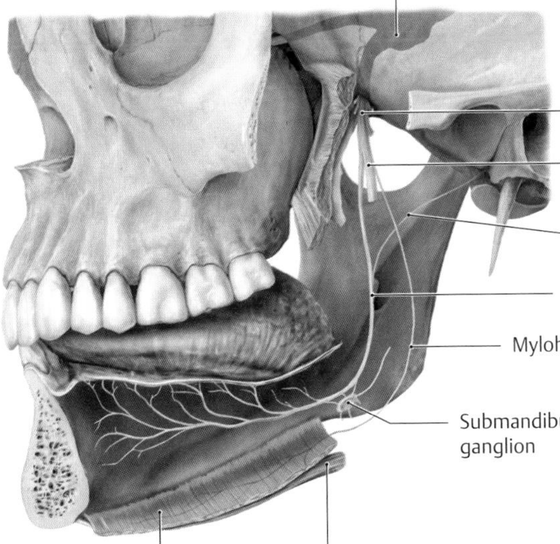

Trigeminal ganglion

Mandibular division (CN V₃)

Inferior alveolar n.

Chorda tympani (CN VII)

Lingual n.

Mylohyoid n.

Submandibular ganglion

Mylohyoid

Digastric, anterior belly

A Mylohyoid nerve (CN V₃). Left lateral view with the left half of the mandible removed.

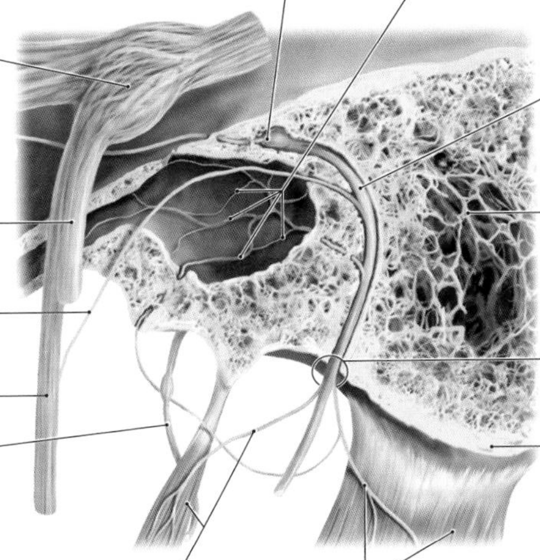

Geniculate ganglion

Tympanic plexus

Trigeminal ganglion

Mandibular division (CN V₃)

Chorda tympani

Lingual n.

Glossopharyngeal n. (CN IX)

Facial n. (CN VII)

Mastoid cells

Stylomastoid foramen

Mastoid process

Stylohyoid branch (with muscle)

Digastric branch (with posterior belly)

B Facial nerve (CN VII). Sagittal section through the right petrous bone at the level of the mastoid process, medial view.

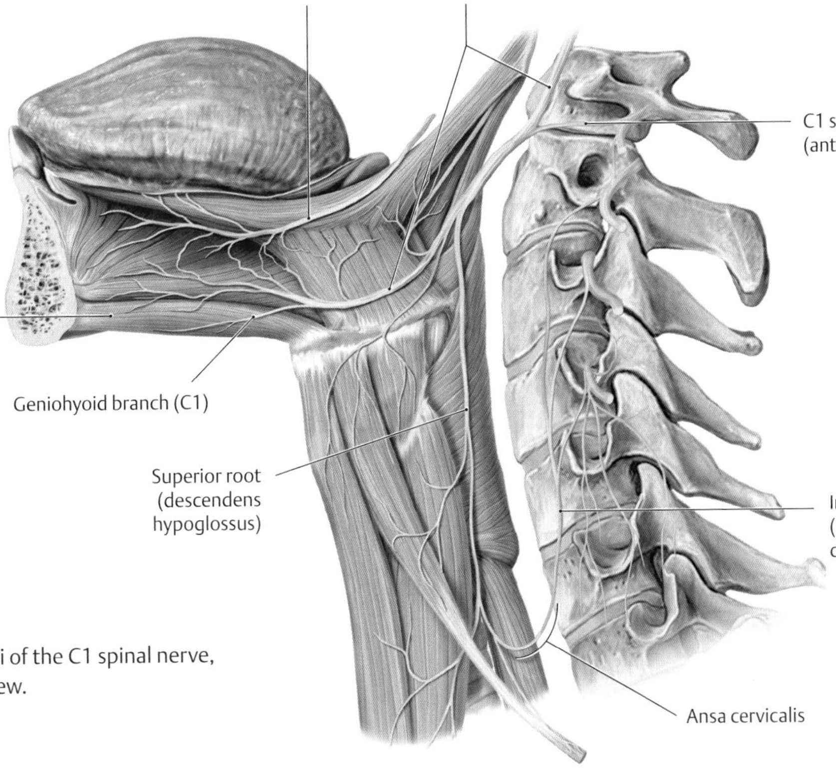

Lingual n.

Hypoglossal n. (CN XII)

C1 spinal n. (anterior ramus)

Geniohyoid

Geniohyoid branch (C1)

Superior root (descendens hypoglossus)

Inferior root (descendens cervicalis)

Ansa cervicalis

C Anterior rami of the C1 spinal nerve, left lateral view.

Tongue

 The dorsum of the tongue is covered by a highly specialized mucosa that supports its sensory functions (taste and fine tactile discrimination; see p. 616). The tongue is endowed with a very powerful muscular body to support its motor properties during mastication, swallowing, and speaking.

Fig. 36.20 Structure of the tongue
The V-shaped sulcus terminalis divides the tongue into an anterior (oral, presulcal) and a posterior (pharyngeal, postsulcal) part.

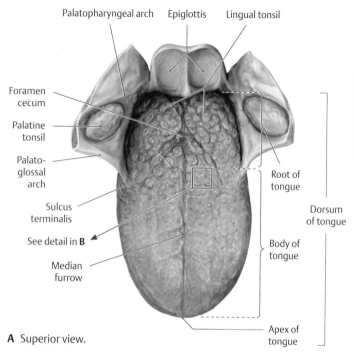

A Superior view.

B Lingual papillae, sectional block diagram. The connective tissue between the mucosal surface and musculature contains many small seromucous glands (not shown).

Fig. 36.21 Muscles of the tongue
The extrinsic lingual muscles (genioglossus, hyoglossus, palatoglossus, and styloglossus) have bony attachments and move the tongue as a whole. The intrinsic lingual muscles (superior and inferior longitudinal muscles, transverse muscle, and vertical muscle) have no bony attachments and alter the shape of the tongue.

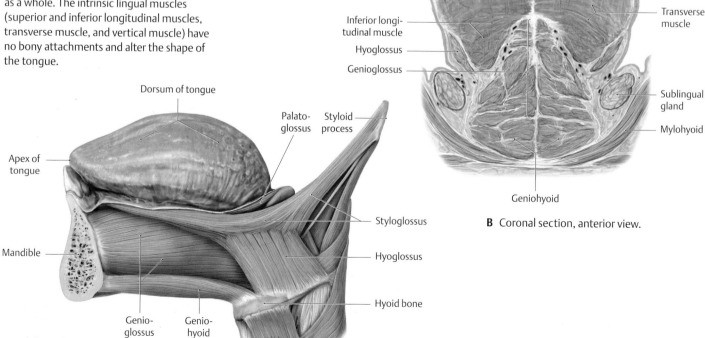

A Left lateral view.

B Coronal section, anterior view.

Fig. 36.22 **Somatosensory and taste innervation of the tongue**

Anterior view.

Fig. 36.23 **Neurovasculature of the tongue**

The lingual muscles receive somatomotor innervation from the hypoglossal nerve (CN XII), with the exception of the palatoglossus (supplied by the vagus nerve, CN X).

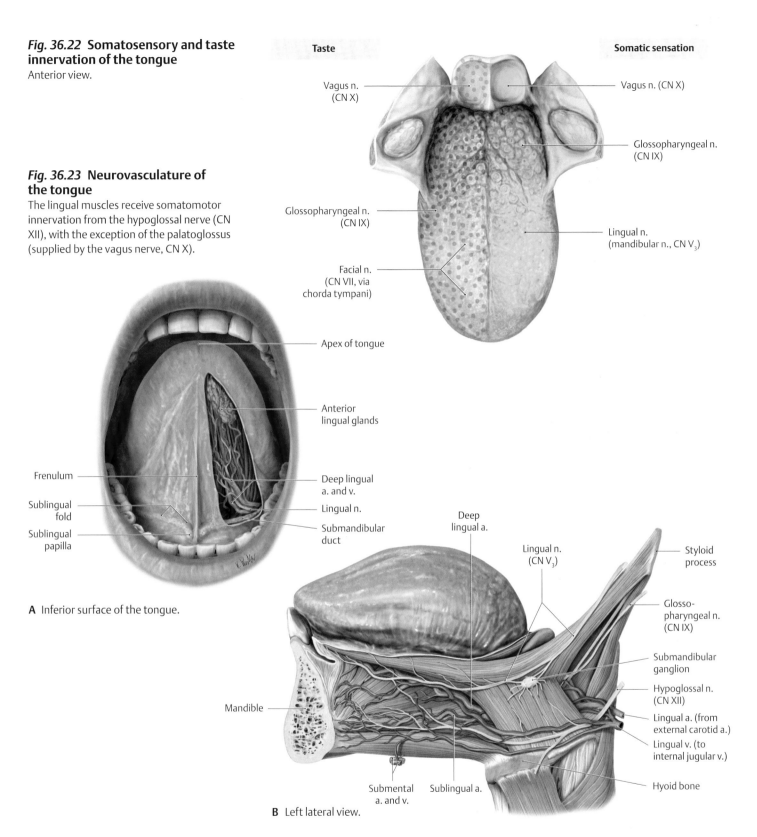

Taste

Vagus n. (CN X)

Glossopharyngeal n. (CN IX)

Facial n. (CN VII, via chorda tympani)

Somatic sensation

Vagus n. (CN X)

Glossopharyngeal n. (CN IX)

Lingual n. (mandibular n., CN V₃)

Apex of tongue

Anterior lingual glands

Frenulum

Sublingual fold

Sublingual papilla

Deep lingual a. and v.

Lingual n.

Submandibular duct

A Inferior surface of the tongue.

Deep lingual a.

Lingual n. (CN V₃)

Styloid process

Glosso-pharyngeal n. (CN IX)

Submandibular ganglion

Hypoglossal n. (CN XII)

Lingual a. (from external carotid a.)

Lingual v. (to internal jugular v.)

Hyoid bone

Mandible

Submental a. and v.

Sublingual a.

B Left lateral view.

✳ Clinical

Unilateral hypoglossal nerve palsy

Damage to the hypoglossal nerve causes paralysis of the genioglossus muscle on the affected side. The healthy (innervated) genioglossus on the unaffected side will therefore dominate. Upon protrusion, the tongue will deviate *toward* the paralyzed side.

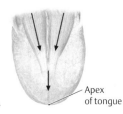

A Active protrusion with an intact hypoglossal nerve.

Apex of tongue

B Active protrusion with a unilateral hypoglossal nerve lesion.

Paralyzed genioglossus on affected side

Topography of the Oral Cavity & Salivary Glands

The oral cavity is located below the nasal cavity and anterior to the pharynx. It is bounded by the hard and soft palates, the tongue and muscles of the oral floor, and the uvula.

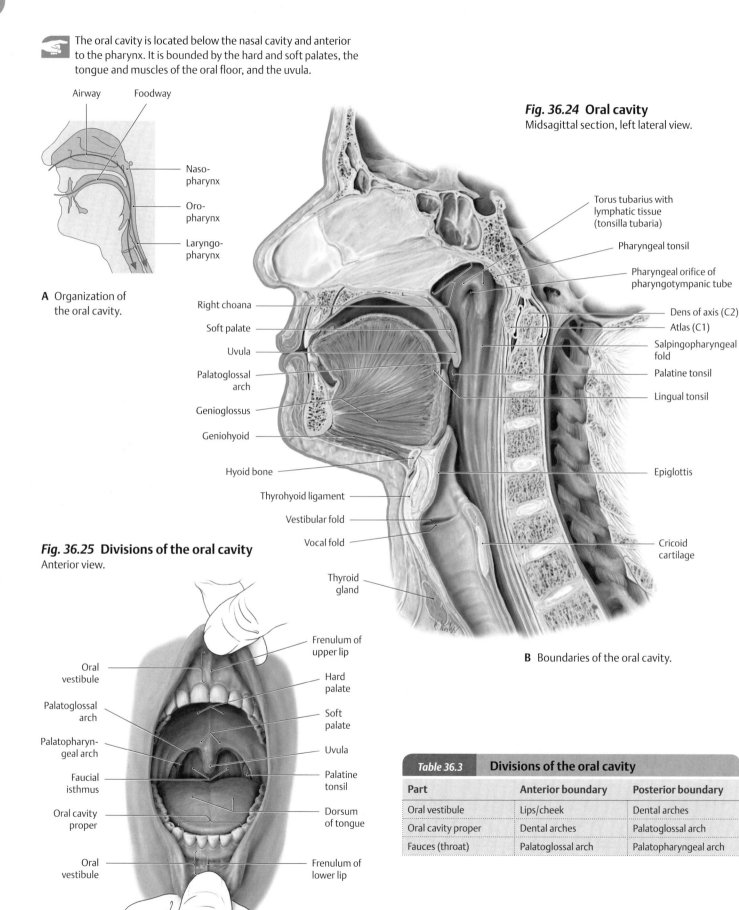

Airway   Foodway

Naso-
pharynx

Oro-
pharynx

Laryngo-
pharynx

A Organization of the oral cavity.

Fig. 36.24 Oral cavity
Midsagittal section, left lateral view.

Torus tubarius with lymphatic tissue (tonsilla tubaria)

Pharyngeal tonsil

Pharyngeal orifice of pharyngotympanic tube

Right choana

Soft palate

Uvula

Palatoglossal arch

Genioglossus

Geniohyoid

Hyoid bone

Thyrohyoid ligament

Vestibular fold

Vocal fold

Thyroid gland

Dens of axis (C2)

Atlas (C1)

Salpingopharyngeal fold

Palatine tonsil

Lingual tonsil

Epiglottis

Cricoid cartilage

B Boundaries of the oral cavity.

Fig. 36.25 Divisions of the oral cavity
Anterior view.

Oral vestibule

Palatoglossal arch

Palatopharyn-geal arch

Faucial isthmus

Oral cavity proper

Oral vestibule

Frenulum of upper lip

Hard palate

Soft palate

Uvula

Palatine tonsil

Dorsum of tongue

Frenulum of lower lip

Table 36.3	Divisions of the oral cavity	
Part	**Anterior boundary**	**Posterior boundary**
Oral vestibule	Lips/cheek	Dental arches
Oral cavity proper	Dental arches	Palatoglossal arch
Fauces (throat)	Palatoglossal arch	Palatopharyngeal arch

The three large, paired salivary glands are the parotid, submandibular, and sublingual glands. The parotid gland is a purely serous (watery) salivary gland. The sublingual gland is predominantly mucous; the submandibular gland is a mixed seromucous gland.

Fig. 36.26 Salivary glands

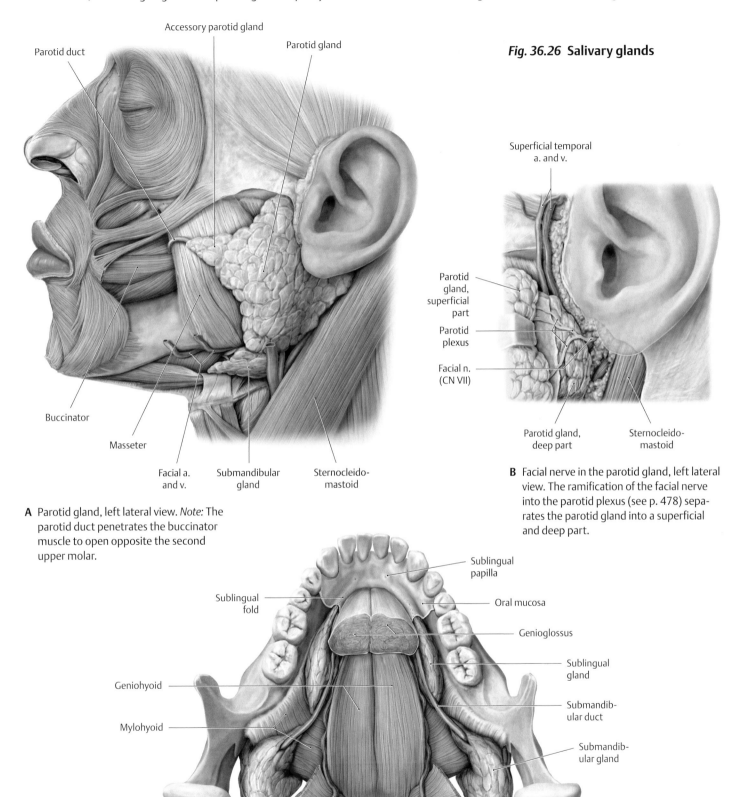

A Parotid gland, left lateral view. *Note:* The parotid duct penetrates the buccinator muscle to open opposite the second upper molar.

Parotid duct
Accessory parotid gland
Parotid gland
Buccinator
Masseter
Facial a. and v.
Submandibular gland
Sternocleido-mastoid

B Facial nerve in the parotid gland, left lateral view. The ramification of the facial nerve into the parotid plexus (see p. 478) separates the parotid gland into a superficial and deep part.

Superficial temporal a. and v.
Parotid gland, superficial part
Parotid plexus
Facial n. (CN VII)
Parotid gland, deep part
Sternocleido-mastoid

C Submandibular and sublingual glands, superior view with tongue removed.

Sublingual papilla
Oral mucosa
Genioglossus
Sublingual gland
Submandibular duct
Submandibular gland
Hyoglossus
Stylohyoid
Hyoid bone
Lingual a.
Mylohyoid
Geniohyoid
Sublingual fold

Tonsils & Pharynx

***Fig. 36.27* Tonsils**

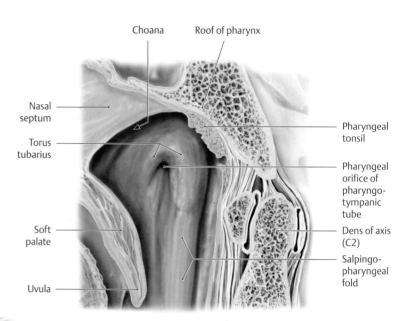

A Palatine tonsils, anterior view.

B Pharyngeal tonsils. Sagittal section through the roof of the pharynx.

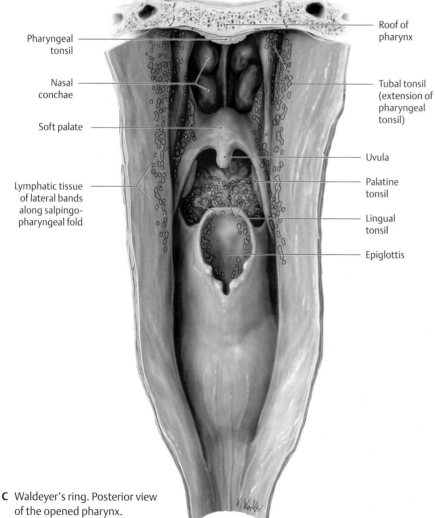

C Waldeyer's ring. Posterior view of the opened pharynx.

Table 36.4	Structures in Waldeyer's ring	
Tonsil		**#**
Pharyngeal tonsil		1
Tubal tonsils		2
Palatine tonsils		2
Lingual tonsil		1
Lateral bands		2

Tonsil infections

Abnormal enlargement of the palatine tonsils due to severe viral or bacterial infection can result in obstruction of the oropharynx, causing difficulty swallowing.

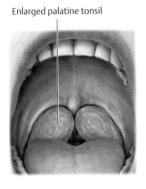

Enlarged palatine tonsil

Particularly well developed in young children, the pharyngeal tonsil begins to regress at 6 to 7 years of age. Abnormal enlargement is common, with the tonsil bulging into the nasopharynx and obstructing air passages, forcing the child to "mouth breathe."

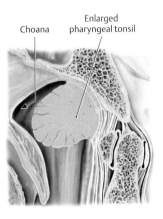

Choana

Enlarged pharyngeal tonsil

Fig. 36.28 **Pharyngeal mucosa**

Posterior view of the opened pharynx. The anterior portion of the muscular tube contains three openings: choanae (to the nasal cavity), faucial isthmus (to the oral cavity), and aditus (to the laryngeal inlet).

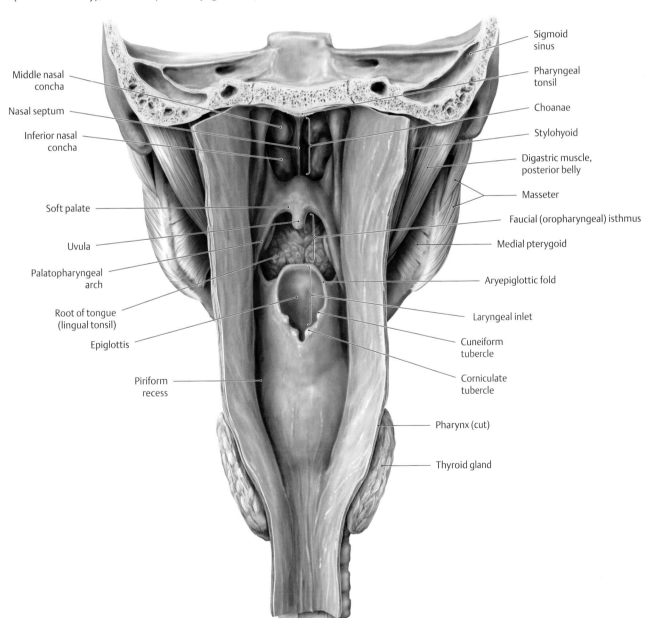

Middle nasal concha

Nasal septum

Inferior nasal concha

Soft palate

Uvula

Palatopharyngeal arch

Root of tongue (lingual tonsil)

Epiglottis

Piriform recess

Sigmoid sinus

Pharyngeal tonsil

Choanae

Stylohyoid

Digastric muscle, posterior belly

Masseter

Faucial (oropharyngeal) isthmus

Medial pterygoid

Aryepiglottic fold

Laryngeal inlet

Cuneiform tubercle

Corniculate tubercle

Pharynx (cut)

Thyroid gland

Pharyngeal Muscles

Fig. 36.29 Pharyngeal muscles: Left lateral view

The pharyngeal musculature consists of the pharyngeal constrictors and the relatively weak pharyngeal elevators.

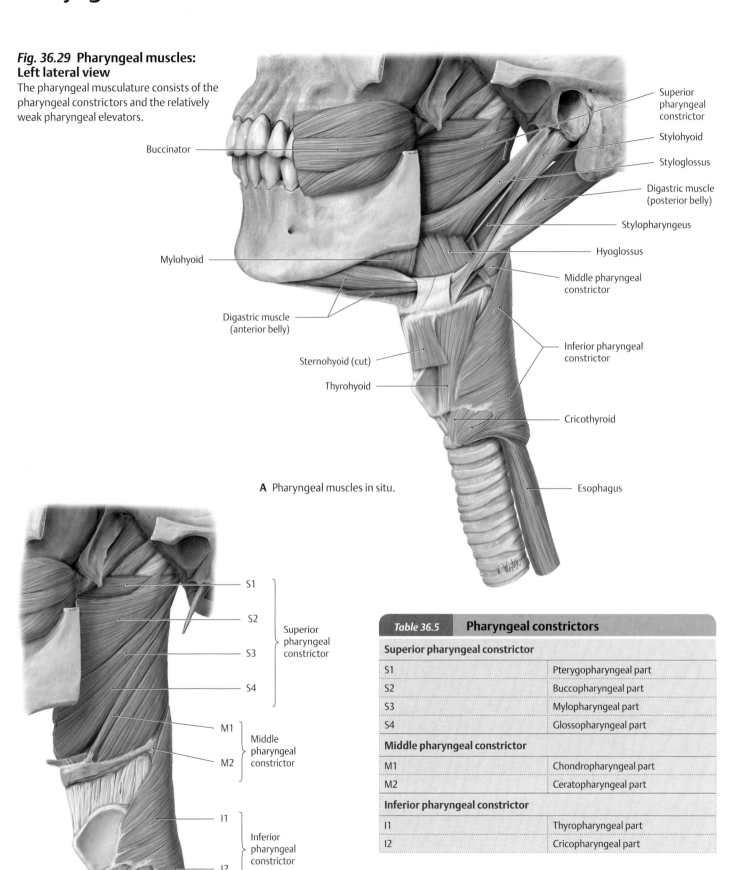

Buccinator

Mylohyoid

Digastric muscle (anterior belly)

Sternohyoid (cut)

Thyrohyoid

Superior pharyngeal constrictor

Stylohyoid

Styloglossus

Digastric muscle (posterior belly)

Stylopharyngeus

Hyoglossus

Middle pharyngeal constrictor

Inferior pharyngeal constrictor

Cricothyroid

Esophagus

A Pharyngeal muscles in situ.

S1
S2
S3
S4

Superior pharyngeal constrictor

M1
M2

Middle pharyngeal constrictor

I1
I2

Inferior pharyngeal constrictor

B Subdivisions of the pharyngeal constrictors.

Table 36.5	Pharyngeal constrictors
Superior pharyngeal constrictor	
S1	Pterygopharyngeal part
S2	Buccopharyngeal part
S3	Mylopharyngeal part
S4	Glossopharyngeal part
Middle pharyngeal constrictor	
M1	Chondropharyngeal part
M2	Ceratopharyngeal part
Inferior pharyngeal constrictor	
I1	Thyropharyngeal part
I2	Cricopharyngeal part

Fig. 36.30 **Pharyngeal muscles: Posterior view**

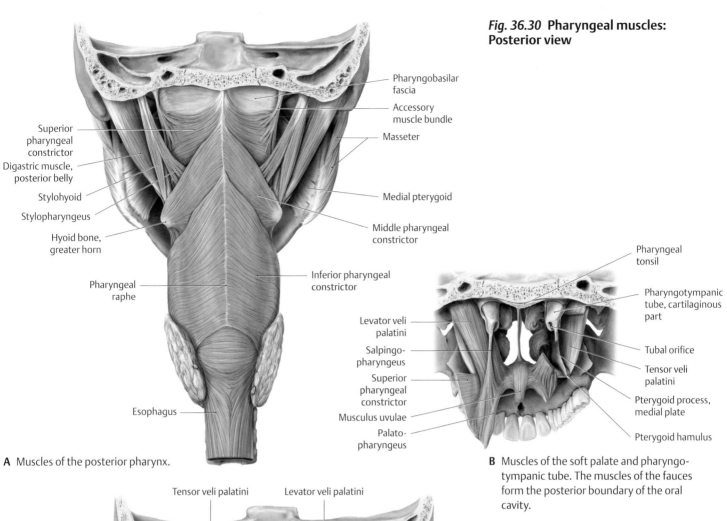

Pharyngobasilar fascia

Accessory muscle bundle

Masseter

Medial pterygoid

Middle pharyngeal constrictor

Superior pharyngeal constrictor

Digastric muscle, posterior belly

Stylohyoid

Stylopharyngeus

Hyoid bone, greater horn

Pharyngeal raphe

Inferior pharyngeal constrictor

Esophagus

A Muscles of the posterior pharynx.

Pharyngeal tonsil

Pharyngotympanic tube, cartilaginous part

Tubal orifice

Tensor veli palatini

Pterygoid process, medial plate

Pterygoid hamulus

Levator veli palatini

Salpingo-pharyngeus

Superior pharyngeal constrictor

Musculus uvulae

Palato-pharyngeus

B Muscles of the soft palate and pharyngo-tympanic tube. The muscles of the fauces form the posterior boundary of the oral cavity.

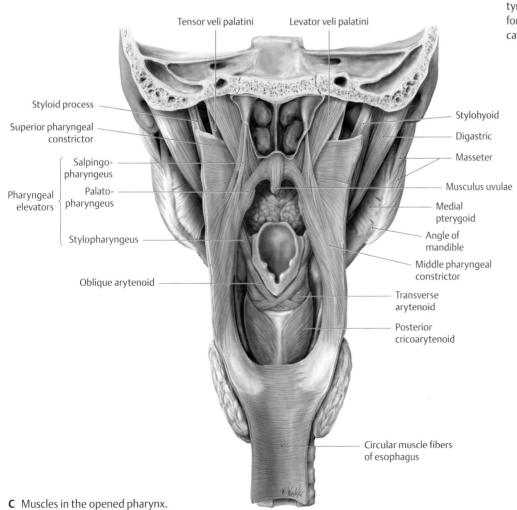

Tensor veli palatini

Levator veli palatini

Stylohyoid

Digastric

Masseter

Musculus uvulae

Medial pterygoid

Angle of mandible

Middle pharyngeal constrictor

Transverse arytenoid

Posterior cricoarytenoid

Styloid process

Superior pharyngeal constrictor

Pharyngeal elevators
- Salpingo-pharyngeus
- Palato-pharyngeus
- Stylopharyngeus

Oblique arytenoid

Circular muscle fibers of esophagus

C Muscles in the opened pharynx.

Neurovasculature of the Pharynx

Fig. 36.31 Neurovasculature in the parapharyngeal space
Posterior view. *Removed:* Vertebral column and posterior structures.

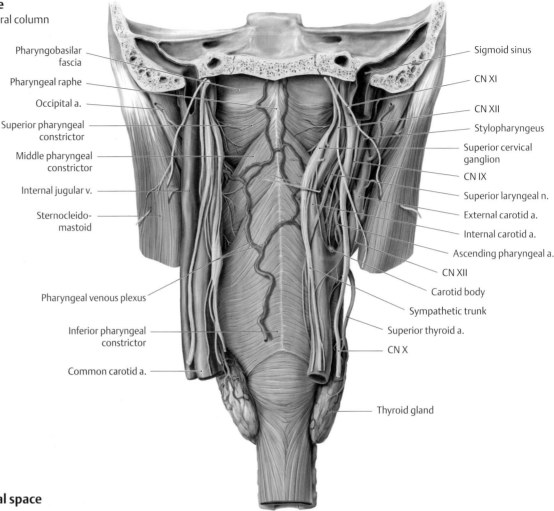

Pharyngobasilar fascia
Pharyngeal raphe
Occipital a.
Superior pharyngeal constrictor
Middle pharyngeal constrictor
Internal jugular v.
Sternocleidomastoid
Pharyngeal venous plexus
Inferior pharyngeal constrictor
Common carotid a.

Sigmoid sinus
CN XI
CN XII
Stylopharyngeus
Superior cervical ganglion
CN IX
Superior laryngeal n.
External carotid a.
Internal carotid a.
Ascending pharyngeal a.
CN XII
Carotid body
Sympathetic trunk
Superior thyroid a.
CN X
Thyroid gland

Fig. 36.32 Parapharyngeal space
Transverse section, superior view.

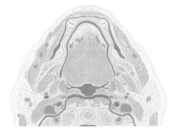

A Parapharyngeal space. The parapharyngeal space consists of a retropharyngeal (green) and a lateropharyngeal space. The lateropharyngeal space is further subdivided into an anterior (yellow) and a posterior (orange) part. Note the deep layer of cervical fascia (prevertebral lamina, red).

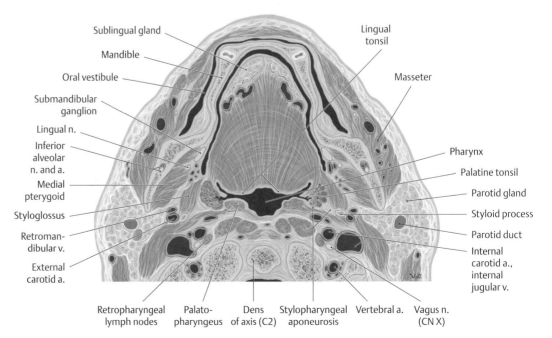

Sublingual gland
Mandible
Oral vestibule
Submandibular ganglion
Lingual n.
Inferior alveolar n. and a.
Medial pterygoid
Styloglossus
Retromandibular v.
External carotid a.

Lingual tonsil
Masseter
Pharynx
Palatine tonsil
Parotid gland
Styloid process
Parotid duct
Internal carotid a., internal jugular v.

Retropharyngeal lymph nodes
Palatopharyngeus
Dens of axis (C2)
Stylopharyngeal aponeurosis
Vertebral a.
Vagus n. (CN X)

B Superior view of the transverse section at the level of the tonsillar fossa.

Fig. 36.33 Neurovasculature of the opened pharynx
Posterior view.

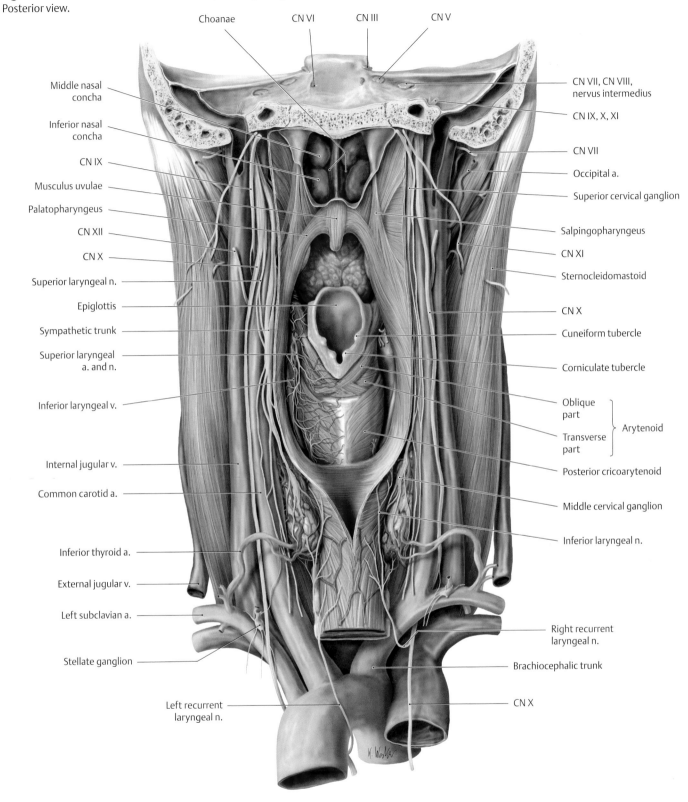

Choanae | CN VI | CN III | CN V

Middle nasal concha
Inferior nasal concha
CN IX
Musculus uvulae
Palatopharyngeus
CN XII
CN X
Superior laryngeal n.
Epiglottis
Sympathetic trunk
Superior laryngeal a. and n.
Inferior laryngeal v.
Internal jugular v.
Common carotid a.
Inferior thyroid a.
External jugular v.
Left subclavian a.
Stellate ganglion
Left recurrent laryngeal n.

CN VII, CN VIII, nervus intermedius
CN IX, X, XI
CN VII
Occipital a.
Superior cervical ganglion
Salpingopharyngeus
CN XI
Sternocleidomastoid
CN X
Cuneiform tubercle
Corniculate tubercle
Oblique part
Transverse part } Arytenoid
Posterior cricoarytenoid
Middle cervical ganglion
Inferior laryngeal n.
Right recurrent laryngeal n.
Brachiocephalic trunk
CN X

CN III = Oculomotor n., CN V = Trigeminal n., CN VI = Abducent n.,
CN VII = Facial n., CN VIII = Vestibulocochlear n., CN IX = Glossopharyngeal n.,
CN X = Vagus n., CN XI = Accessory n., CN XII = Hypoglossal n.
See Chapter 31 for the cranial nerves.

Bones & Ligaments of the Neck

Fig. 37.1 Boundaries of the neck
Left lateral view.

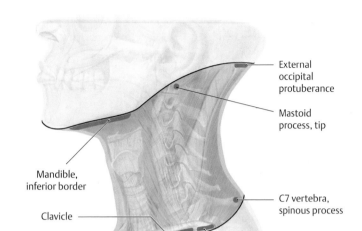

Fig. 37.2 Bony structures of the neck
Left lateral view.

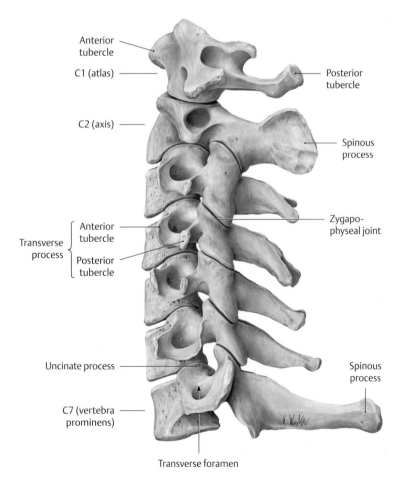

A Cervical spine. The seven vertebrae of the cervical spine are specialized for bearing the weight of the head.

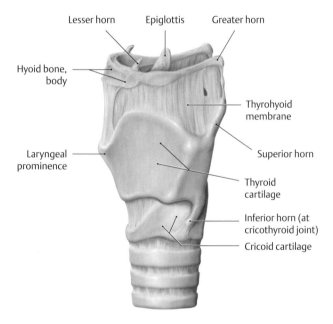

B Hyoid bone and larynx. The hyoid bone provides a site for bony attachment for the supra- and infrahyoid muscles. *Note:* The larynx is suspended from the hyoid bone, primarily by the thyrohyoid membrane.

Fig. 37.3 Ligaments of the cervical spine

Midsagittal section, viewed from the left side.
For the ligaments of the craniovertebral
joints, see p. 16.

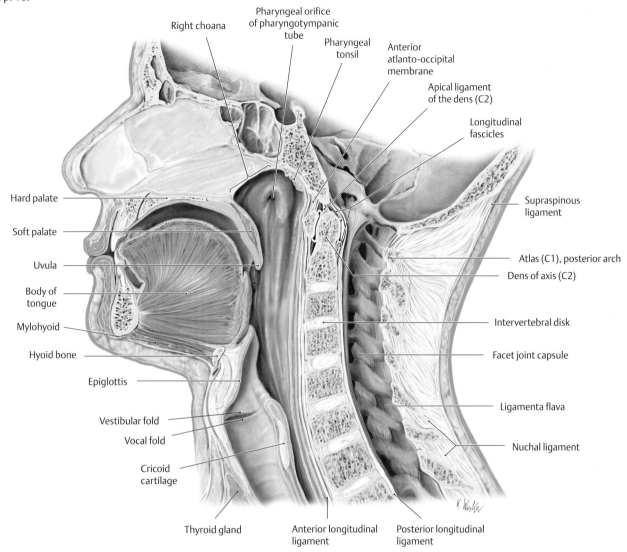

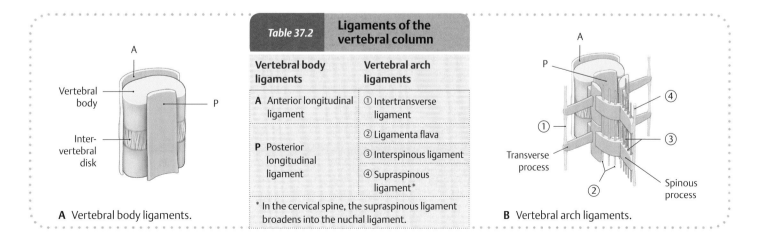

A Vertebral body ligaments.

Table 37.2	Ligaments of the vertebral column	
Vertebral body ligaments	**Vertebral arch ligaments**	
A Anterior longitudinal ligament	① Intertransverse ligament	
P Posterior longitudinal ligament	② Ligamenta flava	
	③ Interspinous ligament	
	④ Supraspinous ligament*	
* In the cervical spine, the supraspinous ligament broadens into the nuchal ligament.		

B Vertebral arch ligaments.

Muscle Facts (I)

From a topographical standpoint, there are six major muscle groups in the neck. Functionally, however, the platysma belongs to the muscles of facial expression, the trapezius belongs to the muscles of the shoulder girdle, and the nuchal muscles belong to the intrinsic back muscles. The suboccipital muscles (short nuchal and cranioverbal joint muscles) are included in this chapter with the deep muscles of the neck.

Table 37.3	**Classification of neck muscles**				
I	**Superficial neck muscles**		**III**	**Suprahyoid muscles**	
	Platysma, sternocleidomastoid, trapezius	Fig. 37.4		Digastric, geniohyoid, mylohyoid, stylohyoid	Fig. 37.7A
II	**Nuchal muscles (intrinsic back muscles)**		**IV**	**Infrahyoid muscles**	
	⑥ Semispinalis capitis ⑦ Semispinalis cervicis	See p. 32		Sternohyoid, sternothyroid, thyrohyoid, omohyoid	Fig. 37.7B
	⑧ Splenius capitis ⑨ Splenius cervicis		**V**	**Prevertebral muscles**	
	⑩ Longissimus capitis ⑪ Longissimus cervicis	See p. 30		Longus capitis, longus coli, rectus capitis anterior and lateralis	Fig. 37.9A
	⑫ Iliocostalis cervicis		**VI**	**Lateral (deep) neck muscles**	
	Suboccipital muscles (short nuchal and cranioverbal joint muscles)	Fig. 37.9C		Anterior, middle, and posterior scalenes	Fig. 37.9B

Fig. 37.4 **Superficial neck muscles**
See Table 37.4 for details.

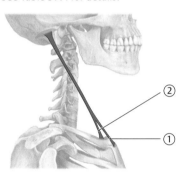

A Sternocleidomastoid.

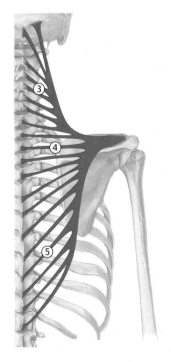

B Trapezius.

Fig. 37.5 **Nuchal muscles**

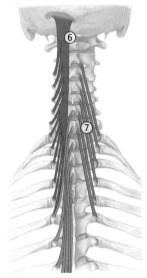

A Semispinalis.

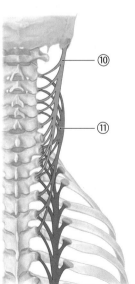

B Splenius.

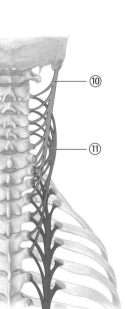

C Longissimus.

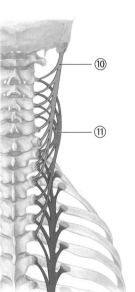

D Iliocostalis.

Fig. 37.6 Superficial musculature of the neck

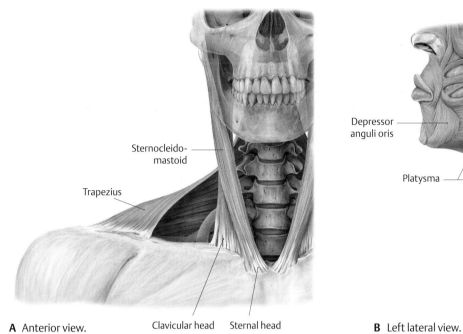

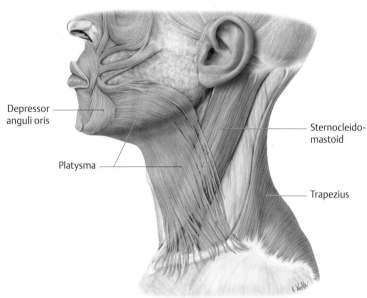

A Anterior view.

B Left lateral view.

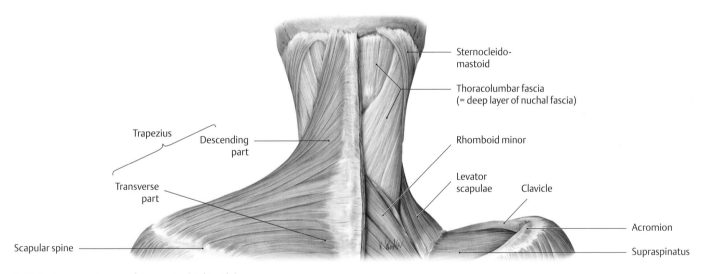

C Posterior view. *Removed:* Trapezius (right side).

Table 37.4	Superficial neck muscles				
Muscle		**Origin**	**Insertion**	**Innervation**	**Action**
Platysma		Skin over lower neck and upper lateral thorax	Mandible (inferior border), skin over lower face and angle of mouth	Cervical branch of facial n. (CN VII)	Depresses and wrinkles skin of lower face and mouth, tenses skin of neck, aids forced depression of mandible
Sternocleido-mastoid	① Sternal head	Sternum (manubrium)	Temporal bone (mastoid process), occipital bone (superior nuchal line)	*Motor:* Accessory n. (CN IX)	*Unilateral:* Tilts head to same side, rotates head to opposite side
	② Clavicular head	Clavicle (medial one third)		*Pain and proprioception:* Cervical plexus (C2, C3)	*Bilateral:* Extends head, aids in respiration when head is fixed
Trapezius	③ Descending part*	Occipital bone, spinous processes of C1–C7	Clavicle (lateral one third)		Draws scapula obliquely upward, rotates glenoid cavity inferiorly

* The transverse ④ and ascending ⑤ parts are described on p. 276.

Muscle Facts (II)

Table 37.5	Suprahyoid muscles

The suprahyoid muscles are also considered accessory muscles of mastication.

Muscle		Origin	Insertion		Innervation	Action
Digastric	① ⓐ Anterior belly	Mandible (digastric fossa)	Via an intermediate tendon with a fibrous loop	Hyoid bone (body)	Mylohyoid n. (from CN V₃)	Elevates hyoid bone (during swallowing), assists in opening mandible
	① ⓑ Posterior belly	Temporal bone (mastoid notch, medial to mastoid process)			Facial n. (CN VII)	
② Stylohyoid		Temporal bone (styloid process)	Via a split tendon			
③ Mylohyoid		Mandible (mylohyoid line)	Via median tendon of insertion (mylohyoid raphe)		Mylohyoid n. (from CN V₃)	Tightens and elevates oral floor, draws hyoid bone forward (swallowing), assists in opening mandible and moving it side to side (mastication)
④ Geniohyoid		Mandible (inferior mental spine)	Directly		Anterior ramus of C1 (via CN XII)	Draws hyoid bone forward (swallowing), assists in opening mandible

Fig. 37.7 **Supra- and infrahyoid muscles**

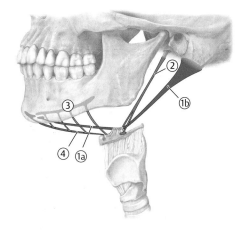

A Suprahyoid muscles, left lateral view.

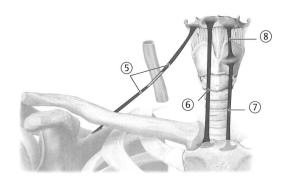

B Infrahyoid muscles, anterior view.

Table 37.6	Infrahyoid muscles

Muscle	Origin	Insertion	Innervation	Action
⑤ Omohyoid	Scapula (superior border)	Hyoid bone (body)	Ansa cervicalis of cervical plexus (C1–C3)	Depresses (fixes) hyoid, draws larynx and hyoid down for phonation and terminal phases of swallowing*
⑥ Sternohyoid	Manubrium and sternoclavicular joint (posterior surface)			
⑦ Sternothyroid	Manubrium (posterior surface)	Thyroid cartilage (oblique line)	Ansa cervicalis (C2–C3)	
⑧ Thyrohyoid	Thyroid cartilage (oblique line)	Hyoid bone (body)	C1 via hypoglossal n. (CN XII)	Depresses and fixes hyoid, raises the larynx during swallowing

* The omohyoid also tenses the cervical fascia (with an intermediate tendon).

Fig. 37.8 **Supra- and infrahyoid muscles**

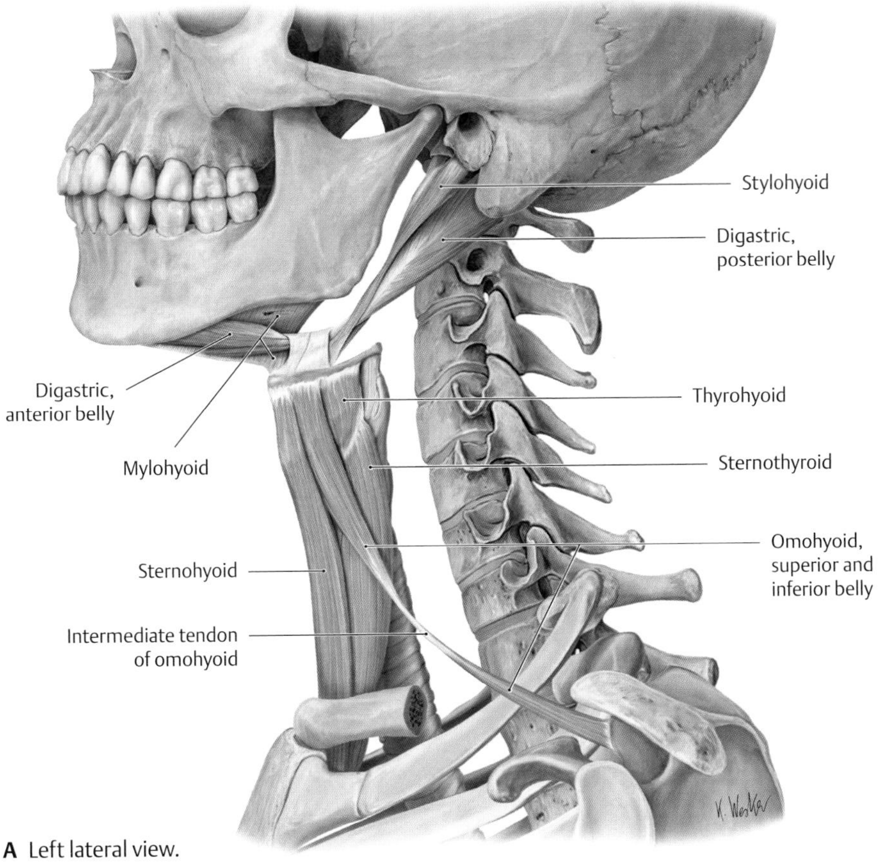

Stylohyoid

Digastric,
posterior belly

Digastric,
anterior belly

Mylohyoid

Thyrohyoid

Sternothyroid

Sternohyoid

Omohyoid,
superior and
inferior belly

Intermediate tendon
of omohyoid

A Left lateral view.

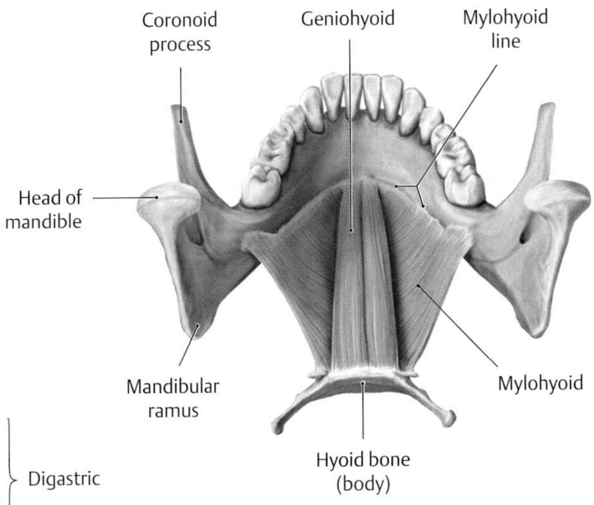

Coronoid
process

Geniohyoid

Mylohyoid
line

Head of
mandible

Mandibular
ramus

Mylohyoid

Hyoid bone
(body)

B Mylohyoid and geniohyoid (oral floor),
posterosuperior view.

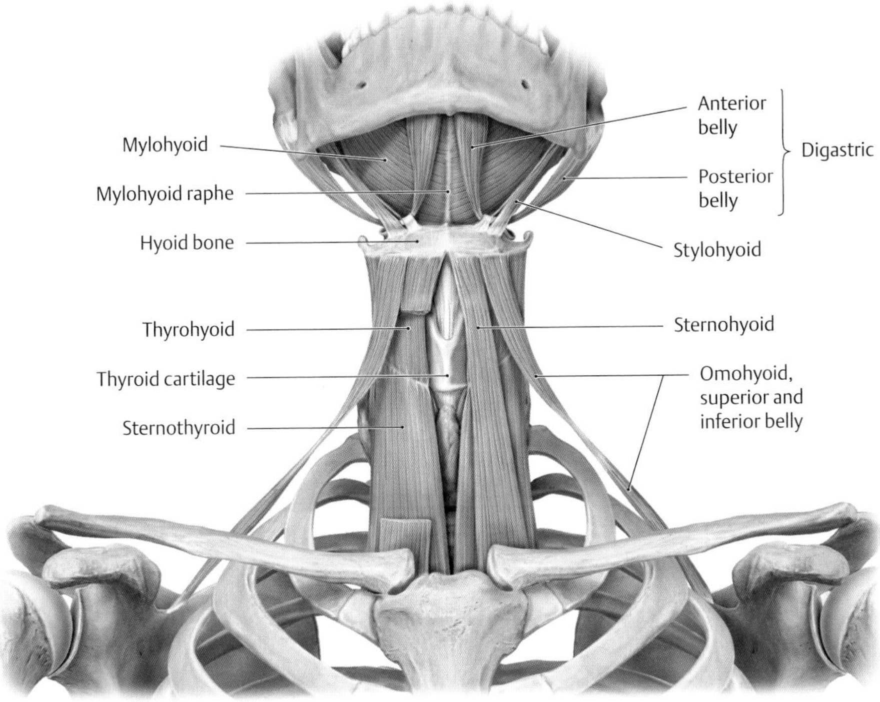

Mylohyoid

Mylohyoid raphe

Hyoid bone

Anterior
belly

Posterior
belly

Digastric

Stylohyoid

Thyrohyoid

Sternohyoid

Thyroid cartilage

Sternothyroid

Omohyoid,
superior and
inferior belly

C Anterior view. The sternohyoid has been cut
(right).

Muscle Facts (III)

Fig. 37.9 Deep muscles of the neck

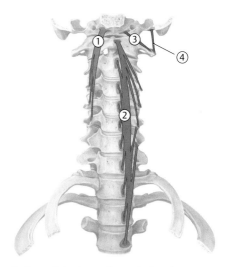

A Prevertebral muscles, anterior view.

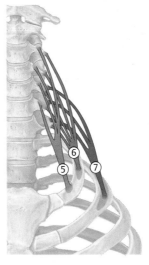

B Scalene muscles, anterior view.

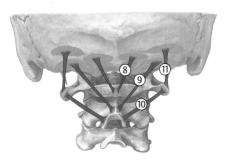

C Suboccipital muscles, posterior view.

Table 37.7	Deep muscles of the neck				
Muscle		**Origin**	**Insertion**	**Innervation**	**Action**
Prevertebral muscles					
① Longus capitis		C3–C6 (anterior tubercles of transverse processes)	Occipital bone (basilar part)	Direct branches from cervical plexus (C1–C3)	Flexion of head at atlanto-occipital joints
② Longus colli	Vertical (intermediate) part	C5–T3 (anterior surfaces of vertebral bodies)	C2–C4 (anterior surfaces)	Direct branches from cervical plexus (C2–C6)	*Unilateral:* Tilts and rotates cervical spine to opposite side *Bilateral:* Forward flexion of cervical spine
	Superior oblique part	C3–C5 (anterior tubercles of transverse processes)	Atlas (anterior tubercle)		
	Inferior oblique part	T1–T3 (anterior surfaces of vertebral bodies)	C5–C6 (anterior tubercles of transverse processes)		
③ Rectus capitis anterior		C1 (lateral mass)	Occipital bone (basilar part)	Anterior rami of C1 and C2	*Unilateral:* Lateral flexion at the atlanto-occipital joint *Bilateral:* Flexion at the atlanto-occipital joint
④ Rectus capitis lateralis		C1 (transverse process)	Occipital bone (basilar part, lateral to occipital condyles)		
Scalene muscles					
⑤ Scalenus anterior		C3–C6 (anterior tubercles of transverse processes)	1st rib (scalene tubercle)	Direct branches from cervical and brachial plexuses (C3–C8)	*With ribs mobile:* Elevates upper ribs (during forced inspiration) *With ribs fixed:* Bends cervical spine to same side (unilateral), flexes neck (bilateral)
⑥ Scalenus medius		C1–C2 (transverse processes), C3–C7 (posterior tubercles of transverse processes)	1st rib (posterior to groove for subclavian artery)		
⑦ Scalenus posterior		C5–C7 (posterior tubercles of transverse processes)	2nd rib (outer surface)		
Suboccipital muscles (short nuchal and craniovertebral joint muscles)					
⑧ Rectus capitis posterior minor		C1 (posterior tubercle)	Occipital bone (inner third of inferior nuchal line)	Posterior ramus of C1 (suboccipital n.)	*Unilateral:* Rotates head to same side *Bilateral:* Extends head
⑨ Rectus capitis posterior major		C2 (spinous process)	Occipital bone (middle third of inferior nuchal line)		
⑩ Obliquus capitis inferior			C1 (transverse process)		
⑪ Obliquus capitis superior		C1 (transverse process)	Occipital bone (above insertion of rectus capitis posterior major)		*Unilateral:* Tilts head to same side, rotates it to opposite side *Bilateral:* Extends head

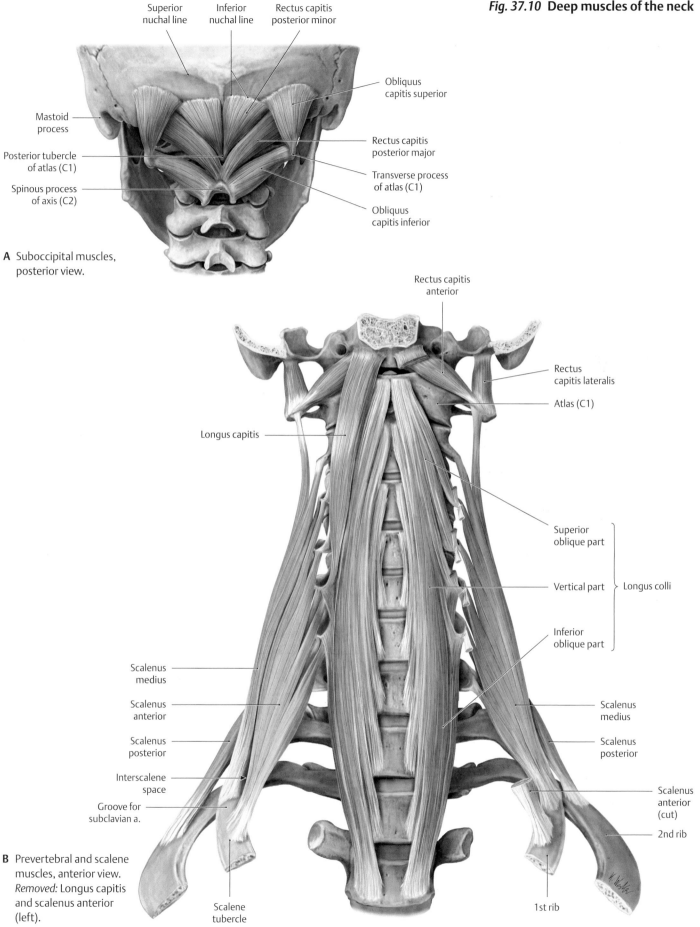

Fig. 37.10 Deep muscles of the neck

Superior nuchal line

Inferior nuchal line

Rectus capitis posterior minor

Obliquus capitis superior

Mastoid process

Rectus capitis posterior major

Posterior tubercle of atlas (C1)

Transverse process of atlas (C1)

Spinous process of axis (C2)

Obliquus capitis inferior

A Suboccipital muscles, posterior view.

Rectus capitis anterior

Rectus capitis lateralis

Atlas (C1)

Longus capitis

Superior oblique part

Vertical part — Longus colli

Inferior oblique part

Scalenus medius

Scalenus anterior

Scalenus medius

Scalenus posterior

Scalenus posterior

Interscalene space

Groove for subclavian a.

Scalenus anterior (cut)

2nd rib

B Prevertebral and scalene muscles, anterior view. *Removed:* Longus capitis and scalenus anterior (left).

Scalene tubercle

1st rib

Arteries & Veins of the Neck

Fig. 37.11 Arteries of the neck
Left lateral view. The structures of the neck are primarily supplied by the external carotid artery (anterior branches) and the subclavian artery (vertebral artery, thyrocervical trunk, and costocervical trunk).

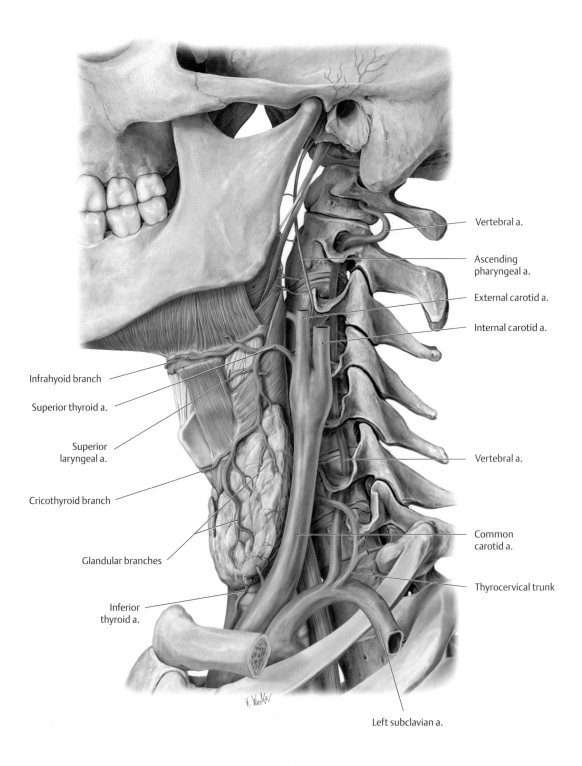

Vertebral a.

Ascending pharyngeal a.

External carotid a.

Internal carotid a.

Infrahyoid branch

Superior thyroid a.

Superior laryngeal a.

Vertebral a.

Cricothyroid branch

Common carotid a.

Glandular branches

Thyrocervical trunk

Inferior thyroid a.

Left subclavian a.

Fig. 37.12 Veins of the neck

Left lateral view. The principal veins of the neck are the internal, external, and anterior jugular veins.

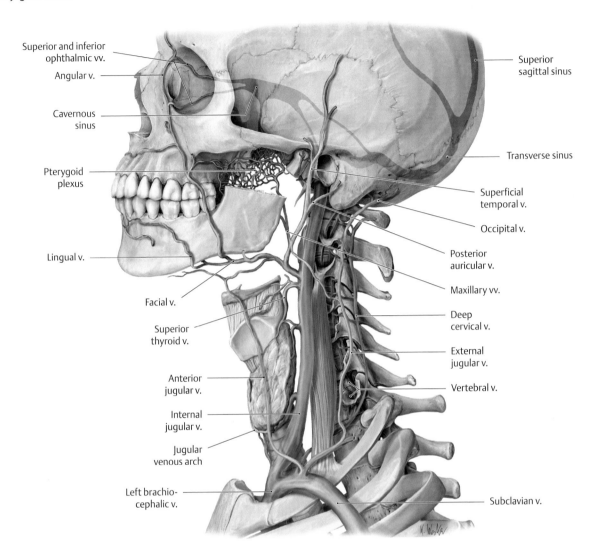

- Superior and inferior ophthalmic vv.
- Angular v.
- Cavernous sinus
- Pterygoid plexus
- Lingual v.
- Facial v.
- Superior thyroid v.
- Anterior jugular v.
- Internal jugular v.
- Jugular venous arch
- Left brachio-cephalic v.
- Superior sagittal sinus
- Transverse sinus
- Superficial temporal v.
- Occipital v.
- Posterior auricular v.
- Maxillary vv.
- Deep cervical v.
- External jugular v.
- Vertebral v.
- Subclavian v.

Clinical

Impeded blood flow and veins of the neck

When clinical factors (e.g., chronic lung disease, mediastinal tumors, or infections) impede the flow of blood to the right heart, blood dams up in the superior vena cava and, consequently, the jugular veins. This causes conspicuous swelling in the jugular (and sometimes more minor) veins.

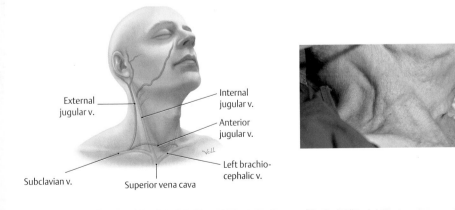

- External jugular v.
- Subclavian v.
- Superior vena cava
- Internal jugular v.
- Anterior jugular v.
- Left brachio-cephalic v.

Innervation of the Neck

Table 37.8	Branches of the spinal nerves in the neck

Posterior (dorsal) ramus

	Nerve	Sensory function	Motor function
C1	Suboccipital n.	No C1 dermatome	Innervate intrinsic nuchal muscles
C2	Greater occipital n.	Innervate C2 dermatome	
C3	3rd occipital n.	Innervate C3 dermatome	

Anterior (ventral) ramus

	Sensory branches	Sensory function	Motor branches	Motor function
C1	—	—	Form ansa cervicalis (motor part of cervical plexus)	Innervate infrahyoid muscles (except thyrohyoid)
C2	Lesser occipital n.	Form sensory part of cervical plexus, innervate anterior and lateral neck		
C2–C3	Great auricular n.			
	Transverse cervical n.			
C3–C4	Supraclavicular nn.		Contribute to phrenic n.*	Innervate diaphragm and pericardium*

*The anterior roots of C3–C5 combine to form the phrenic nerve (see p. 54).

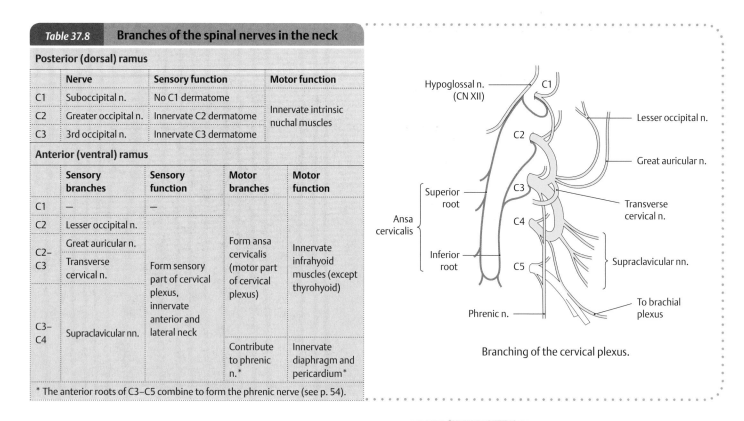

Branching of the cervical plexus.

Fig. 37.13 Innervation of the nuchal region

Posterior view.

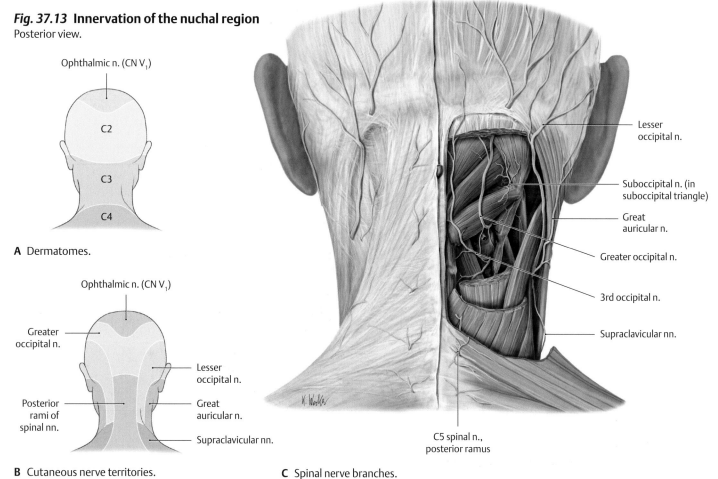

A Dermatomes.

B Cutaneous nerve territories.

C Spinal nerve branches.

Fig. 37.14 Sensory innervation of the anterolateral neck

Left lateral view.

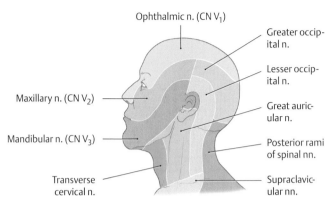

A Cutaneous nerve territories. Trigeminal nerve (orange), posterior rami (blue), anterior rami (yellow).

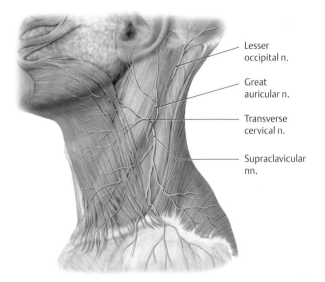

B Sensory branches of the cervical plexus.

Fig. 37.15 Motor innervation of the anterolateral neck

Left lateral view.

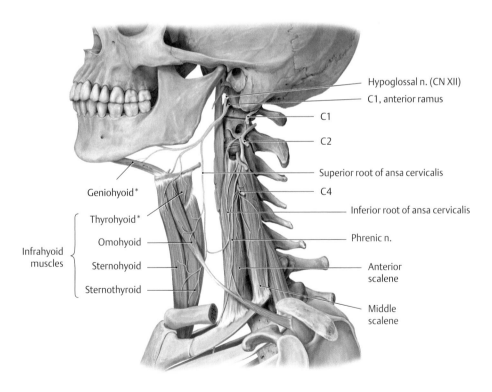

* Innervated by the anterior ramus of C1 (distributed by the hypoglossal n.).

Larynx: Cartilage & Structure

Fig. 37.16 Laryngeal cartilages

Left lateral view. The larynx consists of five laryngeal cartilages: epiglottic, thyroid, cricoid, and the paired arytenoid and corniculate cartilages. They are connected to each other, the trachea, and the hyoid bone by elastic ligaments.

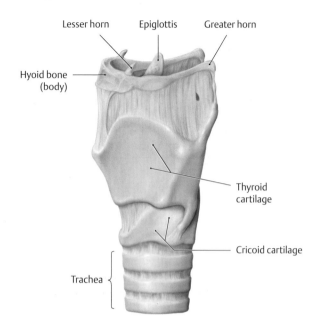

Fig. 37.17 Epiglottic cartilage

The elastic epiglottic cartilage comprises the internal skeleton of the epiglottis, providing resilience to return it to its initial position after swallowing.

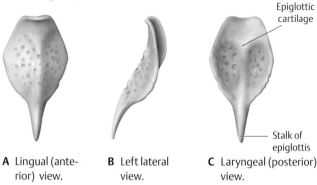

A Lingual (anterior) view. **B** Left lateral view. **C** Laryngeal (posterior) view.

Fig. 37.18 Thyroid cartilage

Left oblique view.

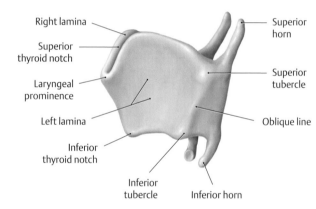

Fig. 37.19 Cricoid cartilage

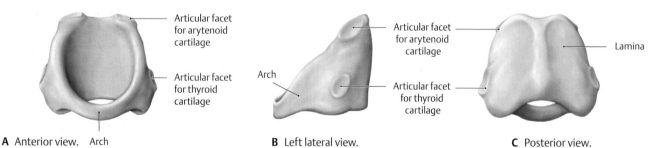

A Anterior view. Arch

B Left lateral view.

C Posterior view.

Fig. 37.20 Arytenoid and corniculate cartilages

Right cartilages.

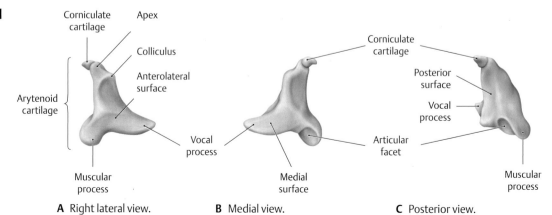

A Right lateral view. **B** Medial view. **C** Posterior view.

Fig. 37.21 **Structure of the larynx**

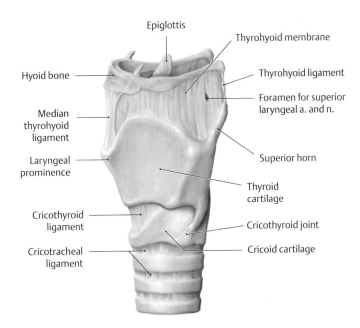

A Left anterior oblique view.

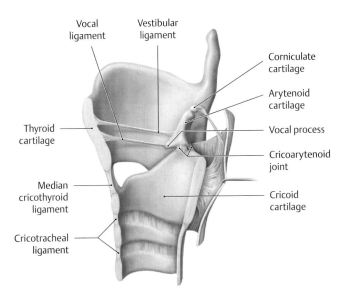

B Sagittal section, viewed from the left medial aspect. The arytenoid cartilage alters the position of the vocal folds during phonation.

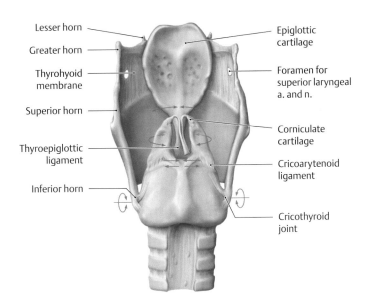

C Posterior view. Arrows indicate the directions of movement in the various joints.

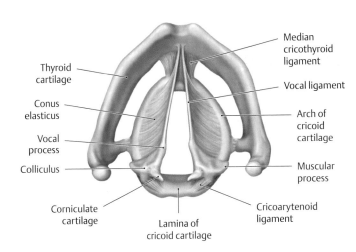

D Superior view.

Larynx: Muscles & Levels

Fig. 37.22 Laryngeal muscles

The laryngeal muscles move the laryngeal cartilages relative to one another, affecting the tension and/or position of the vocal folds. Muscles that move the larynx as a whole (infra- and suprahyoid muscles) are described on p. 562.

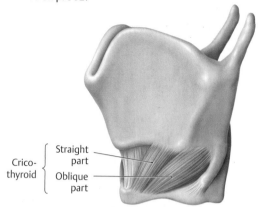

A Extrinsic laryngeal muscles, left lateral oblique view.

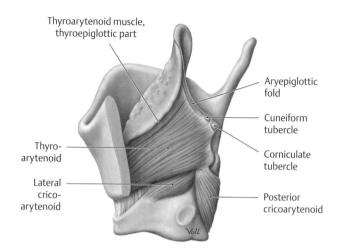

B Intrinsic laryngeal muscles, left lateral view. *Removed:* Thyroid cartilage (left half). *Revealed:* Epiglottis and external thyroarytenoid muscle.

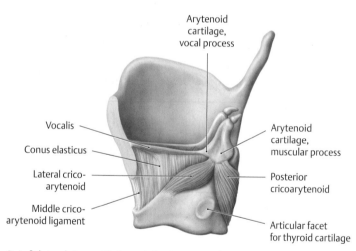

C Left lateral view with the epiglottis removed.

D Posterior view.

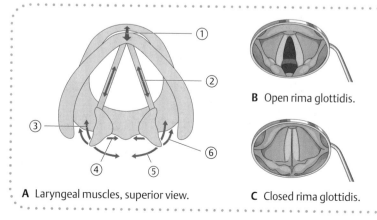

A Laryngeal muscles, superior view.

B Open rima glottidis.

C Closed rima glottidis.

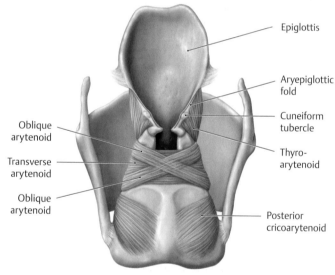

Table 37.9	Actions of the laryngeal muscles	
Muscle	**Action**	**Effect on rima glottidis**
① Cricothyroid m.*	Tightens the vocal folds	None
② Vocalis m.		
③ Thyroarytenoid m.	Adducts the vocal folds	Closes
④ Transverse arytenoid m.		
⑤ Posterior cricoarytenoid m.	Abducts the vocal folds	Opens
⑥ Lateral cricoarytenoid m.	Adducts the vocal folds	Closes

* The cricothyroid is the only extrinsic laryngeal muscle.

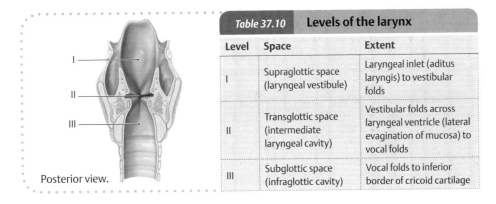

Table 37.10	Levels of the larynx	
Level	**Space**	**Extent**
I	Supraglottic space (laryngeal vestibule)	Laryngeal inlet (aditus laryngis) to vestibular folds
II	Transglottic space (intermediate laryngeal cavity)	Vestibular folds across laryngeal ventricle (lateral evagination of mucosa) to vocal folds
III	Subglottic space (infraglottic cavity)	Vocal folds to inferior border of cricoid cartilage

Posterior view.

Fig. 37.23 Cavity of the larynx

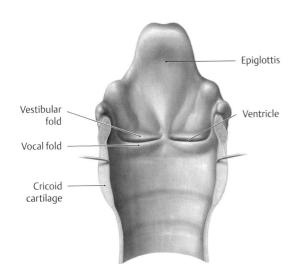

A Posterior view with the larynx splayed open.

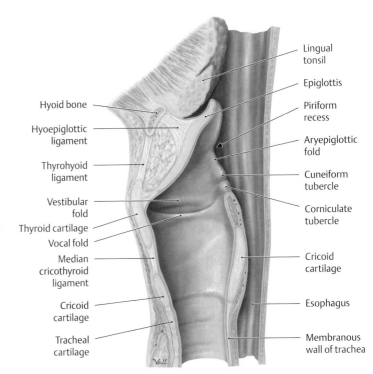

B Midsagittal section viewed from the left side.

Fig. 37.24 Vestibular and vocal folds

Coronal section, superior view.

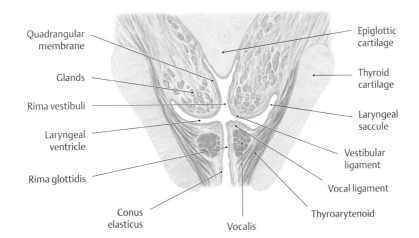

Neurovasculature of the Larynx, Thyroid & Parathyroids

Fig. 37.25 **Thyroid and parathyroid glands**

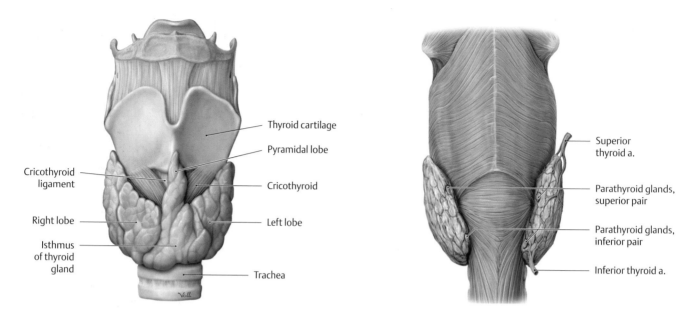

Thyroid cartilage

Pyramidal lobe

Cricothyroid ligament

Cricothyroid

Right lobe

Left lobe

Isthmus of thyroid gland

Trachea

A Thyroid gland, anterior view.

Superior thyroid a.

Parathyroid glands, superior pair

Parathyroid glands, inferior pair

Inferior thyroid a.

B Thyroid and parathyroid glands, posterior view.

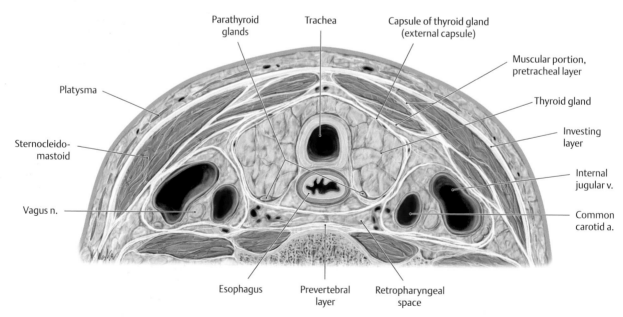

Parathyroid glands

Trachea

Capsule of thyroid gland (external capsule)

Platysma

Muscular portion, pretracheal layer

Thyroid gland

Sternocleido-mastoid

Investing layer

Internal jugular v.

Vagus n.

Common carotid a.

Esophagus

Prevertebral layer

Retropharyngeal space

C Topographical relations of the thyroid and parathyroid glands. See p. 577 for the layers of cervical fascia.

Fig. 37.26 **Arteries and nerves**
Anterior view.

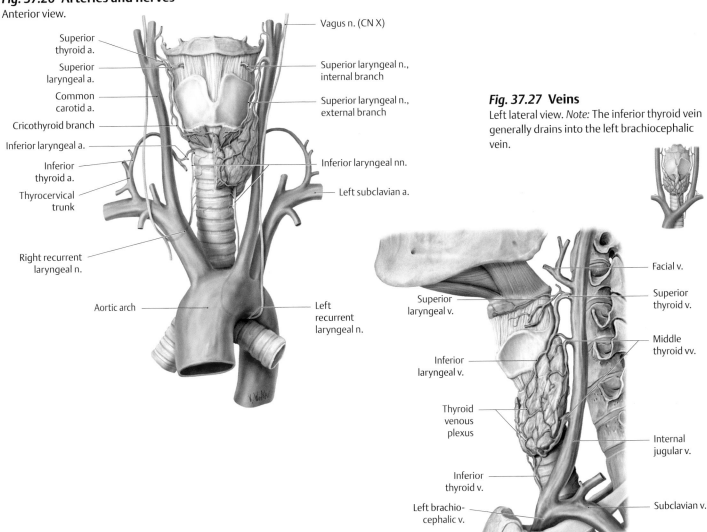

- Vagus n. (CN X)
- Superior thyroid a.
- Superior laryngeal a.
- Common carotid a.
- Cricothyroid branch
- Inferior laryngeal a.
- Inferior thyroid a.
- Thyrocervical trunk
- Superior laryngeal n., internal branch
- Superior laryngeal n., external branch
- Inferior laryngeal nn.
- Left subclavian a.
- Right recurrent laryngeal n.
- Aortic arch
- Left recurrent laryngeal n.

Fig. 37.27 **Veins**
Left lateral view. *Note:* The inferior thyroid vein generally drains into the left brachiocephalic vein.

- Superior laryngeal v.
- Inferior laryngeal v.
- Thyroid venous plexus
- Inferior thyroid v.
- Left brachio-cephalic v.
- Facial v.
- Superior thyroid v.
- Middle thyroid vv.
- Internal jugular v.
- Subclavian v.

Fig. 37.28 **Neurovasculature**
Left lateral view.

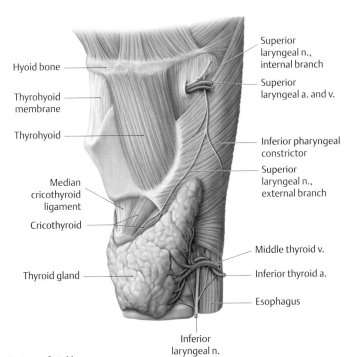

- Hyoid bone
- Thyrohyoid membrane
- Thyrohyoid
- Median cricothyroid ligament
- Cricothyroid
- Thyroid gland
- Superior laryngeal n., internal branch
- Superior laryngeal a. and v.
- Inferior pharyngeal constrictor
- Superior laryngeal n., external branch
- Middle thyroid v.
- Inferior thyroid a.
- Esophagus
- Inferior laryngeal n.

A Superficial layer.

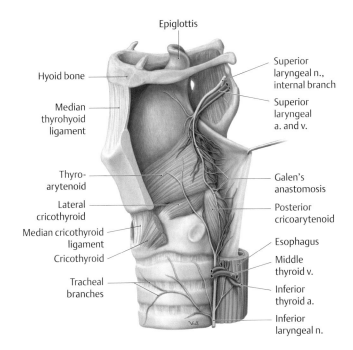

- Epiglottis
- Hyoid bone
- Median thyrohyoid ligament
- Thyro-arytenoid
- Lateral cricothyroid
- Median cricothyroid ligament
- Cricothyroid
- Tracheal branches
- Superior laryngeal n., internal branch
- Superior laryngeal a. and v.
- Galen's anastomosis
- Posterior cricoarytenoid
- Esophagus
- Middle thyroid v.
- Inferior thyroid a.
- Inferior laryngeal n.

B Deep layer. *Removed:* Cricothyroid muscle and left lamina of thyroid cartilage. *Retracted:* Pharyngeal mucosa.

Topography of the Neck: Regions & Fascia

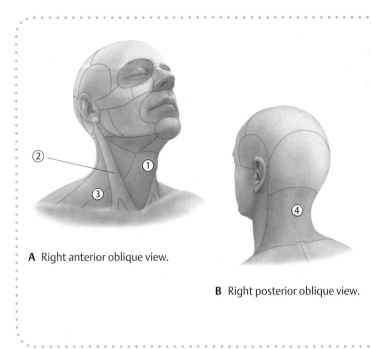

A Right anterior oblique view.

B Right posterior oblique view.

Table 37.11		Regions of the neck
Region	**Divisions**	**Contents**
① Anterior cervical region (triangle)	Submandibular (digastric) triangle	Submandibular gland and lymph nodes, hypoglossal n. (CN XII), facial a. and v.
	Submental triangle	Submental lymph nodes
	Muscular triangle	Sternothyroid and sternohyoid muscles, thyroid and parathyroid glands
	Carotid triangle	Carotid bifurcation, carotid body, hypoglossal (CN XII) and vagus (CN X) nn.
② Sternocleidomastoid region*		Sternocleidomastoid, carotid a., internal jugular v., vagus n. (CN X), jugular lymph nodes
③ Lateral cervical region (posterior triangle)	Omoclavicular (subclavian) triangle	Subclavian a., subscapular a., supraclavicular l.n.
	Occipital triangle	Accessory n. (CN XI), trunks of brachial plexus, transverse cervical a., cervical plexus (posterior branches)
④ Posterior cervical region		Nuchal muscles, vertebral a., cervical plexus

* The sternocleidomastoid region also contains the lesser supraclavicular fossa.

Fig. 37.29 **Cervical regions**

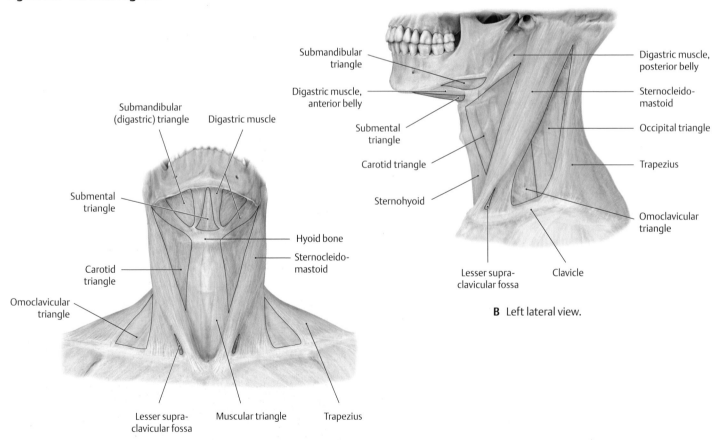

A Anterior view.

B Left lateral view.

Table 37.12	Deep cervical fascia			

The deep cervical fascia is divided into four layers that enclose the structures of the neck.

Layer	Lamina	Type of fascia	Description
① Investing layer	Superficial lamina	Muscular	Envelopes entire neck; splits to enclose sternocleidomastoid and trapezius muscles
Pretracheal layer	② Pretracheal lamina		Encloses infrahyoid muscles
	③ Visceral fascia	Visceral	Surrounds thyroid gland, larynx, trachea, pharynx, and esophagus
④ Prevertebral layer	Prevertebral lamina	Muscular	Surrounds cervical vertebral column and associated muscles
⑤ Carotid sheath		Neurovascular	Encloses common carotid artery, internal jugular vein, and vagus nerve

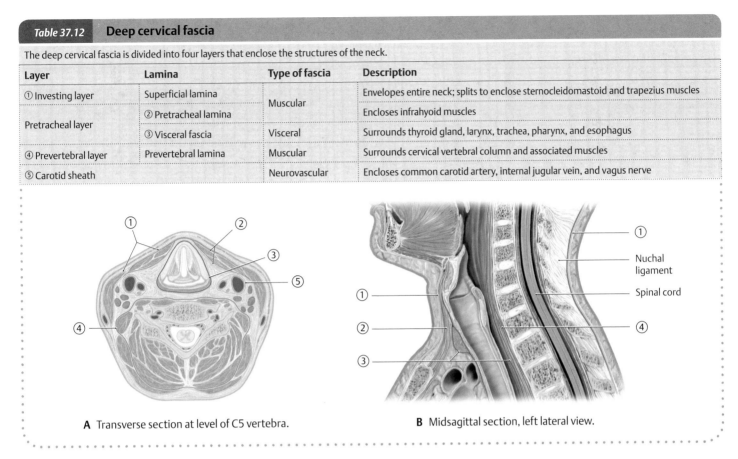

A Transverse section at level of C5 vertebra.

B Midsagittal section, left lateral view.

Fig. 37.30 Deep cervical fascial layers
Anterior view.

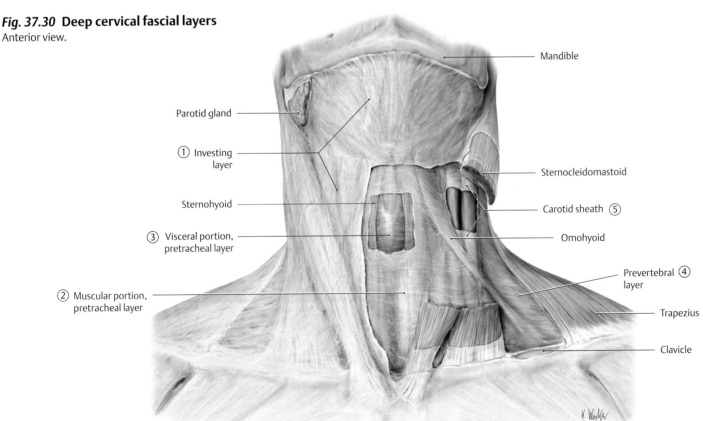

Topography of the Anterior Cervical Region

Fig. 37.31 **Anterior cervical triangle**
Anterior view.

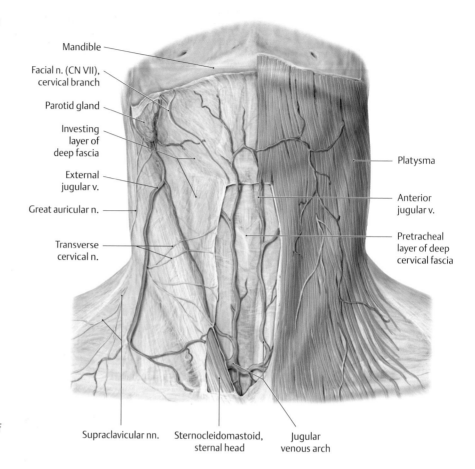

A Superficial layer. *Removed:* Subcutaneous platysma (right side) and investing layer of deep cervical fascia (center).

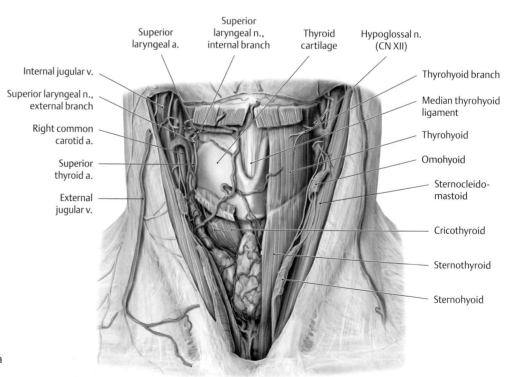

B Deep layer. *Removed:* Pretracheal lamina (middle layer of cervical fascia).

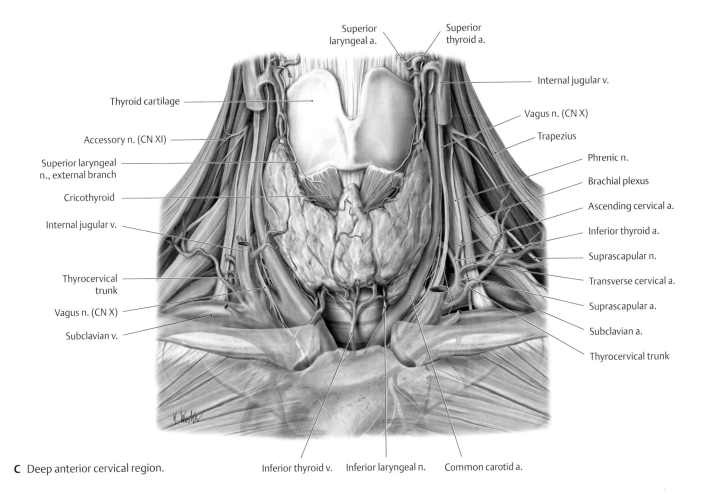

C Deep anterior cervical region.

Superior laryngeal a.

Superior thyroid a.

Thyroid cartilage

Accessory n. (CN XI)

Superior laryngeal n., external branch

Cricothyroid

Internal jugular v.

Thyrocervical trunk

Vagus n. (CN X)

Subclavian v.

Internal jugular v.

Vagus n. (CN X)

Trapezius

Phrenic n.

Brachial plexus

Ascending cervical a.

Inferior thyroid a.

Suprascapular n.

Transverse cervical a.

Suprascapular a.

Subclavian a.

Thyrocervical trunk

Inferior thyroid v.

Inferior laryngeal n.

Common carotid a.

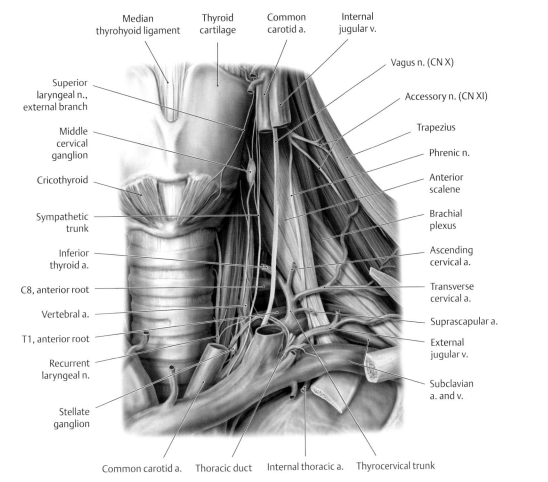

D Root of the neck.

Median thyrohyoid ligament

Thyroid cartilage

Common carotid a.

Internal jugular v.

Superior laryngeal n., external branch

Middle cervical ganglion

Cricothyroid

Sympathetic trunk

Inferior thyroid a.

C8, anterior root

Vertebral a.

T1, anterior root

Recurrent laryngeal n.

Stellate ganglion

Common carotid a.

Thoracic duct

Internal thoracic a.

Thyrocervical trunk

Vagus n. (CN X)

Accessory n. (CN XI)

Trapezius

Phrenic n.

Anterior scalene

Brachial plexus

Ascending cervical a.

Transverse cervical a.

Suprascapular a.

External jugular v.

Subclavian a. and v.

579

Topography of the Anterior & Lateral Cervical Regions

Fig. 37.32 **Carotid triangle**
Right lateral view.

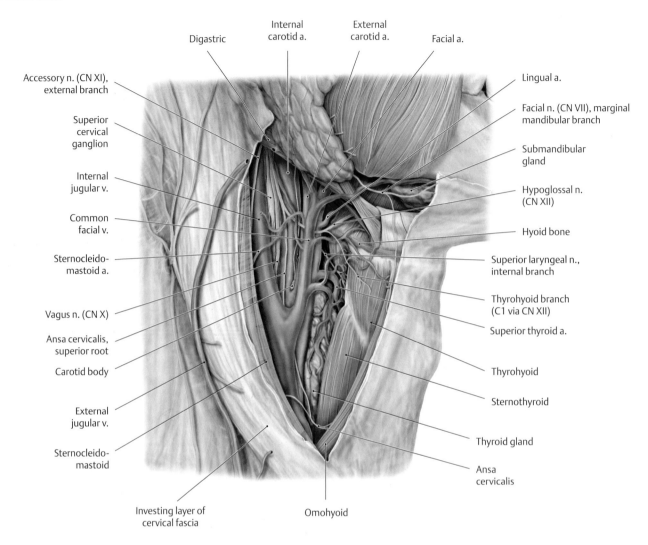

Accessory n. (CN XI), external branch

Superior cervical ganglion

Internal jugular v.

Common facial v.

Sternocleido-mastoid a.

Vagus n. (CN X)

Ansa cervicalis, superior root

Carotid body

External jugular v.

Sternocleido-mastoid

Investing layer of cervical fascia

Omohyoid

Digastric

Internal carotid a.

External carotid a.

Facial a.

Lingual a.

Facial n. (CN VII), marginal mandibular branch

Submandibular gland

Hypoglossal n. (CN XII)

Hyoid bone

Superior laryngeal n., internal branch

Thyrohyoid branch (C1 via CN XII)

Superior thyroid a.

Thyrohyoid

Sternothyroid

Thyroid gland

Ansa cervicalis

Fig. 37.33 **Deep lateral cervical region**
Right lateral view with sternocleidomastoid windowed.

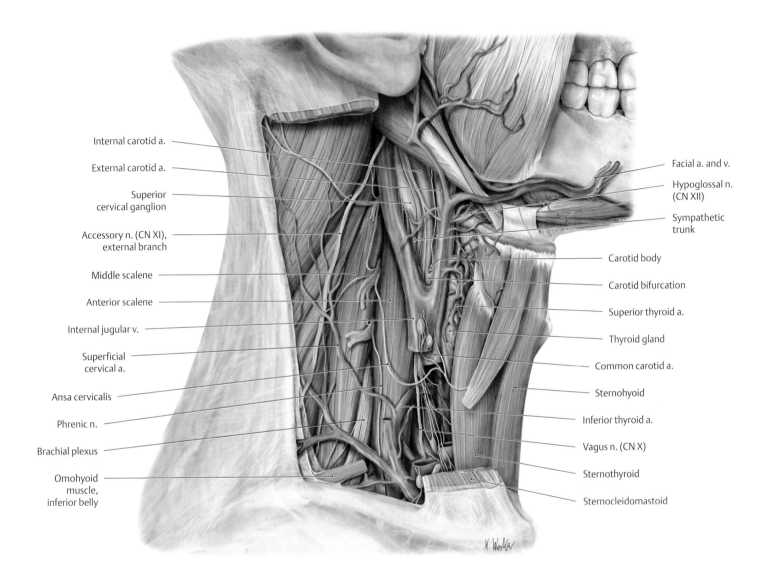

Internal carotid a.

External carotid a.

Superior cervical ganglion

Accessory n. (CN XI), external branch

Middle scalene

Anterior scalene

Internal jugular v.

Superficial cervical a.

Ansa cervicalis

Phrenic n.

Brachial plexus

Omohyoid muscle, inferior belly

Facial a. and v.

Hypoglossal n. (CN XII)

Sympathetic trunk

Carotid body

Carotid bifurcation

Superior thyroid a.

Thyroid gland

Common carotid a.

Sternohyoid

Inferior thyroid a.

Vagus n. (CN X)

Sternothyroid

Sternocleidomastoid

Topography of the Lateral Cervical Region

Fig. 37.34 **Lateral cervical region**
Right lateral view. The contents of the deep lateral cervical region are found in Fig. 37.33.

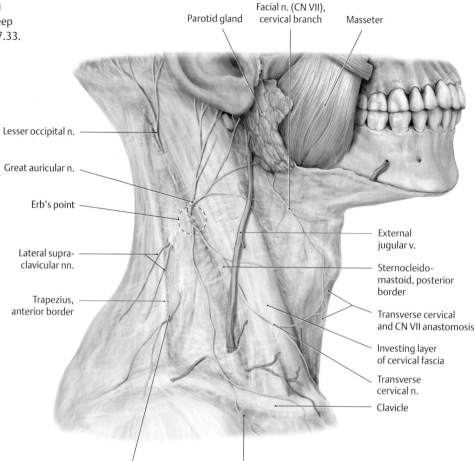

Parotid gland — Facial n. (CN VII), cervical branch — Masseter

Lesser occipital n.

Great auricular n.

Erb's point

Lateral supra-clavicular nn.

Trapezius, anterior border

External jugular v.

Sternocleido-mastoid, posterior border

Transverse cervical and CN VII anastomosis

Investing layer of cervical fascia

Transverse cervical n.

Clavicle

A Subcutaneous layer.

Intermediate supra-clavicular nn.

Medial supra-clavicular nn.

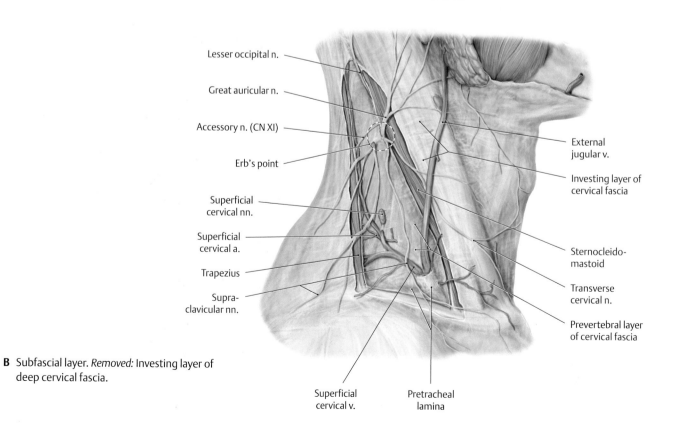

Lesser occipital n.

Great auricular n.

Accessory n. (CN XI)

Erb's point

Superficial cervical nn.

Superficial cervical a.

Trapezius

Supra-clavicular nn.

External jugular v.

Investing layer of cervical fascia

Sternocleido-mastoid

Transverse cervical n.

Prevertebral layer of cervical fascia

B Subfascial layer. *Removed:* Investing layer of deep cervical fascia.

Superficial cervical v.

Pretracheal lamina

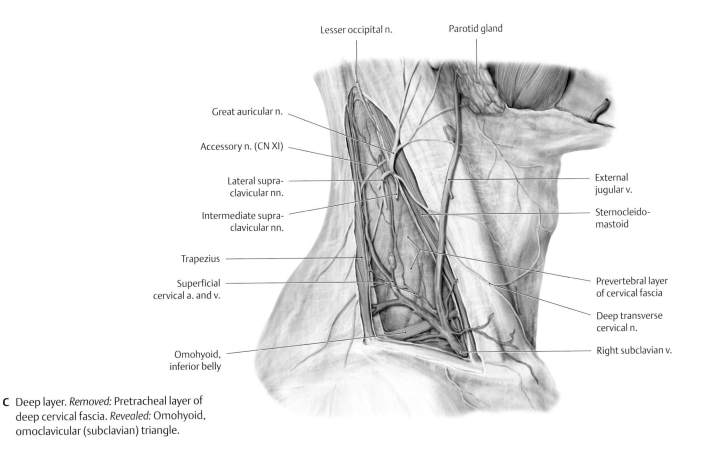

Lesser occipital n.

Parotid gland

Great auricular n.

Accessory n. (CN XI)

Lateral supra-
clavicular nn.

Intermediate supra-
clavicular nn.

Trapezius

Superficial
cervical a. and v.

Omohyoid,
inferior belly

External
jugular v.

Sternocleido-
mastoid

Prevertebral layer
of cervical fascia

Deep transverse
cervical n.

Right subclavian v.

C Deep layer. *Removed:* Pretracheal layer of
deep cervical fascia. *Revealed:* Omohyoid,
omoclavicular (subclavian) triangle.

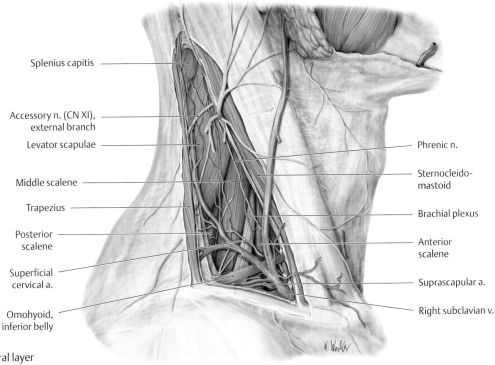

Splenius capitis

Accessory n. (CN XI),
external branch

Levator scapulae

Middle scalene

Trapezius

Posterior
scalene

Superficial
cervical a.

Omohyoid,
inferior belly

Phrenic n.

Sternocleido-
mastoid

Brachial plexus

Anterior
scalene

Suprascapular a.

Right subclavian v.

K. Wesker

D Deepest layer. *Removed:* Prevertebral layer
of deep cervical fascia. *Revealed:* Muscular
floor of posterior triangle, brachial plexus
and phrenic nerve.

Topography of the Posterior Cervical Region

Fig. 37.35 Occipital and posterior cervical regions

Posterior view. Subcutaneous layer (left), subfascial layer (right). The occiput is technically a region of the head, but it is included here due to the continuity of the vessels and nerves from the neck.

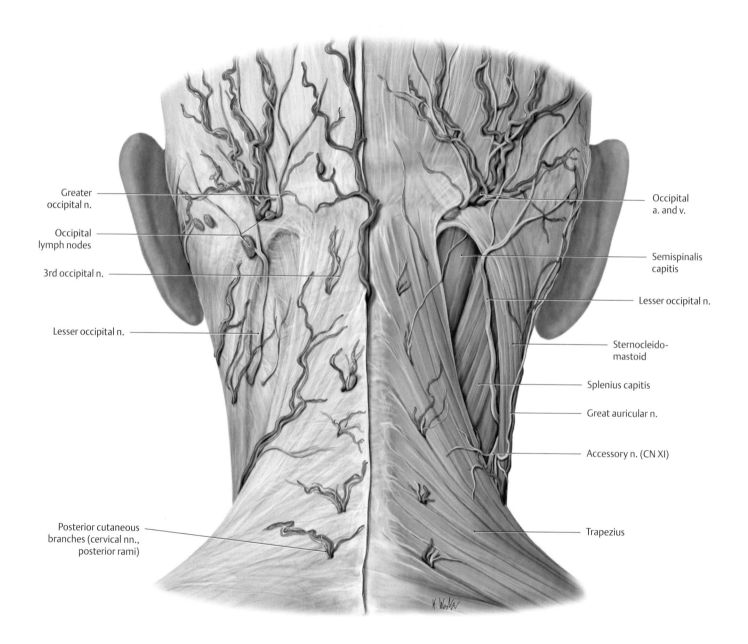

Greater occipital n.

Occipital lymph nodes

3rd occipital n.

Lesser occipital n.

Posterior cutaneous branches (cervical nn., posterior rami)

Occipital a. and v.

Semispinalis capitis

Lesser occipital n.

Sternocleido-mastoid

Splenius capitis

Great auricular n.

Accessory n. (CN XI)

Trapezius

Fig. 37.36 **Suboccipital triangle**

Right side, posterior view. The suboccipital triangle is bounded by the suboccipital muscles (rectus capitis posterior major and obliquus capitis superior and inferior) and contains the vertebral artery. The left and right vertebral arteries pass through the atlanto-occipital membrane and combine to form the basilar artery.

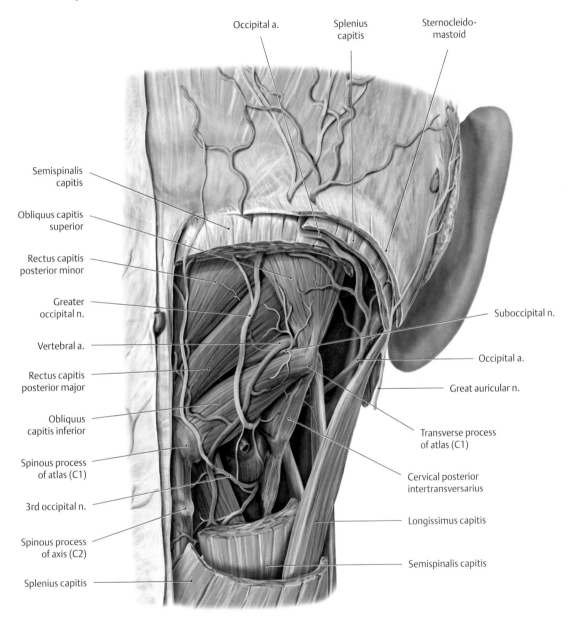

Occipital a.

Splenius capitis

Sternocleido-mastoid

Semispinalis capitis

Obliquus capitis superior

Rectus capitis posterior minor

Greater occipital n.

Vertebral a.

Rectus capitis posterior major

Obliquus capitis inferior

Spinous process of atlas (C1)

3rd occipital n.

Spinous process of axis (C2)

Splenius capitis

Suboccipital n.

Occipital a.

Great auricular n.

Transverse process of atlas (C1)

Cervical posterior intertransversarius

Longissimus capitis

Semispinalis capitis

Lymphatics of the Neck

Fig. 37.37 **Lymphatic drainage regions**
Right lateral view.

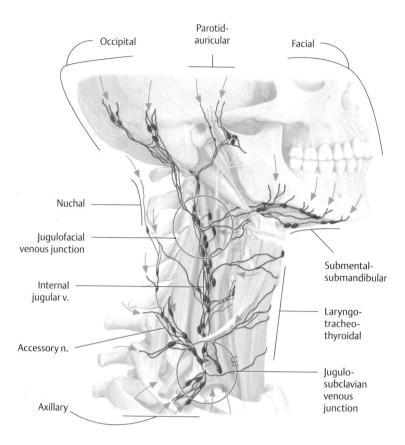

Labels on figure: Occipital, Parotid-auricular, Facial, Nuchal, Jugulofacial venous junction, Internal jugular v., Accessory n., Axillary, Submental-submandibular, Laryngo-tracheo-thyroidal, Jugulo-subclavian venous junction

---

⚕ Clinical

Tumor metastasis

Lymph from the entire body is channeled to the left and right jugulosubclavian junctions (red circles). Gastric carcinoma may metastasize to the left supraclavicular group of lymph nodes, producing an enlarged *sentinel node* (see pp. 73, 231). Systemic lymphomas may also spread to the cervical lymph nodes by this pathway.

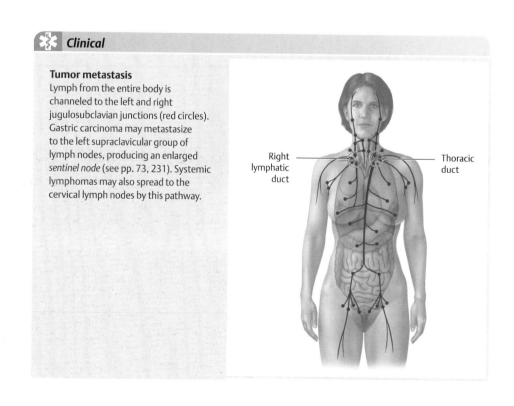

Labels on figure: Right lymphatic duct, Thoracic duct

Fig. 37.38 Superficial cervical lymph nodes
Right lateral view.

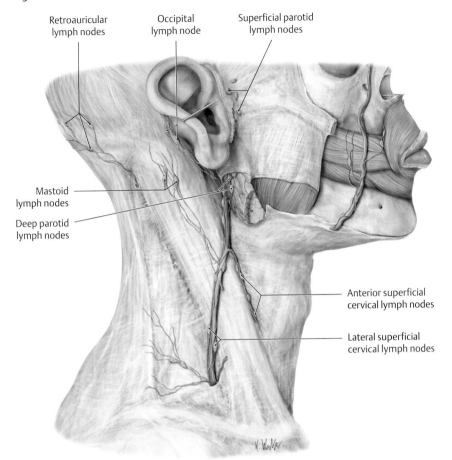

Retroauricular lymph nodes

Occipital lymph node

Superficial parotid lymph nodes

Mastoid lymph nodes

Deep parotid lymph nodes

Anterior superficial cervical lymph nodes

Lateral superficial cervical lymph nodes

Table 37.13	Superficial cervical lymph nodes	
Lymph nodes (l.n.)	**Drainage region**	
Retroauricular l.n.	Occiput	
Occipital l.n.		
Mastoid l.n.		
Superficial parotid l.n.	Parotid-auricular region	
Deep parotid l.n.		
Anterior superficial cervical l.n.	Sternocleidomastoid region	
Lateral superficial cervical l.n.		

Fig. 37.39 Deep cervical lymph nodes
Right lateral view.

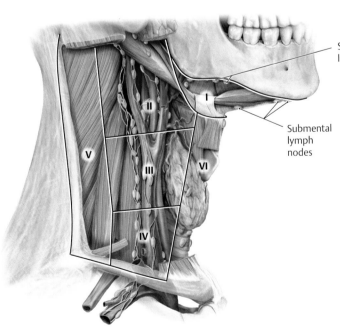

Submandibular lymph nodes

Submental lymph nodes

Table 37.14	Deep cervical lymph nodes		
Level	**Lymph nodes (l.n.)**		**Drainage region**
I	Submental l.n.		Face
	Submandibular l.n.		
II	Lateral jugular l.n. group	Upper lateral group	Nuchal region, laryngo-tracheo-thyroidal region
III		Middle lateral group	
IV		Lower lateral group	
V	L.n. in posterior cervical triangle		Nuchal region
VI	Anterior cervical l.n.		Laryngo-tracheo-thyroidal region

Surface Anatomy

Fig. 38.1 Surface anatomy of the skull and nuchal region

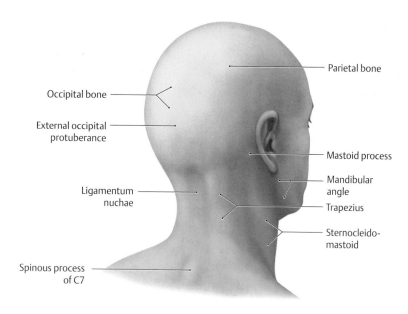

Parietal bone

Occipital bone

External occipital protuberance

Ligamentum nuchae

Spinous process of C7

Mastoid process

Mandibular angle

Trapezius

Sternocleido-mastoid

A Surface anatomy. Right posterolateral view.

Q1: Injecting a bolus of anesthetic two thirds of the way up the posterior border of the sternocleidomastoid would accomplish what task?

Q2: What palpable bony landmark would you use to auscultate the venous blood in the confluence of the sinuses?

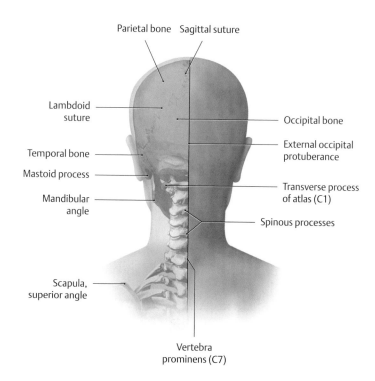

Parietal bone   Sagittal suture

Lambdoid suture

Temporal bone

Mastoid process

Mandibular angle

Occipital bone

External occipital protuberance

Transverse process of atlas (C1)

Spinous processes

Scapula, superior angle

Vertebra prominens (C7)

B Palpable bony prominences. Posterior view.

Fig. 38.2 Surface anatomy of the face and neck

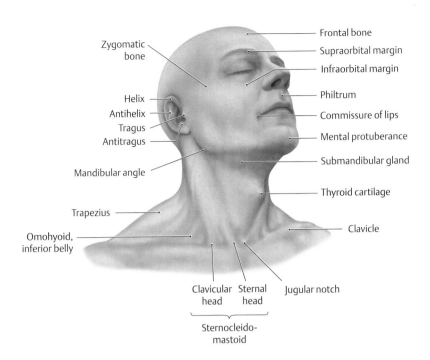

Zygomatic bone

Helix
Antihelix
Tragus
Antitragus

Mandibular angle

Trapezius

Omohyoid, inferior belly

Frontal bone
Supraorbital margin
Infraorbital margin
Philtrum
Commissure of lips
Mental protuberance
Submandibular gland
Thyroid cartilage
Clavicle

Clavicular head   Sternal head   Jugular notch

Sternocleido-mastoid

A Surface anatomy. Right anterolateral view.

Q3: What are the boundaries of the lateral cervical triangle (posterior triangle)? Name two structures within this region that supply motor innervation to the muscles of the upper limb.

Q4: What are the boundaries of the carotid triangle? Name one non-vascular component of the vertical neurovascular bundle within the carotid sheath located in the carotid triangle.

Q5: What is the anatomical structure referred to as the "Adam's apple"?

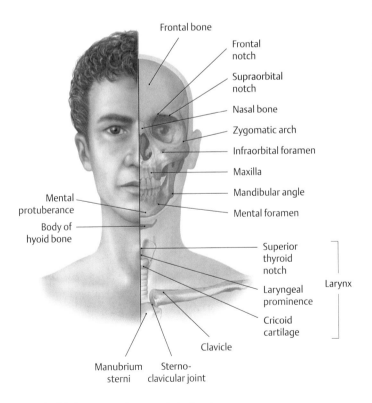

Frontal bone
Frontal notch
Supraorbital notch
Nasal bone
Zygomatic arch
Infraorbital foramen
Maxilla
Mandibular angle
Mental foramen

Mental protuberance
Body of hyoid bone

Superior thyroid notch
Laryngeal prominence
Cricoid cartilage

Larynx

Clavicle

Manubrium sterni   Sterno-clavicular joint

B Palpable bony prominences. Anterior view.

See answers beginning on p. 626.

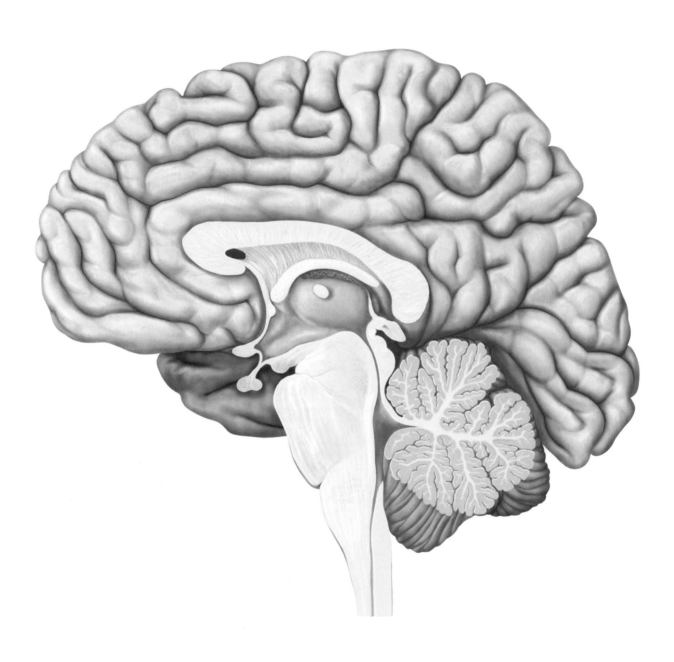

Neuroanatomy

Nervous System: Overview

Fig. 39.1 Central and peripheral nervous systems

The nervous system is divided into the central (CNS) and peripheral (PNS) nervous systems. The CNS consists of the brain and spinal cord, which comprise a functional unit. The PNS consists of the nerves emerging from the brain and spinal cord (cranial and spinal nerves, respectively).

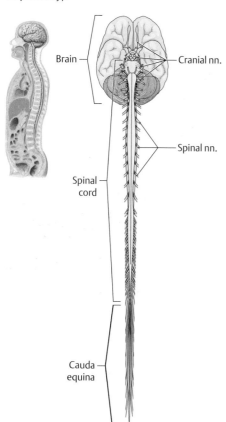

Fig. 39.2 Neurons (nerve cells)

The nervous system is composed of neurons (nerve cells) and supporting neuroglial cells, which vastly outnumber them (10 to 1). Each neuron contains a cell body (soma) with one axon (projecting segment) and one or more dendrites (receptor segments). The release of neurotransmitters at synapses creates an excitatory or inhibitory postsynaptic potential at the target neuron. If this exceeds the depolarization threshold of the neuron, the axon "fires," initiating the release of a transmitter from its presynaptic knob (bouton).

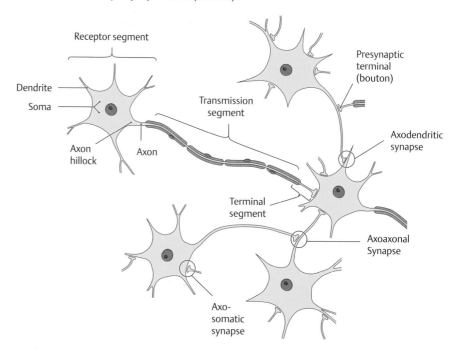

Fig. 39.4 Gray and white matter in the CNS

Nerve cell bodies appear gray in gross inspection, whereas nerve cell processes (axons) and their insulating myelin sheaths appear white.

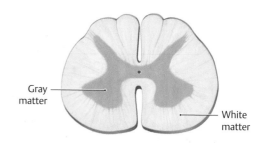

A Coronal section through the brain.

Fig. 39.3 Myelination

Certain glial cells with lipid-rich membranes may myelinate axons (nerve fibers). Myelination electrically insulates axons, thereby increasing impulse conduction speed. In the CNS, one oligodendrocyte myelinates multiple axons; in the PNS, one Schwann cell myelinates one axon.

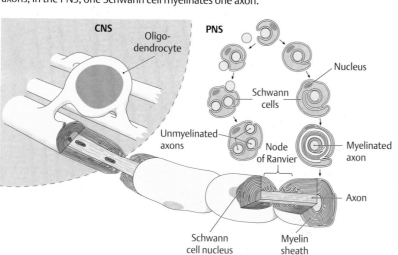

B Transverse section through the spinal cord.

Table 39.1	Development of the brain			
	Primary vesicle	**Region**		**Structure**
Neural tube	Pros-encephalon (forebrain)	Telencephalon (cerebrum)		Cerebral cortex, white matter, and basal ganglia
		Diencephalon		Epithalamus (pineal), dorsal thalamus, subthalamus, and hypothalamus
	Mesencephalon (midbrain)*			Tectum, tegmentum, and cerebral peduncles
	Rhombencephalon (hindbrain)	Metencephalon	Cerebellum	Cerebellar cortex, nuclei, and peduncles
			Pons*	Nuclei and fiber tracts
		Myelencephalon	Medulla oblongata*	

* The mesencephalon, pons, and medulla oblongata are collectively known as the brainstem.

Fig. 39.5 Embryonic development of the brain
Left lateral view.

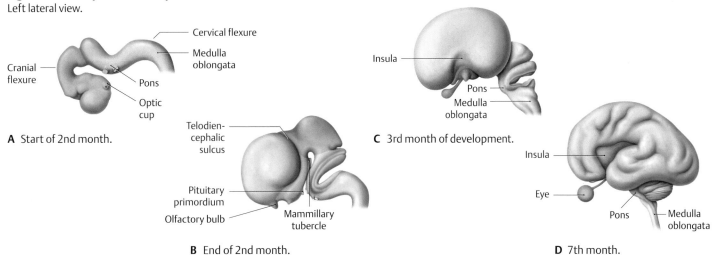

A Start of 2nd month.

B End of 2nd month.

C 3rd month of development.

D 7th month.

Fig. 39.6 Adult brain
See Fig. 39.12 for lobes of the cerebrum. CN = cranial nerve.

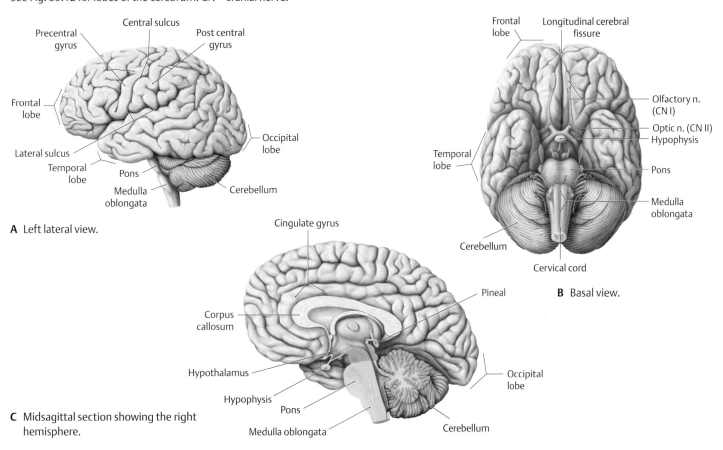

A Left lateral view.

B Basal view.

C Midsagittal section showing the right hemisphere.

Telencephalon

Fig. 39.7 Divisions of the telencephalon

Coronal section, anterior view. The telencephalon is divided into the cerebral cortex, white matter, and basal ganglia. The cerebral cortex is further divided into the allocortex and isocortex (neocortex).

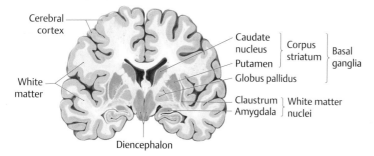

Fig. 39.8 White matter

A special preparation technique was used to show the fiber structure of the superficial layer of white matter.

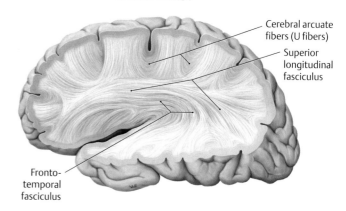

A Lateral view of left hemisphere.

Fig. 39.9 Basal ganglia

Transverse section, superior view. The basal ganglia are an essential component of the motor system (see p. 615).

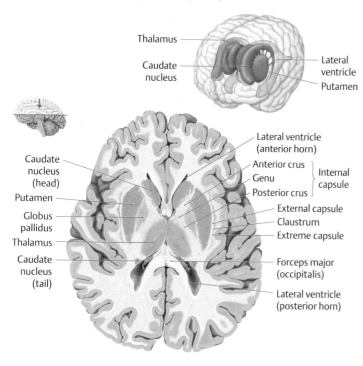

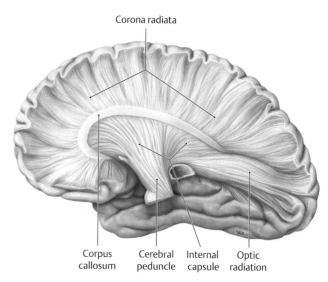

B Medial view of right hemisphere.

Fig. 39.10 Allocortex

The three-layered allocortex consists of the olfactory cortex (blue) and the hippocampus (pink).

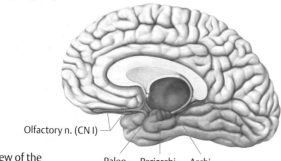

A Medial view of the right hemisphere.

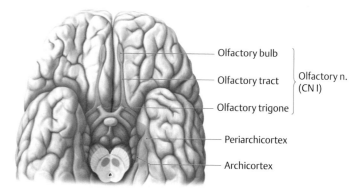

B Basal view.

Fig. 39.11 **Isocortex: Columnar organization**

Morphological considerations divide the isocortex into six horizontal layers; functional considerations divide it into cortical columns.

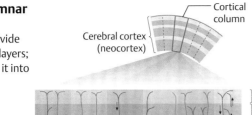

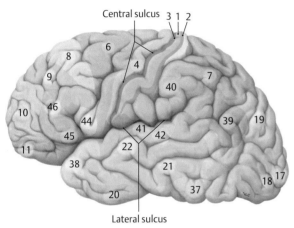

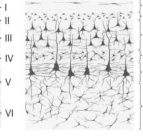

	Layers
Molecular layer (I)	
External granular layer (II)	
External pyramidal layer (III)	
Internal granular layer (IV)	**Layers**
Internal pyramidal layer (V)	
Multiform layer (VI)	

A Histology of the isocortex.

B Brodmann (cortical) areas, lateral view of the left cerebral hemisphere.

C Brodmann (cortical) areas, medial view of the right cerebral hemisphere.

Fig. 39.12 **Lobes in the cerebral hemispheres**

The isocortex also may be functionally divided into association areas (lobes).

Frontal lobe
Parietal lobe
Temporal lobe
Occipital lobe
Insular lobe (insula)
Limbic lobe (limbus)

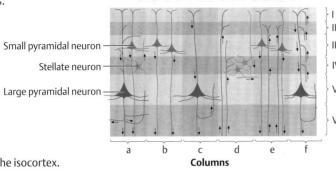

A Lateral view of the left hemisphere.

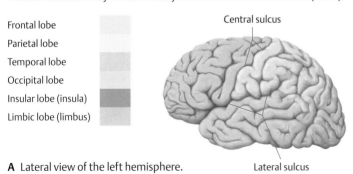

C Medial view of the right hemisphere.

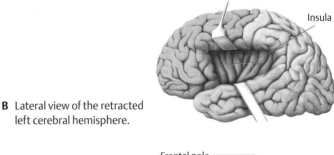

B Lateral view of the retracted left cerebral hemisphere.

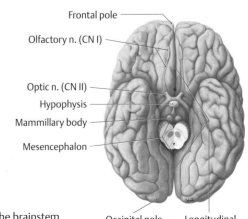

D Basal view with the brainstem removed.

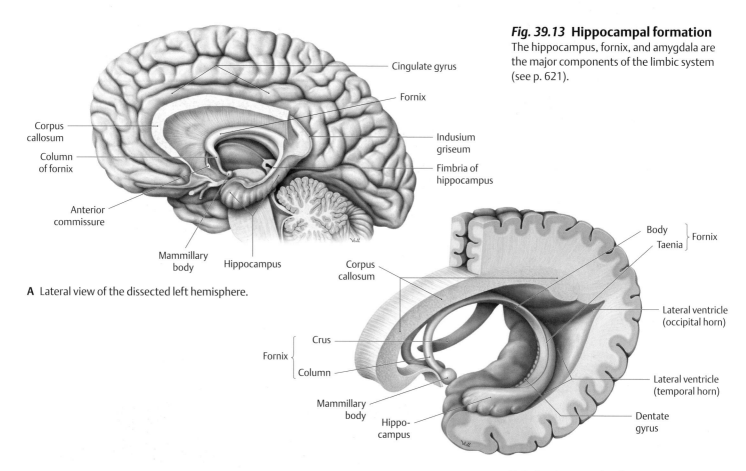

Fig. 39.13 Hippocampal formation

The hippocampus, fornix, and amygdala are the major components of the limbic system (see p. 621).

A Lateral view of the dissected left hemisphere.

B Left anterosuperior view.

Fig. 39.14 Diencephalon

Midsagittal section, medial view of the right hemisphere. The major components of the diencephalon are the thalamus, hypothalamus, and hypophysis (anterior lobe). See p. 598 for the extracted diencephalon.

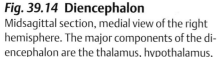

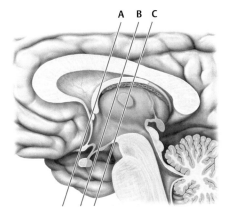

Fig. 39.15 Telencephalon and diencephalon: Internal structure
Coronal section.

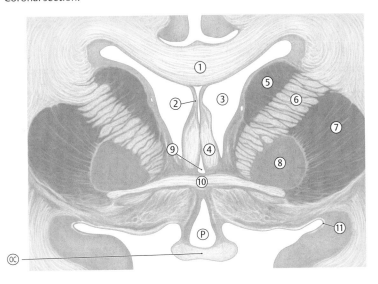

A Level of the optic chiasm.

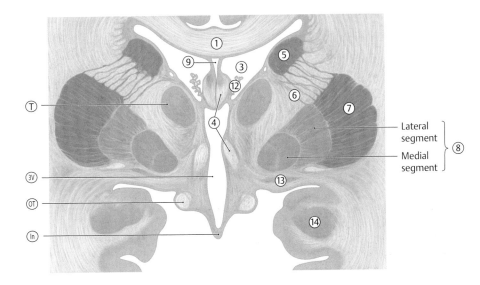

B Level of the tuber cinereum.

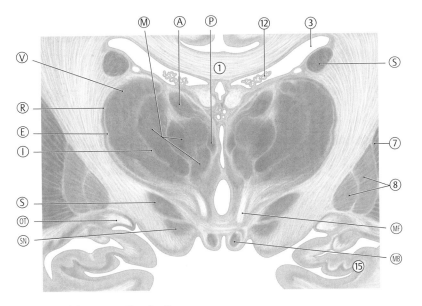

C Level of the mammillary bodies.

Table 39.2	Structures of the diencephalon	
Ⓟ	Preoptic recess	
ⓄⒸ	Optic chiasm	
③Ⓥ	3rd ventricle	
ⓄⓉ	Optic tract	
ⓘₙ	Infundibulum	
Ⓣ	Thalamus (with thalamic nuclei):	
	Ⓡ	Reticular nucleus of thalamus
	Ⓔ	External medullary lamina
	Ⓥ	Ventrolateral thalamic nuclei
	Ⓘ	Internal medullary lamina
	Ⓜ	Medial thalamic nuclei
	Ⓐ	Anterior thalamic nuclei
	Ⓟ	Paraventricular nuclei
Ⓢ	Subthalamic nucleus	
ⓈⓃ*	Substantia nigra	
ⓂⒻ	Mammillothalamic fasciculus	
ⓂⒷ	Mammillary body	

*Actually a structure of the mesencephalon.

Table 39.3	Structures of the telencephalon
①	Corpus callosum
②	Septum pellucidum
③	Lateral ventricle
④	Fornix
⑤	Caudate nucleus
⑥	Internal capsule
⑦	Putamen
⑧	Globus pallidus
⑨	Cavum septi pellucidi
⑩	Anterior commissure
⑪	Lateral olfactory stria
⑫	Choroid plexus
⑬	Basal ganglia
⑭	Amygdala
⑮	Hippocampus

Diencephalon, Brainstem & Cerebellum

Fig. 39.16 Diencephalon, brainstem, and cerebellum
Left lateral view.

Thalamus
Lateral geniculate body
Pulvinar
Quadrigeminal plate
Anterior lobe
Primary fissure
Optic n. (CN II)
Infundibulum
Mammillary body
Cerebral peduncle
Pons
Flocculus
Medulla oblongata
Horizontal fissure
Posterior lobe
Posterolateral fissure
Tonsil

A Isolated structures.

Corpus callosum
Fornix
Choroid plexus
Pineal
Quadrigeminal plate
Anterior commissure
Central lobule
Primary fissure
Hypothalamus
Optic chiasm
Infundibulum
Adenohypophysis
Neurohypophysis
Lingula
Horizontal fissure
Superior medullary velum
Olive
4th ventricle
Choroid plexus
Nodule
Prebiventral fissure

B Midsagittal section.

Fig. 39.17 Cerebellum

Median part
Lateral parts

Horizontal fissure
Anterior lobe
Primary fissure
Culmen
Quadrangular lobule
Simple lobule
Superior semilunar lobule
Vermis
Posterior lobe
Folium vermis

A Superior view.

Fig. 39.18 Cerebellar peduncles
Tracts of afferent (sensory) or efferent (motor) axons enter or leave the cerebellum through cerebellar peduncles. Afferent axons originate in the spinal cord, vestibular organs, inferior olive, and pons. Efferent axons originate in the cerebellar nuclei.

Superior medullary velum
Central lobule
Lingula
Superior cerebellar peduncle
Middle cerebellar peduncle
Inferior cerebellar peduncle
4th ventricle
Horizontal fissure
Uvula vermis
Nodule
Flocculus
Flocculo-nodular lobe
Pyramid of vermis
Vallecula
Tonsil
Peduncle of flocculus
Intermediate parts

Superior cerebellar peduncle
Inferior cerebellar peduncle
Anterior spinocerebellar tract
Middle cerebellar peduncle
Trigeminal n. (CN V)
Vestibulocochlear n. (CN VIII)
Facial n. (CN VII)
Central tegmental tract
Olive

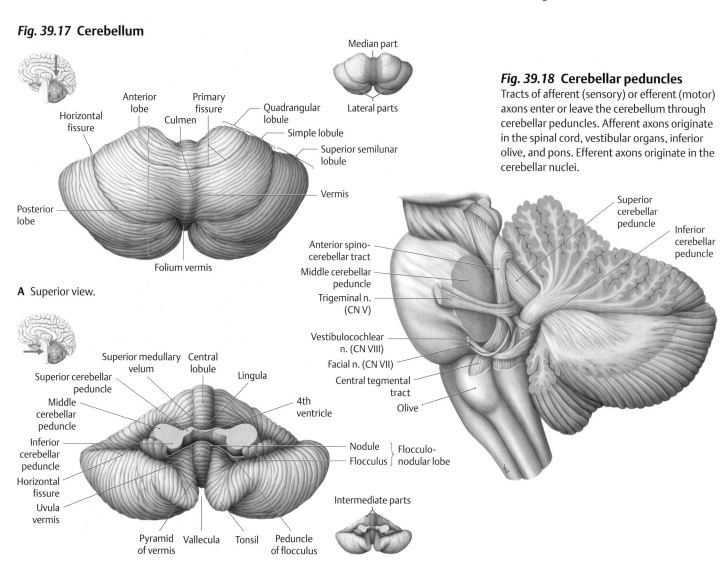

B Anterior view.

Fig. 39.19 **Brainstem**

The brainstem is the site of emergence and entry of the 10 pairs of true cranial nerves (CN III–XII). See p. 470 for an overview of the cranial nerves and their nuclei.

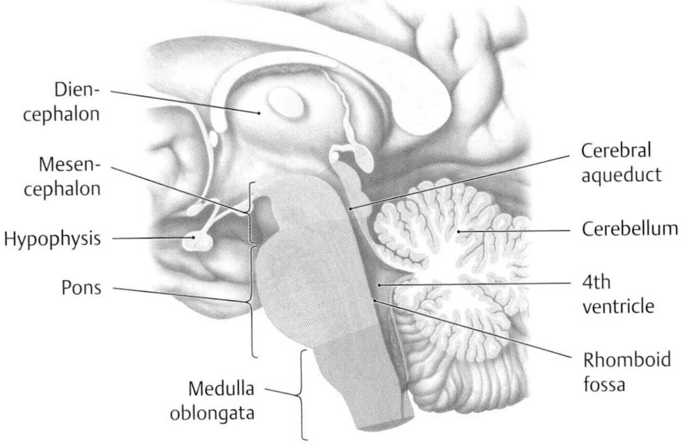

Dien-
cephalon
Mesen-
cephalon
Hypophysis
Pons
Medulla
oblongata
Cerebral
aqueduct
Cerebellum
4th
ventricle
Rhomboid
fossa

A Levels of the brainstem.

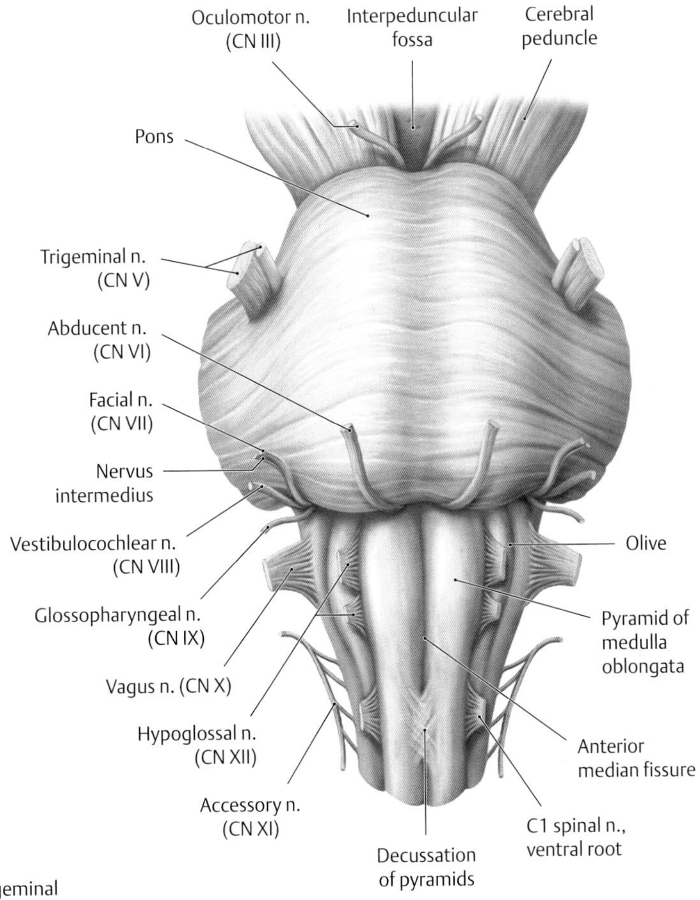

Oculomotor n.
(CN III)
Interpeduncular
fossa
Cerebral
peduncle
Pons
Trigeminal n.
(CN V)
Abducent n.
(CN VI)
Facial n.
(CN VII)
Nervus
intermedius
Vestibulocochlear n.
(CN VIII)
Glossopharyngeal n.
(CN IX)
Vagus n. (CN X)
Hypoglossal n.
(CN XII)
Accessory n.
(CN XI)
Decussation
of pyramids
C1 spinal n.,
ventral root
Anterior
median fissure
Pyramid of
medulla
oblongata
Olive

B Anterior view.

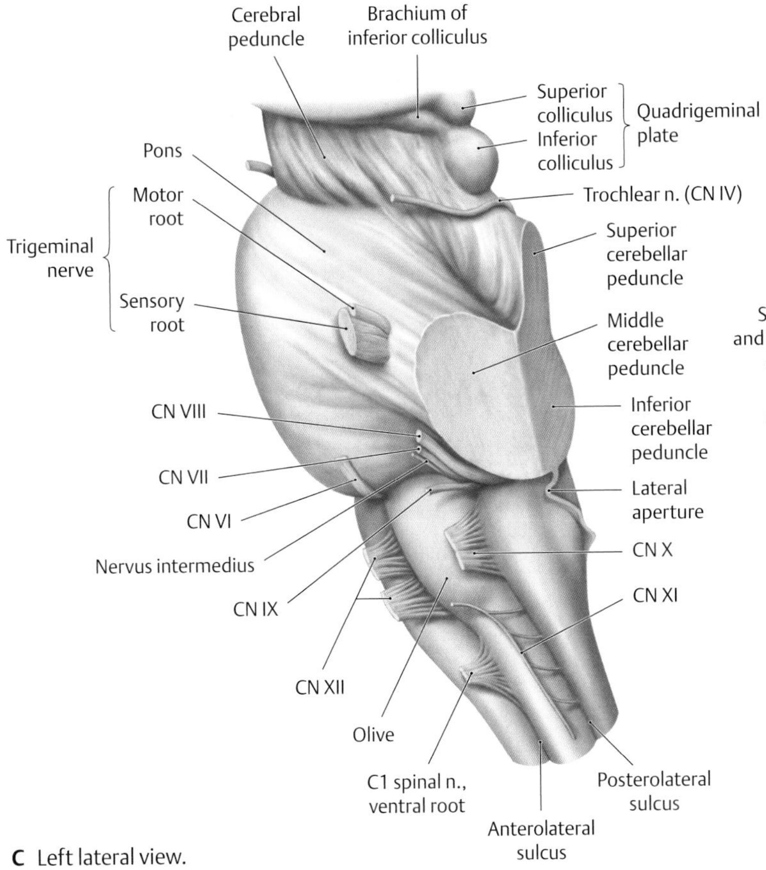

Cerebral
peduncle
Brachium of
inferior colliculus
Superior
colliculus
Inferior
colliculus
Quadrigeminal
plate
Pons
Trigeminal
nerve
Motor
root
Sensory
root
Trochlear n. (CN IV)
Superior
cerebellar
peduncle
Middle
cerebellar
peduncle
Inferior
cerebellar
peduncle
CN VIII
CN VII
CN VI
Nervus intermedius
CN IX
CN XII
Olive
Lateral
aperture
CN X
CN XI
C1 spinal n.,
ventral root
Anterolateral
sulcus
Posterolateral
sulcus

C Left lateral view.

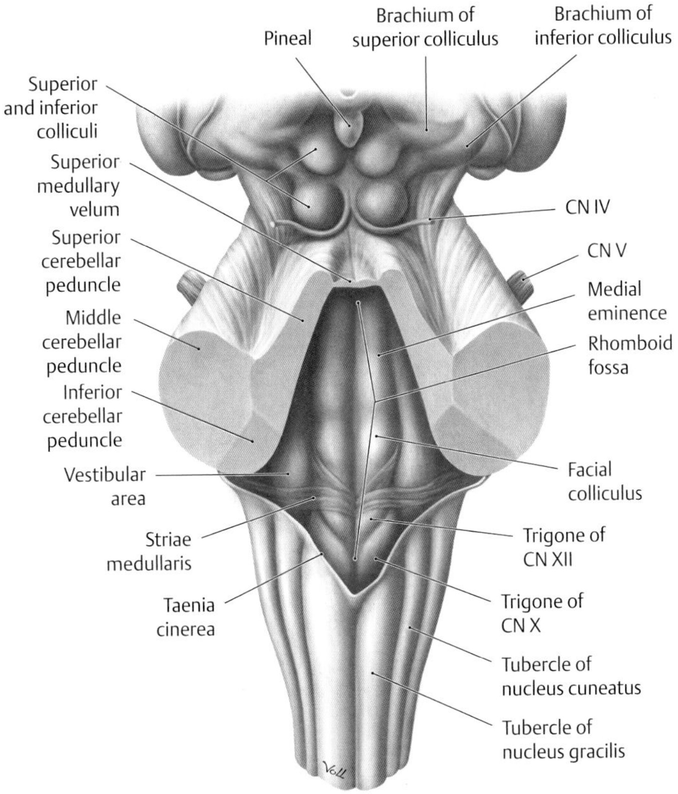

Pineal
Brachium of
superior colliculus
Brachium of
inferior colliculus
Superior
and inferior
colliculi
Superior
medullary
velum
Superior
cerebellar
peduncle
Middle
cerebellar
peduncle
Inferior
cerebellar
peduncle
Vestibular
area
Striae
medullaris
Taenia
cinerea
CN IV
CN V
Medial
eminence
Rhomboid
fossa
Facial
colliculus
Trigone of
CN XII
Trigone of
CN X
Tubercle of
nucleus cuneatus
Tubercle of
nucleus gracilis

D Posterior view.

Spinal Cord

Fig. 39.20 Spinal cord and segments

The spinal cord consists of 31 segments innervating a specific area in the trunk or limbs (see Fig. 39.22). Afferent (sensory) posterior rootlets and efferent (motor) anterior rootlets form the posterior and anterior roots, respectively. The two roots fuse to form a mixed spinal nerve, which then divides into various branches.

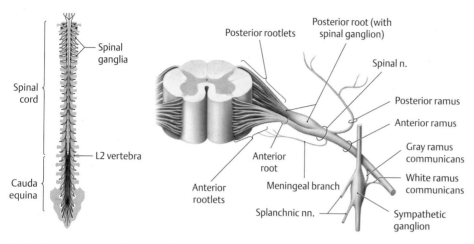

A Spinal cord, posterior view.

B Spinal cord segment, anterior view.

Fig. 39.21 Spinal cord in situ

Posterior view with vertebral canal windowed.

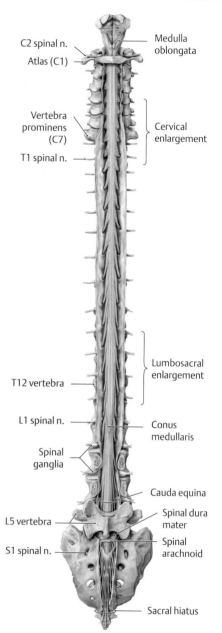

Fig. 39.22 Segmental innervation and spinal cord lesions

The spinal cord is divided into four major regions: cervical, thoracic, lumbar, and sacral. Spinal cord segments are numbered by the exit points of their associated spinal nerves. (*Note:* This does not necessarily correlate numerically with the nearest skeletal element.)

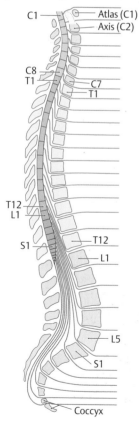

Spinal cord segment	Vertebra

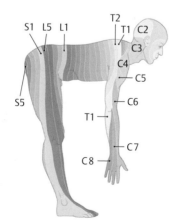

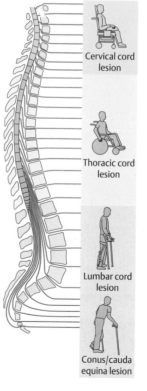

A Spinal cord segments.

B Dermatomes. Each spinal cord segment innervates a particular skin area (dermatome).

C Spinal cord lesions.

Fig. 39.23 Spinal cord in situ: Transverse section

Superior view.

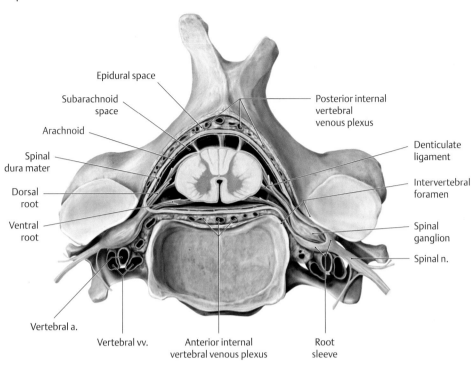

Labels (clockwise from upper left): Epidural space · Subarachnoid space · Arachnoid · Spinal dura mater · Dorsal root · Ventral root · Posterior internal vertebral venous plexus · Denticulate ligament · Intervertebral foramen · Spinal ganglion · Spinal n. · Root sleeve · Anterior internal vertebral venous plexus · Vertebral vv. · Vertebral a.

A Spinal cord at level of C4 vertebra.

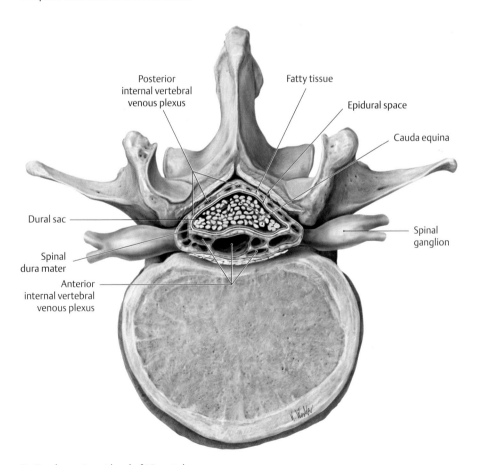

Labels: Posterior internal vertebral venous plexus · Fatty tissue · Epidural space · Cauda equina · Spinal ganglion · Anterior internal vertebral venous plexus · Spinal dura mater · Dural sac

B Cauda equina at level of L2 vertebra.

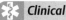
✦ Clinical

Lumbar puncture

A needle introduced into the dural sac (lumbar cistern) generally slips past the spinal nerve roots without injuring the spinal cord. Cerebrospinal fluid (CSF) samples are therefore taken between the L3 and L4 vertebrae (2), once the patient has leaned forward to separate the spinous processes of the lumbar spine.

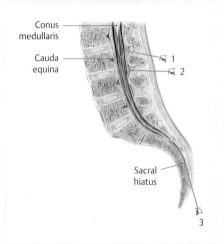

Labels: Conus medullaris · Cauda equina · 1 · 2 · Sacral hiatus · 3

Anesthesia

Lumbar anesthesia may be administered in a similar fashion (2). Epidural anesthesia is administered by placing a catheter in the epidural space without penetrating the dural sac (1). This may also be done by passing a needle through the sacral hiatus (3).

Fig. 39.24 Cauda equina

In adults, the spinal cord ends at approximately the level of L1. Below this, ventral and dorsal roots course through the vertebral canal, uniting in the intervertebral foramen to form the spinal nerve (see p. 36).

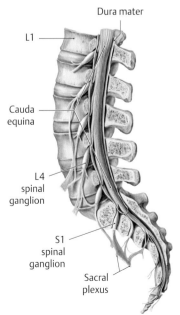

Labels: Dura mater · L1 · Cauda equina · L4 spinal ganglion · S1 spinal ganglion · Sacral plexus

Meninges

 The brain and spinal cord are covered by membranes called meninges. The meninges are composed of three layers: dura mater (dura), arachnoid (arachnoid membrane), and pia mater.

The subarachnoid space, located between the arachnoid and pia, contains cerebrospinal fluid (CSF, see p. 604). See p. 601 for the coverings of the spinal cord.

Fig. 39.25 Meninges
See p. 606 for the veins of the brain.

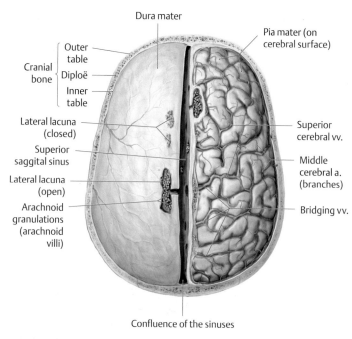

A Superior view. Left side: Dura mater (outer layer). Right side: Pia mater (inner layer). Arachnoid granulations (protrusions of the arachnoid) are sites for reabsorption of CSF.

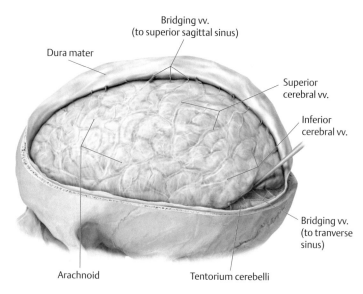

B Arachnoid (middle layer), left anterior oblique view.

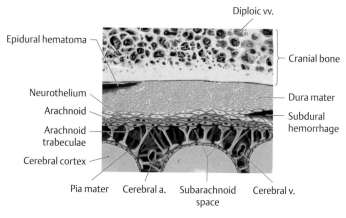

C Layers of the meninges, coronal section, anterior view.

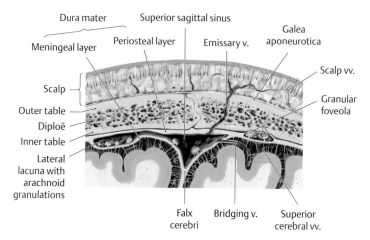

D Dura mater and calvarium, coronal section, anterior view.

Clinical

Extracerebral hemorrhages

Bleeding between the bony calvarium and the soft tissue of the brain (extracerebral hemorrhage) exerts pressure on the brain. A rise of intracranial pressure may damage brain tissue both at the bleeding site and in more remote brain areas. Three types of intracranial hemorrhage are distinguished based on the relationship to the dura mater. See p. 608 for the arteries of the brain.

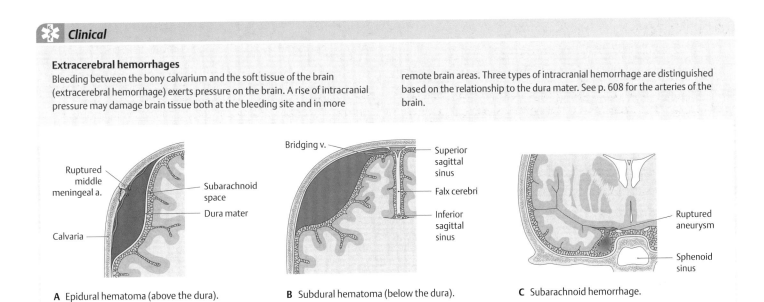

A Epidural hematoma (above the dura).

B Subdural hematoma (below the dura).

C Subarachnoid hemorrhage.

Fig. 39.26 Dural septa

Left anterior oblique view. The major dural reflections are the falx cerebri, tentorium cerebelli, and falx cerebelli (not shown). The dural septa separate the regions of the brain from each other.

Fig. 39.27 Innervation of the dura mater

Superior view. *Removed:* Tentorium cerebelli (right side).

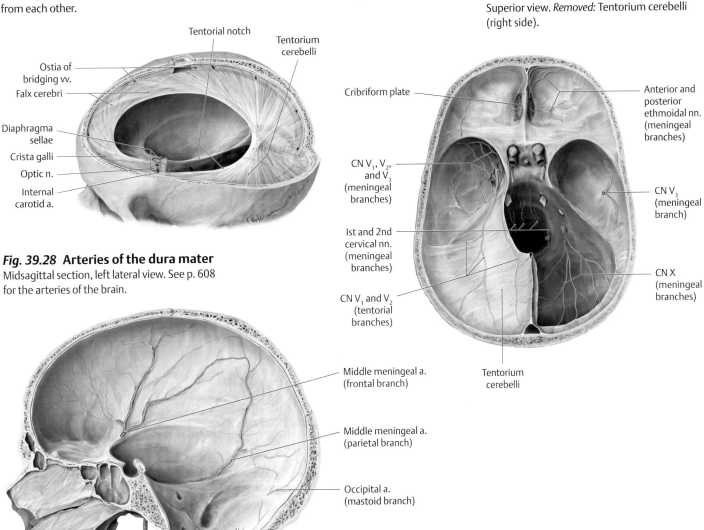

Fig. 39.28 Arteries of the dura mater

Midsagittal section, left lateral view. See p. 608 for the arteries of the brain.

Ventricles & CSF Spaces

Fig. 39.29 Circulation of cerebrospinal fluid (CSF)
The brain and spinal cord are suspended in CSF. Produced in the choroid plexus, CSF occupies the subarachnoid space and ventricles of the brain.

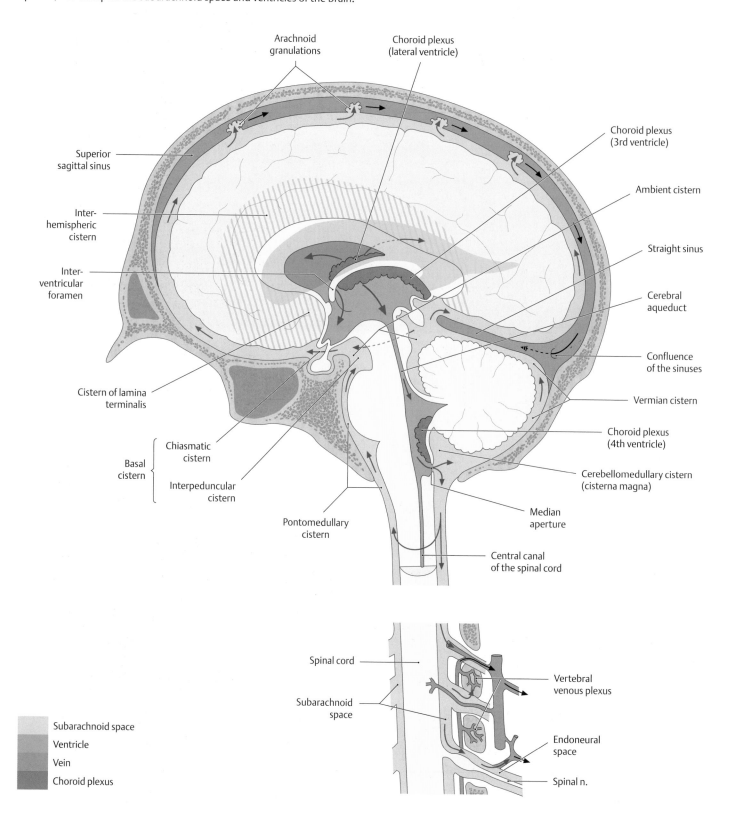

Arachnoid granulations

Choroid plexus (lateral ventricle)

Choroid plexus (3rd ventricle)

Superior sagittal sinus

Ambient cistern

Inter-hemispheric cistern

Straight sinus

Inter-ventricular foramen

Cerebral aqueduct

Confluence of the sinuses

Cistern of lamina terminalis

Vermian cistern

Basal cistern
- Chiasmatic cistern
- Interpeduncular cistern

Choroid plexus (4th ventricle)

Cerebellomedullary cistern (cisterna magna)

Median aperture

Pontomedullary cistern

Central canal of the spinal cord

Spinal cord

Vertebral venous plexus

Subarachnoid space

Endoneural space

Spinal n.

Subarachnoid space

Ventricle

Vein

Choroid plexus

Fig. 39.30 Ventricular system

The ventricular system is a continuation of the central spinal canal into the brain. Cast specimens are used to demonstrate the connections between the four ventricular cavities.

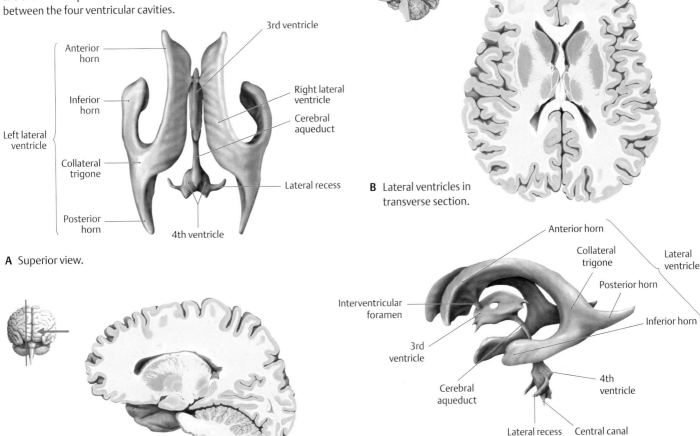

A Superior view.

B Lateral ventricles in transverse section.

C Left lateral ventricle in sagittal section.

D Left lateral view.

Fig. 39.31 Ventricular system in situ

Left lateral view.

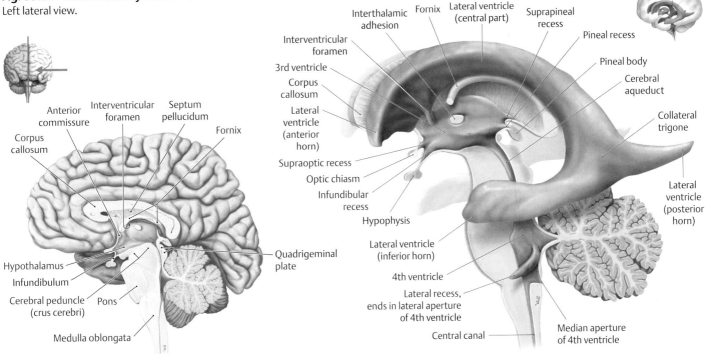

A 3rd and 4th ventricles in the midsagittal section.

B Ventricular system with neighboring structures.

Dural Sinuses & Veins of the Brain

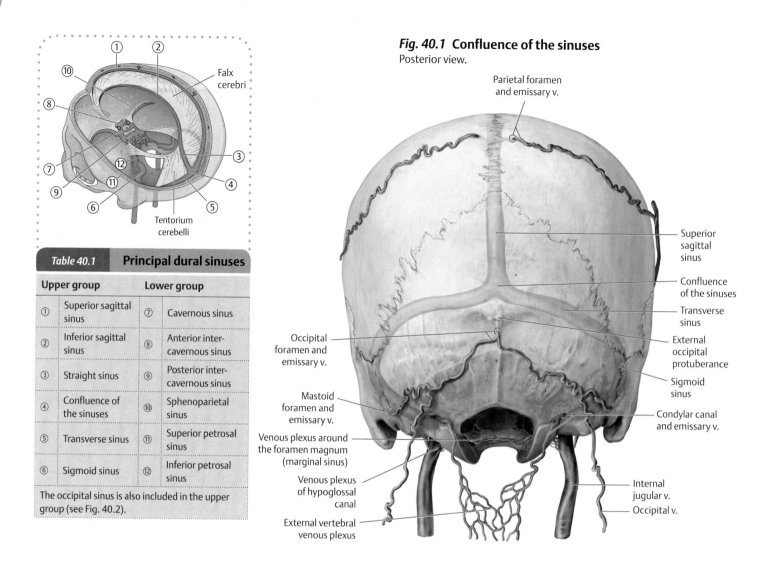

Fig. 40.1 Confluence of the sinuses
Posterior view.

Table 40.1		Principal dural sinuses	
Upper group		**Lower group**	
①	Superior sagittal sinus	⑦	Cavernous sinus
②	Inferior sagittal sinus	⑧	Anterior inter-cavernous sinus
③	Straight sinus	⑨	Posterior inter-cavernous sinus
④	Confluence of the sinuses	⑩	Sphenoparietal sinus
⑤	Transverse sinus	⑪	Superior petrosal sinus
⑥	Sigmoid sinus	⑫	Inferior petrosal sinus

The occipital sinus is also included in the upper group (see Fig. 40.2).

Fig. 40.2 Superficial cerebral veins

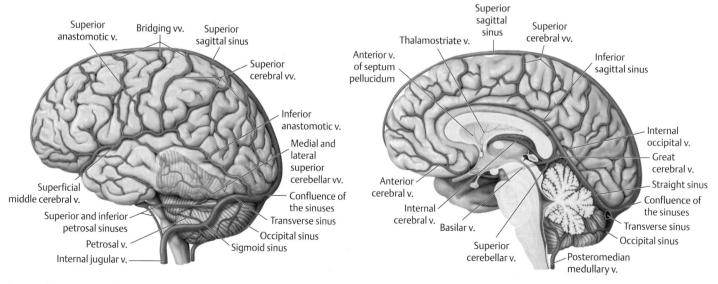

A Lateral view of the left hemisphere.

B Medial view of the right hemisphere.

Fig. 40.3 Basal cerebral venous system
Basal view.

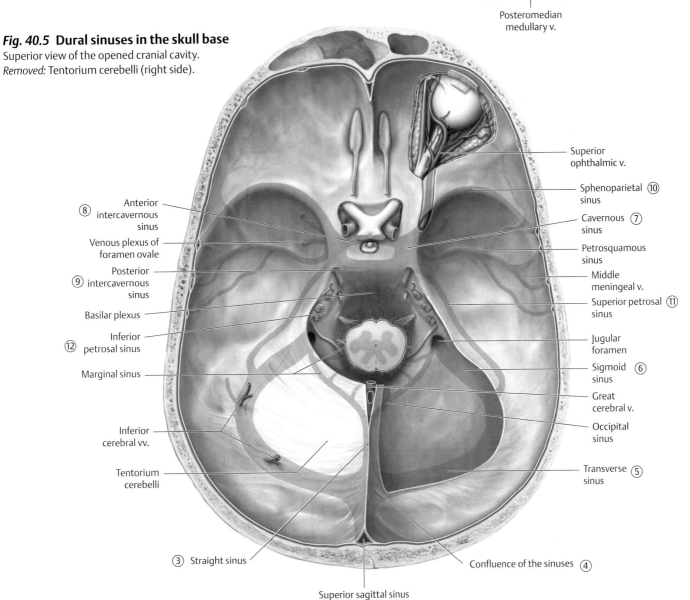

Anterior communicating v.

Interpeduncular v.

Inferior choroidal v.

Basilar v.

Posterior venous confluence

Superficial middle cerebral v.

Anterior cerebral v.

Deep middle cerebral v.

Internal cerebral v.

Great cerebral v.

Fig. 40.4 Veins of the brainstem
Basal view.

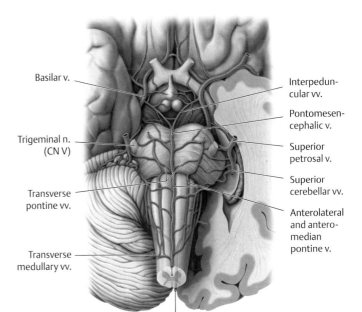

Basilar v.

Trigeminal n. (CN V)

Transverse pontine vv.

Transverse medullary vv.

Interpeduncular vv.

Pontomesencephalic v.

Superior petrosal v.

Superior cerebellar vv.

Anterolateral and anteromedian pontine v.

Posteromedian medullary v.

Fig. 40.5 Dural sinuses in the skull base
Superior view of the opened cranial cavity.
Removed: Tentorium cerebelli (right side).

⑧ Anterior intercavernous sinus

Venous plexus of foramen ovale

⑨ Posterior intercavernous sinus

Basilar plexus

⑫ Inferior petrosal sinus

Marginal sinus

Inferior cerebral vv.

Tentorium cerebelli

Superior ophthalmic v.

Sphenoparietal ⑩ sinus

Cavernous ⑦ sinus

Petrosquamous sinus

Middle meningeal v.

Superior petrosal ⑪ sinus

Jugular foramen

Sigmoid ⑥ sinus

Great cerebral v.

Occipital sinus

Transverse ⑤ sinus

③ Straight sinus

Confluence of the sinuses ④

Superior sagittal sinus ①

Arteries of the Brain

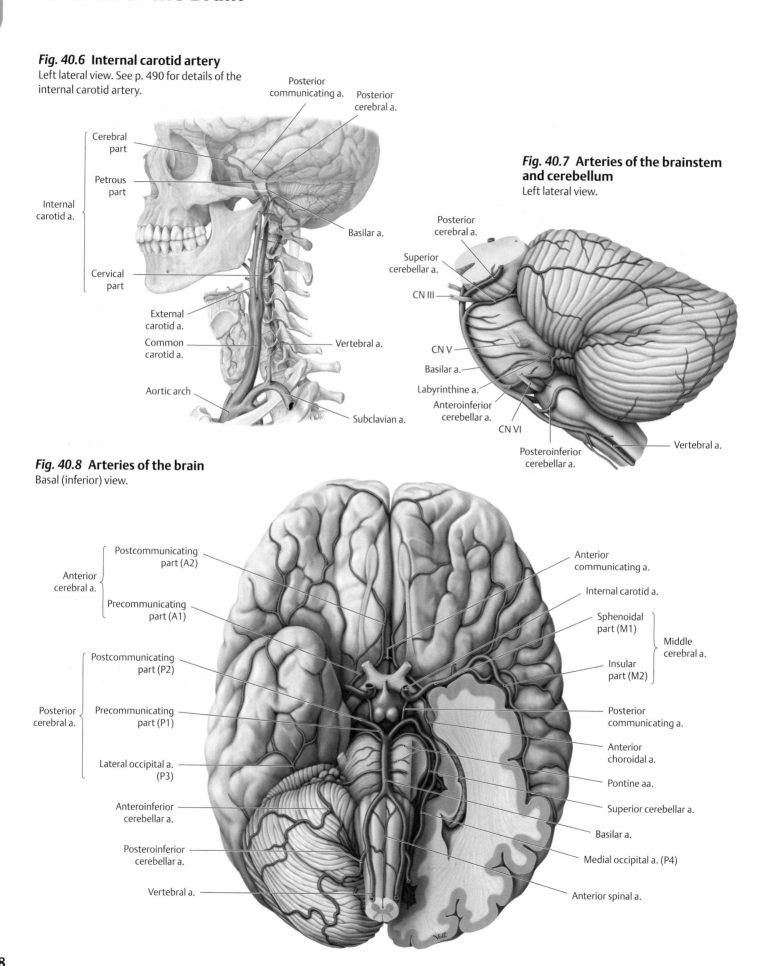

Fig. 40.6 Internal carotid artery
Left lateral view. See p. 490 for details of the internal carotid artery.

- Posterior communicating a.
- Posterior cerebral a.
- Cerebral part
- Petrous part
- Internal carotid a.
- Cervical part
- Basilar a.
- External carotid a.
- Common carotid a.
- Vertebral a.
- Aortic arch
- Subclavian a.

Fig. 40.7 Arteries of the brainstem and cerebellum
Left lateral view.

- Posterior cerebral a.
- Superior cerebellar a.
- CN III
- CN V
- Basilar a.
- Labyrinthine a.
- Anteroinferior cerebellar a.
- CN VI
- Posteroinferior cerebellar a.
- Vertebral a.

Fig. 40.8 Arteries of the brain
Basal (inferior) view.

- Anterior cerebral a.
  - Postcommunicating part (A2)
  - Precommunicating part (A1)
- Posterior cerebral a.
  - Postcommunicating part (P2)
  - Precommunicating part (P1)
  - Lateral occipital a. (P3)
- Anteroinferior cerebellar a.
- Posteroinferior cerebellar a.
- Vertebral a.
- Anterior communicating a.
- Internal carotid a.
- Middle cerebral a.
  - Sphenoidal part (M1)
  - Insular part (M2)
- Posterior communicating a.
- Anterior choroidal a.
- Pontine aa.
- Superior cerebellar a.
- Basilar a.
- Medial occipital a. (P4)
- Anterior spinal a.

Fig. 40.9 Cerebral arteries

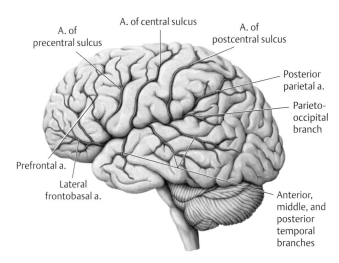

A Middle cerebral artery. Lateral view of the left hemisphere.

- A. of precentral sulcus
- A. of central sulcus
- A. of postcentral sulcus
- Posterior parietal a.
- Parieto-occipital branch
- Prefrontal a.
- Lateral frontobasal a.
- Anterior, middle, and posterior temporal branches

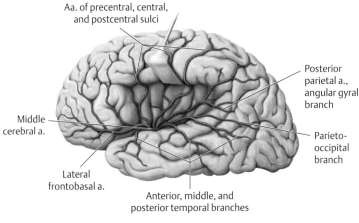

B Middle cerebral artery. Left lateral view with the lateral sulcus retracted.

- Aa. of precentral, central, and postcentral sulci
- Posterior parietal a., angular gyral branch
- Middle cerebral a.
- Parieto-occipital branch
- Lateral frontobasal a.
- Anterior, middle, and posterior temporal branches

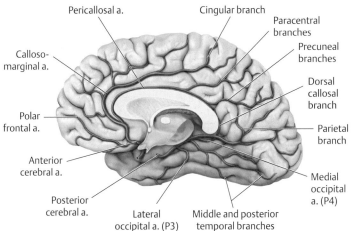

C Anterior and posterior cerebral arteries. Medial view of the right hemisphere.

- Pericallosal a.
- Cingular branch
- Paracentral branches
- Precuneal branches
- Calloso-marginal a.
- Dorsal callosal branch
- Polar frontal a.
- Parietal branch
- Anterior cerebral a.
- Posterior cerebral a.
- Medial occipital a. (P4)
- Lateral occipital a. (P3)
- Middle and posterior temporal branches

Fig. 40.10 Cerebral arteries: Distribution areas

The central gray and white matter have a complex blood supply (yellow) that includes the anterior choroidal artery.

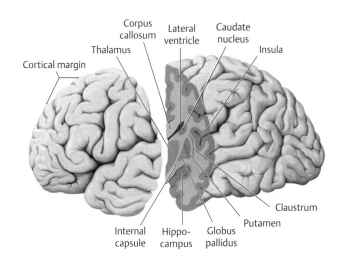

- Corpus callosum
- Lateral ventricle
- Caudate nucleus
- Insula
- Thalamus
- Cortical margin
- Claustrum
- Putamen
- Internal capsule
- Hippo-campus
- Globus pallidus

☐ Anterior cerebral a.
☐ Middle cerebral a.
☐ Posterior cerebral a.

A Lateral view of the left hemisphere.

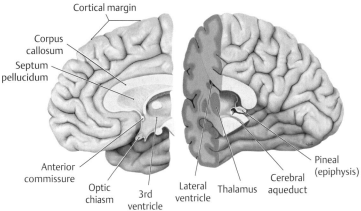

- Cortical margin
- Corpus callosum
- Septum pellucidum
- Anterior commissure
- Optic chiasm
- 3rd ventricle
- Lateral ventricle
- Thalamus
- Cerebral aqueduct
- Pineal (epiphysis)

B Medial view of the right hemisphere.

Arteries & Veins of the Spinal Cord

Like the spinal cord itself, the arteries and veins of the spinal cord consist of multiple horizontal systems (blood vessels of the spinal cord segments) that are integrated into a vertical system.

Fig. 40.11 Arteries of the spinal cord

The unpaired anterior and paired posterior spinal arteries typically arise from the vertebral arteries. As they descend within the vertebral canal, the spinal arteries are reinforced by anterior and posterior segmental medullary arteries. Depending on the spinal level, these reinforcing branches may arise from the vertebral, ascending or deep cervical, posterior intercostal, lumbar, or lateral sacral arteries.

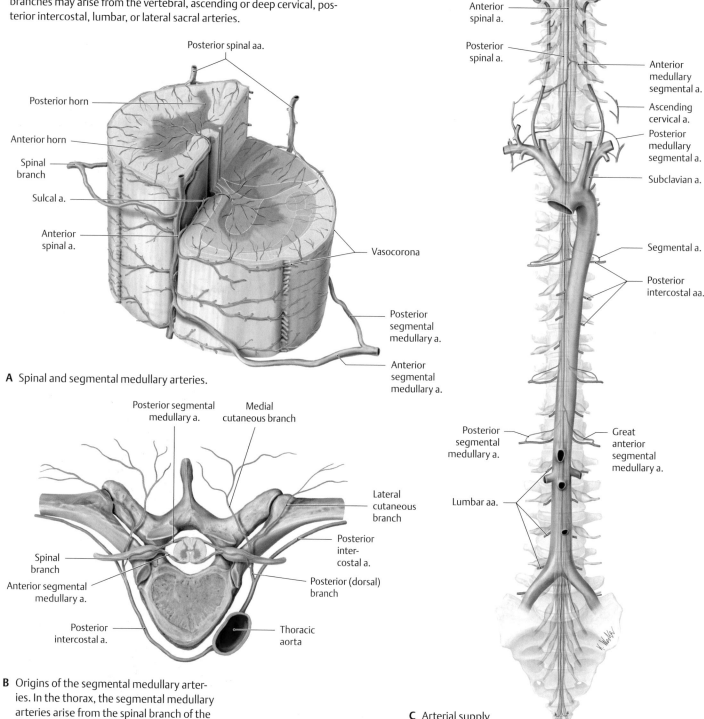

A Spinal and segmental medullary arteries.

B Origins of the segmental medullary arteries. In the thorax, the segmental medullary arteries arise from the spinal branch of the posterior intercostal arteries (see p. 34).

C Arterial supply system.

Fig. 40.12 Veins of the spinal cord

The interior of the spinal cord drains via venous plexuses into an anterior and a posterior spinal vein. The radicular and spinal veins connect the veins of the spinal cord with the internal vertebral venous plexus. The intervertebral and basivertebral veins connect the internal and external venous plexuses, which drain into the azygos system.

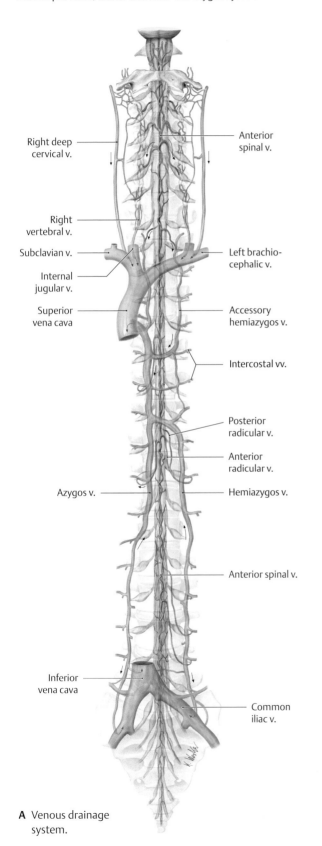

A Venous drainage system.

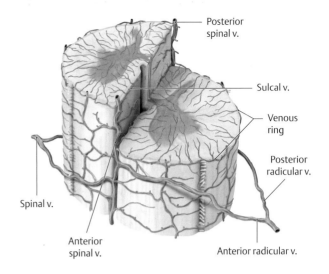

B Spinal and radicular veins.

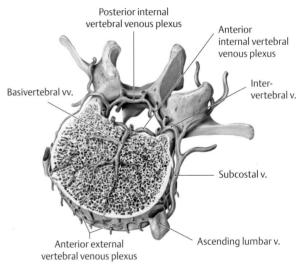

C Vertebral venous plexuses.

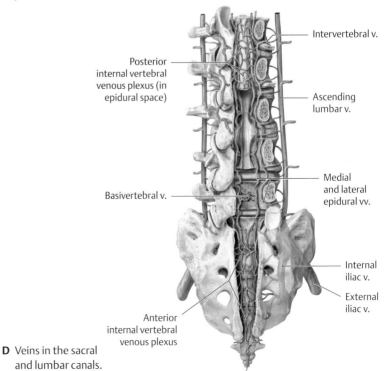

D Veins in the sacral and lumbar canals.

Circuitry

Fig. 41.1 Divisions of the nervous system

Direction of information flow divides nerve fibers into two types: afferent (sensory) fibers, which transmit impulses toward the central nervous system (CNS), and efferent (motor) fibers, which transmit impulses away. The nervous system may also be divided into a somatic and an autonomic part. The somatic nervous system mediates interaction with the environment, whereas the autonomic (visceral) nervous system coordinates the function of the internal organs.

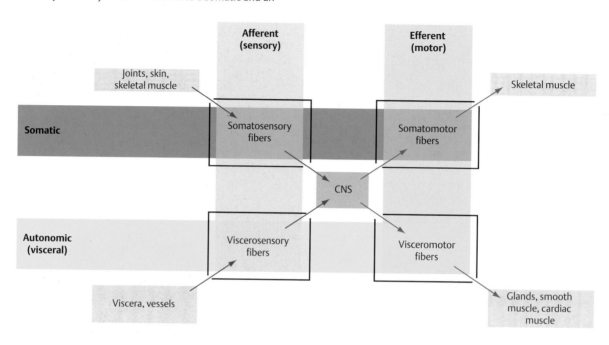

Fig. 41.2 Organization of the gray matter

Left oblique anterosuperior view. The gray matter of the spinal cord is divided into three columns (horns). Afferent (blue) and efferent (red) neurons within these columns are clustered according to function.

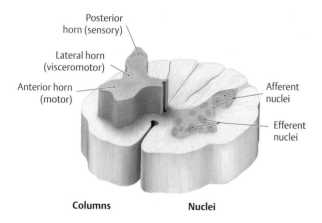

Fig. 41.3 Muscle innervation

Indicator muscles are innervated by motor neurons in the anterior horn of one spinal cord segment. Most muscles (multisegmental muscles) receive innervation from a motor column, a vertical arrangement of motor nuclei spanning several segments.

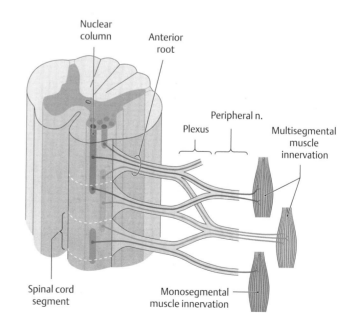

Fig. 41.4 Reflexes

Muscular function at the unconscious (reflex) level is controlled by the gray matter of the spinal cord.

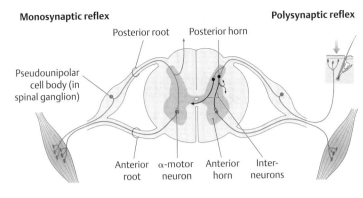

Monosynaptic reflex   **Polysynaptic reflex**

A Polysynaptic reflexes may be mediated by receptors inside of or remote from the muscle (i.e., skin); these receptors act via interneurons to stimulate muscle contraction.

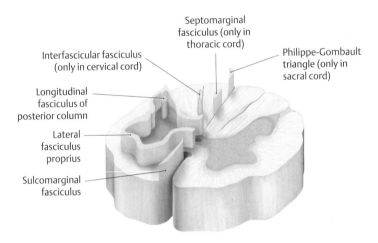

B Principal intrinsic fascicles of the spinal cord. The intrinsic fascicles are the conduction apparatus of the intrinsic circuits, allowing axons to ascend and descend to coordinate spinal reflexes for multisegmental muscles.

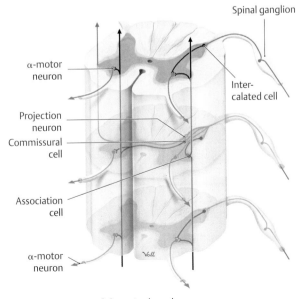

C Intrinsic circuits of the spinal cord.

Fig. 41.5 Sensory and motor systems

The sensory system (see p. 614) and motor system (see p. 615) are so functionally interrelated they may be described as one (sensorimotor system).

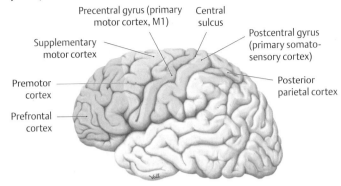

A Cortical areas of the sensorimotor system. Lateral view of the left hemisphere.

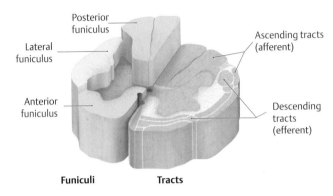

Funiculi   **Tracts**

B White matter of the spinal cord. The white matter of the spinal cord contains ascending tracts (afferent, see p. 614) and descending tracts (efferent, see p. 615), which are the CNS equivalent of peripheral nerves.

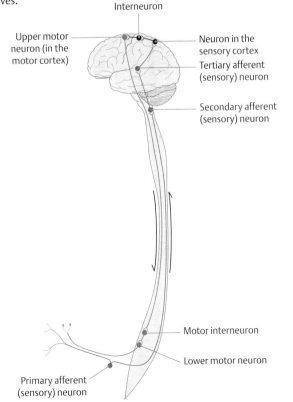

C Overview of sensorimotor integration.

613

Sensory & Motor Pathways

Fig. 41.6 **Sensory pathways (ascending tracts)**

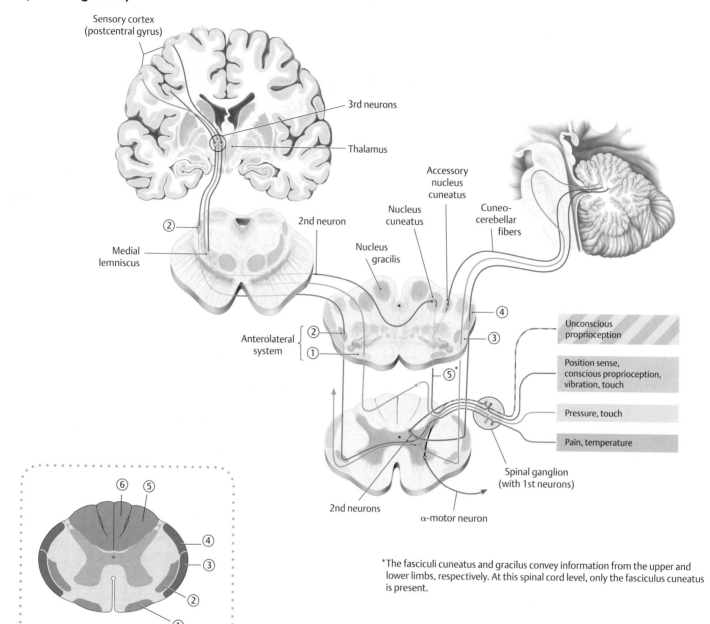

Sensory cortex (postcentral gyrus)

3rd neurons

Thalamus

2nd neuron

Accessory nucleus cuneatus

Nucleus cuneatus

Cuneo-cerebellar fibers

Nucleus gracilis

Medial lemniscus

②

Anterolateral system

②

①

④

③

⑤*

Unconscious proprioception

Position sense, conscious proprioception, vibration, touch

Pressure, touch

Pain, temperature

Spinal ganglion (with 1st neurons)

2nd neurons

α-motor neuron

⑥ ⑤

④

③

②

①

*The fasciculi cuneatus and gracilus convey information from the upper and lower limbs, respectively. At this spinal cord level, only the fasciculus cuneatus is present.

	Table 41.1		Ascending tracts of the spinal cord		
	Tract	**Location**	**Function**		**Neurons**
①	Anterior spino-thalamic tract	Anterior funiculus	Pathway for crude touch and pressure sensation		1st afferent neurons located in spinal ganglia; contain 2nd neurons and cross in the anterior commissure
②	Lateral spino-thalamic tract	Anterior and lateral funiculi	Pathway for pain, temperature, tickle, itch, and sexual sensation		
③	Anterior spino-cerebellar tract	Lateral funiculus	Pathway for unconscious coordination of motor activities (unconscious proprioception, automatic processes, e.g., jogging, riding a bike) to the cerebellum		Projection (2nd) neurons receive proprioceptive signals from 1st afferent fibers originating at the 1st neurons of spinal ganglia
④	Posterior spino-cerebellar tract				
⑤	Fasciculus cuneatus	Posterior funiculus	Pathway for position sense (conscious proprioception) and fine cutaneous sensation (touch, vibration, fine pressure sense, two-point discrimination)	Conveys information from *upper* limb (not present below T3)	Cell bodies of 1st neuron located in spinal ganglion; pass uncrossed to the dorsal column nuclei
⑥	Fasciculus gracilis*			Conveys information from *lower* limb	

Pyramidal (corticospinal) tract

Extrapyramidal motor system

Fig. 41.7 Motor pathways (descending tracts)

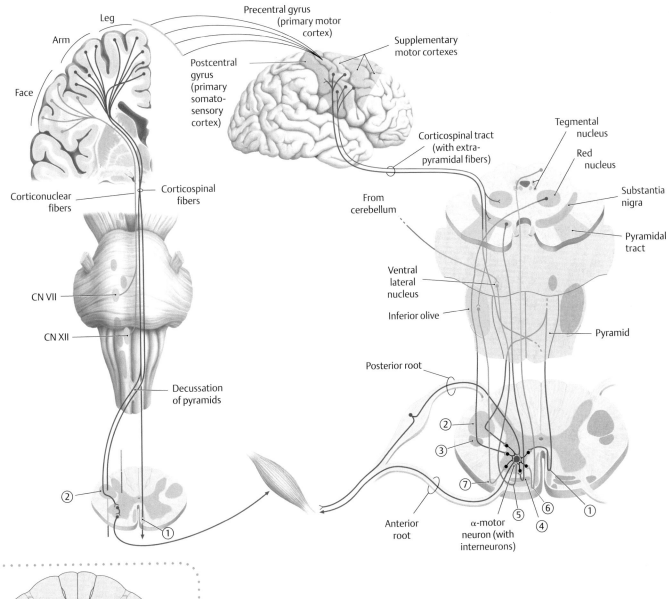

Leg

Arm

Face

Precentral gyrus (primary motor cortex)

Supplementary motor cortexes

Postcentral gyrus (primary somato-sensory cortex)

Corticonuclear fibers

Corticospinal fibers

Corticospinal tract (with extra-pyramidal fibers)

Tegmental nucleus

Red nucleus

Substantia nigra

Pyramidal tract

From cerebellum

Ventral lateral nucleus

Inferior olive

Pyramid

CN VII

CN XII

Decussation of pyramids

Posterior root

②
③
⑦
α-motor neuron (with interneurons)
⑤ ⑥ ④ ①

Anterior root

②

①

②
③

④

① ⑥ ⑤

Table 41.2 **Descending tracts of the spinal cord**

Tract			Function	
Pyramidal tract	①	Anterior corticospinal tract	Most important pathway for voluntary motor function	Originates in the motor cortex *Corticonuclear* fibers to motor nuclei of cranial nerves *Corticospinal* fibers to motor cells in anterior horn of the spinal cord *Corticoreticular* fibers to nuclei of the reticular formation
	②	Lateral corticospinal tract		
Extrapyramidal motor system	③	Rubrospinal tract	Pathway for automatic and learned motor processes (e.g., walking, running, cycling)	
	④	Reticulospinal tract		
	⑤	Vestibulospinal tract		
	⑥	Tectospinal tract		
	⑦	Olivospinal tract		

Sensory Systems (I)

Fig. 41.8 Visual system: Overview

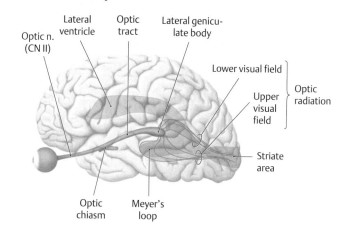

A Left lateral view.

Fig. 41.9 Visual pathways

90% of optic nerve fibers terminate in the lateral geniculate body on neurons that project to the striate area (visual cortex). This forms the geniculate pathway, responsible for conscious visual perception. The remaining 10% travel along the medial root of the optic tract, forming the non-geniculate pathway. This pathway plays an important role in the unconscious regulation of vision-related processes and reflexes.

B Inferior view.

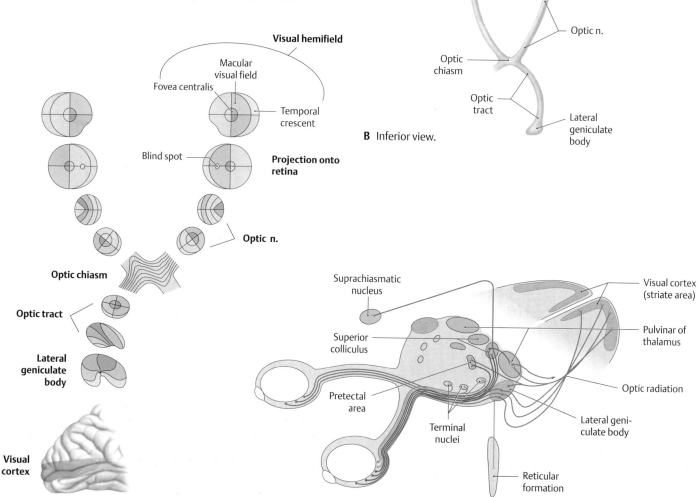

A Geniculate pathway. Left visual hemifield.

B Non-geniculate pathway.

Lesions of the visual pathway

Visual field defects and lesion sites are here illustrated for the left visual pathway.

1 Unilateral lesion of optic n.

   Blindness in affected eye

2 Lesion of optic chiasm

   Bitemporal hemianopia ("blinders")

3 Unilateral lesion of optic tract

   Contralateral homonymous hemianopia

4 Unilateral lesion of optic radiation in Meyer's loop (anterior temporal lobe)

   Contralateral upper quadrantanopia ("pie-in-the-sky")

5 Unilateral lesion of optic radiation, medial part

   Contralateral lower quadrantanopia

6 Lesion of occipital lobe

   Homonymous hemianopia

7 Lesion of occipital pole (cortical areas)

   Homonymous hemianopic central scotoma

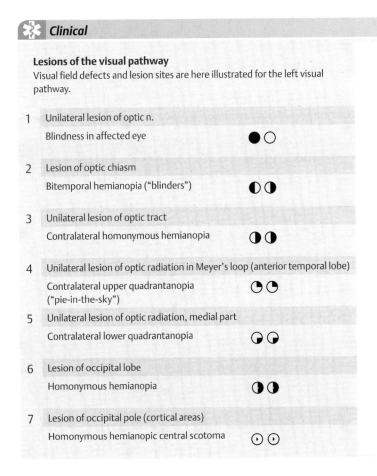

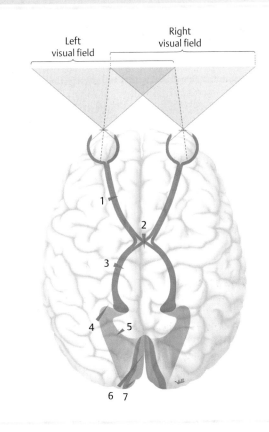

Fig. 41.10 Reflexes of the visual system

The reflexes of the visual system are mediated by the optic (afferent) and oculomotor (efferent) nerves.

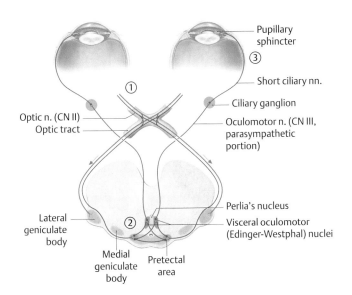

A Pupillary light reflex.

① Incoming light is transmitted via the optic nerve.

② Large amounts of light are transmitted to the pretectal area, bypassing the geniculate pathway.

③ The neurons of the visceral oculomotor nucleus synapse on the ciliary ganglion, which induces contraction of the pupillary sphincter.

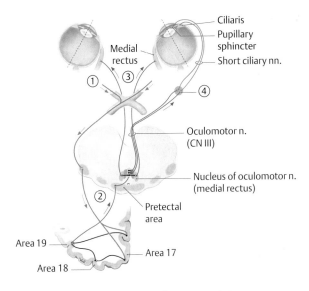

B Pathways for convergence and accommodation.

① Light is received from an approaching object.

② Information is relayed via the primary (17) and secondary (19) visual cortexes to the nuclei of the oculomotor nerve.

③ Convergence: Constriction of the medial rectus muscles converges the visual axes of the eyes, keeping the approaching image on the fovea centralis, the point of maximum visual acuity.

④ Accommodation: The curvature of the lens is increased via contraction of the ciliary muscles. The sphincter pupillae also contracts.

Sensory Systems (II)

Fig. 41.11 Balance

Human balance is regulated by the visual, proprioceptive, and vestibular systems. All three systems send afferent fibers to the vestibular nuclei, which then distribute them to the spinal cord (motor support), cerebellum (fine motor function), and brainstem (oculomotor function). Proprioception ("position sense") is the perception of limb position in space. *Note:* Efferents to the thalamus and cortex control spatial sense; efferents to the hypothalamus regulate vomiting in response to vertigo.

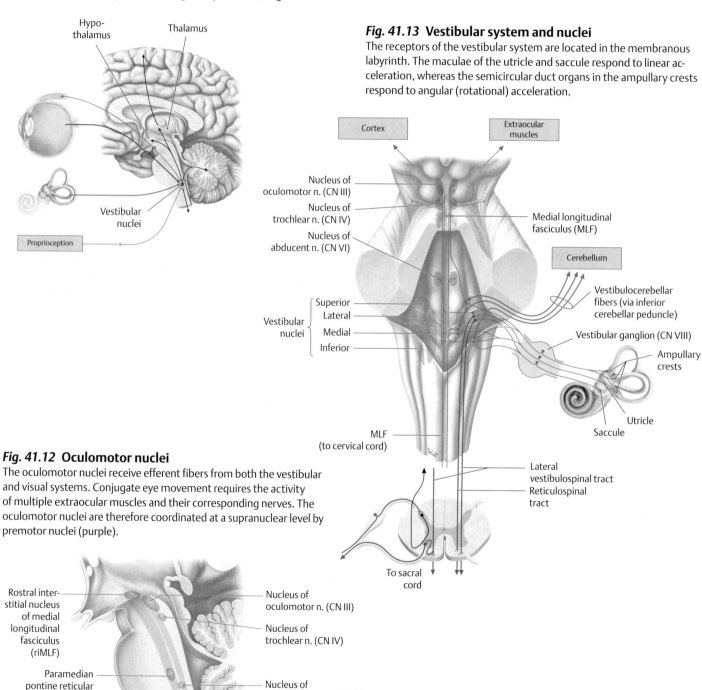

Fig. 41.13 Vestibular system and nuclei

The receptors of the vestibular system are located in the membranous labyrinth. The maculae of the utricle and saccule respond to linear acceleration, whereas the semicircular duct organs in the ampullary crests respond to angular (rotational) acceleration.

Fig. 41.12 Oculomotor nuclei

The oculomotor nuclei receive efferent fibers from both the vestibular and visual systems. Conjugate eye movement requires the activity of multiple extraocular muscles and their corresponding nerves. The oculomotor nuclei are therefore coordinated at a supranuclear level by premotor nuclei (purple).

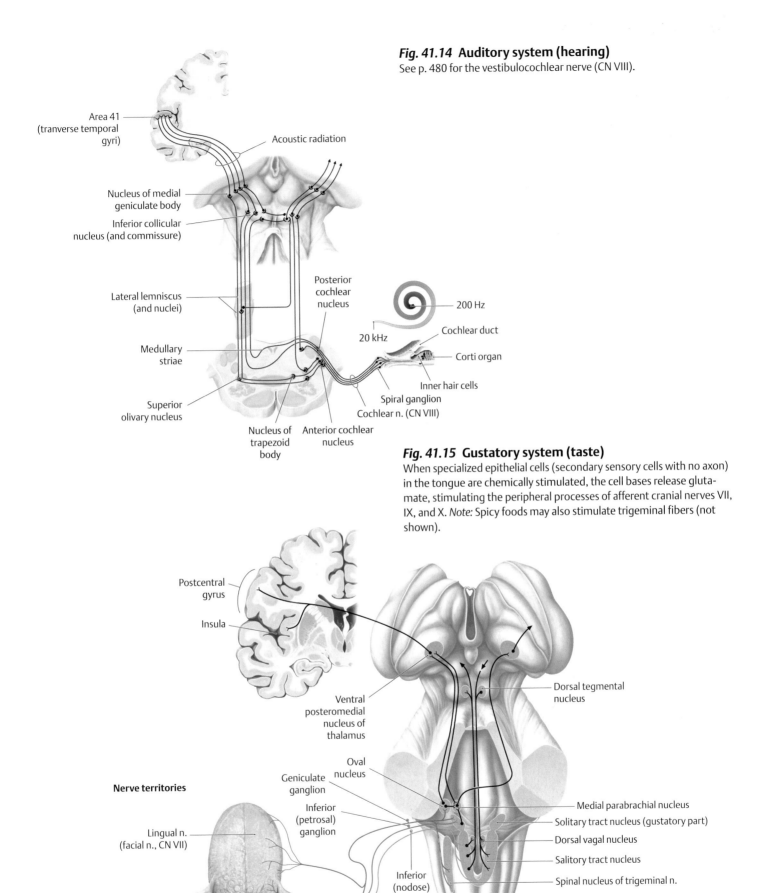

Fig. 41.14 Auditory system (hearing)

See p. 480 for the vestibulocochlear nerve (CN VIII).

Area 41
(tranverse temporal
gyri)

Acoustic radiation

Nucleus of medial
geniculate body

Inferior collicular
nucleus (and commissure)

Lateral lemniscus
(and nuclei)

Posterior
cochlear
nucleus

200 Hz

20 kHz

Cochlear duct

Corti organ

Medullary
striae

Inner hair cells

Spiral ganglion

Cochlear n. (CN VIII)

Superior
olivary nucleus

Nucleus of
trapezoid
body

Anterior cochlear
nucleus

Fig. 41.15 Gustatory system (taste)

When specialized epithelial cells (secondary sensory cells with no axon) in the tongue are chemically stimulated, the cell bases release glutamate, stimulating the peripheral processes of afferent cranial nerves VII, IX, and X. *Note:* Spicy foods may also stimulate trigeminal fibers (not shown).

Postcentral
gyrus

Insula

Ventral
posteromedial
nucleus of
thalamus

Dorsal tegmental
nucleus

Nerve territories

Oval
nucleus

Geniculate
ganglion

Inferior
(petrosal)
ganglion

Lingual n.
(facial n., CN VII)

Medial parabrachial nucleus

Solitary tract nucleus (gustatory part)

Dorsal vagal nucleus

Salitory tract nucleus

Glossopharyngeal
n. (CN IX)

Inferior
(nodose)
ganglion

Spinal nucleus of trigeminal n.

Vagus n.
(CN X)

Sensory Systems (III)

Fig. 41.16 Olfactory system (smell)

The olfactory system is the only sensory system not relayed in the thalamus before reaching the cortex (the prepiriform area is considered the primary olfactory cortex). The olfactory system is linked to other brain areas and can therefore evoke complex emotional and behavioral responses (mediated by the hypothalamus, thalamus, and limbic system): noxious smells induce nausea; appetizing smells evoke salivation.

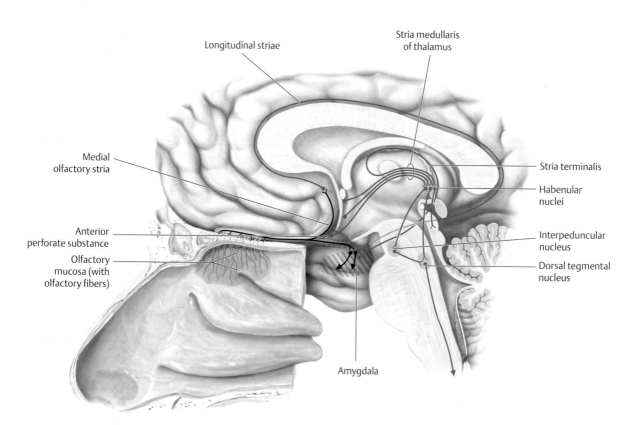

A Olfactory system, inferior view.

*Structure is deep to the surface of the brain.

B Olfactory system with nuclei, left lateral view of midsagittal section.

The limbic system, which exchanges and integrates information between the telencephalon, diencephalon, and mesencephalon, regulates drive and affective behavior. It plays a crucial role in memory and learning.

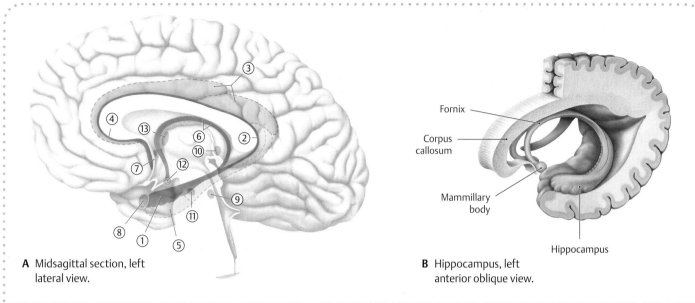

A Midsagittal section, left lateral view.

B Hippocampus, left anterior oblique view.

Table 41.4		Structures of the limbic system			

Outer arc		**Inner arc***		**Subcortical nuclei**	
①	Parahippocampal gyrus	⑤	Hippocampal formation (hippocampus, entorhinal area of parahippocampal gyrus)	⑧	Amygdala
②	Indusium griseum	⑥	Fornix	⑨	Dorsal tegmental nuclei
③	Subcallosal (paraolfactory) area	⑦	Septal area (septum)	⑩	Habenular nuclei
				⑪	Interpeduncular nuclei
④	Cingulate (limbic) gyrus		Paraterminal gyrus	⑫	Mammillary bodies
				⑬	Anterior thalamic nuclei

* The inner arc also contains the diagonal band of Broca (not shown).

Fig. 41.17 Limbic system nuclei

This neuronal circuit (Papez circuit) establishes a connection between information stored at the conscious and unconscious level.

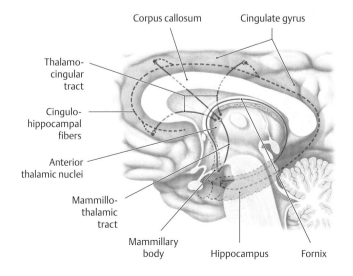

Fig. 41.18 Limbic regulation of the peripheral autonomic nervous system

The limbic system receives afferent feedback signals from its target organs. See p. 623 for the autonomic nervous system.

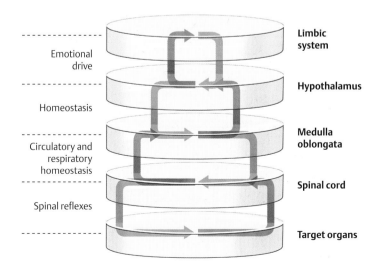

Autonomic Nervous System

Fig. 42.1 Autonomic nervous system circuitry

The autonomic nervous system innervates smooth muscle, cardiac muscle, and glands. It is divided into the sympathetic (red) and parasympathetic (blue) nervous systems, which often act in antagonistic ways to regulate blood flow, secretions, and organ function. Green: Afferent. Purple: Efferent.

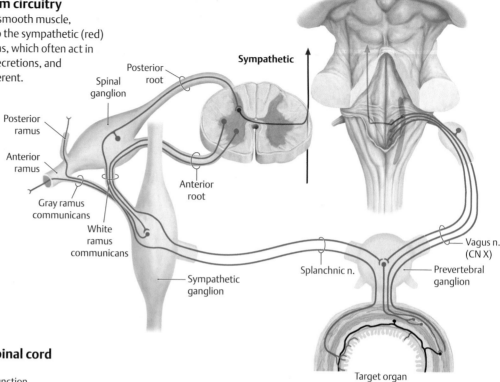

Fig. 42.2 Autonomic tracts in the spinal cord

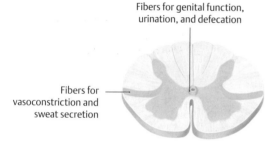

Fig. 42.4 Blood pressure regulation

Sympathetic fibers may release norepinephrine, inducing the α1 receptor to mediate contraction of the vascular smooth muscle (thus increasing blood pressure). Circulating epinephrine acts on the β2 receptors to induce vasodilation (decreasing blood pressure). *Note:* Parasympathetic fibers do not terminate on blood vessels.

Fig. 42.3 Regulatory effects of the autonomic neurotransmitters

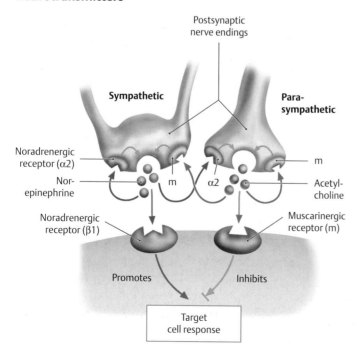

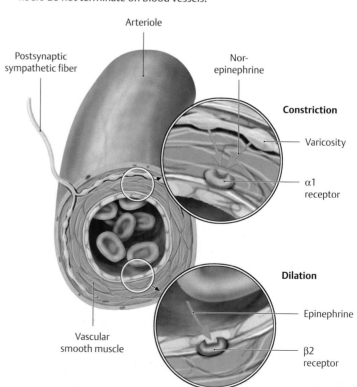

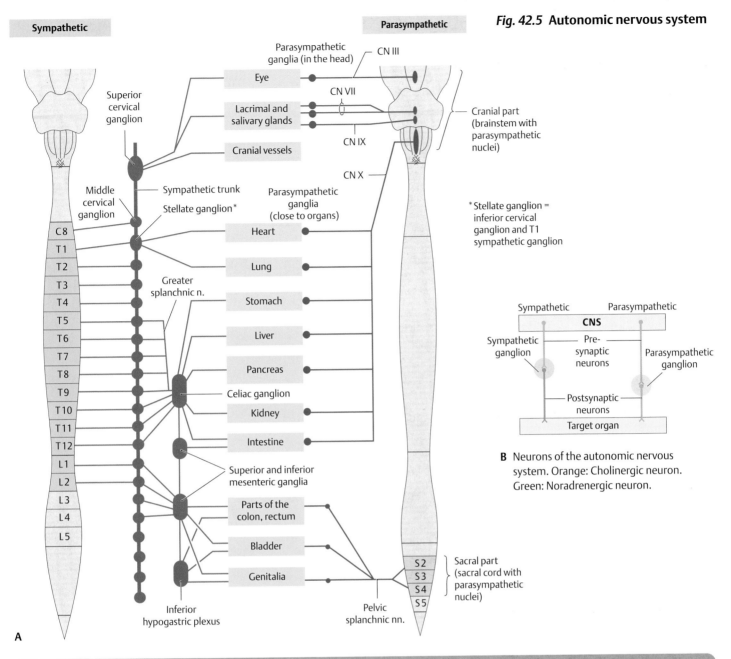

Fig. 42.5 **Autonomic nervous system**

Sympathetic

Parasympathetic

Parasympathetic ganglia (in the head) — CN III

Eye

Superior cervical ganglion

CN VII

Lacrimal and salivary glands

Cranial vessels

CN IX

Cranial part (brainstem with parasympathetic nuclei)

Middle cervical ganglion

Sympathetic trunk

Stellate ganglion*

CN X

Parasympathetic ganglia (close to organs)

* Stellate ganglion = inferior cervical ganglion and T1 sympathetic ganglion

C8
T1
T2
T3
T4
T5
T6
T7
T8
T9
T10
T11
T12
L1
L2
L3
L4
L5

Heart

Lung

Greater splanchnic n.

Stomach

Liver

Pancreas

Celiac ganglion

Kidney

Intestine

Superior and inferior mesenteric ganglia

Parts of the colon, rectum

Bladder

Genitalia

Inferior hypogastric plexus

Pelvic splanchnic nn.

S2
S3
S4
S5

Sacral part (sacral cord with parasympathetic nuclei)

CNS

Sympathetic — Parasympathetic

Sympathetic ganglion — Pre-synaptic neurons — Parasympathetic ganglion

Postsynaptic neurons

Target organ

B Neurons of the autonomic nervous system. Orange: Cholinergic neuron. Green: Noradrenergic neuron.

A

Table 42.1		Effects of the sympathetic and parasympathetic nervous systems	
Organ (organ system)		**Sympathetic NS effect**	**Parasympathetic NS effect**
Gastro-intestinal tract	Longitudinal and circular muscle fibers	↓ motility	↑ motility
	Sphincter muscles	Contraction	Relaxation
	Glands	↓ secretions	↑ secretions
Splenic capsule		Contraction	
Liver		↑ glycogenolysis/gluconeogenesis	No effect
Pancreas	Endocrine pancreas	↓ insulin secretion	
	Exocrine pancreas	↓ secretion	↑ secretion
Bladder	Detrusor vesicae	Relaxation	Contraction
	Functional bladder sphincter	Contraction	
Seminal vesicle		Contraction (ejaculation)	No effect
Vas deferens			
Uterus		Contraction or relaxation, depending on hormonal status	
Arteries		Vasoconstriction	Vasodilation of the arteries of the penis and clitoris (erection)

NS = nervous system. See also p. 244.

Appendix

Answers to Surface Anatomy Questions

Back (pp. 40–41)

Q1: The superior boundaries of Michaelis' rhomboid run from the spinous process of L4 to the posterior superior iliac spines. The rhomboid then follows the curve of the iliac crest to the anal cleft.

Q2: The inferior angle of the scapula is at the level of the T7 spinous process. The iliac crest is at the level of the L4 spinous process. See p. 40 for palpable bony landmarks.

Thorax (pp. 120–121)

Q1: After careful inspection, undertake a systematic palpation of each breast. Palpate the tissue of each breast by quadrant in the following sequence: inferior lateral, inferior medial, superior medial, and superior lateral. Palpate the axilla to examine the axillary tail of breast tissue. The majority of lymph drainage from the breast is to the axillary lymph nodes. The parasternal lymph nodes, which run along the internal thoracic vessels, drain the medial portions of the breast. See p. 64 for the axillary lymph nodes.

Q2: The aortic and pulmonary valves are best auscultated at the 2nd right and left intercostal spaces, respectively. Locate the 2nd intercostal spaces by finding the usually palpable sternal angle (the junction between the manubrium and body of the sternum). The 2nd ribs attach to the sternum at the sternal angle. The tricuspid (right atrioventricular) and bicuspid (left atrioventricular) valves are best auscultated at the left 5th intercostal space. If the ribs are visible/palpable, the 5th rib can be found by counting up from below (the lowest rib at the midclavicular line is the 10th rib). See p. 87 for auscultation sites; see p. 120 for reference lines in the thorax.

Abdomen & Pelvis (pp. 248–249)

Q1: Use a vertical and a horizontal line through the umbilicus (at approximately the level of L4) to divide the abdomen and pelvis into right and left upper and lower quadrants (see p. 140).

LUQ	Liver, stomach, transverse colon, small intestine, spleen, pancreas, duodenum, descending colon, left kidney and suprarenal gland, left ureter.
RUQ	Liver, stomach, transverse colon, small intestine, gallbladder, pancreas, duodenum, ascending colon, right kidney and suprarenal gland, right ureter.
LLQ	Small intestine, descending colon, left ureter, urinary bladder, reproductive organs.
RLQ	Small intestine, ascending colon (with cecum and vermiform appendix), right ureter, urinary bladder, reproductive organs.

Q2: *Direct* inguinal hernias are most common in middle-aged or older males and are believed to be caused by "wear and tear." They typically occupy the medial portion of the inguinal canal (having exited the abdomen through the inguinal triangle). They may also exit via the superficial inguinal ring. Rarely, they enter the scrotum. *Indirect* hernias are seen in male children and young adults and are believed to have a congenital basis. They generally exit via the deep inguinal ring and thus may occupy the entire length of the inguinal canal. They may also exit via the superficial inguinal ring, and occasionally enter the scrotum. See p. 133 for inguinal hernias.

Upper Limb (pp. 350–353)

Q1: The medial and lateral antebrachial cutaneous nerves are both vulnerable during intravenous punctures in the cubital fossa. The medial nerve is a direct branch from the medial cord of the brachial plexus; the lateral nerve is the cutaneous component of the musculatocutaneous nerve (lateral cord). See p. 339 for the cubital region.

Q2: With the elbow joint in flexion, the ulnar collateral ligament can be palpated using the olecranon, the medial and lateral epicondyles, and the coronoid process. The radial collateral ligament can be palpated using the lateral epicondyle. See p. 284 for the collateral ligaments of the elbow.

Q3: In the wrist, the flexor carpi ulnaris tendon runs laterally to the ulnar artery and nerve until the ulnar tunnel. The median nerve is located between the palpable tendons of palmaris longus and flexor carpi radialis. The radial artery is slightly lateral to the flexor carpi radialis tendon. See p. 342 for the topography of the carpal region.

Q4: Tenderness at the base of the anatomic snuffbox suggests a fracture of the scaphoid. See p. 347 for the anatomic snuffbox; see p. 299 for scaphoid fractures.

Lower Limb (pp. 450–451)

Q1: The head of the femur is located directly behind the femoral artery. The femoral artery emerges below the midpoint of the inguinal ligament. See p. 436 for the inguinal region.

Q2: The sciatic nerve can be located as it exits the greater sciatic foramen by identifying the midpoint between the posterior superior iliac spine and the ischial tuberosity. In the gluteal region (see pp. 438–439), the sciatic nerve passes just medial to the midpoint of a line connecting the greater trochanter of the femur and the ischial tuberosity. The common fibular nerve can be palpated on the lateral border of the popliteal fossa as it courses along the medial border of the biceps femoris tendon (see p. 442). At the ankle, the tibial nerve is located midway between the palpable medial malleolus and the calcaneal (Achilles') tendons (see p. 442).

Head & Neck (pp. 588–589)

Q1: A bolus of anesthetic injected approximately two thirds of the way up the posterior border of the sternocleidomastoid would serve as a nerve block for the cervical plexus.

Q2: The confluence of the sinuses is found deep to the external occipital protuberance. See p. 608 for the dural sinuses.

Q3: The lateral cervical (posterior) triangle is bounded by the sternocleidomastoid and trapezius muscles and the clavicle. It contains the (spinal) accessory nerve (CN XI) and the brachial plexus. See p. 576 for the triangles of the neck. See p. 582 for the contents of the lateral cervical triangle.

Q4: The carotid triangle is bounded by the sternohyoid, posterior belly of the digastric, and sternocleidomastoid. It contains the vagus nerve (CN X). See p. 576 for the triangles of the neck. See p. 580 for the contents of the carotid triangle.

Q5: The thyroid cartilage (see p. 570) is commonly referred to as the "Adam's apple."

Index

Note: *Italicized* page numbers represent clinical applications. Tabular material is indicated by a "t" following the page number.